# WORLD MALARIA REPORT

2019

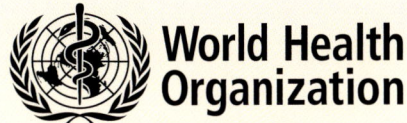

World malaria report 2019

ISBN 978-92-4-156572-1

© **World Health Organization 2019**

Some rights reserved. This work is available under the Creative Commons Attribution-NonCommercial-ShareAlike 3.0 IGO licence (CC BY-NC-SA 3.0 IGO; https://creativecommons.org/licenses/by-nc-sa/3.0/igo).

Under the terms of this licence, you may copy, redistribute and adapt the work for non-commercial purposes, provided the work is appropriately cited, as indicated below. In any use of this work, there should be no suggestion that WHO endorses any specific organization, products or services. The use of the WHO logo is not permitted. If you adapt the work, then you must license your work under the same or equivalent Creative Commons licence. If you create a translation of this work, you should add the following disclaimer along with the suggested citation: "This translation was not created by the World Health Organization (WHO). WHO is not responsible for the content or accuracy of this translation. The original English edition shall be the binding and authentic edition".

Any mediation relating to disputes arising under the licence shall be conducted in accordance with the mediation rules of the World Intellectual Property Organization.

**Suggested citation.** World malaria report 2019. Geneva: World Health Organization; 2019. Licence: CC BY-NC-SA 3.0 IGO.

**Cataloguing-in-Publication (CIP) data.** CIP data are available at http://apps.who.int/iris.

**Sales, rights and licensing.** To purchase WHO publications, see http://apps.who.int/bookorders. To submit requests for commercial use and queries on rights and licensing, see http://www.who.int/about/licensing.

**Third-party materials.** If you wish to reuse material from this work that is attributed to a third party, such as tables, figures or images, it is your responsibility to determine whether permission is needed for that reuse and to obtain permission from the copyright holder. The risk of claims resulting from infringement of any third-party-owned component in the work rests solely with the user.

**General disclaimers.** The designations employed and the presentation of the material in this publication do not imply the expression of any opinion whatsoever on the part of WHO concerning the legal status of any country, territory, city or area or of its authorities, or concerning the delimitation of its frontiers or boundaries. Dotted and dashed lines on maps represent approximate border lines for which there may not yet be full agreement.

The mention of specific companies or of certain manufacturers' products does not imply that they are endorsed or recommended by WHO in preference to others of a similar nature that are not mentioned. Errors and omissions expected, the names of proprietary products are distinguished by initial capital letters.

All reasonable precautions have been taken by WHO to verify the information contained in this publication. However, the published material is being distributed without warranty of any kind, either expressed or implied. The responsibility for the interpretation and use of the material lies with the reader. In no event shall WHO be liable for damages arising from its use.

Map production: WHO Global Malaria Programme and WHO Public Health Information and Geographic Systems.

Layout: DesignIsGood.info

Please consult the WHO Global Malaria Programme website for the most up-to-date version of all documents (https://www.who.int/malaria)

Printed in France

# Contents

| | |
|---|---|
| Foreword | iv |
| Acknowledgements | vii |
| Abbreviations | xi |
| This year's report at a glance | xii |
| 1. Introduction | 1 |
| 2. Regional and global trends in burden of malaria cases and deaths | 4 |
|    2.1  Estimated number of malaria cases by WHO region, 2000–2018 | 4 |
|    2.2  Malaria case incidence rate | 7 |
|    2.3  Estimated number of malaria deaths and mortality rate by WHO region, 2010–2018 | 9 |
|    2.4  Progress towards the GTS milestones for malaria morbidity and mortality | 11 |
| 3. Maternal, infant and child health consequences of malaria | 14 |
|    3.1  Prevalence of exposure to malaria infection during pregnancy, correlation with maternal anaemia and contribution to low birthweight | 15 |
|    3.2  Prevalence and burden of malaria-related anaemia in children aged under 5 years | 19 |
|    3.3  Protecting the mother and child | 21 |
| 4. High burden to high impact approach | 24 |
|    4.1  HBHI initiation activities | 24 |
|    4.2  Burden of malaria cases and deaths | 26 |
|    4.3  Malaria prevention | 28 |
|    4.4  Malaria diagnosis and treatment | 30 |
|    4.5  Malaria funding | 31 |
| 5. Malaria elimination and prevention of re-establishment | 32 |
|    5.1  E-2020 initiative | 32 |
|    5.2  Greater Mekong subregion | 34 |
| 6. Investments in malaria programmes and research | 36 |
|    6.1  Funding for malaria control and elimination | 36 |
|    6.2  Investments in malaria R&D | 40 |
|    6.3  Procurement and distributions of ITNs | 42 |
|    6.4  Deliveries of RDTs | 44 |
|    6.5  Deliveries of ACTs | 45 |
| 7. Preventing malaria | 46 |
|    7.1  Population at risk covered with ITNs | 46 |
|    7.2  Population at risk protected by IRS | 48 |
|    7.3  Pregnant women receiving three or more doses of IPTp | 50 |
|    7.4  Seasonal malaria chemoprevention | 51 |
| 8. Diagnostic testing and treatment | 52 |
|    8.1  Prevalence of fever in children aged under 5 years | 52 |
|    8.2  Numbers of children with fever brought for care | 53 |
|    8.3  Parasitological testing of febrile children | 54 |
|    8.4  Treatment of febrile children with antimalarial drugs | 58 |
|    8.5  Use of ACT for the treatment of febrile children | 59 |
|    8.6  Integrated community case management | 60 |
| 9. Malaria surveillance | 62 |
|    9.1  Strengthening national surveillance systems | 62 |
|    9.2  Malaria modules | 62 |
|    9.3  Assessment of national surveillance systems | 65 |
| 10. Responding to biological threats to the fight against malaria | 68 |
|    10.1  *Pf-hrp2/3* gene deletions | 68 |
|    10.2  Parasite resistance – status of antimalarial drug efficacy (2010–2018) | 69 |
|    10.3  Vector resistance to insecticides | 72 |
| 11. Conclusion | 76 |
| References | 78 |
| Annexes | 83 |

# Foreword

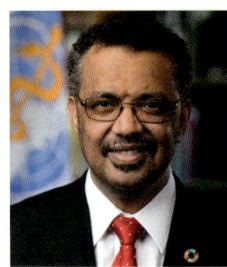

**Dr Tedros Adhanom Ghebreyesus**
Director-General
World Health Organization

## Leaving no one behind in the march to a malaria-free world

The scourge of malaria continues to strike hardest against pregnant women and children in Africa. The *World malaria report 2019* includes a special section focused on the burden and consequences of the disease among these two most at-risk groups. It delivers a clear message: we must all do more to protect the most vulnerable in the fight against a disease that continues to claim more than 400 000 lives every year.

Malaria in pregnancy compromises the mother's health and puts her at greater risk of death. It impacts the health of the fetus, leading to prematurity and low birthweight, major contributors to neonatal and infant mortality. Last year, some 11 million pregnant women in sub-Saharan Africa were infected with malaria and, consequently, nearly 900 000 children were born with a low birthweight.

To protect pregnant women in Africa, WHO recommends the use of insecticide-treated mosquito nets (ITNs) and preventive antimalarial medicines. This report shows progress on both fronts. Still, nearly 40% of pregnant woman did not sleep under an ITN in 2018 and two thirds did not receive the recommended three or more doses of preventive therapy.

Among children, efforts to expand access to preventive antimalarial medicines are bearing fruit. In Africa's Sahel sub-region, WHO recommends seasonal malaria chemoprevention during the peak transmission season. More than 60% of children living in areas eligible for this preventive therapy received it in 2018.

Sierra Leone is to be commended for becoming the first country in Africa to roll out intermittent preventive treatment in infants, another WHO-recommended approach for protecting young children in malaria-affected areas.

Still, access to care for children showing signs of a fever remains too low. Country surveys show that nearly 40% of febrile children in sub-Saharan Africa are not taken for care with a trained medical provider.

At least 10 countries that are part of the WHO "E-2020 initiative" are on track to reach the 2020 elimination milestone of our global malaria strategy. In 2015, all of these countries were malaria endemic; now they have either achieved zero indigenous malaria cases or are nearing the finish line.

However, in recent years, global progress in reducing new malaria cases has levelled off. Most worrying of all, malaria is on the rise across some high-burden countries in Africa.

Critical milestones of our global malaria strategy are likely to be missed.

In 2018, WHO and the RBM Partnership to End Malaria launched "High burden to high impact", a new approach to prevent disease and save lives in the countries hardest hit by malaria. Replacing a "one size fits all" strategy, the approach calls for using the most effective tools in a more targeted way. I am very pleased to note that two countries – India and Uganda – have reported substantial reductions in malaria cases in 2018 over the previous year.

In September, I issued a "Malaria Challenge", calling for greater investment in the research and development of transformative new tools, technologies and approaches to accelerate progress in beating back this disease.

Through a WHO-coordinated pilot progamme, Ghana, Kenya and Malawi recently introduced the world's first malaria vaccine in selected areas. Evidence and experience from the programme will inform policy decisions on the vaccine's potential wider use in Africa. With support from the Global Fund to Fight AIDS, Tuberculosis and Malaria and from Unitaid, other promising tools are being tested, such as new types of ITNs and tools that target outdoor-biting mosquitoes.

Achieving our common vision of a malaria-free world will also require enhanced action in other critical areas. We need affordable, people-centred health services. We need reliable and accurate surveillance and response systems. We need strategies that are tailored to local malaria-transmission settings.

Stepped-up financing for the malaria response is essential. In 2018, total funding for malaria control and elimination reached an estimated US$ 2.7 billion, falling far short of the US$ 5 billion funding target of our global strategy.

Through resolute, robust financing, political leadership and universal health coverage, we can defeat this disease once and for all.

# Acknowledgements

We are very grateful to the numerous people who contributed to the production of the *World malaria report 2019*. The following people collected and reviewed data from both malaria endemic and malaria free countries and areas:

Ahmad Mureed Muradi, Naimullah Safi and Mohammad Shoaib Tamim (Afghanistan); Lammali Karima and Houria Khelifi (Algeria); Fernanda Francisco Guimaraes and Fernanda Isabel Martins Da Graça Do Espirito Santo Alves (Angola); Malena Basilio and Yael Provecho (Argentina); Raja Alsaloom and Hasan Shuaib (Bahrain); Mya Ngon, Anjan Kumar Saha and Sabera Sultana (Bangladesh); Kim Bautista (Belize); Telesphore Houansou and Théophile Migan (Benin); Tobgyel Drukpa, Rinzin Namgay, Phurpa Tenzin and Sonam Wangdi (Bhutan); Raúl Marcelo Manjón Tellería (Bolivia [Plurinational State of]); Kentse Moakofhi and Mpho Mogopa (Botswana); Cássio Roberto Leonel Peterka, Edília Sâmela Freitas Santos and Anderson Coutinho da Silva (Brazil); Laurent Moyenga and Yacouba Savadogo (Burkina Faso); Dismas Baza and Félicien Ndayizeye (Burundi); Carolina Cardoso da Silva Leite Gomes and António Lima Moreira (Cabo Verde); Tol Bunkea, Say Chy and Jean-Olivier Guintran (Cambodia); Abomabo Moïse Hugue René and Alexis Tougordi (Cameroon); Aristide Désiré Komangoya-Nzonzo and Christophe Ndoua (Central African Republic); Mahamat Idriss Djaskano and Daoudongar Honoré Djimrassengar (Chad); Wei Ding, Yao Ruan and Li Zhang (China); Eduin Pachón Abril (Colombia); Mohamed Issa Ibrahim and Ahamada Nassuri (Comoros); Hermann Judicaël Ongouo and Jean-Mermoz Youndouka (Congo); Teresita Solano Chinchilla (Costa Rica); Ehui Anicet Parfait Katche and N'goran Raphaël N'Dri (Côte d'Ivoire); Kim Yun Chol, Nam Ju O and Gagan Sonal (Democratic People's Republic of Korea); Patrick Bahizi Bizoza, Eric Mukomena and Bacary Sambou (Democratic Republic of the Congo); Mohamed Elhakim, Hawa Hassan Guessod and Angela Anna de Tommasi (Djibouti); Dianelba Valdez (Dominican Republic); Jaen Carlos Cagua and Mauricio Vallejo (Ecuador); Jaime Enrique Alemán Escobar (El Salvador); Angela Katherine Lao Seoane and Mathilde Riloha Rivas (Equatorial Guinea); Selam Mihreteab and Assefash Zehaie (Eritrea); Kevin Makadzange and Zulisile Zulu (Eswatini); Henock Ejigu, Mebrahtom Haile and Bekele Worku (Ethiopia); Alice Sanna (French Guiana); Ghislaine Nkone Asseko and Okome Nze Gyslaine (Gabon); Momodou Kalleh and Sharmila Lareef-Jah (Gambia); Keziah Malm and Felicia Owusu-Antwi (Ghana); Ericka Lidia Chávez Vásquez (Guatemala); Siriman Camara and Nouman Diakité (Guinea); Inacio Alveranga and Paulo Djatá (Guinea-Bissau); Horace Cox (Guyana); Antoine Darlie (Haiti); Engels Banegas, Jessica Henriquez, Carlos Miranda, Jose Orlinder Nicolas, Raoul O'Connor and Nely Romero (Honduras); Neeraj Dhingra and Roop Kumari (India); Nancy Dian Anggraeni and Herdiana Basri (Indonesia); Leila Faraji and Ahmad Raeisi (Iran [Islamic Republic of]); Nizar Maswadi (Jordan); James Kiarie and Josephine Njoroge (Kenya); Phonephet Butphomvihane, Chitsavang Chanthavisouk and Viengxay Vanisaveth (Lao People's Democratic Republic); Najib Achi (Lebanon); Levi Hinneh and Moses Jeuronlon (Liberia); Solo Harimalala Rajaobary and Henintsoa Rabarijaona Ratovo (Madagascar); Wilfred Dodoli and Austin Albert Gumbo (Malawi); Jenarun Jelip (Malaysia); Sidibe Boubacar and Idrissa Cissé (Mali); Sidina Mohamed Ghoulam and Saidou Niang (Mauritania); Frédéric Pagès (Mayotte); José Cruz Rodríguez Martínez and Gustavo Sánchez Tejeda (Mexico); Eva de Carvalho and Guidion Mathe (Mozambique); Badri Thapa, Aung Thi and Tet Toe Tun (Myanmar); Clothilde Narib and Wilma Soroses (Namibia); Subhash Lakhe and Bibek Kumar Lal (Nepal); Cristhian Toledo (Nicaragua); Fatima Aboubakar and Hadiza Jackou (Niger); Audu Bala-Mohammed and Lynda Ozor (Nigeria); Muhammad Suleman Memon (Pakistan); Lizbeth Cerezo (Panama); John Deli (Papua New Guinea); Cynthia Viveros (Paraguay); Karim Pardo Ruiz (Peru); Gawrie Galappaththy and Maria Santa Portillo (Philippines); Byoung-Hak Jeon (Republic of Korea); Michee Kabera and Daniel Ngamije (Rwanda); Claudina Augusto da Cruz and Anastácio Pires (Sao Tome and Principe); Mohammed Hassan Al-Zahrani (Saudi Arabia); Ndella Diakhate and Medoune Ndiop (Senegal);

Louise Ganda and Samuel Juana Smith (Sierra Leone); John Leaburi (Solomon Islands); Fahmi Isse Yusuf (Somalia); Mary Anne Groepe and Bridget Shandukani (South Africa); Moses Mutebi Nganda and Harriet Akello Pasquale (South Sudan); Manjula Danansuriya, H.D.B. Herath and Navaratnasingam Janakan (Sri Lanka); Mariam Adam, Doha Elnazir and Abdalla Ibrahim (Sudan); Loretta Hardjopawiro (Suriname); Deyer Gopinath and Suravadee Kitchakarn (Thailand); Maria do Rosario de Fatima Mota, Rajesh Pandav and Manel Yapabandara (Timor-Leste); Kokou Mawule Davi and Tchassama Tchadjobo (Togo); Bayo Fatunmbi, Charles Katureebe, Paul Mbaka and Damian Rutazaana (Uganda); Anna Mahendeka, Irene Mwoga and Ritha Njau (United Republic of Tanzania [mainland]); Mohamed Haji Ali, Irene Mwoga and Ritha Njau (United Republic of Tanzania [Zanzibar]); Johnny Nausien (Vanuatu); Licenciada América Rivero (Venezuela [Bolivarian Republic of]); Dai Tran Cong and Nguyen Quy Anh (Viet Nam); Adel Aljasari and Moamer Mohammed Badi (Yemen); Japhet Chiwaula and Fred Masaninga (Zambia); and Jasper Pasipamire and Ottias Tapfumanei (Zimbabwe).

We are grateful to Patrick Walker and Oliver Watson (Imperial College) for their contribution to the analysis of exposure to malaria infection during pregnancy and attributable low birthweight. Paul Milligan (London School of Hygiene and Tropical Medicine) for his contribution to updating the section on seasonal malaria chemoprevention with the most up-to-date information on implementation and coverage. Manjiri Bhawalkar (Global Fund to Fight AIDS, Tuberculosis and Malaria [Global Fund]) supplied information on financial disbursements from the Global Fund. Adam Aspden (United Kingdom of Great Britain and Northern Ireland [United Kingdom] Department for International Development) and Adam Wexler (Kaiser Family Foundation) provided information on financial contributions for malaria control from the United Kingdom and the United States of America, respectively. Policy Cures Research used its G-FINDER data in the analysis of financing for malaria research and development, and wrote the associated section. John Milliner (Milliner Global Associates) provided information on long-lasting insecticidal nets delivered by manufacturers. Dr Samir Bhatt (Imperial College) and the Malaria Atlas Project (MAP,[1] University of Oxford, led by Professor Peter Gething), with the support of the Bill & Melinda Gates Foundation, produced estimates of insecticide-treated mosquito net (ITN) coverage for African countries using data from household surveys, ITN deliveries by manufacturers, ITNs distributed by national malaria programmes (NMPs) and ITN coverage indicators. They also produced estimates of *Plasmodium falciparum* parasite prevalence in sub-Saharan Africa. MAP's work was managed and coordinated by Dr Dan Weiss. Tom McLean and Jason Richardson (Innovative Vector Control Consortium [IVCC]) provided national indoor residual spraying coverage and implementation data complementary to reported country information. Melanie Renshaw (African Leaders Malaria Alliance) provided information on the status of national insecticide resistance monitoring and management plans. Christen Fornadel (US President's Malaria Initiative) provided insecticide resistance data and Gildas Yahouedo assisted with data compilation from publications. Colin Mathers (World Health Organization [WHO] Department of Health Statistics and Information Systems) prepared estimates of malaria mortality in children aged under 5 years, on behalf of the Child Health Epidemiology Reference Group. John Painter, Anna Bowen and Julie Gutman (US Centers for Disease Control and Prevention) provided data analysis and interpretation for the section on intermittent preventive treatment in pregnancy.

The following WHO staff in regional and subregional offices assisted in the design of data collection forms; the collection and validation of data; and the review of epidemiological estimates, country profiles, regional profiles and sections:

- Birkinesh Amenshewa, Ebenezer Sheshi Baba, Magaran Bagayoko, Steve Banza Kubenga and Jackson Sillah (WHO Regional Office for Africa [AFRO]);
- Spes Ntabangana (AFRO/Inter-country Support Team [IST] Central Africa);
- Khoti Gausi (AFRO/IST East and Southern Africa);

---

[1] https://map.ox.ac.uk/

# Acknowledgements

- Abderrahmane Kharchi Tfeil (AFRO/IST West Africa);
- Maria Paz Ade, Janina Chavez, Rainier Escalada, Valerie Mize, Roberto Montoya, Eric Ndofor and Prabhjot Singh (WHO Regional Office for the Americas);
- Samira Al-Eryani and Ghasem Zamani (WHO Regional Office for the Eastern Mediterranean);
- Elkhan Gasimov and Elena Chulkova (WHO Regional Office for Europe);
- Risintha Premaratne and Neena Valecha (WHO Regional Office for South-East Asia); and
- James Kelley (WHO Regional Office for the Western Pacific).

The maps for country and regional profiles were produced by MAP's ROAD-MAPII team (led by Mike Thorn); map production was led and coordinated by Jen Rozier, with help from Lisa Chestnutt and Joe Harris. ROAD-MAPII is supported by the Bill & Melinda Gates Foundation.

We are also grateful to Kevin Marsh (University of Oxford), Arantxa Roca-Feltrer (Malaria Consortium), Larry Slutsker (PATH) and Robert Snow (KEMRI Wellcome Trust), who graciously reviewed all sections and provided substantial comments for improvement; Ana Balcazar Moreno, Egle Granziera and Claudia Nannini (WHO) for legal review; Martha Quiñones (WHO consultant), Amélie Latour (WHO consultant) and Laurent Bergeron (WHO) for the translation into Spanish and French, respectively, of the foreword and key points; Claude Cardot and the DesignIsGood team for the design and layout of the report; Lushomo (Cape Town, South Africa) for the report cover; and Hilary Cadman and the Cadman Editing Services team for technical editing of the report.

On behalf of the WHO Global Malaria Programme (GMP), the publication of the *World malaria report 2019* was coordinated by Abdisalan Noor. Significant contributions were made by Laura Anderson, John Aponte, Maru Aregawi, Amy Barrette, Nelly Biondi, Lucia Fernandez Montoya, Beatriz Galatas, Peter Olumese, Edith Patouillard, Salim Sadruddin and Ryan Williams, in close collaboration with Yuen Ching Chan and Tamara Ehler (WHO consultants). Laurent Bergeron (WHO GMP) provided programmatic support for overall management of the project. The editorial committee for the report comprised Pedro Alonso, Andrea Bosman, Jan Kolaczinski, Kimberly Lindblade, Leonard Ortega, Pascal Ringwald and David Schellenberg from the WHO GMP. Additional reviews were received from colleagues in the GMP: Jane Cunningham, Xiao Hong Li, Charlotte Rasmussen, Silvia Schwarte, Erin Shutes, Saira Stewart and Amanda Tiffany. Report layout, design and production were coordinated by Laurent Bergeron.

Funding for the production of this report was gratefully received from the Bill & Melinda Gates Foundation; the Global Fund; Luxembourg's Ministry of Foreign and European Affairs – Directorate for Development Cooperation and Humanitarian Affairs; the Spanish Agency for International Development Cooperation; Unitaid; and the United States Agency for International Development.

# Abbreviations

| | | | |
|---|---|---|---|
| ACT | artemisinin-based combination therapy | IPTi | intermittent preventive treatment in infants |
| AIDS | acquired immunodeficiency syndrome | IPTp | intermittent preventive treatment in pregnancy |
| AL | artemether-lumefantrine | IQR | interquartile range |
| ANC | antenatal care | IRS | indoor residual spraying |
| AQ | amodiaquine | ITN | insecticide-treated mosquito net |
| AS | artesunate | LBW | low birthweight |
| AS-SP | artesunate-sulfadoxine-pyrimethamine | LLIN | long-lasting insecticidal net |
| AS-AQ | artesunate-amodiaquine | MEOC | Malaria Elimination Oversight Committee |
| AS-MQ | artesunate-mefloquine | MIS | malaria indicator survey |
| AS-PY | artesunate-pyronaridine | MPAC | Malaria Policy Advisory Committee |
| CHW | community health worker | NMP | national malaria programme |
| CI | confidence interval | OECD | Organisation for Economic Co-operation and Development |
| CQ | chloroquine | P. | *Plasmodium* |
| DHA | dihydroartemisinin | PBO | piperonyl butoxide |
| DHIS2 | District Health Information Software2 | PPQ | piperaquine |
| DHS | demographic and health survey | PQ | primaquine |
| E-2020 | eliminating countries for 2020 | RAcE | Rapid Access Expansion Programme |
| Global Forum | Global Forum of Malaria-Eliminating Countries | R&D | research and development |
| Global Fund | Global Fund to Fight AIDS, Tuberculosis and Malaria | RBM | Roll Back Malaria |
| GMP | Global Malaria Programme | RDT | rapid diagnostic test |
| GMS | Greater Mekong subregion | SDG | Sustainable Development Goal |
| GPW13 | WHO's 13th General Programme of Work | SMC | seasonal malaria chemoprevention |
| GTS | *Global technical strategy for malaria 2016–2030* | SP | sulfadoxine-pyrimethamine |
| Hb | haemoglobin | TES | therapeutic efficacy study |
| HBHI | high burden to high impact | UNICEF | United Nations Children's Fund |
| HIV | human immunodeficiency virus | United Kingdom | United Kingdom of Great Britain and Northern Ireland |
| HMIS | health management information system | USA | United States of America |
| HRP2 | histidine-rich protein 2 | WHO | World Health Organization |
| iCCM | integrated community case management | | |
| iDES | integrated drug efficacy surveillance | | |

# This year's report at a glance

## REGIONAL AND GLOBAL TRENDS IN BURDEN OF MALARIA CASES AND DEATHS

### Malaria cases

- In 2018, an estimated 228 million cases of malaria occurred worldwide (95% confidence interval [CI]: 206–258 million), compared with 251 million cases in 2010 (95% CI: 231–278 million) and 231 million cases in 2017 (95% CI: 211–259 million).

- Most malaria cases in 2018 were in the World Health Organization (WHO) African Region (213 million or 93%), followed by the WHO South-East Asia Region with 3.4% of the cases and the WHO Eastern Mediterranean Region with 2.1%.

- Nineteen countries in sub-Saharan Africa[1] and India carried almost 85% of the global malaria burden. Six countries accounted for more than half of all malaria cases worldwide: Nigeria (25%), the Democratic Republic of the Congo (12%), Uganda (5%), and Côte d'Ivoire, Mozambique and Niger (4% each).

- The incidence rate of malaria declined globally between 2010 and 2018, from 71 to 57 cases per 1000 population at risk. However, from 2014 to 2018, the rate of change slowed dramatically, reducing to 57 in 2014 and remaining at similar levels through to 2018.

- The WHO South-East Asia Region continued to see its incidence rate fall – from 17 cases of the disease per 1000 population at risk in 2010 to five cases in 2018 (a 70% decrease). In the WHO African Region, case incidence levels also declined from 294 in 2010 to 229 in 2018, representing a 22% reduction. All other WHO regions recorded either little progress or an increase in incidence rate. The WHO Region of the Americas recorded a rise, largely due to increases in malaria transmission in the Bolivarian Republic of Venezuela.

- Between 2015 and 2018, only 31 countries, where malaria is still endemic, reduced case incidence significantly and were on track to reduce incidence by 40% or more by 2020. Without accelerated change, the *Global technical strategy for malaria 2016–2030* (GTS) milestones for morbidity in 2025 and 2030 will not be achieved.

- *Plasmodium falciparum* is the most prevalent malaria parasite in the WHO African Region, accounting for 99.7% of estimated malaria cases in 2018, as well as in the WHO South-East Asia Region (50%), the WHO Eastern Mediterranean Region (71%) and the WHO Western Pacific Region (65%).

- Globally, 53% of the *P. vivax* burden is in the WHO South-East Asia Region, with the majority being in India (47%). *P. vivax* is the predominant parasite in the WHO Region of the Americas, representing 75% of malaria cases.

### Malaria deaths

- In 2018, there were an estimated 405 000 deaths from malaria globally, compared with 416 000 estimated deaths in 2017, and 585 000 in 2010.

- Children aged under 5 years are the most vulnerable group affected by malaria. In 2018, they accounted for 67% (272 000) of all malaria deaths worldwide.

---

[1] The full list of sub-Saharan countries is available at https://unstats.un.org/unsd/methodology/m49; for all analyses conducted in this report and pertaining to malaria endemic sub-Saharan countries, Sudan is also included.

- The WHO African Region accounted for 94% of all malaria deaths in 2018. Although this region was home to the highest number of malaria deaths in 2018, it also accounted for 85% of the 180 000 fewer global malaria deaths reported in 2018 compared with 2010.
- Nearly 85% of global malaria deaths in 2018 were concentrated in 20 countries in the WHO African Region and India; Nigeria accounted for almost 24% of all global malaria deaths, followed by the Democratic Republic of the Congo (11%), the United Republic of Tanzania (5%), and Angola, Mozambique and Niger (4% each).
- In 2018, only the WHO African Region and the WHO South-East Asia Region showed reductions in malaria deaths compared with 2010. The WHO African Region had the largest absolute reduction in malaria deaths, from 533 000 in 2010 to 380 000 in 2018. Despite these gains, the malaria mortality reduction rate has also slowed since 2016.

## MATERNAL, INFANT AND CHILD HEALTH CONSEQUENCES OF MALARIA

- In 2018, about 11 million pregnancies in moderate and high transmission sub-Saharan African countries would have been exposed to malaria infection.
- In 2018, prevalence of exposure to malaria infection in pregnancy was highest in the West African subregion and Central Africa (each with 35%), followed by East and Southern Africa (20%). About 39% of these were in the Democratic Republic of the Congo and Nigeria.
- The 11 million pregnant women exposed to malaria infections in 2018 delivered about 872 000 children with low birthweight (16% of all children with low birthweight in these countries), with West Africa having the highest prevalence of low birthweight children due to malaria in pregnancy.
- Between 2015 and 2018 in 21 moderate to high malaria burden countries in the WHO African Region, the prevalence of anaemia in children under 5 years with a positive rapid diagnostic test (RDT) was double that of children with a negative RDT. In the children who were positive for malaria, 9% had severe anaemia and 54% had moderate anaemia; in contrast, in the children without malaria, only 1% had severe anaemia and 31% had moderate anaemia.
- The countries with the highest percentage of severe anaemia among children aged under 5 years who were positive for malaria were Senegal (26%), Mali (16%), Guinea (14%) and Mozambique (12%). For most other countries, severe anaemia ranged from 5% to 10%.
- Overall, about 24 million children were estimated to be infected with *P. falciparum* in 2018 in sub-Saharan Africa, and an estimated 1.8 million of them were likely to have severe anaemia.

## HIGH BURDEN TO HIGH IMPACT APPROACH

- There were about 155 million malaria cases in the 11 high burden to high impact (HBHI) countries in 2018, compared with 177 million in 2010. The Democratic Republic of the Congo and Nigeria accounted for 84 million (54%) of total cases.
- Of the 10 highest burden countries in Africa, Ghana and Nigeria reported the highest absolute increases in cases of malaria in 2018 compared with 2017. The burden in 2018 was similar to that of 2017 in all other countries, apart from in Uganda and India, where there were reported reductions of 1.5 and 2.6 million malaria cases, respectively, in 2018 compared with 2017.
- Malaria deaths reduced from about 400 000 in 2010 to about 260 000 in 2018, the largest reduction being in Nigeria, from almost 153 000 deaths in 2010 to about 95 000 deaths in 2018.

- By 2018, in all of the 11 HBHI countries, at least 40% of the population at risk were sleeping under long-lasting insecticidal nets (LLINs), the highest percentage being in Uganda (80%) and the lowest in Nigeria (40%).
- Only Burkina Faso and the United Republic of Tanzania were estimated as having more than half of pregnant women receiving three doses of intermittent preventive treatment in pregnancy (IPTp3) in 2018. In Cameroon, Nigeria and Uganda, the estimated coverage was about 30% or less.
- Six countries in Africa's Sahel subregion implemented seasonal malaria chemoprevention (SMC) in 2018; a mean total of 17 million children, out of the 26 million targeted, were treated per SMC cycle.
- The percentage of children aged under 5 years with fever seeking treatment varied from 58% in Mali to 82% in Uganda. In the Democratic Republic of the Congo and Mali, more than 40% of children were not brought for care at all. Testing was also worryingly low in children who were brought for care, with 30% or less being tested in Cameroon, the Democratic Republic of the Congo and Nigeria.
- Except for India, direct domestic investment remains very low relative to international funding in the HBHI countries.

## MALARIA ELIMINATION AND PREVENTION OF RE-ESTABLISHMENT

- Globally, the elimination net is widening, with more countries moving towards zero indigenous cases: in 2018, 49 countries reported fewer than 10 000 such cases, up from 46 countries in 2017 and 40 countries in 2010. The number of countries with fewer than 100 indigenous cases – a strong indicator that elimination is within reach – increased from 17 countries in 2010, to 25 countries in 2017 and 27 countries in 2018.
- Paraguay and Uzbekistan were awarded WHO certification of elimination in 2018, with Algeria and Argentina achieving certification in early 2019. In 2018, China, El Salvador, Iran, Malaysia and Timor-Leste reported zero indigenous cases.
- One of the key GTS milestones for 2020 is elimination of malaria in at least 10 countries that were malaria endemic in 2015. At the current rate of progress, it is likely that this milestone will be reached.
- In 2016, WHO identified 21 countries with the potential to eliminate malaria by the year 2020. WHO is working with the governments in these countries – known as "E-2020 countries" – to support their elimination acceleration goals.
- Although 10 E-2020 countries remain on track to achieve their elimination goals, Comoros and Costa Rica reported increases in indigenous malaria cases in 2018 compared with 2017.
- In the six countries of the Greater Mekong subregion (GMS) – Cambodia, China (Yunnan Province), Lao People's Democratic Republic, Myanmar, Thailand and Viet Nam – the reported number of malaria cases fell by 76% between 2010 and 2018, and malaria deaths fell by 95% over the same period. In 2018, Cambodia reported no malaria related deaths for the first time in the country's history.

# INVESTMENTS IN MALARIA PROGRAMMES AND RESEARCH

- In 2018, an estimated US$ 2.7 billion was invested in malaria control and elimination efforts globally by governments of malaria endemic countries and international partners – a reduction from the US$ 3.2 billion that was invested in 2017. The amount invested in 2018 fell short of the US$ 5.0 billion estimated to be required globally to stay on track towards the GTS milestones.
- Nearly three quarters of investments in 2018 were spent in the WHO African Region, followed by the WHO Region of the Americas (7%), the WHO South-East Asia Region (6%), and the WHO Eastern Mediterranean Region and the WHO Western Pacific Region (5% each).
- In 2018, 47% of total funding for malaria was invested in low-income countries, 43% in lower-middle-income countries and 11% in upper-middle-income countries. International funding represented the major source of funding in low-income and lower-middle-income countries, at 85% and 61%, respectively. Domestic funding has remained stable since 2010.
- Of the US$ 2.7 billion invested in 2018, US$ 1.8 billion came from international funders. Governments of malaria endemic countries contributed 30% of total funding (US$ 900 million) in 2018, a figure unchanged from 2017. Two thirds of domestically sourced funds were invested in malaria control activities carried out by national malaria programmes (NMPs), with the remaining share estimated as the cost of patient care.
- As in previous years, the United States of America (USA) was the largest international source of malaria financing, providing US$ 1.0 billion (37%) in 2018. Country members of the Development Assistance Committee together accounted for US$ 300 million (11%). The United Kingdom of Great Britain and Northern Ireland contributed around US$ 200 million (7%).
- Of the US$ 2.7 billion invested in 2018, US$ 1.0 billion was channelled through the Global Fund to Fight AIDS, Tuberculosis and Malaria.
- Although funding for malaria has remained relatively stable since 2010, the level of investment in 2018 is far from what is required to reach the first two milestones of the GTS; that is, a reduction of at least 40% in malaria case incidence and mortality rates globally by 2020, compared with 2015 levels.
- US$ 663 million was invested in basic research and product development for malaria in 2018, an increase of US$ 18 million compared with 2017.
- Funding for drug research and development (R&D) increased to the highest level ever recorded, from US$ 228 million in 2017 to US$ 252 million in 2018. This increase was a result of private sector industry investment in several Phase II trials of new chemical entities with the potential for single-exposure radical cure.

## Deliveries of malaria commodities

### Insecticide-treated mosquito nets

- Between 2016 and 2018, a total of 578 million insecticide-treated mosquito nets (ITNs), mainly LLINs, were reported by manufacturers as having been delivered globally, with 50% going to Côte d'Ivoire, the Democratic Republic of the Congo, Ethiopia, Ghana, India, Nigeria, Uganda and the United Republic of Tanzania.
- In 2018 about 197 million ITNs were delivered by manufacturers, of which more than 87% were delivered to countries in sub-Saharan Africa.
- Globally, 80% of ITNs were distributed through mass distribution campaigns, 10% in antenatal care facilities and 6% as part of immunization programmes.

### Rapid diagnostic tests

- An estimated 412 million RDTs were sold globally in 2018.
- In 2018, 259 million RDTs were distributed by NMPs. Most RDTs (64%) were tests that detected *P. falciparum* only and were supplied to sub-Saharan Africa.

**Artemisinin-based combination therapy**

- An estimated 3 billion treatment courses of artemisinin-based combination therapy (ACT) were procured by countries over the period 2010–2018. An estimated 63% of these procurements were reported to have been made for the public sector.
- In 2018, 214 million ACT treatment courses were delivered by NMPs, of which 98% were in the WHO African Region.

# PREVENTING MALARIA

## Vector control

- Half of people at risk of malaria in sub-Saharan Africa are sleeping under an ITN; in 2018, 50% of the population were protected by this intervention, an increase from 29% in 2010. Furthermore, the percentage of the population with access to an ITN increased from 33% in 2010 to 57% in 2018. However, coverage has improved only marginally since 2015 and has been at a standstill since 2016.
- Households with at least one ITN for every two people increased to 72% in 2018, from 47% in 2010. However, this figure represents only a modest increase over the past 3 years, and remains far from the target of universal coverage.
- Fewer people at risk of malaria are being protected by indoor residual spraying (IRS), a prevention method that involves spraying the inside walls of dwellings with insecticides. Globally, IRS protection declined from a peak of 5% in 2010 to 2% in 2018, with declining trends seen across all WHO regions apart from the WHO Eastern Mediterranean Region.
- Although IRS coverage dropped from 180 million people at risk protected globally in 2010 to 93 million in 2018, the 2018 figure was a decrease of 13 million compared with 2017.
- The declines in IRS coverage may be due to the switch from pyrethroids to more expensive insecticides in response to increasing pyrethroid resistance, or changes in operational strategies (e.g. at-risk populations decreasing in countries aiming for elimination of malaria).

## Preventive therapies

- To protect women in areas of moderate and high malaria transmission in Africa, WHO recommends IPTp with the antimalarial drug sulfadoxine-pyrimethamine (SP). Among 36 African countries that reported on IPTp coverage levels in 2018, an estimated 31% of eligible pregnant women received the recommended three or more doses of IPTp, compared with 22% in 2017 and 2% in 2010, indicating considerable improvements in country uptake.
- About 18% of women who use antenatal care services at least once do not receive any IPTp, representing a missed opportunity that, if harnessed, could considerably and rapidly improve IPTp coverage.
- In 2018, 19 million children in 12 countries in Africa's Sahel subregion were protected through SMC programmes. All targeted children received treatment in Cameroon, Guinea, Guinea-Bissau and Mali. However, about 12 million children who could have benefited from this intervention were not covered, mainly due to a lack of funding.

# DIAGNOSTIC TESTING AND TREATMENT

### Accessing care

- Prompt diagnosis and treatment is the most effective way to prevent a mild case of malaria from developing into severe disease and death. Based on national household surveys completed in 20 countries in sub-Saharan Africa between 2015 and 2018, a median of 42% (interquartile range [IQR]: 34–49%) of children with a fever (febrile) were taken to a trained medical provider for care in the public sector compared with 10% (IQR: 8–22%) in the formal private sector and 3% (IQR: 2–7%) in the informal private sector.
- A high proportion of febrile children did not receive any medical attention (median: 36%, IQR: 28–45%). Poor access to health care providers or lack of awareness of malaria symptoms among caregivers are among the contributing factors.

### Diagnosing malaria

- The percentage of patients suspected of having malaria who are seen in public health facilities and tested with either an RDT or microscopy, rose from 38% in 2010 to 85% in 2018.
- In 71% of moderate to high transmission countries in sub-Saharan Africa, the percentage of suspected cases tested with any parasitological test was greater than 80% in 2018.
- According to 19 nationally representative household surveys conducted between 2015 and 2018 in sub-Saharan Africa, the median percentage of febrile children brought for care who received a finger or heel stick (suggesting that a malaria diagnostic test may have been performed) was greater in the public sector (median: 66%, IQR: 49–75%) than in the formal private sector (median: 40%, IQR: 16–46%) or the informal private sector (median: 9%, IQR: 5–22%).
- According to 61 surveys conducted in 29 sub-Saharan African countries between 2010 and 2018, the percentage of children with a fever that received a diagnostic test before antimalarial treatment in the public health sector increased from a median of 48% (IQR: 30–62%) in 2010–2013 to a median of 76% (IQR: 60–86%) in 2015–2018.

### Treating malaria

- Based on 20 household surveys conducted in sub-Saharan Africa in 2015–2018, the median percentage of febrile children who were treated with any antimalarial drug was higher in the public sector (median: 48%, IQR: 30–69%) than in the formal private sector (median: 40%, IQR: 21–51%) or the informal private sector (median: 18%, IQR: 10–29%).
- Data from 20 national surveys conducted in sub-Saharan Africa show that for the period 2015–2018, an estimated 47% (IQR: 29–69%) of febrile children brought for treatment for malaria in the public health sector received antimalarial drugs, compared with 59% (IQR: 53–84%) among those visiting a community health worker and 49% (IQR: 19–55%) in the formal medical private sector.
- Based on 19 surveys, antimalarial treatments among febrile children who received antimalarial medicine were slightly more likely to be ACTs if treatment was sought in the public sector (median: 80%, IQR: 45–94%) than in the formal private sector (median: 77%, IQR: 43–87%) or the informal private sector (median: 60%, IQR: 40–84%).
- To bridge the treatment gap among children, WHO recommends the uptake of integrated community case management (iCCM). This approach promotes integrated management of common life-threatening conditions in children – malaria, pneumonia and diarrhoea – at health facility and community levels. In 2018, 30 countries were implementing iCCM at different levels, with only a few implementing nationally.

## MALARIA SURVEILLANCE SYSTEMS

- Pillar 3 of the GTS is to transform malaria surveillance into a core intervention. To understand whether malaria surveillance systems are fit for purpose, WHO recommends the regular monitoring and evaluation of surveillance systems.
- The Global Malaria Programme (GMP), in collaboration with the University of Oslo, has developed standardized malaria modules in District Health Information Software2 (DHIS2) for aggregate and case-based collection of routine data with associated data elements, dashboards of key epidemiological and data quality indicators, reports and a curriculum for facility-level data analysis to facilitate data analysis and interpretation.
- As of October 2019, 23 countries have installed the WHO aggregate malaria module and another six installations are planned over the next year. Five countries have already developed and integrated their own malaria module into DHIS2.
- WHO has been working in coordination with national health management information systems (HMIS) departments of ministries of health, in particular the HBHI countries, to establish structured dynamic databases known as data repositories. The GMP has developed an easily adaptable repository structure in DHIS2, with guidance on relevant data elements and indicators, their definitions and computation to cover key thematic areas. So far, work to develop these databases has started in Gambia, Ghana, Mozambique, Nigeria, Uganda and the United Republic of Tanzania.
- WHO also encourages countries to implement surveillance system assessments. An example of such an assessment and its role in improving surveillance systems is illustrated through a case study of Mozambique.

## RESPONDING TO BIOLOGICAL THREATS TO THE FIGHT AGAINST MALARIA

### *Pfhrp2/3* gene deletions

- Deletions in the *pfhrp2* and *pfhrp3* (*pfhrp2/3*) genes of the parasite renders parasites undetectable by RDTs based on histidine-rich protein 2 (HRP2). The prevalence of dual *pfhrp2* and *pfhrp3* among symptomatic patients reached as high as 80% in Eritrea and Peru.
- WHO has recommended that countries with reports of *pfhrp2/3* deletions or neighbouring countries should conduct representative baseline surveys among suspected malaria cases to determine whether the prevalence of *pfhrp2/3* deletions causing false negative RDT results has reached a threshold for RDT change (>5% *pfhrp2* deletions causing false negative RDT results).
- WHO is tracking published reports of *pfhrp2/3* deletions using the Malaria Threat Map mapping tool. To date, 28 countries have reported *pfhrp2* deletions.

### Drug resistance

- *PfKelch13* mutations have been identified as molecular markers of partial artemisinin resistance. *PfKelch13* mutations associated with artemisinin resistance are widespread in the GMS, and have also been detected at a significant prevalence (over 5%) in Guyana, Papua New Guinea and Rwanda. In the case of Rwanda, the presence of *PfKelch13* mutations does not affect efficacy of first-line treatment.
- In the WHO Western Pacific Region, artemisinin resistance has been confirmed in Cambodia, Lao People's Democratic Republic and Viet Nam through several studies conducted between 2001

and 2018. Treatment efficacy for *P. vivax* remains high across all countries where treatment failure rates are below 10%.

- In the WHO African Region the efficacy rates of artemether-lumefantrine (AL), artesunate-amodiaquine (AS-AQ) and dihydroartemisinin-piperaquine (DHA-PPQ) for *P. falciparum* were more than 98%, and efficacy has remained high over time.

- Treatment efficacy with first-line treatment remains high for *P. falciparum* and *P. vivax* in the WHO Region of the Americas.

- In the WHO South-East Asia Region, the presence of molecular markers of artemisinin resistance has been reported in Bangladesh, India, Myanmar and Thailand. With the exception of Myanmar, failure rates of *P. falciparum* to first-line ACTs were found to be above 10% and were as high as 93% in Thailand. For *P. vivax* most countries continue to demonstrate high efficacy of chloroquine (CQ), except for Myanmar and Timor-Leste.

- In the WHO Eastern Mediterranean Region, high failure rates of treatment with artesunate-sulfadoxine-pyrimethamine (AS-SP) for *P. falciparum* in Somalia and Sudan led to a change in first-line treatment policy to AL. For *P. vivax* there is high treatment efficacy with AL and CQ in all countries where a therapeutic efficacy study (TES) has been conducted.

## Insecticide resistance

- From 2010 through 2018, some 81 countries reported data on insecticide resistance monitoring to WHO.

- Of the 81 malaria endemic countries that provided data for 2010–2018, resistance to at least one of the four insecticide classes in one malaria vector from one collection site was detected in 73 countries, an increase of five countries compared with the previous reporting period 2010–2017. In 26 countries, resistance was reported to all main insecticide classes.

- Resistance to pyrethroids – the only insecticide class currently used in ITNs – is widespread and was detected in at least one malaria vector in more than two thirds of the sites tested, and was highest in the WHO African Region and in the WHO Eastern Mediterranean Region.

- Resistance to organochlorines was detected for at least one malaria vector in almost two thirds of the sites. Resistance to carbamates and organophosphates was less prevalent and was detected in 31% and 26% of the tested sites, respectively. Prevalence was highest for carbamates in the WHO South-East Asia Region and for organophosphates in the WHO South-East Asia Region and in the WHO Western Pacific Region.

- All the standard insecticide resistance data reported to WHO are included in the WHO Global Insecticide Resistance database, and are available for exploration via the Malaria Threats Map. This online tool was extended in 2019 to cover invasive mosquito species, and currently shows the geographical extent of reports on the detection of *Anopheles stephensi*.

- To guide resistance management, countries should develop and implement a national plan for insecticide-resistance monitoring and management, drawing on the WHO *Framework for a national plan for monitoring and management of insecticide resistance in malaria vector*. In 2018, a total of 45 countries reported having completed plans for resistance monitoring and management and 36 were currently in the process of developing them.

- NMPs and their partners should consider the deployment of pyrethroid-piperonyl butoxide nets in geographical areas where the main malaria vectors meet the criteria recommended by WHO in 2017, rather than being based on whether the whole country meets the criteria.

# Avant-propos

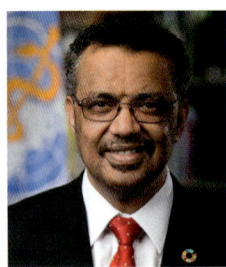

**Dr Tedros Adhanom Ghebreyesus**
Directeur général
de l'Organisation mondiale de la Santé (OMS)

### N'oublier personne sur la voie d'un monde sans paludisme

Le fléau du paludisme continue de toucher plus lourdement les femmes enceintes et les enfants en Afrique. Le *Rapport sur le paludisme dans le monde 2019* comporte donc une section spéciale sur le poids de cette maladie et ses conséquences sur ces deux groupes les plus à risque. Le message qu'il délivre est très clair : nous devons tous faire davantage pour protéger les plus vulnérables contre une maladie responsable de plus de 400 000 décès chaque année.

Le paludisme pendant la grossesse nuit à la santé de la mère et l'expose à un risque accru de décès. Il a un impact sur la santé du fœtus, entraînant prématurité et insuffisance pondérale à la naissance qui sont les principales causes de mortalité néonatale et infantile. L'an passé, environ 11 millions de femmes enceintes en Afrique subsaharienne ont présenté une infection palustre et, par conséquent, près de 900 000 enfants un faible poids à la naissance.

Pour protéger les femmes enceintes en Afrique, l'OMS recommande l'utilisation de moustiquaires imprégnées d'insecticide (MII) et de médicaments antipaludiques préventifs. Ce rapport fait état de progrès sur les deux fronts. Pourtant, près de 40 % des femmes enceintes n'ont pas dormi sous MII en 2018 et les deux tiers n'ont pas reçu le minimum de trois doses de traitement préventif comme il est recommandé.

En ce qui concerne les enfants, les efforts déployés pour améliorer l'accès aux médicaments antipaludiques préventifs portent leurs fruits. En Afrique, dans la sous-région du Sahel, l'OMS recommande la chimioprévention du paludisme saisonnier durant la période de pic de transmission. Plus de 60 % des enfants vivant dans des zones éligibles à ce traitement préventif en ont bénéficié en 2018.

La Sierra Leone peut être citée en exemple ; en effet, elle est devenue le premier pays d'Afrique à déployer le traitement préventif intermittent chez les nourrissons, une autre approche recommandée par l'OMS pour protéger les enfants en bas âge dans les zones touchées par le paludisme.

Chez les enfants présentant des signes de fièvre, l'accès aux soins reste néanmoins trop faible. En Afrique subsaharienne, les enquêtes nationales indiquent que près de 40 % des enfants ayant eu de la fièvre n'ont pas été orientés vers un prestataire médical formé.

Au moins 10 pays participant à l'« Initiative E-2020 » de l'OMS sont en passe d'atteindre l'objectif d'élimination du paludisme d'ici à 2020 défini dans notre stratégie mondiale de lutte contre le paludisme. En 2015, la maladie était endémique dans tous ces pays ; aujourd'hui, soit ils n'enregistrent aucun cas de paludisme indigène, soit ils sont tout proches de l'objectif.

Toutefois, les progrès réalisés au niveau mondial en termes de baisse de l'incidence du paludisme ont ralenti ces dernières années. Plus préoccupant encore, le paludisme progresse dans quelques pays d'Afrique où il pèse déjà lourdement.

Il est probable que des objectifs essentiels de notre stratégie mondiale de lutte contre le paludisme ne seront pas atteints.

En 2018, l'OMS et le Partenariat RBM pour en finir avec le paludisme ont lancé « *High burden to high impact* » (« D'une charge élevée à un fort impact »), une nouvelle approche visant à prévenir la maladie et à sauver des vies dans les pays les plus durement touchés par le paludisme. Se substituant à une stratégie « universelle », cette approche encourage l'utilisation des outils les plus efficaces de façon plus ciblée. Je suis ravi de constater que deux pays, l'Inde et l'Ouganda, ont rapporté une baisse substantielle du nombre de cas de paludisme en 2018 par rapport à l'année précédente.

En septembre, j'ai publié un « Malaria Challenge », préconisant d'investir davantage dans la recherche et le développement d'outils, de technologies et d'approches de transformation innovants afin d'accélérer les progrès réalisés pour vaincre cette maladie.

Grâce à un programme pilote coordonné par l'OMS, le Ghana, le Kenya et le Malawi ont récemment introduit dans certaines régions le premier vaccin antipaludique au monde. Les données et les expériences tirées de ce programme éclaireront les décisions politiques sur une utilisation éventuellement plus large du vaccin en Afrique. Grâce au soutien du Fonds mondial de lutte contre le sida, la tuberculose et le paludisme et d'Unitaid, d'autres outils prometteurs sont en phase de test, notamment de nouveaux types de moustiquaires imprégnées d'insecticide, ainsi que des outils ciblant les moustiques exophages.

Pour concrétiser notre vision commune d'un monde sans paludisme, nous allons également devoir renforcer notre action dans d'autres domaines essentiels. Nous avons besoin de services de santé abordables et axés sur les populations. Nous avons également besoin de systèmes de surveillance et de riposte qui soient fiables et précis. Enfin, nous devons définir des stratégies parfaitement adaptées aux conditions locales de transmission du paludisme.

Augmenter le financement de la lutte contre le paludisme est également indispensable. En 2018, le financement total du contrôle et de l'élimination du paludisme a atteint US$ 2,7 milliards, bien en deçà de l'objectif de US$ 5 milliards défini dans le cadre de notre stratégie mondiale.

Grâce à un financement solide et résolu, à un véritable leadership politique et à une couverture de santé universelle, nous pourrons venir à bout de cette maladie une fois pour toutes.

# Le rapport de cette année en un clin d'œil

## POIDS DU PALUDISME AU NIVEAU MONDIAL ET RÉGIONAL : ÉVOLUTION DU NOMBRE DE CAS ET DE DÉCÈS

### Cas de paludisme

- Au niveau mondial, le nombre de cas de paludisme est estimé à 228 millions en 2018 (intervalle de confiance [IC] de 95 % : 206-258 millions), contre 251 millions en 2010 (IC de 95 % : 231-278 millions) et 231 millions en 2017 (IC de 95 % : 211-259 millions).
- La plupart des cas (213 millions ou 93 %) ont été enregistrés en 2018 dans la région Afrique de l'OMS, loin devant la région Asie du Sud-Est (3,4 %) et la région Méditerranée orientale (2,1 %).
- Dix-neuf pays d'Afrique subsaharienne[1] et l'Inde ont concentré quasiment 85 % du nombre total de cas de paludisme dans le monde. Six pays, à eux seuls, ont enregistré plus de la moitié des cas : le Nigéria (25 %), la République démocratique du Congo (12 %), l'Ouganda (5 %), ainsi que la Côte d'Ivoire, le Mozambique et le Niger (4 % chacun).
- Au niveau mondial, l'incidence du paludisme a reculé entre 2010 et 2018, passant de 71 cas pour 1 000 habitants exposés au risque de paludisme à 57 pour 1 000. Néanmoins, cette baisse a considérablement ralenti entre 2014 et 2018, l'incidence ayant diminué à 57 pour 1 000 en 2014 pour rester à un niveau similaire jusqu'en 2018.
- Dans la région Asie du Sud-Est de l'OMS, l'incidence du paludisme continue à baisser, de 17 cas pour 1 000 habitants exposés au risque de paludisme en 2010 à 5 pour 1 000 en 2018 (soit une baisse de 70 %). De même, l'incidence du paludisme a diminué dans la région Afrique de l'OMS, avec 294 cas pour 1 000 en 2010 contre 229 en 2018 (-22 %). Toutes les autres régions de l'OMS ont enregistré des progrès très modestes, voire une hausse de l'incidence. Dans la région Amériques de l'OMS, l'incidence du paludisme a augmenté, principalement à cause d'une transmission accrue au Venezuela (République bolivarienne du).
- Seuls 31 pays dans lesquels le paludisme est encore endémique ont réduit l'incidence du paludisme de manière significative entre 2015 et 2018 et étaient donc en passe d'atteindre une baisse de l'incidence égale à au moins 40 % d'ici 2020. À moins d'un changement rapide, les objectifs de morbidité définis pour 2025 et 2030 dans la *Stratégie technique de lutte contre le paludisme 2016-2030* ([le] GTS) ne seront pas atteints.
- *P. falciparum* est le parasite du paludisme le plus prévalent dans la région Afrique de l'OMS ; il est en effet à l'origine de 99,7 % des cas de paludisme estimés en 2018, tout comme dans les régions Asie du Sud-Est (50 %), Méditerranée orientale (71 %) et Pacifique occidental (65 %).
- Au niveau mondial, 53 % des cas de paludisme à *P. vivax* sont enregistrés dans la région Asie du Sud-Est de l'OMS, avec une majorité des cas en Inde (47 %). *P. vivax* prédomine dans la région Amériques de l'OMS, représentant 75 % des cas de paludisme.

### Mortalité associée

- Au niveau mondial, le nombre de décès dus au paludisme a été estimé à 405 000 en 2018, contre 416 000 en 2017 et 585 000 en 2010.
- Les enfants de moins de 5 ans sont les plus vulnérables face au paludisme. En 2018, ils ont représenté 67 % (272 000) des décès associés au paludisme dans le monde.
- À elle seule, la région Afrique de l'OMS a enregistré 94 % des décès liés au paludisme dans le monde en 2018. Pourtant, elle a aussi représenté 85 % des 180 000 décès en moins dus à la maladie par rapport à 2010.

---

[1] La liste des pays d'Afrique subsaharienne est disponible à l'adresse https://unstats.un.org/unsd/methodology/m49 ; pour toutes les analyses présentées dans ce rapport et liées aux pays d'endémie du paludisme en Afrique subsaharienne, le Soudan est également inclus.

- Près de 85 % des décès dus au paludisme dans le monde en 2018 ont été concentrés dans 20 pays de la région Afrique de l'OMS et en Inde. Le Nigéria a représenté à lui seul près de 24 % de ces décès, suivi par la République démocratique du Congo (11 %), la République-Unie de Tanzanie (5 %), ainsi que l'Angola, le Mozambique et le Niger (4 % chacun).
- Par rapport à 2010, la mortalité liée au paludisme n'a diminué en 2018 que dans les régions Afrique et Asie du Sud-Est de l'OMS. La baisse la plus prononcée du nombre de décès dus au paludisme, en valeur absolue, a été observée dans la région Afrique de l'OMS, qui est passée de 533 000 décès en 2010 à 380 000 en 2018. Malgré ces progrès, la baisse de la mortalité liée au paludisme a ralenti depuis 2016.

## CONSÉQUENCES DU PALUDISME SUR LA SANTÉ MATERNELLE ET INFANTILE

- En 2018, près de 11 millions de femmes enceintes vivant dans des zones de transmission modérée à élevée en Afrique subsaharienne auraient été exposées à une infection palustre.
- Cette même année, la prévalence de l'exposition à l'infection palustre durant la grossesse a été plus forte dans les sous-régions Afrique de l'Ouest et Afrique centrale (chacune avec 35 %), suivies par la sous-région Afrique de l'Est et Afrique australe (20 %). Près de 39 % de cette prévalence a été concentrée en République démocratique du Congo et au Nigéria.
- Les 11 millions de femmes enceintes exposées à une infection palustre en 2018 ont donné naissance à quelque 872 000 enfants présentant un faible poids à la naissance (soit 16 % de tous les enfants avec un faible poids à la naissance dans ces pays). L'Afrique de l'Ouest a enregistré la plus forte prévalence d'insuffisance pondérale (liée au paludisme pendant la grossesse) chez le nouveau-né.
- Entre 2015 et 2018, dans 21 pays de la région Afrique de l'OMS où la transmission du paludisme est modérée à élevée, la prévalence de l'anémie chez les enfants de moins de 5 ans avec un résultat positif à un test de diagnostic rapide (TDR) était deux fois plus élevée que chez les enfants avec un résultat de TDR négatif. Parmi les enfants avec un résultat de test positif, 9 % souffraient d'anémie grave et 54 % d'anémie modérée. À titre de comparaison, 1 % seulement des enfants non infectés par le paludisme souffraient d'anémie grave et 31 % d'anémie modérée.
- Les pays où l'anémie grave chez les enfants de moins de 5 ans présentant un résultat positif à un test de dépistage du paludisme était la plus prévalente étaient les suivants : le Sénégal (26 %), le Mali (16 %), la Guinée (14 %) et le Mozambique (12 %). Dans la plupart des autres pays, l'anémie grave atteignait entre 5 % et 10 %.
- Selon les estimations, près de 24 millions d'enfants d'Afrique subsaharienne ont souffert d'infections palustres à *P. falciparum* en 2018, avec un risque d'anémie grave pour 1,8 million d'entre eux.

## APPROCHE « HIGH BURDEN TO HIGH IMPACT » (D'UNE CHARGE ÉLEVÉE À UN FORT IMPACT)

- Les 11 pays où le paludisme sévit le plus (pays de l'approche HBHI) ont enregistré près de 155 millions de cas en 2018, contre 177 millions en 2010. La République démocratique du Congo et le Nigéria ont cumulé 84 millions de ces cas (54 %).
- Parmi les 10 pays africains de l'approche HBHI, le Ghana et le Nigéria ont rapporté les plus fortes augmentations, en valeur absolue, du nombre de cas en 2018 par rapport à 2017. En 2018, le poids du paludisme dans les autres pays est resté à un niveau similaire à celui de 2017, à l'exception de l'Ouganda et de l'Inde, qui ont rapporté respectivement 1,5 million et 2,6 millions de cas en moins.
- Les décès dus au paludisme ont diminué, passant de près de 400 000 en 2010 à environ 260 000 en 2018. La plus forte baisse a été enregistrée au Nigéria, avec 153 000 décès en 2010 et 95 000 décès en 2018.
- En 2018, dans les 11 pays de l'approche HBHI, au moins 40 % de la population à risque avait dormi sous moustiquaire imprégnée d'insecticide longue durée (MILD). Le pourcentage le plus élevé a été enregistré en Ouganda (80 %), et le plus faible au Nigéria (40 %).

- Selon les estimations, c'est uniquement au Burkina Faso et en République-Unie de Tanzanie que plus de 50 % des femmes enceintes ont reçu trois doses de traitement préventif intermittent pendant la grossesse (TPIp3) en 2018. Au Cameroun, au Nigéria et en Ouganda, le taux de couverture a atteint environ 30 %, voire moins.
- Six pays de la sous-région sahélienne ont mis en œuvre la chimioprévention du paludisme saisonnier (CPS) en 2018. En moyenne, 17 millions d'enfants sur les 26 millions ciblés ont été traités par cycle de CPS.
- Le pourcentage des enfants de moins de 5 ans ayant de la fièvre et sollicitant des soins a varié entre 58 % au Mali et 82 % en Ouganda. En République démocratique du Congo et au Mali, plus de 40 % des enfants n'ont sollicité aucun soin. Tout aussi préoccupant, le taux de dépistage du paludisme a été très faible chez les enfants sollicitant des soins, avec 30 % ou moins d'enfants testés au Cameroun, en République démocratique du Congo et au Nigéria.
- Dans tous les pays de l'approche HBHI à l'exception de l'Inde, les investissements nationaux directs restent très peu élevés par rapport au financement international.

## ÉLIMINATION DU PALUDISME ET PRÉVENTION DE SA RÉAPPARITION

- Au niveau mondial, l'élimination du paludisme progresse. En effet, de plus en plus de pays tendent vers un nombre de cas de paludisme indigène égal à zéro. En 2018, 49 pays ont rapporté moins de 10 000 cas de paludisme indigène, alors qu'ils n'étaient que 46 en 2017 et 40 en 2010. Le nombre de pays comptant moins de 100 cas de paludisme indigène, un bon indicateur que l'élimination de la maladie est proche, est passé de 17 en 2010 à 25 en 2017, puis à 27 en 2018.
- Le Paraguay et l'Ouzbékistan ont été certifiés exempts de paludisme par l'OMS en 2018, alors que l'Algérie et l'Argentine ont obtenu cette certification début 2019. En 2018, la Chine, El Salvador, l'Iran, la Malaisie et le Timor-Leste ont rapporté zéro cas de paludisme indigène.
- Éliminer le paludisme dans au moins 10 pays où il était encore endémique en 2010 est l'un des principaux objectifs intermédiaires du GTS pour 2020. Compte tenu du rythme de progression actuel, il est probable que cet objectif sera atteint.
- En 2016, l'OMS a identifié 21 pays ayant le potentiel pour éliminer le paludisme d'ici 2020. L'OMS travaille avec les gouvernements de ces pays appelés « E-2020 » pour les aider à atteindre leurs objectifs d'élimination.
- Même si 10 de ces pays restent en bonne voie pour atteindre leurs objectifs, les Comores et le Costa Rica ont rapporté une augmentation des cas de paludisme indigène en 2018 par rapport à 2017.
- En revanche, dans les six pays de la sous-région du Grand Mékong (Cambodge, Chine [province du Yunnan], République démocratique populaire lao, Myanmar, Thaïlande et Viet Nam), le nombre de cas de paludisme rapportés a diminué de 76 % entre 2010 et 2018, alors que le nombre de décès dus au paludisme a chuté de 95 % sur la même période. En 2018, le Cambodge n'a rapporté aucun décès dû au paludisme pour la première fois de son histoire.

## INVESTISSEMENTS DANS LES PROGRAMMES ET LA RECHERCHE ANTIPALUDIQUES

- En 2018, US$ 2,7 milliards ont été investis au total par les gouvernements des pays d'endémie et les partenaires internationaux pour le contrôle et l'élimination du paludisme, soit une baisse par rapport aux US$ 3,2 milliards investis en 2017. Les investissements de 2018 sont bien inférieurs aux

- US$ 5 milliards estimés nécessaires à l'échelle mondiale pour rester sur la voie des objectifs du GTS.
- Près des trois quarts des investissements réalisés en 2018 ont été dirigés vers la région Afrique de l'OMS, suivie par les régions Amériques (7 %), Asie du Sud-Est (6 %), Méditerranée orientale et Pacifique occidental (5 % chacune).
- En 2018, 47 % du financement total a été investi dans des pays à faible revenu, 43 % dans des pays à revenu intermédiaire de la tranche inférieure et 11 % dans des pays à revenu intermédiaire de la tranche supérieure. Les fonds internationaux ont représenté la principale source de financement dans les pays à faible revenu et à revenu intermédiaire de la tranche inférieure (respectivement 85 % et 61 %). Les financements nationaux stagnent depuis 2010.
- Sur les US$ 2,7 milliards investis en 2018, US$ 1,8 milliard provenaient de bailleurs de fonds internationaux. En 2018, les gouvernements des pays d'endémie ont contribué à hauteur de 30 % du financement total (US$ 900 millions), un chiffre inchangé par rapport à 2017. Deux tiers des financements nationaux ont été investis dans des activités de contrôle menées par les programmes nationaux de lutte contre le paludisme (PNLP), le tiers restant étant estimé correspondre aux coûts des soins dispensés aux patients.
- Comme les années précédentes, les États-Unis ont été le premier bailleur de fonds international pour les programmes de lutte contre le paludisme, avec US$ 1 milliard en 2018 (37 % du total). Les pays membres du Comité d'aide au développement ont investi au total US$ 300 millions (11 %). Le Royaume-Uni de Grande-Bretagne et d'Irlande du Nord a contribué à hauteur d'environ US$ 200 millions (7 %).
- Sur les US$ 2,7 milliards investis en 2018, US$ 1 milliard ont transité par le Fonds mondial de lutte contre le sida, la tuberculose et le paludisme.
- Même si le financement de la lutte contre le paludisme est relativement stable depuis 2010, les investissements consentis en 2018 sont loin d'atteindre le niveau requis pour réaliser les deux premiers objectifs intermédiaires du GTS, à savoir réduire d'au moins 40 % l'incidence du paludisme et la mortalité associée au plan mondial par rapport à 2015.
- Au total, US$ 663 millions ont été investis en 2018 dans la recherche fondamentale et le développement de produits contre le paludisme, soit une hausse de US$ 18 millions par rapport à 2017.
- Les fonds dédiés à la recherche et au développement (R&D) de médicaments ont atteint un niveau record, passant de US$ 228 millions en 2017 à US$ 252 millions en 2018. Cette augmentation est due aux investissements du secteur industriel privé dans plusieurs essais de phase II sur de nouveaux composants chimiques offrant le potentiel d'une guérison radicale en une prise unique.

## Livraison de produits antipaludiques

### Moustiquaires imprégnées d'insecticide

- Les fabricants de moustiquaires imprégnées d'insecticide (MII) ont indiqué en avoir livré 578 millions dans le monde entre 2016 et 2018, principalement des MILD, dont 50 % en Côte d'Ivoire, en République démocratique du Congo, en Éthiopie, au Ghana, en Inde, au Nigéria, en Ouganda et en République-Unie de Tanzanie.
- En 2018, ces fabricants ont livré environ 197 millions de MII, dont plus de 87 % en Afrique subsaharienne.
- Au niveau mondial, 80 % des MII ont été distribuées gratuitement par le biais de campagnes de distribution de masse, 10 % via des établissements de soins prénataux et 6 % dans le cadre de programmes de vaccination.

### Tests de diagnostic rapide

- En 2018, 412 millions de TDR ont été vendus dans le monde.
- En 2018, 259 millions de TDR ont été distribués par les PNLP. La plupart de ces TDR (64 %) étaient des tests livrés en Afrique subsaharienne et pouvant uniquement détecter le parasite *P. falciparum*.

**Combinaisons thérapeutiques à base d'artémisinine**
- Entre 2010 et 2018, les pays ont acheté 3 milliards de traitements par combinaison thérapeutique à base d'artémisinine (ACT). Au total, 63 % de ces achats auraient été effectués pour le secteur public de la santé.
- En 2018, 214 millions de traitements par ACT ont été distribués par les PNLP, dont 98 % dans la région Afrique de l'OMS.

# PRÉVENTION DU PALUDISME

## Lutte antivectorielle
- En Afrique subsaharienne, la moitié de la population à risque dort sous MII : en 2018, 50 % de la population a donc été protégée par cette intervention, contre 29 % en 2010. Par ailleurs, la part de la population ayant accès à une MII est passée de 33 % en 2010 à 57 % en 2018. Le taux de couverture n'a cependant que très peu augmenté depuis 2015 et il s'est même stabilisé depuis 2016.
- Le pourcentage des ménages disposant d'au moins une MII pour deux membres du foyer est passé de 47 % en 2010 à 72 % en 2018. Ce pourcentage ne représente néanmoins qu'une augmentation très modeste au cours des trois dernières années et reste bien loin de l'objectif de couverture universelle.
- La part de la population à risque protégée par pulvérisation intradomiciliaire d'insecticides à effet rémanent (PID), une mesure préventive qui consiste à pulvériser d'insecticides les murs intérieurs des habitations, a diminué. Au niveau mondial, le taux de couverture de cette intervention a diminué, passant d'un pic de 5 % en 2010 à 2 % en 2018, avec des tendances à la baisse dans toutes les régions de l'OMS, hormis la région Méditerranée orientale.
- Même si la population à risque couverte par cette intervention a chuté de 180 millions en 2010 à 93 millions en 2018, elle est pour 2018 inférieure de 13 millions au niveau de 2017.
- Ce recul de la couverture en PID est sans doute lié au passage des pyréthoïdes à des insecticides plus onéreux en réponse à la résistance aux pyréthoïdes ou à des changements de stratégies opérationnelles (baisse de la population à risque dans les pays en voie d'élimination du paludisme).

## Traitements préventifs
- En Afrique, pour protéger les femmes vivant dans des zones de transmission modérée à élevée, l'OMS recommande le traitement préventif intermittent pendant la grossesse (TPIp) par sulfadoxine-pyriméthamine (SP). Sur 36 pays africains ayant communiqué des données de couverture en TPIp en 2018, 31 % des femmes enceintes éligibles ont reçu au moins trois doses de TPIp (comme recommandé par l'OMS), contre 22 % en 2017 et 2 % en 2010, ce qui traduit des progrès considérables en termes de mise en œuvre au niveau national.
- Toutefois, environ 18 % des femmes s'étant présentées au moins une fois dans un établissement de soins prénataux n'ont reçu aucune dose de TPIp. Si elles avaient été exploitées, ces opportunités de traitement auraient permis d'améliorer considérablement et rapidement la couverture en TPIp.
- En 2018, 19 millions d'enfants vivant dans 12 pays d'Afrique sahélienne ont été protégés par des programmes de CPS. Tous les enfants ciblés ont reçu un traitement au Cameroun, en Guinée, en Guinée-Bissau et au Mali. Cependant, quelque 12 millions d'enfants qui auraient pu bénéficier de cette intervention n'ont pas été couverts, principalement à cause d'un manque de financements.

## DIAGNOSTIC ET TRAITEMENT

### Accès aux soins

- Un diagnostic précoce et un traitement rapide sont les moyens les plus efficaces de prévenir l'aggravation des cas de paludisme et les décès associés. D'après les enquêtes nationales réalisées dans 20 pays d'Afrique subsaharienne entre 2015 et 2018, une médiane de 42 % (écart interquartile [ÉI] : 34 %-49 %) des enfants ayant eu de la fièvre ont sollicité des soins auprès d'un prestataire formé dans un établissement public, contre une médiane de 10 % (ÉI : 8 %-22 %) dans un établissement privé formel et de 3 % (ÉI : 2 %-7 %) dans le secteur privé informel.
- Une part importante des enfants n'ont pas reçu de soins médicaux (médiane de 36 %, ÉI : 28 %-45 %), ce qui s'explique en partie par un accès limité aux prestataires de santé ou un manque de connaissances de la part du personnel soignant.

### Diagnostic

- Le pourcentage de patients suspectés de paludisme et soumis à un test de diagnostic par TDR ou microscopie dans un établissement public est passé de 38 % en 2010 à 85 % en 2018.
- Dans 71 % des pays d'Afrique subsaharienne où la transmission est modérée à élevée, le pourcentage des cas suspectés de paludisme ayant été soumis à un test parasitologique a dépassé 80 % en 2018.
- Sur les 19 enquêtes nationales réalisées auprès des ménages en Afrique subsaharienne entre 2015 et 2018, le pourcentage médian d'enfants fiévreux ayant subi un prélèvement sanguin au doigt ou au talon (laissant penser qu'un test de dépistage du paludisme a été réalisé) a été plus élevé dans le secteur public (médiane de 66 %, ÉI : 49 %-75 %) que dans les établissements privés formels (médiane de 40 %, ÉI : 16 %-46 %) ou dans le secteur privé informel (médiane de 9 %, ÉI : 5 %-22 %).
- Sur 61 enquêtes menées dans 29 pays d'Afrique subsaharienne entre 2010 et 2018, le pourcentage des enfants fiévreux soumis à un test de diagnostic préalablement à tout traitement antipaludique dans un établissement public a augmenté, passant d'une médiane de 48 % (ÉI : 30 %-62 %) sur la période 2010-2013 à une médiane de 76 % (ÉI : 60 %-86 %) sur la période 2015-2018.

### Traitement

- Sur 20 enquêtes nationales réalisées auprès des ménages en Afrique subsaharienne entre 2015 et 2018, le pourcentage médian des enfants fiévreux et ayant reçu un médicament antipaludique a été plus important dans le secteur public (médiane de 48 %, ÉI : 30 %-69 %) que dans le secteur privé formel (médiane de 40 %, ÉI : 21 %-51 %) ou le secteur privé informel (médiane de 18 %, ÉI : 10 %-29 %).
- Entre 2015 et 2018, les données collectées à partir de 20 enquêtes nationales menées en Afrique subsaharienne montrent que 47 % (ÉI : 29 %-69 %) des enfants fiévreux ayant sollicité des soins dans le secteur public ont reçu un traitement antipaludique, contre 59 % (ÉI : 53 %-84 %) auprès d'un agent de santé communautaire et 49 % (ÉI : 19 %-55 %) dans un établissement privé formel.
- D'après 19 enquêtes, la probabilité que les traitements antipaludiques donnés aux enfants fiévreux soient des ACT est légèrement plus élevée si le traitement est sollicité dans le secteur public (médiane de 80 %, ÉI : 45 %-94 %) que s'il l'est dans le secteur privé formel (médiane de 77 %, ÉI : 43 %-87 %) ou le secteur privé informel (médiane de 60 %, ÉI : 40 %-84 %).
- Pour combler les écarts de traitement parmi les enfants, l'OMS recommande la prise en charge intégrée des cas dans la communauté (PEC-C). Cette approche favorise la gestion intégrée des causes de mortalité infantile, à savoir paludisme, pneumonie et diarrhée, au niveau des établissements de santé et de la communauté. En 2018, 30 pays avaient des politiques de PEC-C en place à différents niveaux, mais la mise en œuvre n'était effective au niveau national que dans quelques-uns.

## SYSTÈMES DE SURVEILLANCE DU PALUDISME

- Faire de la surveillance du paludisme une intervention de base est le pilier 3 du GTS. Pour savoir si les systèmes de surveillance du paludisme en place sont adaptés, l'OMS recommande un suivi et une évaluation à intervalles réguliers de ces systèmes.
- En collaboration avec l'Université d'Oslo, le Programme mondial de lutte antipaludique a développé des modules sur le paludisme uniformisés et intégrés à District Health Information Software2 (DHIS2). Ils permettent une collecte basée sur les cas et agrégée des données de routine, ainsi que la mise à disposition d'éléments associés, de tableaux de bord des principaux indicateurs épidémiologiques, d'indicateurs de qualité des données, de rapports et d'un programme d'analyse des données au niveau des établissements en vue de faciliter l'analyse et l'interprétation des données.
- En date du mois d'octobre 2019, 23 pays avaient installé le module agrégé de l'OMS sur le paludisme, et six autres installations étaient planifiées pour 2020. Cinq pays ont déjà développé leur propre module sur le paludisme et l'ont intégré à DHIS2.
- L'OMS travaille conjointement avec les départements chargés des systèmes de gestion de l'information sanitaire de différents ministères de la Santé, en particulier dans les pays de l'approche HBHI, pour établir des bases de données dynamiques structurées, appelées référentiels de données. Le Programme mondial de lutte antipaludique a ainsi développé une structure de référentiel facile à adapter dans DHIS2, ainsi que des directives sur des éléments de données et des indicateurs pertinents, leurs définitions et les calculs en vue de couvrir les domaines thématiques essentiels. À ce jour, le travail de développement de ces bases de données a commencé en Gambie, au Ghana, au Mozambique, au Nigéria, en Ouganda et en République-Unie de Tanzanie.
- L'OMS encourage également les pays à mettre en œuvre des évaluations de leur système de surveillance. L'étude de cas du Mozambique est un parfait exemple de ce genre d'évaluation et de son rôle pour améliorer les systèmes de surveillance.

## RÉPONSES AUX MENACES BIOLOGIQUES EN MATIÈRE DE LUTTE CONTRE LE PALUDISME

### Suppression du gène *pfhrp2/3*

- La suppression des gènes *pfhrp2* et *pfhrp3* (*pfhrp2/3*) du parasite rendent ces derniers indétectables par les TDR basés sur la protéine riche en histidine 2 (HRP2). La prévalence des deux gènes *pfhrp2* et *pfhrp3* chez les patients symptomatiques a atteint jusqu'à 80 % en Érythrée et au Pérou.
- L'OMS a recommandé aux pays rapportant des suppressions des gènes *pfhrp2/3* ou à leurs pays voisins de mener des études de référence représentatives sur les cas suspectés de paludisme, afin de déterminer si la prévalence des suppressions *pfhrp2/3* causant des résultats de TDR négatifs avait atteint un seuil qui nécessite un changement de TDR (suppressions du gène *pfhrp2* > 5 % causant des faux résultats de TDR négatifs).
- L'OMS effectue un suivi des rapports publiés sur les suppressions des gènes *pfhrp2/3* par le biais de l'outil de cartographie Carte des menaces du paludisme. À ce jour, 28 pays ont rapporté des suppressions du gène *pfhrp2*.

### Résistance aux antipaludiques

- Des mutations du gène *PfKelch13* ont été identifiées en tant que marqueurs moléculaires de résistance partielle à l'artémisinine. Ces mutations *PfKelch13* associées à la résistance à l'artémisinine sont répandues dans la sous-région du Grand Mékong et ont également été détectées avec une forte prévalence (plus de 5 %) au Guyana, en Papouasie-Nouvelle-Guinée et au Rwanda. Dans le cas du Rwanda, la présence de mutations *PfKelch13* n'affecte pas l'efficacité des traitements de première intention.

- Dans la région Pacifique occidental de l'OMS, diverses études menées entre 2001 et 2018 ont confirmé une résistance à l'artémisinine au Cambodge, en République démocratique populaire lao et au Viet Nam. L'efficacité du traitement contre les infections à *P. vivax* reste élevée dans tous les pays où le taux d'échec au traitement est inférieur à 10 %.
- Dans la région Afrique de l'OMS, les taux d'efficacité des traitements à base d'artéméther-luméfantrine (AL), d'artésunate-amodiaquine (AS-AQ) et de dihydroartémisinine-pipéraquine (DHA-PPQ) contre les infections à *P. falciparum* ont été supérieurs à 98 %, et l'efficacité n'a jamais faibli au fil du temps.
- L'efficacité des traitements de première intention reste élevée contre les infections à *P. falciparum* et à *P. vivax* dans la région Amériques de l'OMS.
- Dans la région Asie du Sud-Est de l'OMS, la présence de marqueurs moléculaires de résistance à l'artémisinine a été rapportée au Bangladesh, en Inde, au Myanmar et en Thaïlande. À l'exception du Myanmar, les taux d'échec des ACT de première intention contre les infections à *P. falciparum* se sont avérés supérieurs à 10 % et ont même atteint 93 % en Thaïlande. Concernant les infections à *P. vivax*, la plupart des pays continuent d'enregistrer une grande efficacité de la chloroquine (CQ), sauf au Myanmar et au Timor-Leste.
- Dans la région Méditerranée orientale de l'OMS, les taux d'échec importants des traitements à base d'AS-SP contre les infections à *P. falciparum* en Somalie et au Soudan ont induit un changement dans la politique du traitement de première intention en faveur de l'AL. Concernant les infections à *P. vivax*, l'efficacité des traitements à base d'AL et de CQ est élevée dans tous les pays où une étude sur leur efficacité thérapeutique a été menée.

### Résistance aux insecticides

- De 2010 à 2018, quelque 81 pays ont transmis à l'OMS des données de surveillance sur la résistance aux insecticides.
- Sur les 81 pays d'endémie palustre ayant fourni des données pour la période 2010-2018, la résistance à au moins une des quatre classes d'insecticides chez l'un des vecteurs du paludisme sur un site de collecte a été détectée dans 73 pays. Il s'agit là d'une augmentation de cinq pays par rapport à la période précédente de 2010-2017. Dans 26 pays, la résistance a été rapportée à toutes les principales classes d'insecticides.
- La résistance aux pyréthoïdes, la seule classe d'insecticides actuellement utilisés dans les MII, est répandue. Elle a été détectée chez au moins un des vecteurs du paludisme sur plus des deux tiers des sites testés et s'est avérée la plus élevée dans les régions Afrique et Méditerranée orientale de l'OMS.
- La résistance aux organochlorés a été détectée chez au moins un des vecteurs du paludisme sur près des deux tiers des sites. La résistance aux carbamates et aux organophosphorés a été moins prévalente, mais a été détectée, respectivement, sur 31 % et 26 % des sites testés. La résistance la plus prévalente aux carbamates a été détecté dans la région Asie du Sud-Est de l'OMS, et aux organophosphorés dans les régions Asie du Sud-Est et Pacifique occidental de l'OMS.
- Toutes les données standard sur la résistance aux insecticides rapportées à l'OMS sont intégrées à la base de données mondiales de l'OMS sur la résistance aux insecticides, et leur accès à des fins d'exploration est possible via la Carte des menaces du paludisme. Cet outil en ligne a été enrichi en 2019 pour couvrir les espèces de moustiques envahissantes et présente à l'heure actuelle la dimension géographique des rapports sur la détection des espèces *Anopheles stephensi*.
- Pour orienter la gestion de la résistance, les pays doivent développer et mettre en œuvre des plans nationaux de suivi et de gestion de la résistance aux insecticides, en se basant sur le *Cadre conceptuel d'un plan national de suivi et de gestion de la résistance aux insecticides chez les vecteurs du paludisme* élaboré par l'OMS. En 2018, 45 pays ont indiqué avoir établi un plan de suivi et de gestion de la résistance, et 36 en étaient encore à la phase de développement.
- Les PNLP et leurs partenaires devraient envisager de déployer des moustiquaires imprégnées de butoxyde de pipéronyle (PBO) dans les zones géographiques où les principaux vecteurs du paludisme répondent aux critères recommandés par l'OMS en 2017, plutôt qu'en partant du principe que tout le pays doit répondre à ces critères.

# Prefacio

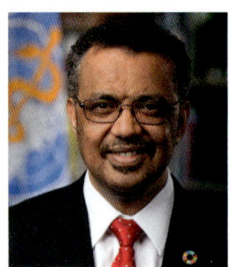

**Dr Tedros Adhanom Ghebreyesus**
Director General
Organización Mundial de la Salud (OMS)

**No dejar a nadie atrás en la marcha hacia un mundo libre de malaria**

El flagelo de la malaria continúa golpeando con más fuerza a las mujeres embarazadas y a los niños en África. El *Informe mundial sobre la malaria 2019* incluye una sección especial centrada en la carga y las consecuencias de la enfermedad entre estos dos grupos de mayor riesgo. Transmite un mensaje claro: todos debemos hacer más para proteger a los más vulnerables en la lucha contra una enfermedad que sigue cobrando más de 400 000 vidas cada año.

La malaria en el embarazo compromete la salud de la madre y la pone en mayor riesgo de muerte. Afecta la salud del feto, lo que lleva a la prematuridad y al bajo peso al nacer, los principales contribuyentes de la mortalidad neonatal e infantil. El año pasado, unos 11 millones de mujeres embarazadas en África subsahariana se infectaron con malaria y, en consecuencia, casi 900 000 niños nacieron con bajo peso al nacer.

Para proteger a las mujeres embarazadas en África, la OMS recomienda el uso de mosquiteros tratados con insecticidas (MTI) y medicamentos antimaláricos preventivos. Este informe muestra el progreso en ambos frentes. Aún así, casi el 40% de las mujeres embarazadas no durmieron bajo un MTI en 2018 y dos tercios no recibieron las tres o más dosis recomendadas de terapia preventiva.

En los niños, los esfuerzos para ampliar el acceso a los medicamentos antipalúdicos preventivos están dando frutos. En la subregión del Sahel de África, la OMS recomienda la quimio-prevención de la malaria estacional durante la temporada alta de transmisión. Más del 60% de los niños que viven en áreas elegibles para esta terapia preventiva la recibieron en 2018.

Se debe elogiar a Sierra Leona por convertirse en el primer país de África en implementar un tratamiento preventivo intermitente en infantes, otro enfoque recomendado por la OMS para proteger a los niños pequeños en las áreas afectadas por la malaria.

Aún así, el acceso a la atención de los niños que muestran signos de fiebre sigue siendo demasiado bajo. Las encuestas de países muestran que casi 40% de los niños febriles en África subsahariana no son atendidos por un proveedor de atención médica capacitado.

Al menos 10 países que forman parte de la "Iniciativa E-2020" de la OMS están en camino de alcanzar la eliminación en 2020, hito de nuestra estrategia mundial contra la malaria. En 2015, todos estos países eran endémicos de malaria; ahora han logrado cero casos autóctonos de malaria o se están acercando a ésta meta.

Sin embargo, en los últimos años, el progreso global de la reducción de nuevos casos de malaria se ha estabilizado. Lo más preocupante de todo es que la malaria está en aumento en algunos países de alta carga en África.

Es probable que se pierdan los hitos críticos de nuestra estrategia global contra la malaria.

En 2018, la OMS y la Alianza para Hacer Retroceder la Malaria lanzaron el nuevo enfoque de "Alta carga a alto impacto", para prevenir la enfermedad y salvar vidas en los países más afectados por la malaria. Reemplazando una estrategia de "talla única", el enfoque requiere el uso de las herramientas más efectivas de una manera más específica. Me complace observar que dos países, India y Uganda, han reportado reducciones sustanciales en los casos de malaria en 2018 comparado con el año anterior.

En septiembre, emití el "Reto de la malaria", que pedía una mayor inversión en investigación y el desarrollo de nuevas herramientas, tecnologías y enfoques transformadores para acelerar el progreso en la lucha contra esta enfermedad.

A través de un programa piloto coordinado por la OMS, Ghana, Kenia y Malawi introdujeron recientemente, en áreas seleccionadas, la primera vacuna contra la malaria del mundo. La evidencia y la experiencia del programa informarán las decisiones de política sobre el posible uso más amplio de la vacuna en África. Con el apoyo del Fondo Mundial para la lucha contra el VIH/SIDA, la tuberculosis y la malaria y del Unitaid, se están probando otras herramientas prometedoras, como nuevos tipos de mosquiteros tratados con insecticidas e intervenciones dirigidas a los mosquitos que pican fuera de las viviendas.

Lograr nuestra visión común de un mundo libre de malaria también requerirá mejorar acciones en otras áreas críticas. Necesitamos servicios de salud asequibles y centrados en las personas. Necesitamos sistemas de vigilancia y respuesta confiables y precisos. Necesitamos estrategias que se adapten a los entornos locales de transmisión de la malaria.

Acelerar el financiamiento para responder a la malaria es esencial. En 2018, el financiamiento total para el control y la eliminación de la malaria alcanzó un estimado de US $ 2.7 mil millones, muy por debajo del objetivo de financiamiento de US $ 5 mil millones de nuestra estrategia global.

A través de una financiación sólida y decidida, liderazgo político y cobertura de salud universal, podemos vencer esta enfermedad de una vez por todas.

# El informe de este año de un vistazo

## TENDENCIAS REGIONALES Y MUNDIALES SOBRE LA CARGA DE CASOS Y MUERTES POR MALARIA

### Casos de malaria

- En 2018, se estima que hubo 228 millones de casos de malaria en todo el mundo (intervalo de confianza [IC] del 95%: 206–258 millones), en comparación con 251 millones de casos en 2010 (IC del 95%: 231–278 millones) y 231 millones de casos en 2017 (IC 95%: 211–259 millones).

- La mayoría de los casos de malaria en 2018 se produjeron en la Región de África de la Organización Mundial de la Salud (OMS) (213 millones o 93%), seguida de la Región de Asia Sudoriental con el 3,4% de los casos y la Región del Mediterráneo Oriental con el 2.1%.

- Diecinueve países en África subsahariana[1] e India sumaron casi el 85% de la carga mundial de malaria. Mas de la mitad de todos los casos de malaria en todo el mundo se concentró en seis países: Nigeria (25%), la República Democrática del Congo (12%), Uganda (5%) y Costa de Marfil, Mozambique y Níger (4% cada uno).

- La tasa de incidencia de la malaria disminuyó a nivel mundial entre 2010 y 2018, de 71 a 57 casos por 1000 habitantes en riesgo. Sin embargo, de 2014 a 2018, la tasa de cambio disminuyó drásticamente, reduciendo a 57 en 2014 y permaneciendo en niveles similares hasta 2018.

- En la Región de Asia Sudoriental de la OMS la tasa de incidencia continúo disminuyendo: de 17 casos por cada 1000 habitantes en riesgo en 2010 a cinco casos en 2018 (una disminución del 70%). En la Región de África, los niveles de incidencia de casos también disminuyeron de 294 en 2010 a 229 en 2018, lo que representa una reducción del 22%. Todas las demás regiones de la OMS registraron poco progreso o un aumento en la tasa de incidencia. La Región de las Américas de la OMS registró un aumento, en gran parte debido a los aumentos en la transmisión de la malaria en la República Bolivariana de Venezuela.

- Entre 2015 y 2018, solo 31 países endémicos redujeron significativamente la incidencia de casos y estaban en camino de reducir la incidencia en un 40% o más en el año 2020. Sin un cambio acelerado, los hitos de la Estrategia Técnica Mundial contra la malaria 2016–2030 (ETM) relacionados con la morbilidad en 2025 y 2030 no se van a lograr.

- *Plasmodium falciparum* es el parásito de la malaria más frecuente en la Región de África de la OMS, representando el 99.7% de los casos estimados de malaria en 2018, así como en la Región de Asia Sudoriental de la OMS (50%), Región del Mediterráneo Oriental (71%) y Región del Pacífico occidental (65%).

- A nivel mundial, el 53% de la carga de *P. vivax* se concentra en la Región de Asia Sudoriental de la OMS, con la mayoría en India (47%). *P. vivax* es el parásito predominante en la Región de las Américas, representando el 75% de los casos de malaria.

### Muertes por malaria

- En 2018, se estimaron 405 000 muertes por malaria en todo el mundo, comparado con 416 000 muertes estimadas en 2017 y 585 000 en 2010.

- Los niños menores de 5 años son el grupo más vulnerable afectado por la malaria. En 2018, este grupo represento el 67% (272 000) de todas las muertes por malaria en todo el mundo.

---

[1] La lista completa de países del África subsahariana puede consultarse en https://unstats.un.org/unsd/methodology/m49; Sudan ha sido incluido como país subsahariano en todos los análisis llevados a cabo para este informe para esta región.

- El 94% de todas las muertes por malaria en 2018 se produjo en la Región de África de la OMS. A pesar de ser la región que albergó la mayor cantidad de muertes por malaria en 2018, también es la región donde se produjo 85% de la reducción de muertes conseguida globalmente en 2018, 180 000 muertes de menos en comparación con 2010.
- Casi el 85% de las muertes por malaria en el mundo en 2018 se concentraron en 20 países de la Región de África de la OMS y la India. Nigeria representó casi el 50% de todas las muertes por malaria en el mundo, seguida de la República Democrática del Congo (11%), la República Unida de Tanzania (5%) y Angola, Mozambique y Níger (4% cada uno).
- En 2018, solo la Región de África de la OMS y la Región de Asia Sudoriental mostraron reducciones en las muertes por malaria en comparación con 2010. La Región de África tuvo la mayor reducción absoluta en las muertes por malaria, de 533 000 en 2010 a 380 000 en 2018. Sin embargo, a pesar de estas ganancias, la tasa de reducción de la mortalidad por malaria en esta región también se ha desacelerado desde 2016.

## CONSECUENCIAS DE LA MALARIA PARA LA SALUD MATERNA, DE LOS INFANTES Y LOS NIÑOS

- En 2018, alrededor de 11 millones de embarazos en países con transmisión de malaria moderada y alta en el África subsahariana, habrían estado expuestas a una infección por malaria.
- En 2018, la prevalencia de exposición a infección por malaria durante el embarazo fue más alta en la subregión de África occidental y África central (cada una con un 35%), seguida de África oriental y Suráfrica (20%). Alrededor del 39% de esta exposición se concentró en la República Democrática del Congo y Nigeria.
- Los 11 millones de mujeres embarazadas expuestas a infecciones por malaria en 2018 dieron a luz a unos 872 000 niños con bajo peso al nacer (16% de todos los niños con bajo peso al nacer en estos países), con África Occidental teniendo la mayor prevalencia de niños con bajo peso al nacer atribuido a malaria durante el embarazo.
- Entre 2015 y 2018 en 21 países con carga de malaria de moderada a alta en la Región de África de la OMS, la prevalencia de anemia en niños menores de 5 años con una prueba de diagnóstico rápido (PDR) positivo fue el doble que la de los niños con una PDR negativa. En los niños con malaria confirmada, el 9% tenía anemia severa y el 54% tenía anemia moderada; en contraste, en los niños sin malaria, solo el 1% tenía anemia severa y el 31% tenía anemia moderada.
- Los países con el mayor porcentaje de anemia severa entre los niños menores de 5 años con malaria confirmada fueron Senegal (26%), Malí (16%), Guinea (14%) y Mozambique (12%). Para la mayoría de los otros países, la anemia severa varió del 5% al 10%.
- En general, se estimó que alrededor de 24 millones de niños estaban infectados con *P. falciparum* en 2018 en África subsahariana, y se estima que 1.8 millones de ellos tenían anemia severa.

## ENFOQUE DE ALTA CARGA A ALTO IMPACTO

- En 2018, hubo alrededor de 155 millones de casos de malaria en los 11 países incluidos en el enfoque alta carga a alto impacto (ACAI), en comparación con 177 millones en 2010. La República Democrática del Congo y Nigeria tuvieron 84 millones (54% del total de casos).
- De los 10 países con mayor carga de malaria en África, Ghana y Nigeria reportaron, en 2018, los aumentos absolutos de casos más altos en comparación con 2017. La carga en 2018 fue similar a la de 2017 en los otros países, exceptuando Uganda e India, donde, en 2018, se reportó una reducción de 1.5 y 2.6 millones de casos, respectivamente en comparación con 2017.

- Las muertes por malaria se redujeron de aproximadamente de 400 000 en 2010 a aproximadamente 260 000 en 2018. La mayor reducción se produjo en Nigeria, donde las casi 153 000 muertes en 2010 pasaron a aproximadamente 95 000 en 2018.
- Para el año 2018, en todos los 11 países del enfoque ACAI, al menos el 40% de la población en riesgo durmió bajo mosquiteros tratados con insecticida de larga duración (MILD), el porcentaje más alto lo tuvo Uganda (80%) y el más bajo Nigeria (40%).
- En Burkina Faso y la República Unida de Tanzania, se estimó que más de la mitad de las mujeres embarazadas recibieron tres dosis de tratamiento preventivo intermitente durante el embarazo (TPI) en 2018. En Camerún, Nigeria y Uganda, la cobertura estimada fue de alrededor del 30% o menos.
- Seis países de la subregión africana del Sahel implementaron la quimio-prevención estacional de malaria (QPE) en 2018; de los 26 millones de niños objetivo, un total de 17 millones de niños, fueron tratados con QPE.
- El porcentaje de niños menores de 5 años con fiebre que buscaron tratamiento varió del 58% en Malí al 82% en Uganda. En la República Democrática del Congo y Malí, más del 40% de los niños no fueron llevados a recibir tratamiento. El porcentaje de niños que fueron diagnosticados también fue preocupantemente bajo entre los niños que fueron sometidos a tratamiento, con un 30% o menos de niños que fueron diagnosticados en Camerún, la República Democrática del Congo y Nigeria.
- A excepción de la India, en los países ACAI la inversión interna directa sigue siendo muy baja en relación con la financiación internacional.

## ELIMINACIÓN DE LA MALARIA Y PREVENCIÓN DEL RESTABLECIMIENTO

- A nivel mundial, la red de eliminación se está ampliando, con más países avanzando hacia el objetivo de cero casos autóctonos: en 2018, 49 países reportaron menos de 10 000 de estos casos, frente a 46 países en 2017 y 40 países en 2010. El número de países con menos de 100 casos autóctonos, -un fuerte indicador de que la eliminación está cerca-, aumentó de 17 países en 2010 a 25 países en 2017 y 27 países en 2018.
- Paraguay y Uzbekistán obtuvieron la certificación de eliminación de la OMS en 2018, y Argelia y Argentina lograron la certificación a principios de 2019. En 2018, China, El Salvador, Irán, Malasia y Timor-Leste reportaron cero casos autóctonos.
- Uno de los hitos clave de la ETM para 2020 es la eliminación de la malaria en al menos 10 países de los que eran endémicos de malaria en 2015. Al ritmo actual de progreso, es probable que se alcance este hito.
- En 2016, la OMS identificó 21 países con el potencial de eliminar la malaria para el año 2020. La OMS está trabajando con los gobiernos de estos países, conocidos como "países E-2020", para apoyar sus objetivos de aceleración de la eliminación.
- Aunque hay 10 países del E-2020 que están en el buen camino para lograr sus objetivos de eliminación, en 2018 Comoros y Costa Rica informaron de aumentos en los casos de malaria autóctonos en comparación con 2017.
- En los seis países de la subregión del Gran Mekong (GM) - Camboya, China (provincia de Yunnan), República Democrática Popular Laos, Myanmar, Tailandia y Vietnam - el número de casos de malaria disminuyó en un 76% entre 2010 y 2018, y las muertes por malaria disminuyeron en un 95% durante el mismo período. En 2018, Camboya, por primera vez en la historia, reportó de que no hubo muertes relacionadas con la malaria denle el país.

# INVERSIONES EN LOS PROGRAMAS DE MALARIA E INVESTIGACIÓN

- En 2018, los gobiernos de los países endémicos de malaria y sus colaboradores internacionales invirtieron aproximadamente $ 2.700 millones en esfuerzos de control y eliminación de la malaria a nivel mundial, menos que los $ 3.200 millones que se invirtieron en 2017. La cantidad invertida en 2018 es insuficiente dado que se estima que se requieren $ 5.0 mil millones para continuar avanzando hacia el complimiento de los objetivos de la ETM.
- Casi tres cuartas partes de las inversiones en 2018 se gastaron en la Región de África de la OMS, seguidas por la Región de las Américas (7%), la Región de Asia Sudoriental (6%), la Región del Mediterráneo Oriental y la Región del Pacífico Occidental (5% cada uno).
- En 2018, el 47% de la financiación total para la malaria se invirtió en países de bajos ingresos, el 43% en países de ingresos bajo a medio y el 11% en países de ingresos medio a alto. La financiación internacional representó la principal fuente de financiación en los países de bajos y de bajo a medios ingresos, con 85% y 61% respectivamente. La financiación interna se ha mantenido estable desde 2010.
- De los $ 2.700 millones de dólares invertidos en 2018, $ 1.800 millones provienen de financiadores internacionales. Los gobiernos de los países endémicos contribuyeron con el 30% de la financiación total ($ 900 millones de dólares) en 2018, una cifra sin cambios desde 2017. Dos tercios de los fondos de origen nacional se invirtieron en actividades de control de la malaria llevadas a cabo por los programas nacionales de malaria (PNM), siendo el resto estimado como el costo de atención a los pacientes.
- Como en años anteriores, los Estados Unidos de América (EE. UU.) Fue la mayor fuente internacional de financiación de la malaria, proporcionando $ 1 mil millones de dólares (37%) en 2018. Los países miembros del Comité de Asistencia para el Desarrollo representaron $ 300 millones (11%). El Reino Unido de Gran Bretaña e Irlanda del Norte contribuyeron con alrededor de $ 200 millones (7%).
- De los $ 2.700 millones de dólares invertidos en 2018, $ 1.000 millones se canalizaron a través del Fondo Mundial de Lucha contra el SIDA, la Tuberculosis y la Malaria.
- Aunque la financiación para la malaria se ha mantenido relativamente estable desde 2010, el nivel de inversión en 2018 está lejos de lo que se requiere para alcanzar los dos primeros hitos de la ETM; es decir, conseguir, para el 2020, una reducción de al menos el 40% en la incidencia de casos de malaria y en las tasas de mortalidad a nivel mundial en comparación con los niveles de 2015.
- Se invirtieron $ 663 millones de dólares en investigación básica y desarrollo de productos para la malaria en 2018, un aumento de $ 18 millones en comparación con 2017.
- La financiación para investigación y desarrollo de medicamentos antimaláricos llego al nivel más alto jamás registrado, de $ 228 millones en 2017 a $ 252 millones de dólares en 2018. Este aumento fue el resultado de la inversión del sector privado en varios ensayos de Fase II de nuevos productos con potencial de curación radical con una dosis única.

## Distribución de productos básicos contra la malaria

### Mosquiteros tratados con insecticida

- Entre 2016 y 2018, de acuerdo con los fabricantes, se entregaron 578 millones de mosquiteros tratados con insecticida (MTI), principalmente MILD, con un 50% destinado a Costa de Marfil, República Democrática del Congo, Etiopía, Ghana, India, Nigeria, Uganda y la República Unida de Tanzania.
- En 2018, los fabricantes entregaron alrededor de 197 millones de MILD, de los cuales más del 87% fueron entregados a países del África subsahariana.
- A nivel mundial, el 85% de los MTI se distribuyeron a través de campañas gratuitas de distribución masiva, el 10% en centros de atención prenatal y el 6% como parte de los programas de inmunización.

**Pruebas de diagnóstico rápido (PDR).**
- Se estima que 412 millones de PDR se vendieron a nivel mundial en 2018.
- En 2018, los PNM distribuyeron 259 millones de PDR. La mayoría de las PDR (64%) fueron pruebas para detectar *P. falciparum* y se suministraron al África subsahariana.

**Terapia combinada basada en artemisinina**
- Se estima que 3,000 millones de tratamientos de terapia combinada basada en artemisinina (TCA) fueron adquiridos por los países durante el período 2010-2018 y que el 63% fue adquirido por el sector público.
- En 2018, los PNM distribuyeron 214 millones de tratamientos con TCA, el 98% fueron en la Región de África de la OMS.

# PREVENCIÓN DE LA MALARIA

## Control de vectores
- La mitad de las personas en riesgo de malaria en África están durmiendo bajo un MTI; en 2018, el 50% de la población estaba protegida por esta intervención, un aumento del 29% comparado con 2010. Además, el porcentaje de la población con acceso a un MTI aumentó del 33% en 2010 al 57% en 2018. Sin embargo, la cobertura mejoró solo marginalmente desde 2015 y se ha estancado desde 2016.
- El porcentaje de hogares con al menos un MTI por cada dos personas aumentaron a 72% en 2018, de 47% en 2010. Sin embargo, esta cifra representa solo un aumento modesto en los últimos 3 años, y sigue estando lejos del objetivo de cobertura universal.
- El número de personas en riesgo de contraer malaria protegidas por el rociado residual intradomiciliar (RRI), un método de prevención que implica el rociado de insecticidas en las paredes interiores de las viviendas, está disminuyendo. A nivel mundial, la protección del RRI disminuyó de un pico del 5% en 2010 al 2% en 2018, año en el que se observaron disminuciones en todas las regiones de la OMS, salvo en la Región del Mediterráneo Oriental.
- Aunque la cobertura del RRI en la Región de África de la OMS cayo de 180 millones de personas en riesgo protegidas en 2010 a 93 millones en 2018, la cobertura disminuyó de 13 millones de personas entre 2017 y 2018.
- La disminución de la cobertura del RRI puede deberse los cambios en los insecticidas usados, la transición de piretroides a insecticidas más caros en respuesta al aumento de la resistencia a los piretroides; o a cambios en las estrategias operativas (por ejemplo, la disminución de las poblaciones en riesgo en los países en vías de eliminación de la malaria).

## Terapias preventivas
- Para proteger a las mujeres en áreas de transmisión de malaria moderada y alta en África, la OMS recomienda TPI con el antimalárico sulfadoxina-pirimetamina (SP). Entre los 36 países africanos que informaron sobre los niveles de cobertura de TPI en 2018, se estima que el 31% de las mujeres embarazadas elegibles recibieron las tres o más dosis recomendadas de TPI, en comparación con el 22% en 2017 y el 0% en 2010, lo que indica mejoras considerables en la implementación de esta intervención en los países.
- Alrededor del 18% de las mujeres que utilizaron los servicios de atención prenatal al menos una vez, no recibieron ninguna dosis de TPI, lo que representa una oportunidad perdida que, si se aprovecha, podría mejorar considerablemente y rápidamente la cobertura de TPI.
- En 2018, 19 millones de niños en 12 países de la subregión del Sahel de África fueron protegidos a través de programas de quimio-prevención estacional (QPE). Todos los niños seleccionados recibieron tratamiento en Camerún, Guinea, Guinea-Bissau y Malí. Sin embargo, unos 12 millones de niños que podrían haberse beneficiado de esta intervención no lo hicieron. Esto es debido principalmente a la falta de fondos.

## PRUEBAS DE DIAGNÓSTICO Y TRATAMIENTO

### Acceso a la atención médica

- El diagnóstico y el tratamiento oportunos son la forma más efectiva de evitar que un caso leve de malaria se convierta en enfermedad grave y que cause la muerte. Según las encuestas nacionales de hogares realizadas en 20 países del África subsahariana entre 2015 y 2018, una mediana del 42% (rango inter-cuartil [RI]: 34-49%) de los niños con fiebre (febriles) fueron trasladados a un proveedor de atención médica capacitado en el sector público, comparado con el 10% (RI: 8-22%) en el sector privado formal y el 3% (RI: 2-7%) en el sector privado informal.
- Una alta proporción de niños febriles no recibió atención médica (mediana: 36%, RI: 28-45%). El pobre acceso a los proveedores de atención médica o la falta de conocimiento de los síntomas de la malaria entre los cuidadores son algunos de los factores que contribuyen a esta falta de atención médica.

### Diagnóstico de la malaria

- El porcentaje de pacientes con sospecha de malaria, que son atendidos en centros de salud pública y examinados con una PDR o microscopía, aumentó del 38% en 2010 al 85% en 2018.
- En 2018, en el 71% de los países con transmisión moderada a alta en el África subsahariana, el porcentaje de casos con sospecha de malaria a quienes se les realizó una prueba parasitológica fue superior al 80%.
- Según 19 encuestas de hogares a nivel nacional, realizadas entre 2015 y 2018 en África subsahariana, el porcentaje promedio de niños febriles que fueron atendidos y recibieron un pinchazo en el dedo o el talón (lo que sugiere que pudo haberse realizado una prueba de diagnóstico de malaria) fue mayor en el sector público (mediana: 66%, RI: 49-75%) que en el sector privado formal (mediana: 40%, RI: 16-46%) o el sector privado informal (mediana: 9%, RI: 5- 22%).
- Según 61 encuestas de hogares realizadas en 29 países del África subsahariana entre 2010 y 2018, el porcentaje de niños con fiebre que recibieron una prueba de diagnóstico antes de recibir tratamiento antimalárico en el sector de la salud pública aumentó de una mediana del 48% (RI: 30 -62%) en 2010-2013, a una mediana del 76% (RI: 60-86%) en 2015-2018.

### Tratamiento de la malaria

- Según 20 encuestas de hogares realizadas en África subsahariana en 2015-2018, el porcentaje medio de niños febriles que fueron tratados con algún medicamento antimalárico fue mayor en el sector público (mediana: 48%, RI: 30-69%) que en el sector privado formal (mediana: 40%, RI: 21-51%) o el sector privado informal (mediana: 18%, RI: 10-29%).
- Los datos de 20 encuestas nacionales realizados en África subsahariana muestran que, para el período 2015-2018, el 47% (RI: 29-69%) de los niños febriles que recibieron tratamiento para la malaria en el sector de la salud pública recibieron tratamiento antimalárico, en comparación con 59% (RI: 53-84%) entre quienes visitan a un trabajador de salud comunitario y 49% (RI: 19-55%) en el sector privado formal.
- Con base en 19 encuestas de hogares, los tratamientos antimaláricos dados a los niños febriles fueron más frecuentemente un TCA cuando se buscó tratamiento en el sector público (mediana: 80%, RI: 45-94%) que en el sector privado formal (mediana: 77%, RI: 43-87%) o el sector privado informal (mediana: 60%, RI: 40-84%).
- Para cerrar la brecha de tratamiento a los niños, la OMS recomienda la adopción del manejo integrado de casos por la comunidad (MICC). Este enfoque promueve el manejo integrado de condiciones de salud que comúnmente amenazan la vida de los niños (malaria, neumonía y diarrea) a nivel de centros de salud y comunitarios. En 2018, 30 países implementaron el MICC en diferentes niveles, con solo unos pocos implementando ésta a nivel nacional.

## SISTEMAS DE VIGILANCIA DE LA MALARIA

- El pilar 3 de la Estrategia Mundial de malaria (ETM) es transformar la vigilancia de malaria en una intervención principal. Para comprender si los sistemas de vigilancia de la malaria son adecuados para su propósito, la OMS recomienda el monitoreo y la evaluación regulares de los sistemas de vigilancia.
- El Programa Global contra la Malaria (PGM), en colaboración con la Universidad de Oslo, ha desarrollado módulos estandarizados de vigilancia de malaria basados en el Software de Información de Salud del Distrito-2 (DHIS2) para la recogida de datos epidemiológicos de rutina, datos de casos individuales y datos de vigilancia entomológica y monitoria de intervenciones de control vectorial. Estos modules incluyen elementos de datos, indicadores de monitoria y de calidad de los datos, tableros estandarizados de interpretación de los datos e informes.
- Hasta octubre de 2019, 23 países han instalado el módulo agregado de malaria de la OMS, otras ocho instalaciones están planificadas para el próximo año y otros cinco países ya han desarrollado e integrado su propio módulo para la vigilancia de malaria en DHIS2.
- La OMS ha estado trabajando en coordinación con los departamentos de Sistemas de Información de Gestión de Salud (SIGS) de los ministerios de salud, en particular de los países ACAI, para establecer bases de datos dinámicas estructuradas conocidas como repositorios de datos. El PGM ha desarrollado una estructura de repositorio standard basada en DHIS2 y fácilmente adaptable, que contiene los elementos de datos e indicadores más relevantes, sus definiciones y computación para cubrir las áreas temáticas clave. Hasta ahora, el trabajo para desarrollar estas bases de datos ha comenzado en Gambia, Ghana, Mozambique, Nigeria, Uganda y la República Unida de Tanzania.
- La OMS también alienta a los países a implementar evaluaciones del sistema de vigilancia. Un ejemplo de estudio de caso de Mozambique ilustra tal evaluación y su papel en la mejora de los sistemas de vigilancia.

## RESPONDIENDO A LOS DESAFÍOS BIOLÓGICAS EN LA LUCHA CONTRA LA MALARIA

### Supresión del gen *Pfhrp2 / 3*

- La supresión de los genes *pfhrp2* y *pfhrp3* (*pfhrp2 / 3*) del parásito hacen que los parásitos sean indetectables por las PDR que se basan en la detección del HRP2. La supresión doble *pfhrp2* y *pfhrp3* entre pacientes sintomáticos ha alcanzado una prevalencia de hasta el 80% en Eritrea y Perú.
- La OMS ha recomendado a los países con evidencia de supresiones de *pfhrp2 / 3*, o los países vecinos, que realicen encuestas representativas entre los casos sospechosos de malaria para determinar si la prevalencia de supresión de *pfhrp2 / 3*, que causan falsos negativos en las PDR, ha alcanzado un umbral que indique la necesidad de cambio de PDR (> 5 % de deleciones en *pfhrp2* causan resultados de falsos negativos en PDR).
- La OMS está rastreando los informes publicados de supresiones *pfhrp2 / 3* utilizando la herramienta de mapeo del Mapa de los Desafíos de la Malaria. Hasta la fecha, 28 países han reportado supresiones de *pfhrp2*.

### Resistencia a los medicamentos antimaláricos

- Las mutaciones de *PfKelch13* se han identificado como marcadores moleculares de resistencia parcial a la artemisinina. Las mutaciones de *PfKelch13* asociadas con la resistencia a la artemisinina están muy extendidas en la subregión del Gran Mekong (GM) y también se han detectado con una prevalencia significativa (más del 5%) en Guyana, Papua Nueva Guinea y Ruanda. En el caso de Ruanda, se ha visto que la presencia de mutaciones *PfKelch13* no afecta la eficacia del tratamiento de primera línea.

- En la Región del Pacífico Occidental de la OMS, la resistencia a la artemisinina se ha confirmado en Camboya, República Democrática Popular Lao y Vietnam a través de varios estudios realizados entre 2001 y 2018. La eficacia del tratamiento para P. vivax sigue siendo alta en todos los países, las tasas de fallo del tratamiento son inferiores al 10 %.
- En la Región de África, las tasas de eficacia de arteméter-lumefantrina (AL), artesunato-amodiaquina (AS-AQ) y dihidroartemisinina-piperaquina (DHA-PPQ) para P. falciparum fueron más del 98%, y la eficacia se ha mantenido alta a lo largo del tiempo.
- En la Región de las Américas, la eficacia del tratamiento para P. falciparum, contratamientos de primera línea, sigue siendo alta.
- En la Región de Asia Sudoriental, se han encontrado marcadores moleculares de resistencia a la artemisinina en Bangladesh, India, Myanmar y Tailandia. Con excepción de Myanmar, las tasas de fallo de los TCA de primera línea para P. falciparum fueron mayores que 10% y llegaron hasta el 93% en Tailandia. Con base a los estudios de eficacia terapéutica reportados, la cloroquina (CQ) sigue siendo altamente eficaz contra P. vivax en la mayoría de los países, excepto en Myanmar y Timor-Leste.
- En la Región del Mediterráneo Oriental, las altas tasas de fallo del tratamiento con AS-SP contra P. falciparum detectadas en Somalia y Sudán llevaron a un cambio en la política de tratamiento de primera línea que ahora es AL. Los estudios de eficacia terapéutica (EET) realizados con AL y CQ contra P. vivax indican una alta eficacia de estos tratamientos.

## Resistencia a los insecticidas

- Desde 2010 hasta 2018, unos 81 países informaron datos a la OMS sobre el monitoreo de la resistencia a los insecticidas.
- De los 81 países endémicos de malaria que proporcionaron datos para 2010-2018, 73 confirmaron la resistencia a al menos una de las cuatro clases de insecticidas en al menos un vector de malaria y un sitio de recolección, un aumento de cinco países en comparación con el período del informe anterior 2010-2017. 26 países, confirmaron la resistencia a las cuatro clases principales de insecticidas.
- La resistencia a los piretroides, la única clase de insecticidas actualmente utilizada en los MTI, es generalizada y se detectó en al menos un vector de malaria en más de dos tercios de los sitios analizados, y fue más alta en la Región de África de la OMS y en la Región del Mediterráneo Oriental.
- La resistencia a los organoclorados fue confirmada en casi un tercio de los sitios de recolección en al menos un vector de malaria. La resistencia a los carbamatos y los organofosforados fue menos prevalente, siendo confirmada en el 31% y 26% de los sitios de recolección testados, respectivamente. La resistencia a los carbamatos fue más prevalente en la región de Asia sudoriental, mientras que la resistencia a los organofosforados fue más prevalente en la región de Asia sudoriental y el Pacífico Oriental.
- Todos los datos estándar de resistencia a los insecticidas proporcionados a la OMS están incluidos en la Base de datos Mundial de Resistencia a los Insecticidas en los Vectores de Malaria de la OMS y están disponibles para su consulta a través del Mapa de los Desafíos de la Malaria. Esta herramienta en línea se extendió en 2019 para cubrir los movimientos de las especies de mosquitos invasoras, y actualmente muestra el alcance geográfico de los informes sobre la detección de *Anopheles stephensi*.
- Para guiar el manejo de la resistencia, los países deben desarrollar e implementar un plan nacional para el monitoreo y manejo de la resistencia a los insecticidas, basándose en el documento *Estructura general de un plan nacional de monitoreo y manejo de la resistencia a insecticidas en vectores del paludismo* de la OMS. En 2018, un total de 45 países informaron haber completado el plan para el monitoreo y manejo de la resistencia y 36 estaban en proceso de desarrollarlo.
- Los PNM y sus socios deberían considerar la distribución de mosquiteros con piretroide y butóxido de piperonilo (PBO) en áreas geográficas concretas donde los principales vectores de la malaria cumplen con los criterios recomendados por la OMS en 2017, en lugar de basarse en si todo el país cumple los criterios.

**FIG. 1.1.**

**Countries with indigenous cases in 2000 and their status by 2018** Countries with zero indigenous cases over at least the past 3 consecutive years are considered as having eliminated malaria. In 2018, China and El Salvador reported zero indigenous cases for the second consecutive year, and Iran (Islamic Republic of), Malaysia and Timor-Leste reported zero indigenous cases for the first time. *Source: WHO database.*

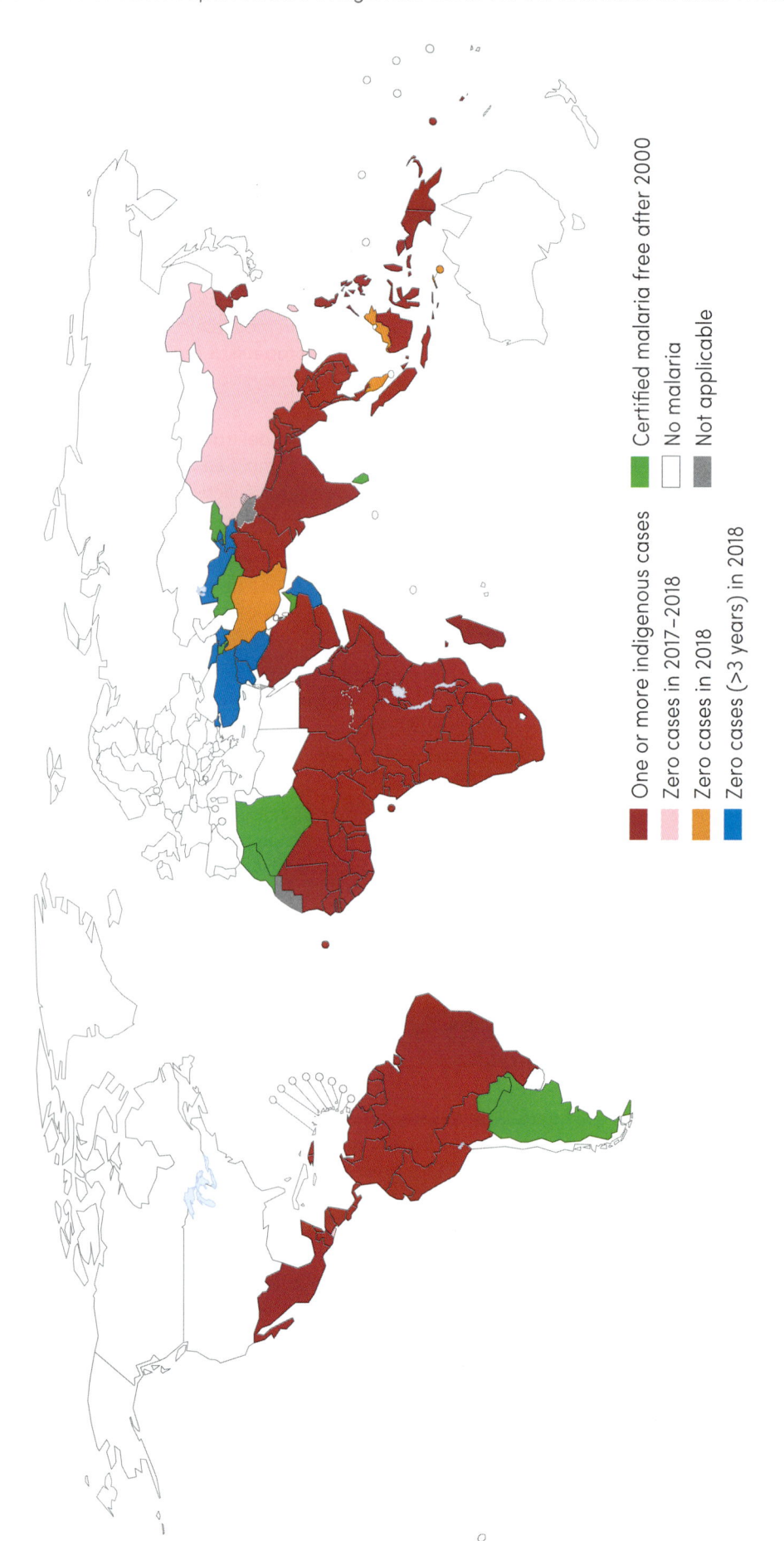

WHO: World Health Organization.

# 1 Introduction

The World Health Organization's (WHO's) *World malaria report 2019* summarizes global progress in the fight against malaria up to the end of 2018. This is the fourth world malaria report since the launch of the *WHO Global technical strategy for malaria 2016–2030* (GTS) (*1*). Key indicators are tracked across several countries (**Fig. 1.1**) and WHO regions against the milestones outlined in the GTS (**Table 1.1**).

**TABLE 1.1.**
**GTS: global targets for 2030 and milestones for 2020 and 2025** Source: GTS (*1*).

### Vision – A world free of malaria

| Pillars | |
|---|---|
| Pillar 1 | Ensure universal access to malaria prevention, diagnosis and treatment |
| Pillar 2 | Accelerate efforts towards elimination and attainment of malaria free status |
| Pillar 3 | Transform malaria surveillance into a core intervention |

| Goals | Milestones | | Targets |
|---|---|---|---|
| | 2020 | 2025 | 2030 |
| 1. Reduce malaria mortality rates globally compared with 2015 | At least 40% | At least 75% | At least 90% |
| 2. Reduce malaria case incidence globally compared with 2015 | At least 40% | At least 75% | At least 90% |
| 3. Eliminate malaria from countries in which malaria was transmitted in 2015 | At least 10 countries | At least 20 countries | At least 35 countries |
| 4. Prevent re-establishment of malaria in all countries that are malaria free | Re-establishment prevented | Re-establishment prevented | Re-establishment prevented |

GTS: *Global technical strategy for malaria 2016–2030.*

# 1 Introduction

**FIG. 1.2.**

**Malaria and the SDGs 2016–2030** Reducing the burden of malaria will contribute to or benefit from progress towards the SDG goals. *Sources: United Nations (3) and Swiss Malaria Group (5).*

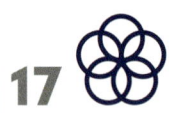

**Goal 17: Partnership for the Goals.** The many **multisectoral partnerships** in place to reduce and eliminate malaria have a positive collateral effect, and also bring progress to other **domains of development**.

**Goal 1: No Poverty.** Sustained investment in health and malaria unlocks the potential of human capital to **generate growth**. A 10% reduction in malaria has been associated with a 0.3% rise in annual GDP. At household level, **reducing malaria protects household income** from lost earnings and the costs of seeking care.

**Goal 2: Zero Hunger.** Sustainable agricultural practices help reduce malaria. People who suffer less from malaria work their fields more consistently, resulting in better harvests and **improved food security**. Well-nourished people, especially children, are better able to fight malaria.

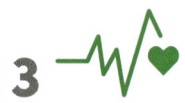

**Goal 3: Good Health and Well-being.** The scale-up of malaria interventions **averted at least 670 million bouts of malaria illness and 4.3 million malaria deaths** between 2001 and 2013. Preventing malaria in pregnancy **reduces maternal mortality and gives newborns a far healthier start in life.** Lowering the burden of malaria makes a substantial contribution to **improvements in child health,** and thus often to a decline in fertility rates, and an associated increase in the investment that parents can make in their children.

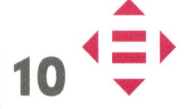

**Goals 10, 16: Reduce Inequality. Promote Peace and Justice.** A targeted response to malaria actively improves the health of the poorest, enabling vulnerable families to **break the vicious cycle of disease and poverty**, and helping to make sure that no one is left behind. Investing in malaria reduction contributes to the creation of more **cohesive, inclusive societies**. Stable countries are more likely to attract international investment and overseas development aid.

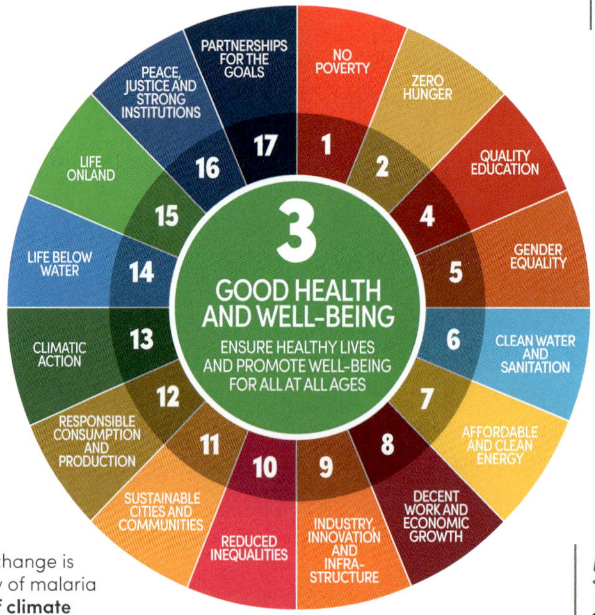

**Goal 4: Quality Education.** Reducing malaria enables children to **attend school regularly and learn more effectively.** This significantly improves their school performance, and later wage-earning capacity. As a mother's or caregiver's level of education increases, so do the chances that their children will access malaria prevention and treatment services and survive childhood.

**Goal 13: Climate Action.** Given that climate change is predicted to increase the range and intensity of malaria transmission, plans to **mitigate the effects of climate change** are likely to include an increased commitment to controlling and eliminating malaria, and vice versa.

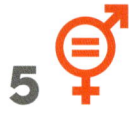

**Goal 5: Gender Equality. Freeing women and school-age girls** from the burden of caring for family members when they fall sick with malaria increases their likelihood of completing school, entering and remaining in the workforce, and participating in public decision-making.

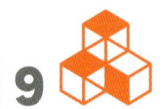

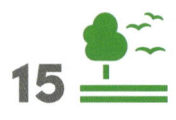

**Goals 9, 11, 15: Infrastructure, Sustainable Cities and Life on Land.** By ensuring that major construction and development projects do not introduce or increase malaria transmission, the benefits of progress can be reaped, while also **protecting human health and ecosystems**. Well-planned infrastructure and improved housing help reduce exposure to mosquitoes, and facilitate greater access to health and malaria services.

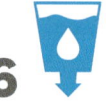

**Goal 6: Clean Water and Sanitation. Drainage of standing water** leads to decreased mosquito breeding and a reduction in the rate of malaria transmission. It also improves water quality, generating further health benefits.

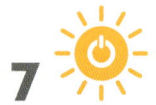

**Goal 7: Affordable and Clean Energy.** In resource-constrained malaria endemic regions, **access to sustainable energy will stimulate prosperity** and increase the adoption of more sophisticated personal protection measures. It will also mean greater access to electric lighting and cooling, enabling people to increase time spent indoors, where vectors are more easily controlled through insecticides, bet nets and temperature. These developments are likely to result in a reduced burden of malaria.

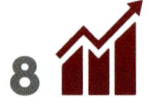

**Goal 8, 12: Decent Work, Economic Growth and Responsible Production.** Reducing malaria creates **healthier, more productive workforces** which can help to attract trade and commerce. When combined with pro-poor policies, these factors **drive job creation, inclusive growth and shared prosperity**. Enterprises that invest in their workers reduce the costs of doing business, increase their **competitiveness** and enhance their reputation.

GDP: gross domestic product; SDG: Sustainable Development Goal.

The report also tracks a set of indicators outlined in the Roll Back Malaria (RBM) advocacy plan, *Action and investment to defeat malaria 2016–2030* (AIM) (*2*) and the Sustainable Development Goals (SDGs) (*3*) – a set of interconnected global goals seen as a plan of action for people, the planet and prosperity (**Fig. 1.2**). The report highlights the various ways investment in the fight against malaria contributes to the SDGs and the aligned WHO "triple billion" targets of the 13th General programme of work (GPW13) (*4*) (**Fig. 1.3**).

The main results, presented in **Sections 2–10**, cover the period 2010–2018. **Section 2** describes the global trends in malaria morbidity and mortality burden. Estimates of the burden of anaemia and its association with malaria – and for the first time in the world malaria report, burden and consequences of malaria during pregnancy – are presented in **Section 3**. The "high burden to high impact" (HBHI) approach and related control activities and funding are described in **Section 4**, while progress towards elimination is presented in **Section 5**. **Section 6** dwells on total funding for malaria control and elimination, for malaria research and for the supply of key commodities to endemic countries. The population-level coverage achieved through these investments is presented in **Section 7** and **Section 8**. **Section 9** focuses on surveillance as an intervention, and **Section 10** describes the threats posed by *Plasmodium falciparum* parasite histidine-rich protein 2 (HRP2) deletions, and by drug and insecticide resistance. The main text is followed by annexes that contain data sources and methods, regional profiles and data tables. Country profiles are presented online (*6*).

**FIG. 1.3.**

**The WHO triple billion targets and the contribution of the fight against malaria** These interconnected targets articulated in the GPW13 aim for one billion more people benefiting from universal health coverage; one billion more people better protected from health emergencies; and one billion more people enjoying better health and well-being. *Source: WHO (2018) (4).*

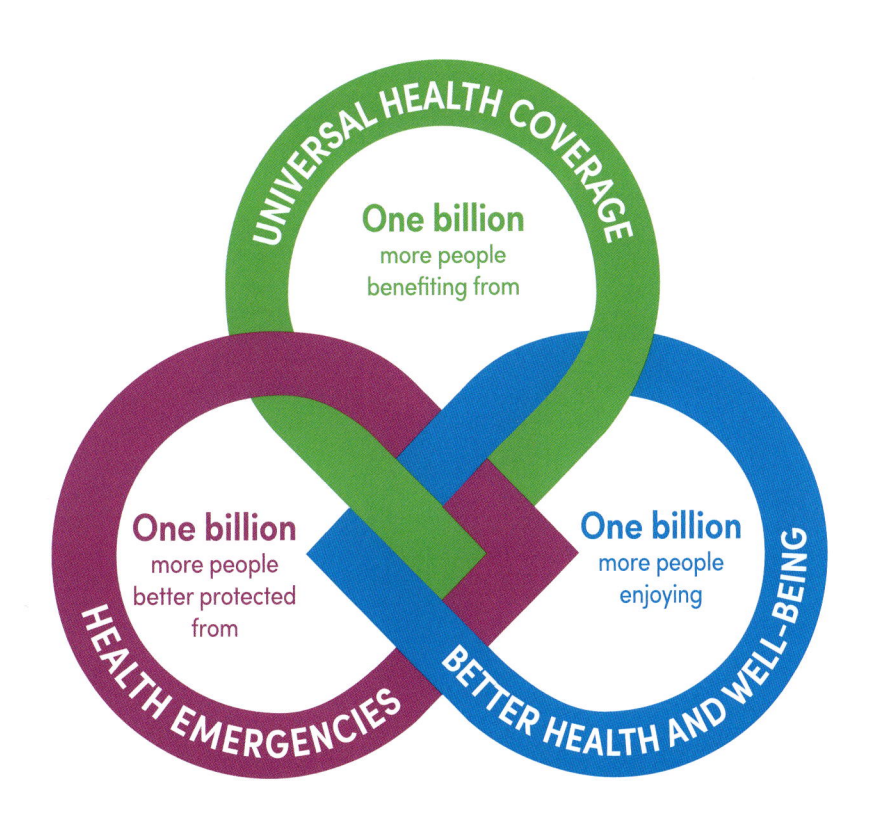

WHO: World Health Organization.

# Regional and global trends in burden of malaria cases and deaths

Assessing progress in reducing the burden of malaria, to track the targets and milestones of the GTS (*1*), is a key mandate of the WHO Global Malaria Programme (GMP). This section of the report reviews the total number of cases and deaths estimated to have occurred between 2010 and 2018. There are several methods for estimating the burden of malaria cases and deaths; the method used depends on the quality of the national surveillance systems and the availability of data over time (**Section 9.1** and **Annex 1**).

## 2.1 ESTIMATED NUMBER OF MALARIA CASES BY WHO REGION, 2000–2018

An estimated 228 million cases of malaria occurred worldwide in 2018 (95% confidence interval [CI]: 206–258 million) compared with 251 million cases in 2010 (95% CI: 231–278 million) and 231 million cases in 2017 (95% CI: 211–259 million) (**Table 2.1**).

The WHO African Region still bears the largest burden of malaria morbidity, with 213 million cases (93%) in 2018, followed by the WHO South-East Asia Region (3.4%) and the WHO Eastern Mediterranean Region (2.1%) (**Table 2.1**). Globally, 3.3% of all estimated cases were caused by *P. vivax*, with 53% of the vivax burden being in the WHO South-East Asia Region (**Table 2.2**). *P. vivax* is the predominant parasite in the WHO Region of the Americas (75%), and is responsible for 50% of cases in the WHO South-East Asia Region and 29% in the WHO Eastern Mediterranean Region (**Table 2.2**).

## TABLE 2.1.

**Estimated malaria cases by WHO region, 2010–2018** Estimated cases are shown with 95% upper and lower CIs. *Source: WHO estimates.*

|  | Number of cases (000) | | | | | | | | |
|---|---|---|---|---|---|---|---|---|---|
|  | 2010 | 2011 | 2012 | 2013 | 2014 | 2015 | 2016 | 2017 | 2018 |
| **African** | | | | | | | | | |
| Lower 95% CI | 199 000 | 194 000 | 190 000 | 185 000 | 181 000 | 184 000 | 189 000 | 192 000 | 191 000 |
| **Estimated total** | **218 000** | **213 000** | **209 000** | **204 000** | **197 000** | **199 000** | **206 000** | **212 000** | **213 000** |
| Upper 95% CI | 245 000 | 237 000 | 233 000 | 229 000 | 218 000 | 219 000 | 229 000 | 240 000 | 244 000 |
| **Americas** | | | | | | | | | |
| Lower 95% CI | 744 | 566 | 541 | 520 | 445 | 525 | 640 | 880 | 867 |
| **Estimated total** | **814** | **611** | **580** | **562** | **477** | **566** | **691** | **944** | **929** |
| Upper 95% CI | 894 | 666 | 627 | 613 | 512 | 611 | 749 | 1 026 | 1 007 |
| **Eastern Mediterranean** | | | | | | | | | |
| Lower 95% CI | 3 300 | 3 400 | 3 200 | 3 000 | 3 100 | 3 000 | 3 800 | 3 800 | 3 700 |
| **Estimated total** | **4 300** | **4 500** | **4 200** | **3 900** | **4 000** | **3 800** | **4 800** | **5 000** | **4 900** |
| Upper 95% CI | 6 300 | 6 500 | 6 000 | 5 300 | 5 500 | 5 200 | 6 400 | 6 800 | 6 800 |
| **South-East Asia** | | | | | | | | | |
| Lower 95% CI | 19 800 | 17 700 | 14 700 | 10 900 | 10 400 | 10 700 | 10 500 | 8 800 | 5 800 |
| **Estimated total** | **25 000** | **21 100** | **18 400** | **13 700** | **13 000** | **13 600** | **14 000** | **11 300** | **7 900** |
| Upper 95% CI | 33 900 | 23 300 | 24 400 | 18 000 | 17 400 | 18 200 | 19 700 | 15 400 | 10 700 |
| **Western Pacific** | | | | | | | | | |
| Lower 95% CI | 1 045 | 922 | 914 | 1 305 | 1 588 | 1 115 | 1 318 | 1 392 | 1 495 |
| **Estimated total** | **1 839** | **1 576** | **1 761** | **2 027** | **2 345** | **1 445** | **1 733** | **1 854** | **1 980** |
| Upper 95% CI | 2 779 | 2 340 | 3 009 | 2 925 | 3 339 | 1 852 | 2 228 | 2 420 | 2 588 |
| **World** | | | | | | | | | |
| Lower 95% CI | 231 000 | 222 000 | 214 000 | 205 000 | 202 000 | 203 000 | 210 000 | 211 000 | 206 000 |
| **Estimated total** | **251 000** | **241 000** | **234 000** | **224 000** | **217 000** | **219 000** | **227 000** | **231 000** | **228 000** |
| Upper 95% CI | 278 000 | 267 000 | 260 000 | 250 000 | 238 000 | 240 000 | 251 000 | 260 000 | 258 000 |
| **Estimated *P. vivax*** | | | | | | | | | |
| Lower 95% CI | 11 700 | 10 600 | 9 400 | 7 200 | 6 300 | 5 900 | 6 400 | 6 200 | 5 900 |
| **Estimated total** | **16 300** | **15 700** | **14 200** | **10 900** | **8 700** | **8 000** | **8 300** | **7 700** | **7 500** |
| Upper 95% CI | 23 700 | 24 100 | 22 300 | 17 200 | 12 300 | 10 900 | 10 900 | 9 800 | 9 300 |

CI: confidence interval; *P. vivax*: *Plasmodium vivax*; WHO: World Health Organization.

## TABLE 2.2.

**Estimated *P. vivax* malaria cases by WHO region, 2018** Estimated cases are shown with 95% upper and lower CI. *Source: WHO estimates.*

|  | Number of cases (000) | | | | | |
|---|---|---|---|---|---|---|
|  | African | Americas | Eastern Mediterranean | South-East Asia | Western Pacific | World |
| **Estimated *P. vivax*** | | | | | | |
| Lower 95% CI | 91 | 657 | 1 171 | 2 860 | 556 | 5 900 |
| **Estimated total** | **704** | **700** | **1 414** | **3 947** | **690** | **7 500** |
| Upper 95% CI | 1 813 | 758 | 1 738 | 5 390 | 858 | 9 300 |
| Percentage of *P. vivax* cases | 0.3 | 75.4 | 28.9 | 50.0 | 34.8 | 3.3 |

CI: confidence interval; *P. vivax*: *Plasmodium vivax*; WHO: World Health Organization.

# 2  Regional and global trends in burden of malaria cases and deaths

Almost 85% of all malaria cases globally were in 19 countries: India and 18 African countries (**Fig. 2.1a**). Over 50% of all cases globally were accounted for by Nigeria (25%), followed by the Democratic Republic of the Congo (12%), Uganda (5%), and Côte d'Ivoire, Mozambique and Niger (4% each). Of these 19 countries, India reported the largest absolute reductions in cases, with 2.6 million fewer cases in 2018 than in 2017, followed by Uganda (1.5 million fewer cases) and Zimbabwe (0.6 million fewer cases).

Notable increases were seen in Ghana (8% increase, 0.5 million more cases) and Nigeria (6% increase, 3.2 million more cases). Changes in the remaining 14 countries were generally small, suggesting a similar burden of cases in 2017 and 2018.

More than 85% of estimated vivax malaria cases in 2018 occurred in just six countries, with India accounting for 47% of all vivax cases globally (**Fig. 2.1b**).

**FIG. 2.1.**

**Estimated country share of (a) total malaria cases and (b) *P. vivax* malaria cases, 2018** *Source: WHO estimates.*

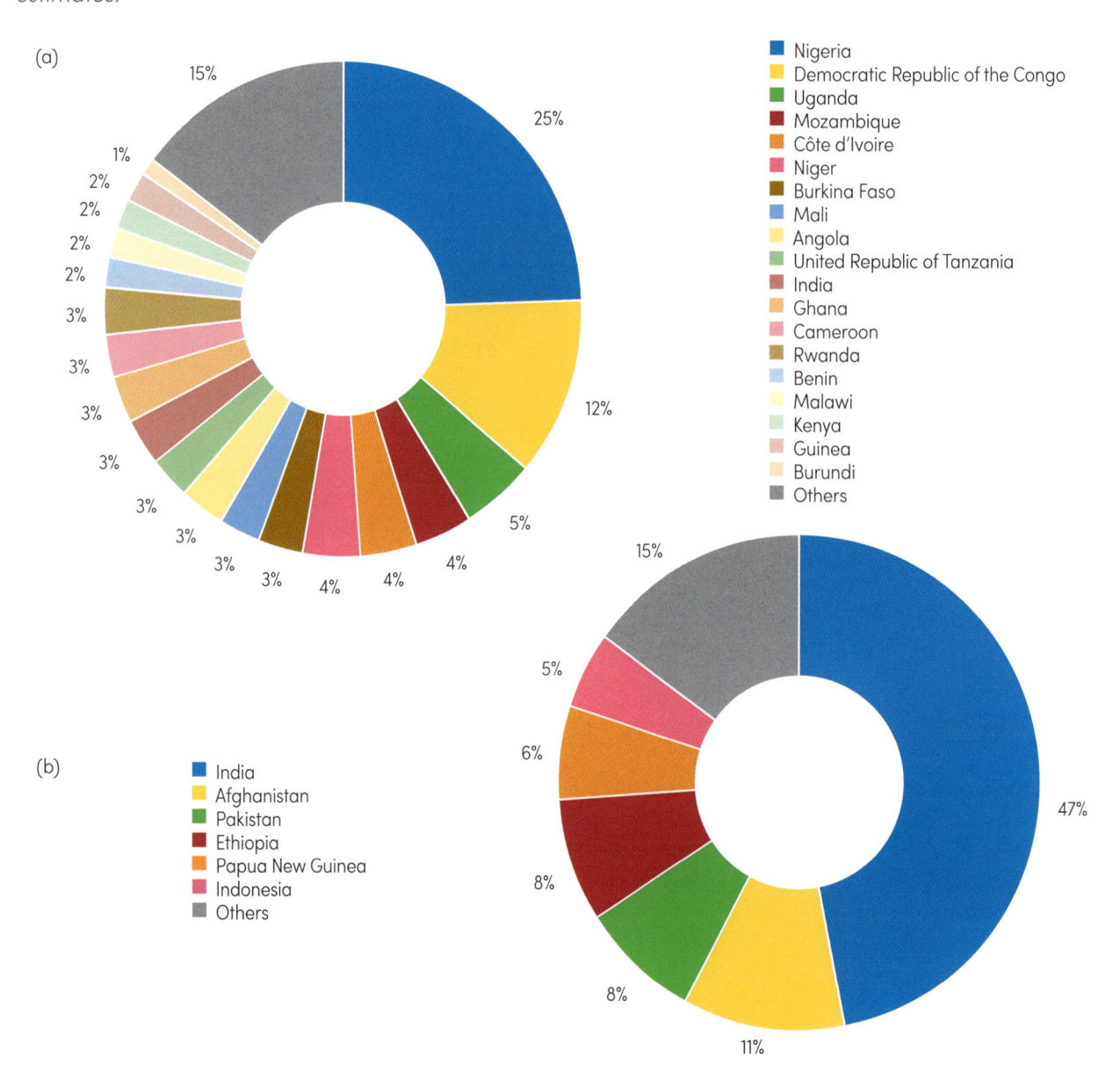

*P. vivax: Plasmodium vivax;* WHO: World Health Organization.

## 2.2 MALARIA CASE INCIDENCE RATE

The global incidence rate (i.e. the number of cases per 1000 population) of malaria reduced between 2010 and 2018; it fell from 71 in 2010 to 57 in 2018 (**Fig. 2.2a**). However, from 2014 to 2018, the rate of change slowed dramatically, reducing from 60 in 2013 to 57 in 2014 and remaining at similar levels through to 2018. In the WHO African Region, case incidence levels declined from 294 in 2010 to 229 in 2018, representing a 22% reduction in incidence, although the rate of change also appeared to slow from 2014.

The WHO Eastern Mediterranean Region and WHO Western Pacific Region saw a slight increase in case incidence between 2010 and 2018, while the WHO Region of the Americas saw a moderate increase, largely due to an increase in cases in Venezuela (Bolivarian Republic of). The highest reductions in incidence, however, were seen in the WHO South-East Asia Region, mainly owing to reductions in India, Indonesia and countries in the Greater Mekong subregion (GMS) (**Fig. 2.2b**). The geographic distribution of malaria case incidence by country is shown in **Fig. 2.3**.

**FIG. 2.2.**

**Trends in malaria case incidence rate (cases per 1000 population at risk) globally and by WHO region, 2010–2018** The WHO European Region has reported zero indigenous cases since 2015. *Source: WHO estimates.*

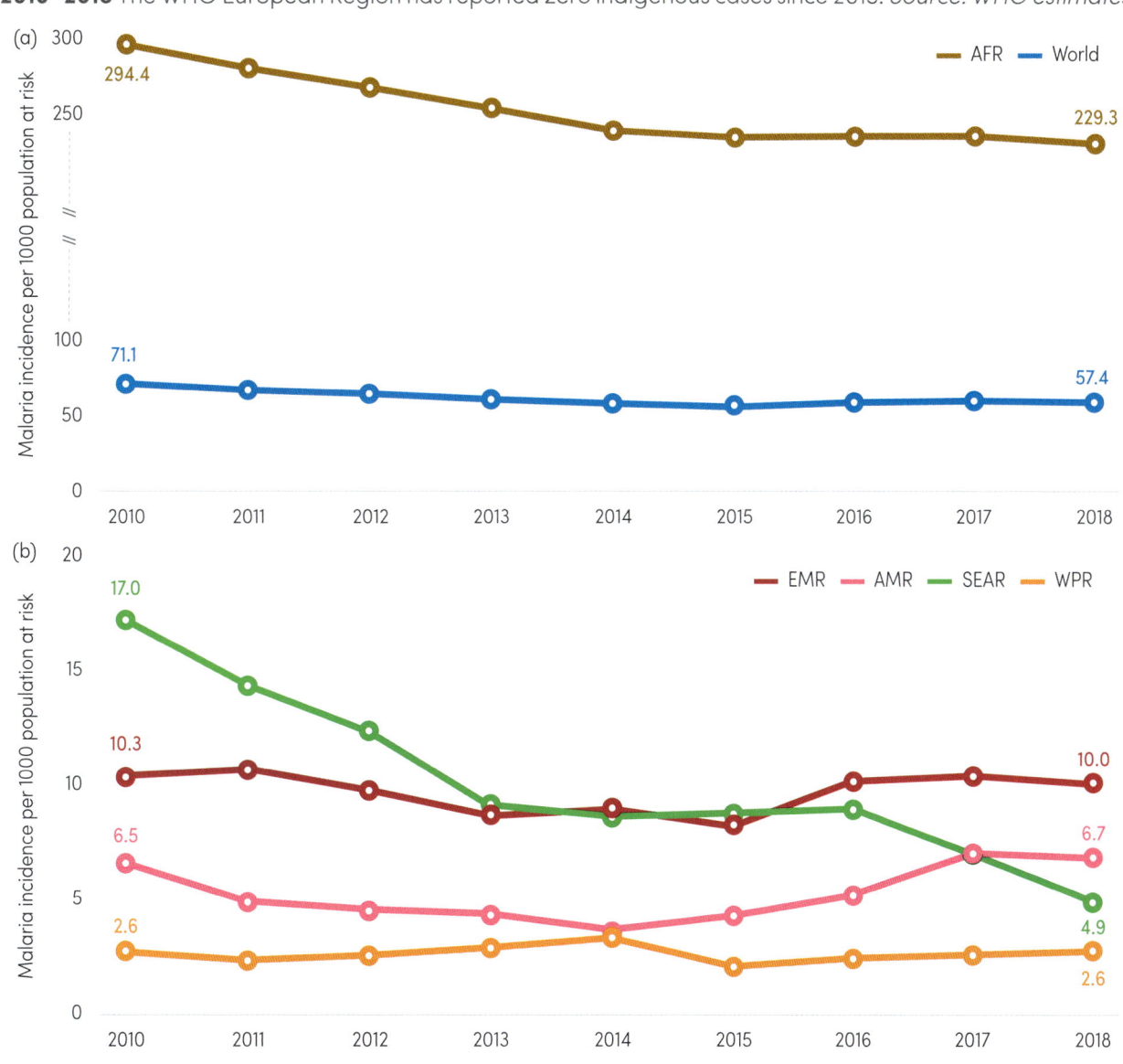

AFR: WHO African Region; AMR: WHO Region of the Americas; EMR: WHO Eastern Mediterranean Region; SEAR: WHO South-East Asia Region; WHO: World Health Organization; WPR: WHO Western Pacific Region.

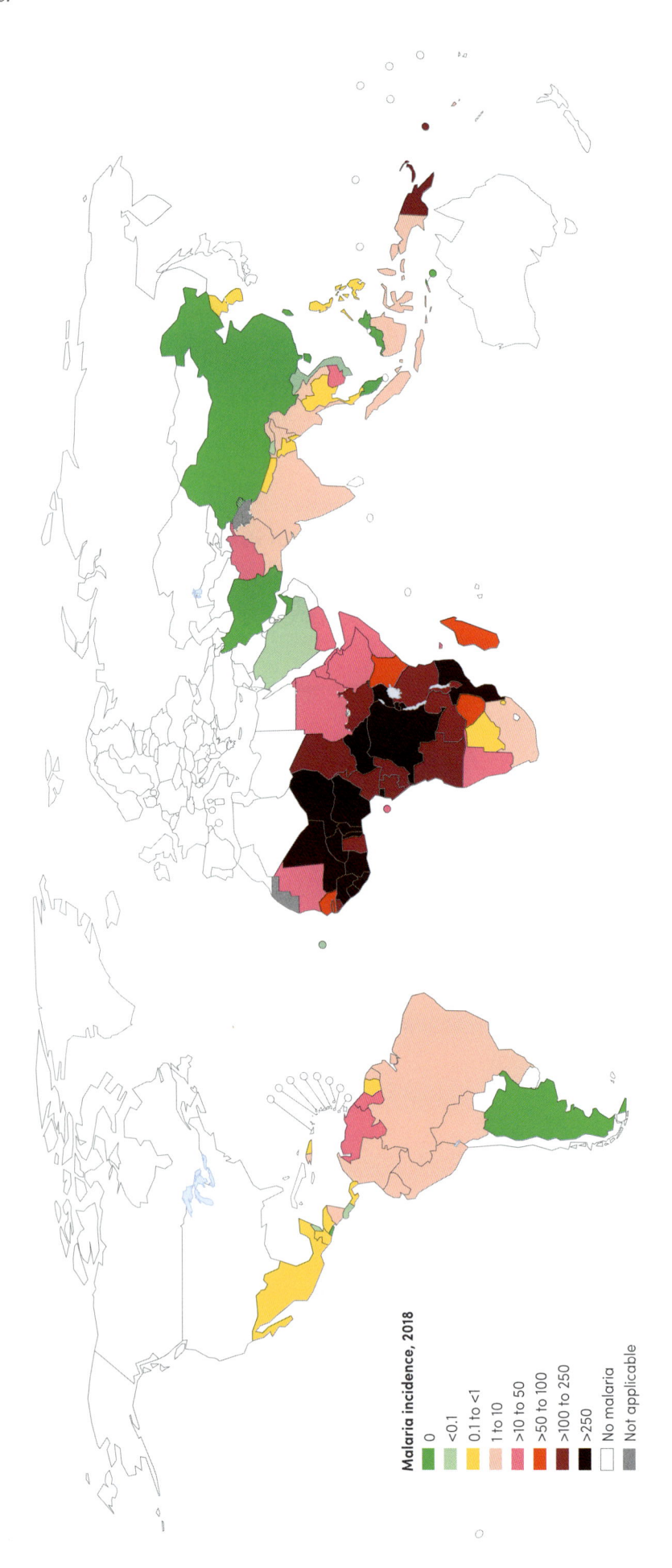

**FIG. 2.3.**
**Map of malaria case incidence rate (cases per 1000 population at risk) by country, 2018** *Source: WHO estimates.*

## 2.3 ESTIMATED NUMBER OF MALARIA DEATHS AND MORTALITY RATE BY WHO REGION, 2010–2018

Between 2010 and 2018, estimated deaths due to malaria globally declined from 585 000 to 405 000 cases (**Table 2.3**). Declines were recorded in all regions apart from the WHO Region of the Americas due to increases in malaria in Venezuela (Bolivarian Republic of) and the WHO Eastern Mediterranean Region due to increases in Somalia, Sudan and Yemen. Estimates of the malaria mortality rate (i.e. deaths per 100 000 population at risk) show that, compared with 2010, only the WHO African Region and the WHO South-East Asia Region had recorded notable reductions by 2018 (**Fig. 2.4** and **Fig. 2.5**). The highest absolute reduction in malaria deaths occurred in the WHO African Region, from 533 000 deaths in 2010 to 380 000 deaths in 2018. The rate of reduction of malaria mortality was slower in the period 2016–2018 than in the period 2010–2015.

**FIG. 2.4.**

**Trends in malaria mortality rate (deaths per 100 000 population at risk), globally and in the WHO African Region, 2010–2018** *Source: WHO estimates.*

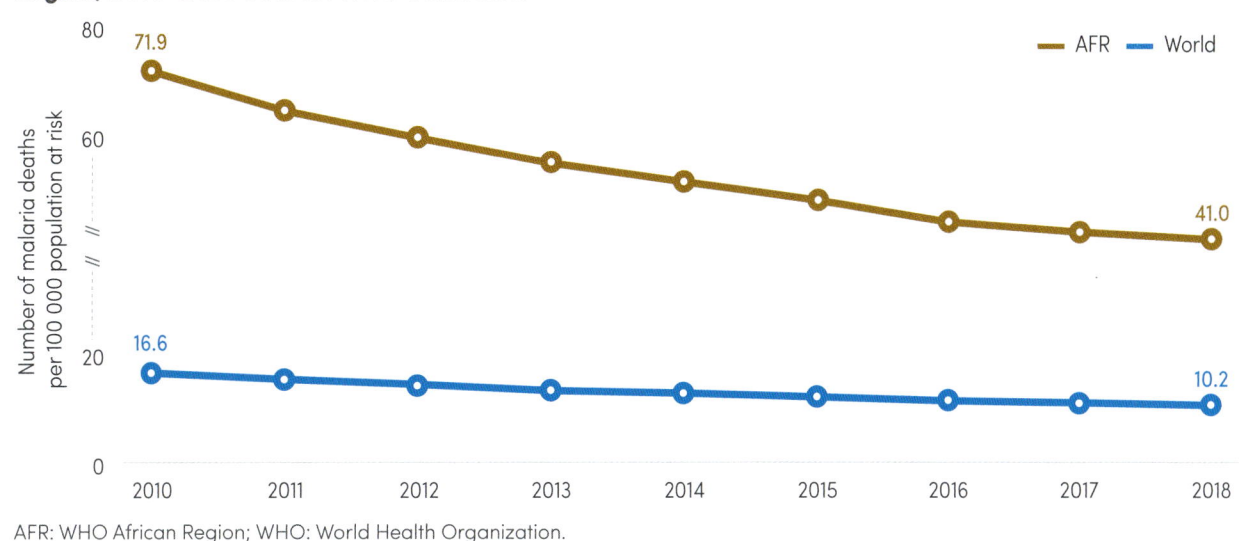

AFR: WHO African Region; WHO: World Health Organization.

**FIG. 2.5.**

**Trends in malaria mortality rate (deaths per 100 000 population at risk) in WHO regions, 2010–2018** *Source: WHO estimates.*

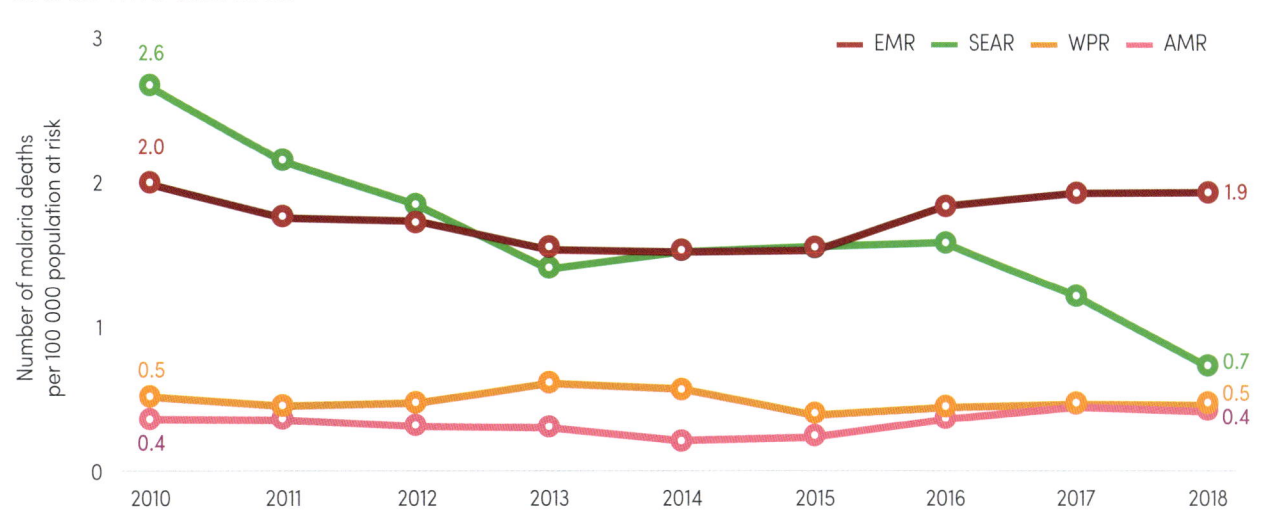

AMR: WHO Region of the Americas; EMR: WHO Eastern Mediterranean Region; SEAR: WHO South-East Asia Region; WHO: World Health Organization; WPR: WHO Western Pacific Region.

# 2  Regional and global trends in burden of malaria cases and deaths

Globally, 272 000 (67%) malaria deaths were estimated to be in children aged under 5 years (**Table 2.3**).

Almost 85% of all deaths in 2018 occurred in 20 countries in the WHO African Region and India, and almost 50% of all malaria deaths globally were accounted for by Nigeria (24%) followed by the Democratic Republic of the Congo (11%), the United Republic of Tanzania (5%), and Niger, Mozambique and Angola (4% each) (**Fig. 2.6**).

## TABLE 2.3.

**Estimated number of malaria deaths by WHO region, 2010–2018** *Source: WHO estimates.*

| | Number of deaths | | | | | | | | |
|---|---|---|---|---|---|---|---|---|---|
| | 2010 | 2011 | 2012 | 2013 | 2014 | 2015 | 2016 | 2017 | 2018 |
| African | 533 000 | 493 000 | 469 000 | 444 000 | 428 000 | 411 000 | 389 000 | 383 000 | 380 000 |
| Americas | 459 | 444 | 392 | 391 | 289 | 324 | 474 | 620 | 577 |
| Eastern Mediterranean | 8 300 | 7 500 | 7 600 | 6 900 | 6 900 | 7 100 | 8 600 | 9 200 | 9 300 |
| European | 0 | 0 | 0 | 0 | 0 | 0 | 0 | 0 | 0 |
| South-East Asia | 39 000 | 32 000 | 28 000 | 21 000 | 24 000 | 25 000 | 25 000 | 20 000 | 12 000 |
| Western Pacific | 3 800 | 3 300 | 3 600 | 4 600 | 4 400 | 2 800 | 3 500 | 3 600 | 3 600 |
| World (total) | 585 000 | 536 000 | 508 000 | 477 000 | 463 000 | 446 000 | 427 000 | 416 000 | 405 000 |
| World (children aged under 5 years) | 450 000 | 406 000 | 377 000 | 348 000 | 334 000 | 311 000 | 290 000 | 278 000 | 272 000 |

WHO: World Health Organization.

## FIG. 2.6.

**Percentage of estimated malaria deaths attributable to the 21 countries with nearly 85% of malaria deaths globally in 2018** *Source: WHO estimates.*

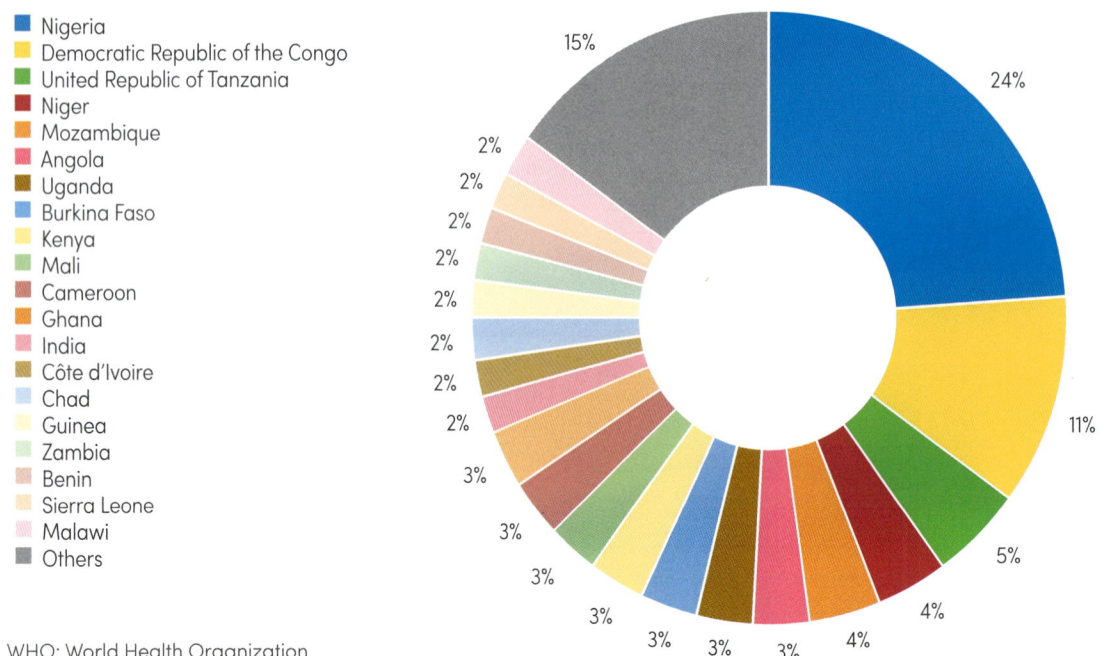

WHO: World Health Organization.

## 2.4 PROGRESS TOWARDS THE GTS MILESTONES FOR MALARIA MORBIDITY AND MORTALITY

The GTS aims for a reduction of 40% of malaria morbidity incidence and mortality rate by 2020 from a 2015 baseline (*1*). To illustrate the level of progress made so far, our analysis shows that if malaria case incidence and mortality rate remained the same as those in 2000, globally there would be 321 million cases and nearly 1 million malaria deaths in 2018 (**Fig. 2.7** and **Fig. 2.8**). Instead, there were an estimated 228 million malaria cases (**Table 2.1**) and 405 000 malaria deaths (**Table 2.3**) in 2018. These represent about 29% fewer cases and 60% fewer deaths in 2018 than would have been the case had levels of malaria incidence and malaria death remained similar to those in 2000.

**FIG. 2.7.**

**Comparison of current estimated malaria cases with expected cases had malaria incidence remained at 2000 levels globally** *Source: WHO estimates.*

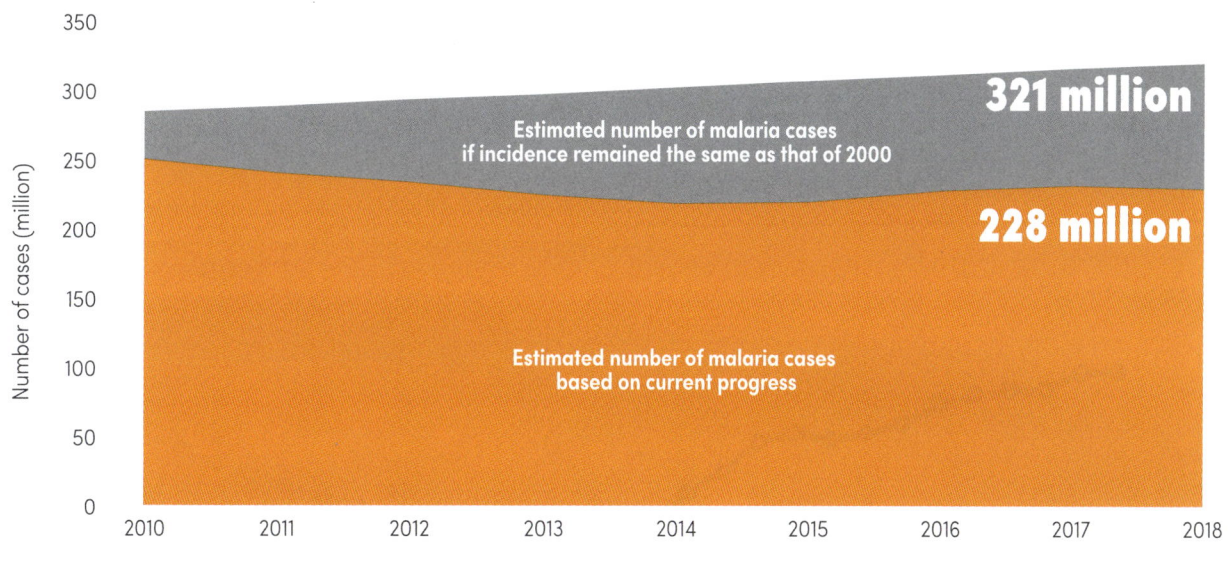

- Estimated number of malaria cases if incidence remained the same as that of 2000: **321 million**
- Estimated number of malaria cases based on current progress: **228 million**

WHO: World Health Organization.

**FIG. 2.8.**

**Comparison of current estimated malaria deaths with expected deaths had malaria incidence remained at 2000 levels globally** *Source: WHO estimates.*

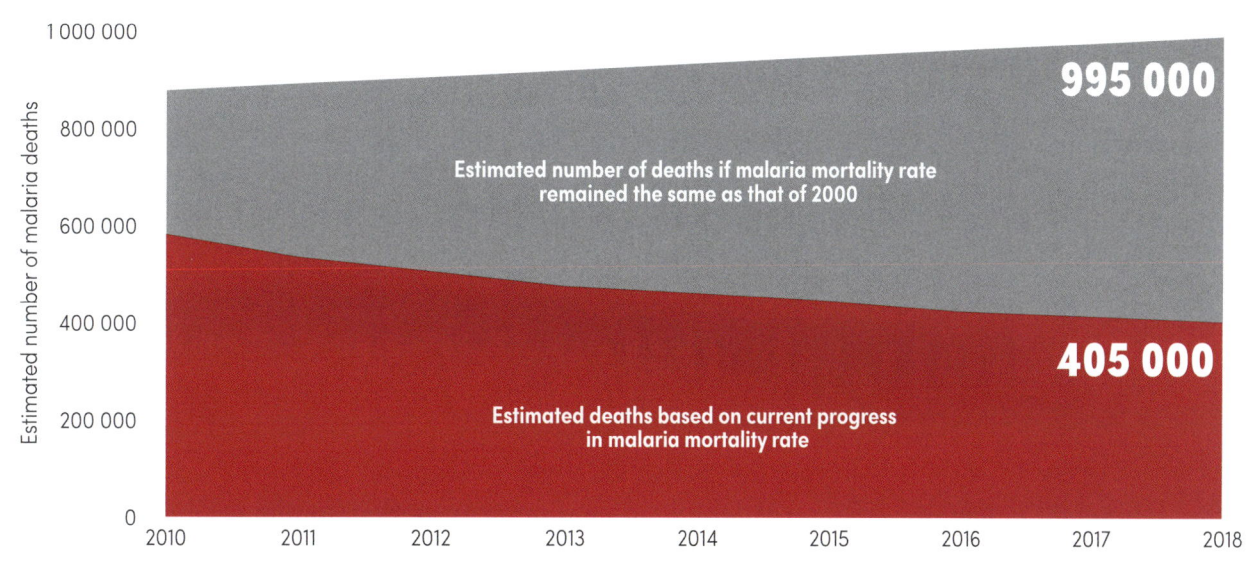

- Estimated number of deaths if malaria mortality rate remained the same as that of 2000: **995 000**
- Estimated deaths based on current progress in malaria mortality rate: **405 000**

WHO: World Health Organization.

# 2 Regional and global trends in burden of malaria cases and deaths

While the gains to date are impressive, the global malaria challenge remains enormous and the level of progress is slowing down. For example, on the current trajectory, globally, the 2020 GTS milestones for morbidity will not be achieved, and without accelerated change, the 2025 and 2030 milestones will not be achieved. A global malaria case incidence of 45 per 1000 population at risk in 2018 would have been required to get the world on target for the 2020 milestones, but current estimated incidence is at 57 cases per 1000 population at risk. If the current trend in incidence is maintained, estimated malaria case incidence (per 1000 population at risk) would be 54 in 2020, 48 in 2025 and 42 in 2030, instead of the 34, 14 and 6 required to achieve the GTS milestones (**Fig. 2.9**).

**FIG. 2.9.**

**Comparison of progress in malaria case incidence considering three scenarios: current trajectory maintained (blue), GTS targets achieved (green) and worst case scenario, that is a return to mean peak past incidence in the period 2000–2007 (red)** *Source: WHO estimates.*

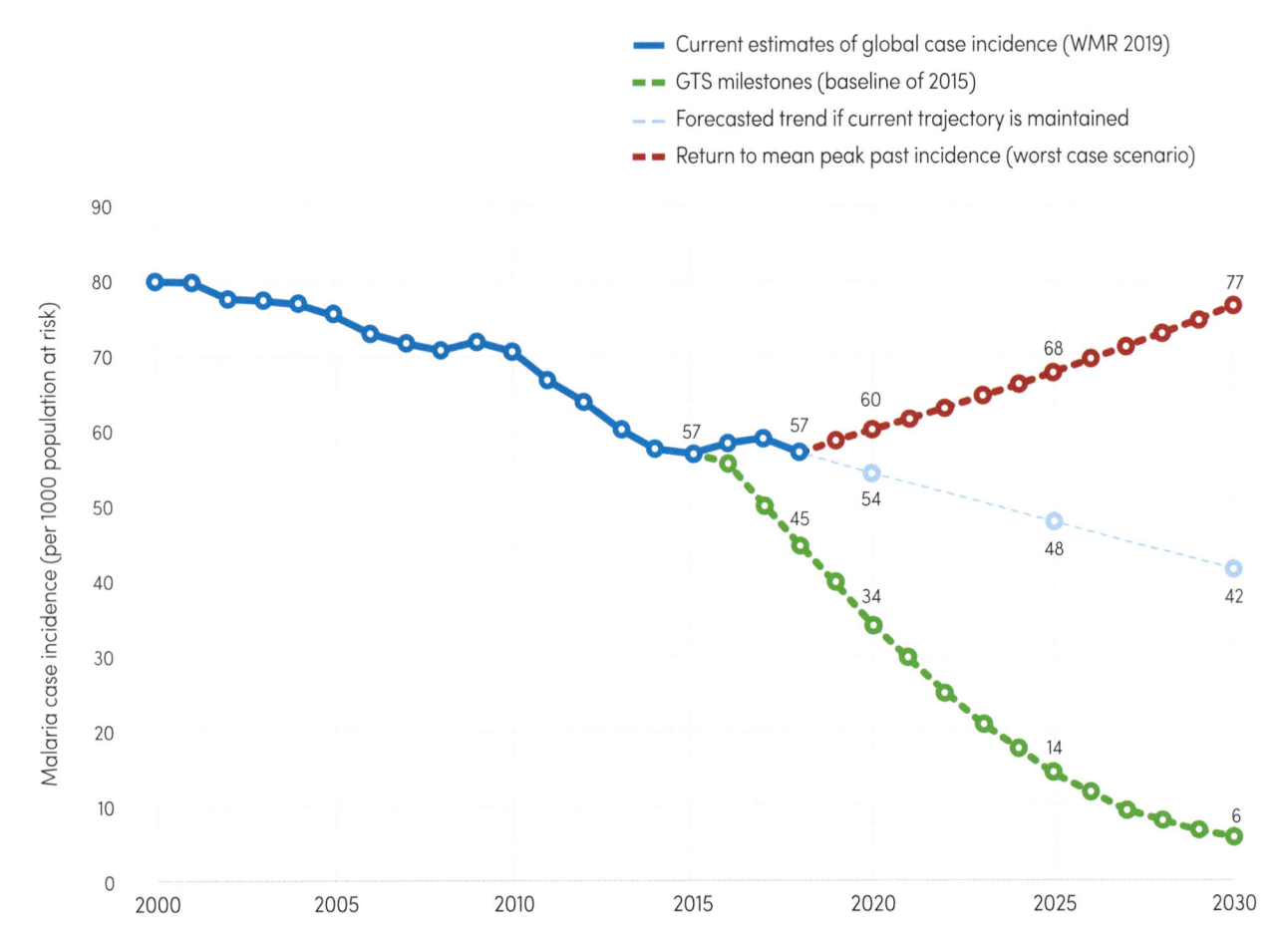

GTS: *Global technical strategy for malaria 2016–2030*; WHO: World Health Organization; WMR: *World Malaria Report*.

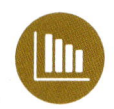

# 3. Maternal, infant and child health consequences of malaria

Malaria infection during pregnancy is a significant public health problem, with substantial risks for the pregnant woman, her fetus and the newborn child. The symptoms and complications of malaria in pregnancy vary according to malaria transmission intensity in the given geographical area, and the individual's level of acquired immunity (*7*). Malaria-associated maternal illness and anaemia, preterm birth and low birthweight newborns are mostly the result of *P. falciparum* infection and occurs predominantly in Africa. Maternal anaemia, of which malaria remains an important contributor, puts the mother at increased risk of death before and after childbirth. This also leads to preterm births and children of low weight at birth, causing problems with child growth and cognitive development, as well as being major risk factors for perinatal, neonatal and infant mortality (*8, 9*).

In moderate and high transmission settings, where levels of acquired immunity tend to be high, *P. falciparum* infection is usually asymptomatic in pregnancy. Nevertheless, parasites may be present in the placenta and contribute to maternal anaemia even in the absence of documented peripheral parasitaemia. Both maternal anaemia and placental parasitaemia can lead to low birthweight, which is an important contributor to infant mortality (*7, 10, 11*). In these settings, the adverse effects of *P. falciparum* infection in pregnancy are most pronounced for women in their first pregnancy. Infection with *P. vivax* leads to chronic anaemia, reducing the birthweight and increasing the risk of neonatal death. For women in their first pregnancy, the reduction in birthweight due to infection with *P. vivax* is about two thirds of the reduction associated with *P. falciparum* (*12, 13*).

In addition to a higher risk of low birthweight, infants once again become susceptible to *P. falciparum* malaria when immunity acquired from the mother starts to wane. Infants are at increased risk of rapid disease progression, severe malaria (especially of the severe anaemia form) and death.

To avert the consequences of malaria infections to pregnant women, fetuses, infants and children, WHO recommends – in combination with vector control, and prompt diagnosis and effective treatment of malaria – the use of intermittent preventive treatment in pregnancy (IPTp) with sulfadoxine-pyrimethamine (SP) as part of antenatal care (ANC) (**Section 7.3**); and intermittent preventive treatment in infants (IPTi) with SP in areas of moderate to high transmission in sub-Saharan Africa. In addition, seasonal malaria chemoprevention (SMC) with amodiaquine plus SP in children aged under 5 years is recommended in Africa's Sahel subregion.

In this section, exposure to malaria infection during pregnancy is estimated, then that estimation is used to compute the risk and prevalence of low birthweight. The correlation between malaria in pregnancy and malaria anaemia is presented, as is the prevalence of anaemia in children aged under 5 years, with or without malaria infection, as measured during household surveys. The analysis is restricted to moderate to high transmission countries in sub-Saharan Africa (**Annex 1**), where burden of malaria in pregnancy, infants and children is greatest.

## 3.1 PREVALENCE OF EXPOSURE TO MALARIA INFECTION DURING PREGNANCY, CORRELATION WITH MATERNAL ANAEMIA AND CONTRIBUTION TO LOW BIRTHWEIGHT

Anaemia is characterized by a decrease in the number of red blood cells in the blood (or a decrease in haemoglobin [Hb] concentration) to a level that impairs the normal physiological capacity of the blood to transport oxygen to cells around the body. WHO defines mild anaemia as a Hb concentration of between 10 g/dL and 10.9 g/dL, moderate anaemia as between 7 g/dL and 9.9 g/dL, and severe anaemia as below 7 g/dL. Deficiency in iron is thought to be the most common cause of anaemia.[1] Maternal anaemia has multiple causes, mainly related to nutrition, infection and genetics (*14*). In malaria endemic countries, malaria is a major cause of anaemia in pregnant women, many of whom also have other conditions, such as HIV and helminths infections and iron deficiency.

Malaria infections cause anaemia through multiple mechanisms; for example, direct destruction of red blood cells, clearance of infected and uninfected red cells by the spleen, and impaired red cell production by bone marrow. Individuals who are anaemic are at a greater risk of mortality, including from malaria. Single or repeated episodes of malaria may result in life-threatening anaemia, metabolic acidosis (*15*) and death. Exposure to malaria infection during pregnancy leads to maternal anaemia, which is associated with higher risk of obstetric haemorrhage and death. WHO estimates of maternal anaemia (Hb concentration of <10.9 g/dL at sea level) by country were obtained for 38 moderate to high malaria transmission countries in sub-Saharan Africa.[2]

Exposure to malaria infection in pregnancy (measured as cumulative prevalence over 40 weeks) was estimated from mathematic models (*16*) that relate estimates of the geographical distribution of *P. falciparum* exposure by age across Africa in 2018 to patterns of infections in placental histology by age and parity (*17*) (**Annex 1**). Fertility rates specific to country, age and gravidity, stratified by urban/rural status, were obtained from demographic health surveys (DHS) and malaria indicator surveys (MIS) where such surveys had been carried out since 2014 and were available from the DHS program website.[3] Countries where surveys were not available were allocated fertility patterns based on survey data from a different country, matched on the basis of total fertility rate (*18*) and geography. The exposure prevalence and the expected number of pregnant women who would have been exposed to infection were computed by country and subregion.

---

[1] Additional important causes of anaemia include infections, other nutritional deficiencies (e.g. in folate, and vitamins B12, A and C), genetic conditions and haemoglobinopathies (e.g. sickle cell disease and thalassaemia), and chronic kidney disease (*10*). Anaemia is highly prevalent globally and is particularly prevalent in sub-Saharan Africa. According to the WHO guidelines for treatment of malaria (*36*), a Hb concentration of less than 5 g/dL in an individual infected with malaria defines severe malaria.

[2] https://apps.who.int/gho/data/node.main.1?lang=en; Maternal anaemia prevalence estimates are presented to 2016 and were kept the same for the 2018 estimates in this report.

[3] https://dhsprogram.com/

# 3 Maternal, infant and child health consequences of malaria

Analysis by subregion showed that the prevalence of exposure to malaria infection in pregnancy was highest in West Africa and Central Africa, each with 35%, followed by East and Southern Africa (20%) (**Fig. 3.1**, **Table 3.1**). Overall prevalence of exposure to malaria infection in pregnancy in moderate to high transmission sub-Saharan Africa was 29%. In total, about 11 million pregnancies would have been exposed to malaria infection in these countries in 2018. About 39% (4.4 million) of these pregnancies were in the Democratic Republic of the Congo and Nigeria.

The analysis shows a positive correlation of maternal anaemia and prevalence of exposure to malaria infection during pregnancy (**Fig. 3.2**). In 20 countries (Benin, Burkina Faso, Burundi, Cameroon, Central

## FIG. 3.1.

**Estimated prevalence of exposure to malaria infection during pregnancy overall and by subregion in 2018 in moderate to high transmission sub-Saharan Africa** *Source: Imperial College, WHO estimates.*

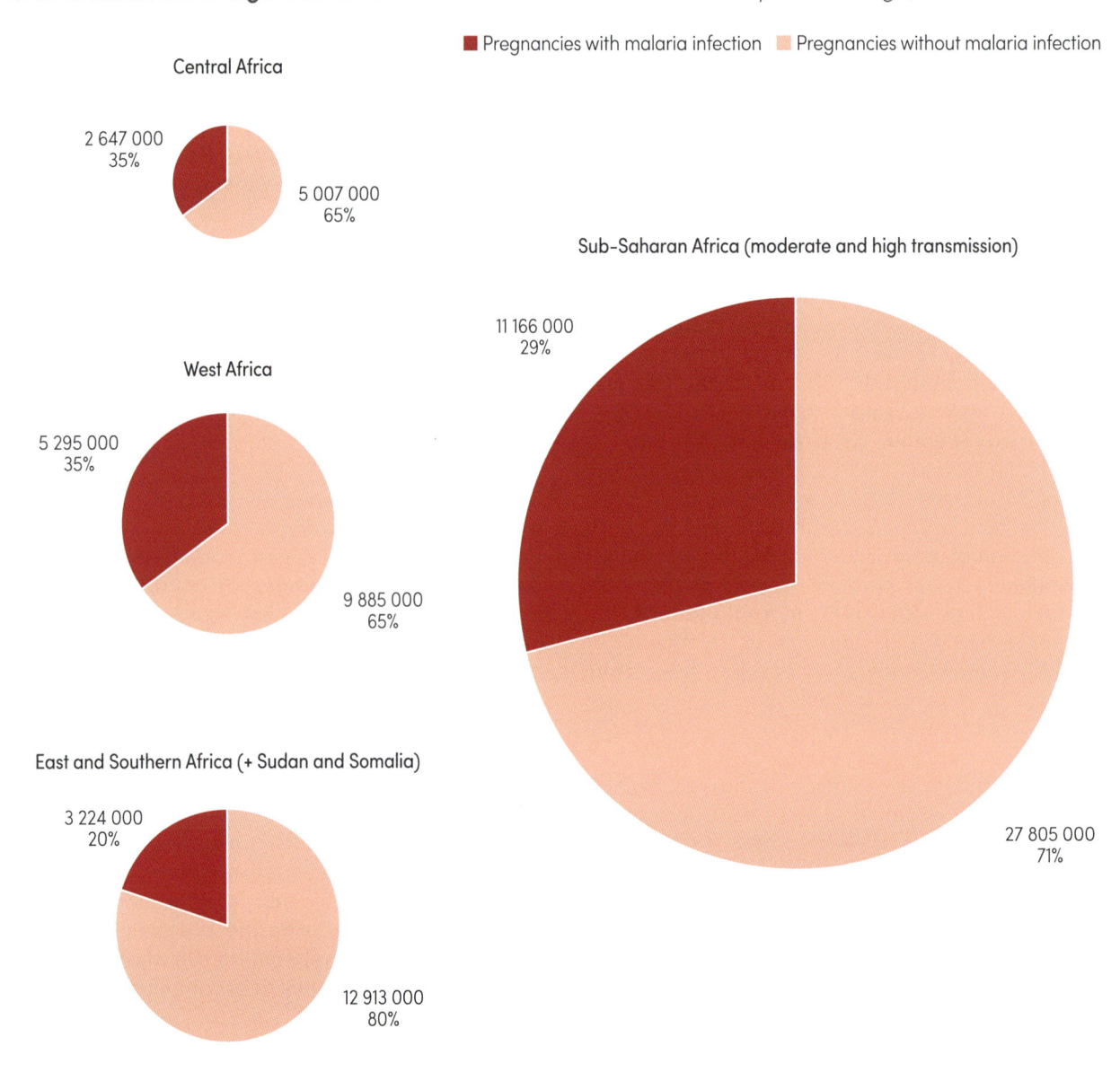

■ Pregnancies with malaria infection  ■ Pregnancies without malaria infection

**Central Africa**
- 2 647 000 — 35%
- 5 007 000 — 65%

**West Africa**
- 5 295 000 — 35%
- 9 885 000 — 65%

**East and Southern Africa (+ Sudan and Somalia)**
- 3 224 000 — 20%
- 12 913 000 — 80%

**Sub-Saharan Africa (moderate and high transmission)**
- 11 166 000 — 29%
- 27 805 000 — 71%

WHO: World Health Organization.

African Republic, Congo, Côte d'Ivoire, the Democratic Republic of the Congo, Equatorial Guinea, Gabon, Ghana, Guinea, Liberia, Malawi, Mozambique, Nigeria, Sierra Leone, South Sudan, Togo and Uganda), prevalence of exposure to malaria infection during pregnancy was 30% or more while maternal anaemia exceeded 40%. Although these countries have some of the highest malaria burden, the results should be interpreted recognizing that in sub-Saharan Africa, iron deficiency, an important cause of maternal anaemia, and malaria infection often coexist, but the relationship between them is complex. Measuring iron status in someone with current or recent past *P. falciparum* malaria infection is complicated by the inflammatory response to malaria infection (19).

## TABLE 3.1.

Estimates of pregnancies, livebirths, low birthweights, exposure to malaria infection in pregnancy and malaria-attributable low birthweights in 2018 in moderate to high transmission sub-Saharan Africa
*Source: Imperial College, WHO estimates.*

| Subregion | Number of pregnancies | Number of children born alive | Number of pregnancies infected during a 40-week gestation period | Number of children born with low birthweight (<2500 g) | Number of children born with low birthweight (<2500 g) due to malaria |
|---|---|---|---|---|---|
| Central Africa | 7 654 000 | 7 187 000 | 2 647 000 | 934 000 | 186 000 |
| West Africa | 15 180 000 | 14 253 000 | 5 295 000 | 2 321 000 | 418 000 |
| East and Southern Africa (+ Sudan and Somalia) | 16 137 000 | 15 174 000 | 3 224 000 | 2 280 000 | 268 000 |
| Sub-Saharan Africa: total | 38 971 000 | 36 614 000 | 11 166 000 | 5 535 000 | 872 000 |

WHO: World Health Organization.

## FIG. 3.2.

Estimated maternal anaemia (20)[a] versus exposure to malaria infection in pregnancy in 2018 in moderate to high transmission countries in sub-Saharan Africa *Source: Imperial College, UNICEF-WHO estimates.*

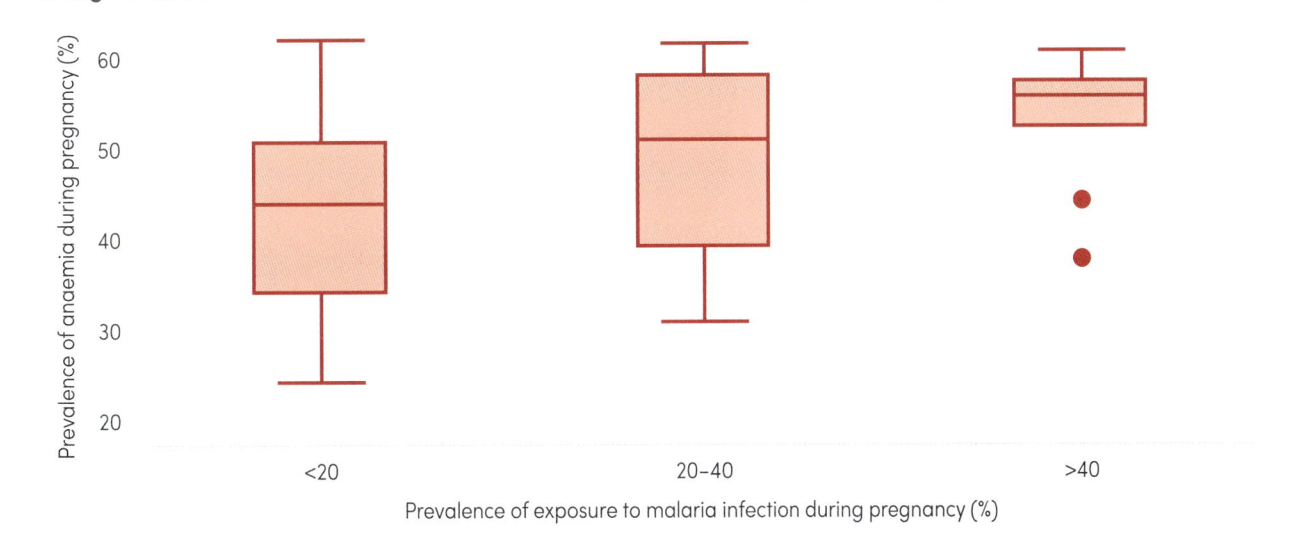

UNICEF: United Nations Children's Fund; WHO: World Health Organization.
[a] Prevalence of all cause low birthweight used in this analysis were those estimated for 2015 as shown in this source.

# 3. Maternal, infant and child health consequences of malaria

Low birthweight is defined as weight at birth of less than 2500 g, regardless of gestational age (*20*). Premature birth (<37 weeks) and growth faltering in the womb are the main reasons for low birthweight. Several factors contribute to these: maternal malnutrition and anaemia; maternal characteristics such as low or high age, parity and poor birth spacing; health problems such as high blood pressure, diabetes and infections; and other risk factors including smoking and alcohol consumption (*20*). Children with low weight at birth not only have a high risk of stunting and poor cognitive development but also are at higher risk of death.

In moderate to high transmission malaria endemic countries, malaria infection during pregnancy and the consequent placental infection are important contributors to low birthweight (*7, 10, 11*). The incremental risk of low birthweight posed by the different categories of placental infection, and the relation between parity-specific and histology-specific placental infection categories and the risk of low birthweight in the absence of other competing "non-malaria" risk factors were computed with data from different transmission settings (*16*).

In 38 moderate to high transmission countries in sub-Saharan Africa, the estimated 11 million (**Table 3.1**) pregnancies exposed to malaria infection in 2018 resulted in about 872 000 children born with low birthweight (**Fig. 3.3**), representing 16% of all children with low birthweight in these countries (**Fig. 3.3**). By subregion, the percentage of low birthweight children due to malaria was, in line with exposure to malaria infection during pregnancy, highest in West Africa (18% of low birthweight children), followed by Central Africa (20%) and East and Southern Africa (12%) (**Fig. 3.3**).

## FIG. 3.3.

**Estimated low birthweights due to exposure to malaria infection during pregnancy overall and by subregion in 2018 in moderate to high transmission sub-Saharan Africa** *Source: Imperial College, WHO estimates.*

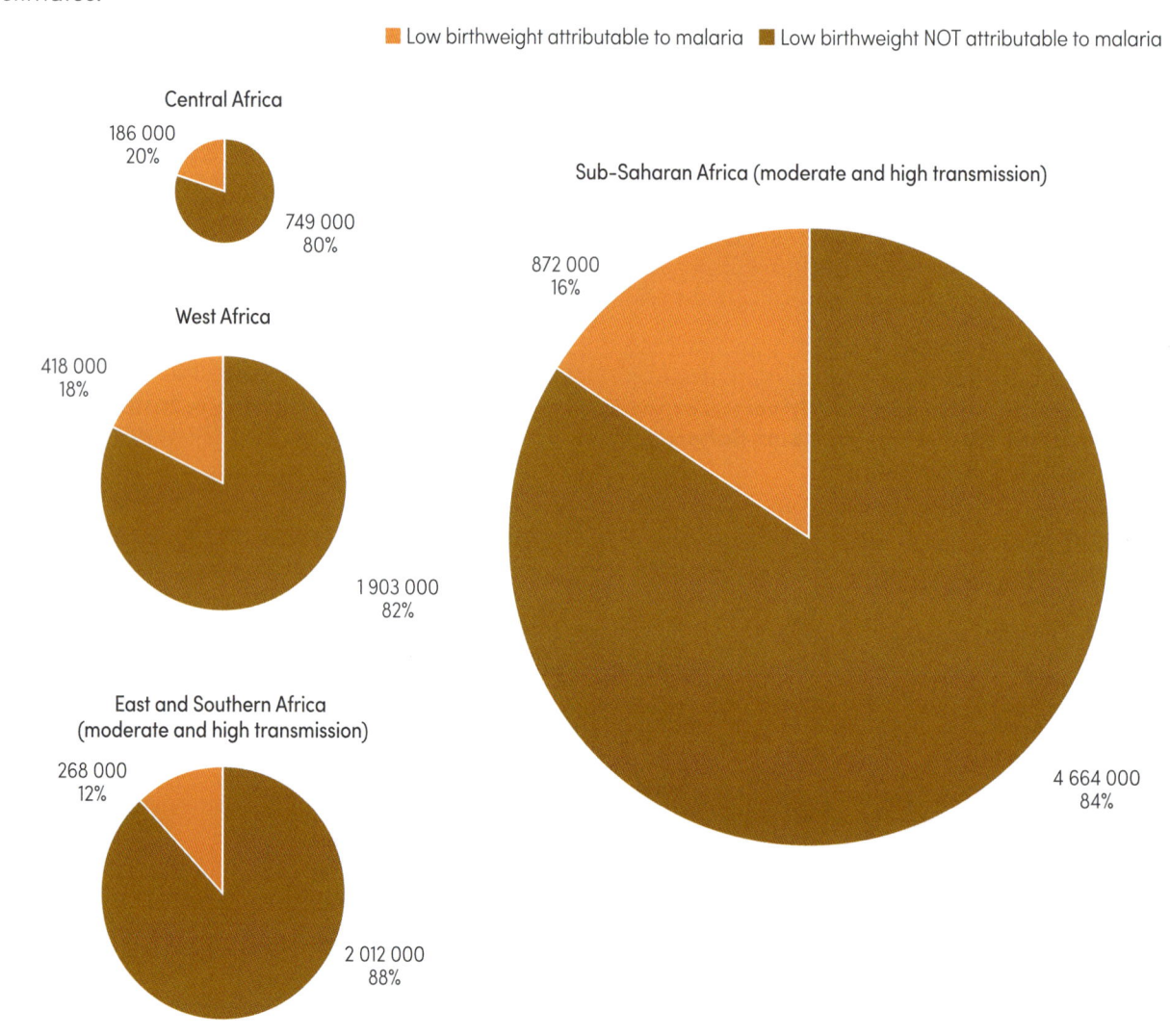

■ Low birthweight attributable to malaria ■ Low birthweight NOT attributable to malaria

**Central Africa**
186 000 — 20%
749 000 — 80%

**West Africa**
418 000 — 18%
1 903 000 — 82%

**East and Southern Africa (moderate and high transmission)**
268 000 — 12%
2 012 000 — 88%

**Sub-Saharan Africa (moderate and high transmission)**
872 000 — 16%
4 664 000 — 84%

WHO: World Health Organization.

## 3.2 PREVALENCE AND BURDEN OF MALARIA-RELATED ANAEMIA IN CHILDREN AGED UNDER 5 YEARS

Data from household surveys implemented in 21 moderate to high malaria burden countries between 2015 and 2018 showed that, among children aged under 5 years, the prevalence of any anaemia was 61%, mild anaemia 25%, moderate anaemia 33% and severe anaemia 3%.

When children were categorized by malaria rapid diagnostic test (RDT) results, overall anaemia was higher in children who were positive for malaria than in those who were negative (**Fig. 3.4**). When anaemia prevalence was further classified, of the children who were positive for malaria, 9% had severe anaemia, 54% had moderate anaemia, 21% had mild anaemia and only 17% had no anaemia. In contrast, among those children who had no malaria, 1% had severe anaemia, 31% had moderate anaemia, 28% had mild anaemia and 40% had no anaemia (**Fig. 3.4**).

### FIG. 3.4.
**Prevalence of severe anaemia (<7 g/dL), moderate anaemia (7-9.9 g/dL) and mild anaemia (10–10.9 g/dL) in children aged under 5 years in sub-Saharan Africa, 2015–2018, by age and malaria infection status**
*Source: Household surveys.*

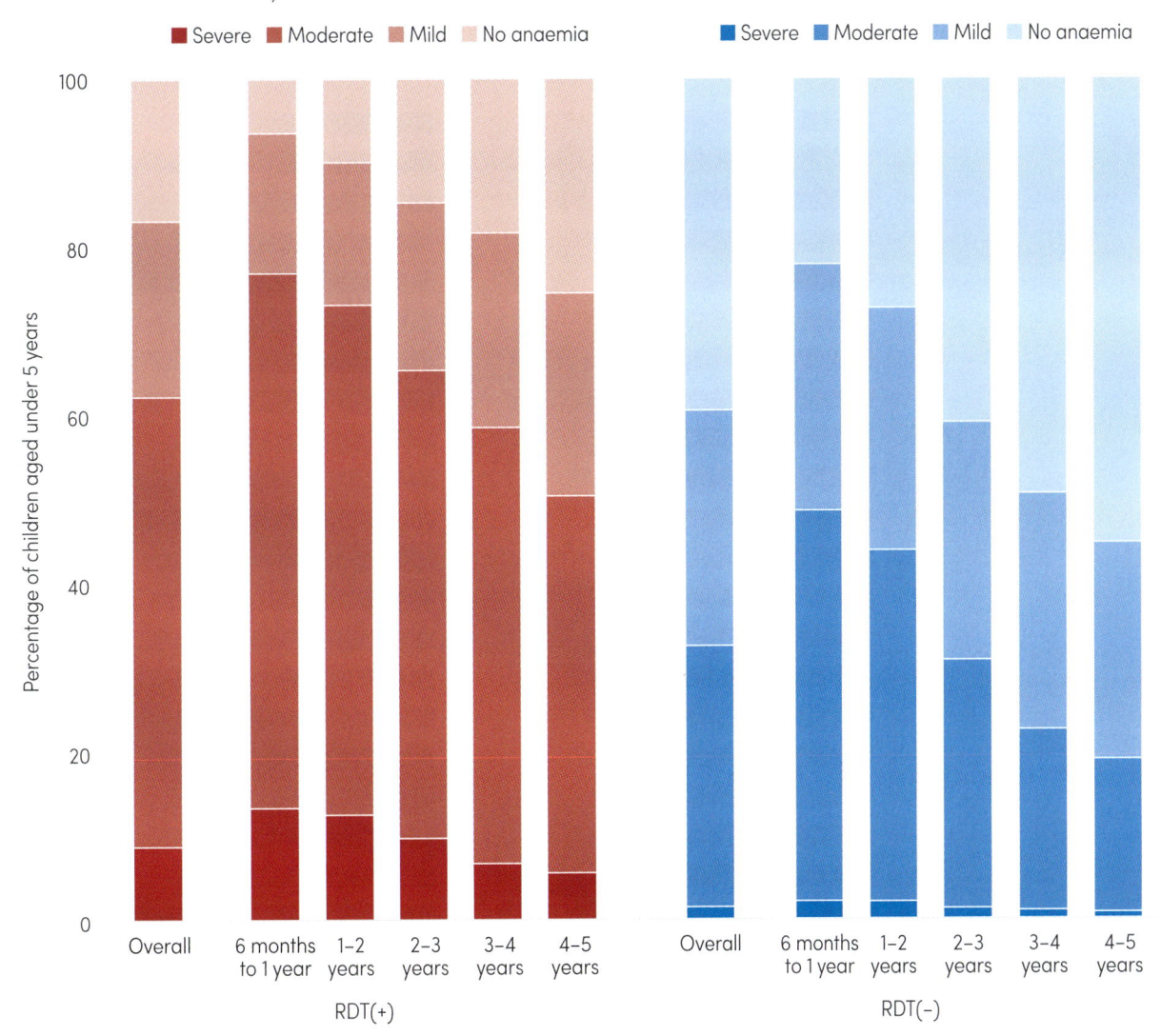

RDT: rapid diagnostic test.

# 3 Maternal, infant and child health consequences of malaria

Analysis by country presents a mixed picture, although in general, higher anaemia prevalence was observed among children infected with malaria than among those who were not (**Fig. 3.5**). For most countries, the percentage of severe anaemia among children aged under 5 years who were positive for malaria ranged from 5% to 10%, except in Mozambique (12%), Guinea (14%), Mali (16%) and Senegal (26%).

The number of children who were likely to be infected with *P. falciparum* in moderate to high transmission countries in sub-Saharan Africa was estimated using spatiotemporal methods applied to community parasite prevalence data obtained from household surveys.[1] The anaemia by infection status derived from household surveys (**Fig. 3.4**, **Fig. 3.5**) were then applied to the estimated number of infections among children aged 1–59 months (**Table 3.2**). Overall, about 24 million children were infected with *P. falciparum* in 2018 in sub-Saharan Africa. Of these, 7.2 million were in Central Africa, 6.1 million in East and Southern Africa, and 10.6 million in West Africa. An estimated 1.8 million were likely to have severe anaemia (Hb <7 g/dL), 12 million had moderate anaemia (7–9.9 g/dL), 5.2 million had mild anaemia (10–10.9 g/dL), and only about 4.8 million had no anaemia.

[1] https://apps.who.int/malaria/maps/threats/

**FIG. 3.5.**

**Prevalence of severe anaemia (<7 g/dL), moderate anaemia (7–9.9 g/dL) and mild anaemia (10–10.9 g/dL) in children aged under 5 years in sub-Saharan Africa, 2015–2018, by country** *Source: Household surveys.*

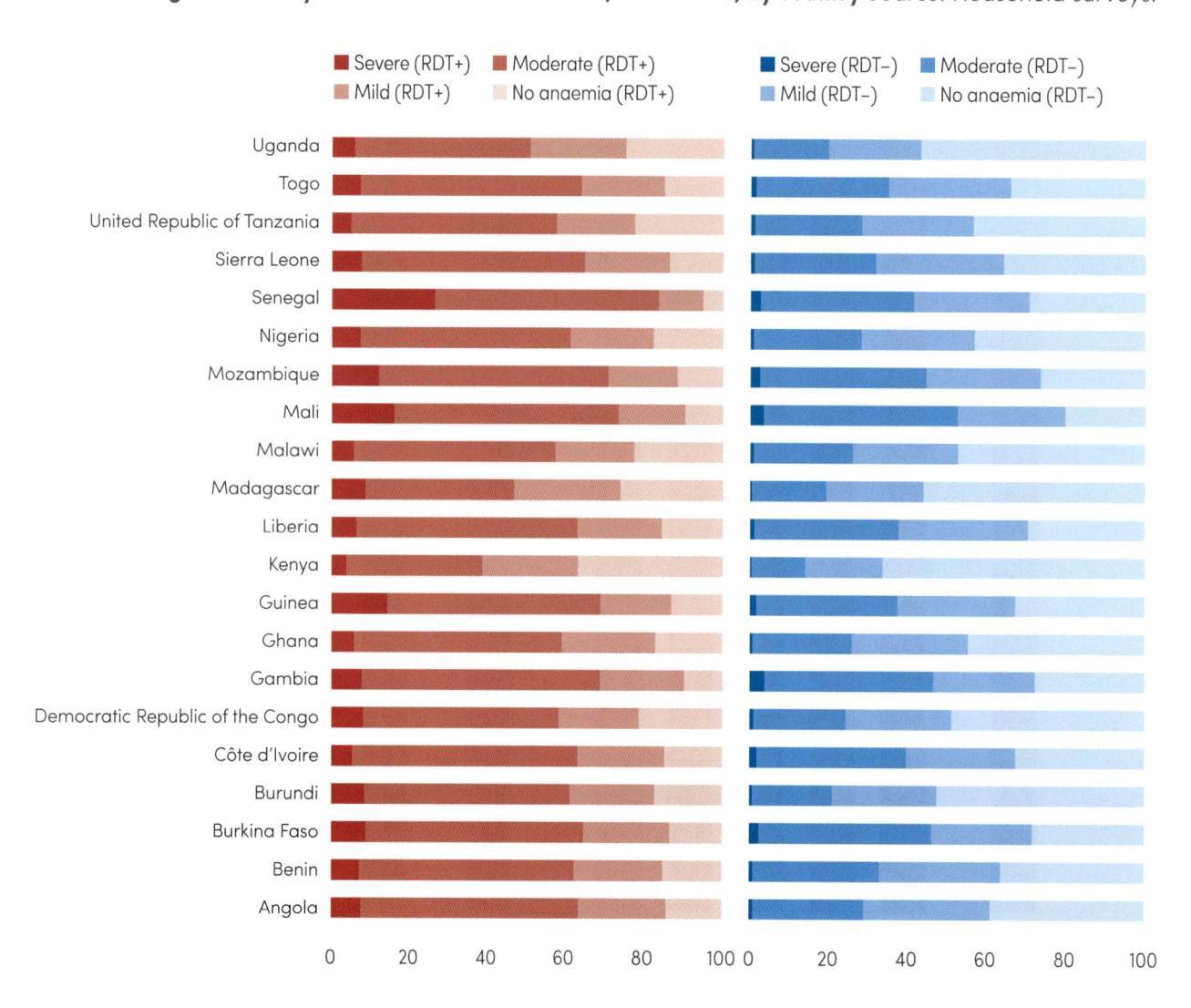

RDT: rapid diagnostic test.

## 3.3 PROTECTING THE MOTHER AND CHILD

The sub-Saharan African countries most affected by malaria-related consequences in pregnancy and early childhood also have some of the highest concentration of other risk factors for unhealthy pregnancies, new-borns and children. Often in these communities, malaria occurs in mothers and children who are already weakened by parasitic, viral and bacterial infections; nutritional deficiencies; and genetic conditions (*21*). Broader determinants, such as socioeconomic status, mother's age, parity and health system factors further threaten the wellbeing of the mother and child, leading to some of the highest levels of maternal, infant and child mortality rates globally (*22*). Addressing these determinants requires a multisectoral approach underpinned by a health system that delivers effective primary health care, both in terms of quality and coverage.

To ensure that mothers and new-borns are protected, long-lasting insecticidal nets (LLINs) are routinely delivered through ANC and expanded programmes for immunization, respectively. About 28 million nets were distributed through these channels in sub-Saharan Africa in 2018. In the same year, about 61% of pregnant women and children slept under a treated mosquito net (**Section 7**). IPTp is now part of the WHO recommended

### TABLE 3.2.

**Estimated number of children aged 1–59 months infected with *P. falciparum* parasites in 2018 by subregion and overall in sub-Saharan Africa,** *Source: WHO estimates.*

| | Total number of children aged 1–59 months infected in 2018 | Number by anaemia level among children aged 1–59 months who were infected in 2018 | | | |
|---|---|---|---|---|---|
| | | Severe (<7 g/dL) | Moderate (7–9.9 g/dL) | Mild (10–10.9 g/dL) | Not anaemic |
| Central Africa | 7 130 000 | 630 000 | 3 800 000 | 1 5000 000 | 1 200 000 |
| East and Southern Africa (+ Sudan and Somalia) | 6 080 000 | 480 000 | 3 200 000 | 1 300 000 | 1 100 000 |
| West Africa | 10 610 000 | 14 253 000 | 5 000 000 | 2 400 000 | 2 500 000 |
| **Sub-Saharan Africa: total** | **23 810 000** | **1 800 000** | **12 000 000** | **5 200 000** | **4 800 000** |

*P. falciparum*: *Plasmodium falciparum*; WHO: World Health Organization.

# 3. Maternal, infant and child health consequences of malaria

ANC package, with an estimated 31% of pregnant women receiving at least three doses of IPTp (**Section 7**). IPTi has been scaled up nationally only in Sierra Leone, despite a WHO recommendation since 2010, following evidence of a significant impact on clinical incidence and severe anaemia in infants. It is recommended for delivery on a schedule that corresponds to that of diphteria, pertussis and tetanus (DPT) and measles vaccines. Management of fever remains inadequate, with nearly 40% of febrile children in sub-Saharan Africa not accessing treatment (**Section 8**). Although integrated community case management (iCCM) is considered an effective strategy in bridging the gap in clinical care for common childhood illnesses, its roll-out in most sub-Saharan African countries remains poor, mainly due to health-financing bottlenecks.

To highlight some of the potential health system quality and coverage issues related to malaria interventions, an analysis of the prevalence of exposure to malaria infection during pregnancy, coverage of four or more ANC visits (ANC4) (22) and use of three or more doses of IPTp during pregnancy (IPTp3) were implemented (**Fig. 3.6**). Countries appear to fall into several categories: those where access to ANC services is a major impediment to increasing coverage of IPTp3 (e.g. Central African Republic, Chad, Niger, Somalia and South Sudan); those where ANC4 coverage is relatively high but quality of care is an issue and few women receive IPTp during ANC visits (e.g. Angola, Cameroon, Congo, Equatorial Guinea, Gabon, Guinea-Bissau, Liberia, Mauritania and Zimbabwe); and those where coverage of both ANC4 and IPTp3 are moderate and the main opportunities are in increasing access (Burkina Faso, Burundi, the Democratic Republic of the Congo, Gambia, Ghana, Mali, Mozambique, Sierra Leone, the United Republic of Tanzania and Zambia).

## FIG. 3.6.

**Country comparison of coverage of ANC4 and IPTp3 in moderate and high transmission sub-Saharan Africa, 2018** Countries in red typeface are those where prevalence of exposure to malaria infection during pregnancy was >20% in 2018. *Source: WHO estimates.*

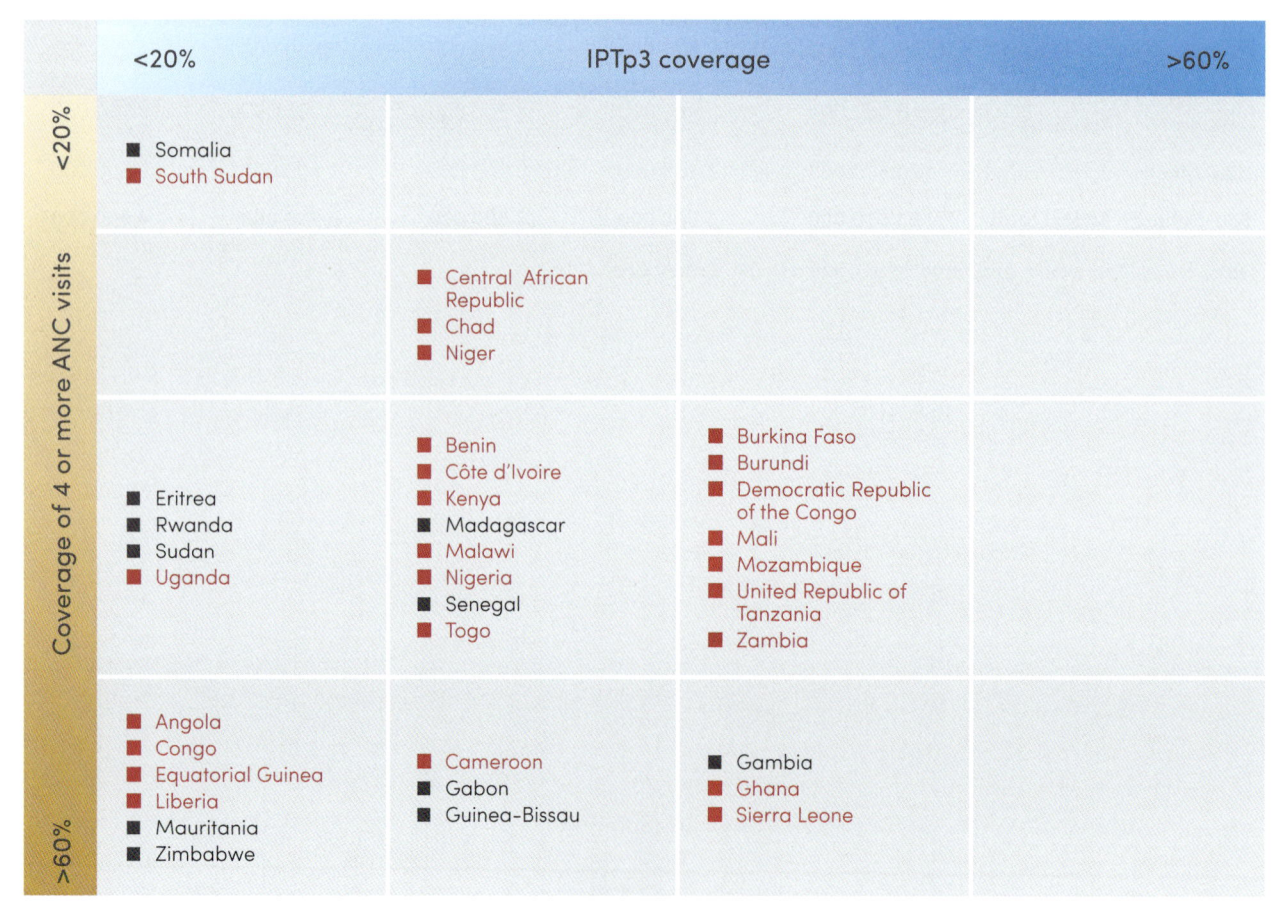

| Coverage of 4 or more ANC visits | IPTp3 coverage <20% | IPTp3 coverage (mid-low) | IPTp3 coverage (mid-high) | IPTp3 coverage >60% |
|---|---|---|---|---|
| <20% | Somalia; South Sudan | | | |
| (mid-low) | | Central African Republic; Chad; Niger | | |
| (mid-high) | Eritrea; Rwanda; Sudan; Uganda | Benin; Côte d'Ivoire; Kenya; Madagascar; Malawi; Nigeria; Senegal; Togo | Burkina Faso; Burundi; Democratic Republic of the Congo; Mali; Mozambique; United Republic of Tanzania; Zambia | |
| >60% | Angola; Congo; Equatorial Guinea; Liberia; Mauritania; Zimbabwe | Cameroon; Gabon; Guinea-Bissau | Gambia; Ghana; Sierra Leone | |

ANC4: 4 or more antenatal care visits; IPTp3: third dose of intermittent preventive treatment in pregnancy; WHO: World Health Organization.

# 4. High burden to high impact approach

In November 2018, WHO and the RBM Partnership to End Malaria launched the *high burden to high impact* (HBHI) country-led approach (*23*) as a mechanism to bring the 11 highest burden countries back on track to achieve the 2025 GTS milestones (*1*). This followed the results of the world malaria reports of 2017 (*24*) and 2018 (*25*), which showed that, globally, progress has stalled in high-burden countries and that the GTS 2020 milestones are, therefore, unlikely to be achieved. These 11 countries (Burkina Faso, Cameroon, the Democratic Republic of the Congo, Ghana, India, Mali, Mozambique, Niger, Nigeria, Uganda and the United Republic of Tanzania) account for 70% of the global estimated case burden and 71% of global estimated deaths.

Many factors contribute to the rising malaria burden in these, and other, high-burden countries, including the underlying intensity of malaria transmission, sociodemographic and epidemiologic risk factors, poor access to care and suboptimal malaria intervention coverage, and funding constraints. Consequently, the approach includes the four key response elements shown in **Fig. 4.1**, which have the aim of supporting countries to address their core country challenges so that they can get back on track towards the GTS milestones.

## 4.1 HBHI INITIATION ACTIVITIES

By November 2019, the HBHI approach had been initiated in Burkina Faso, Cameroon, Democratic Republic of Congo, Ghana, India, Mozambique, Niger, Nigeria and Uganda. The process involved national consultation meetings with in-country stakeholders, key international malaria partners and WHO. Countries implemented self-assessments on various aspects of the four response elements, which formed the basis of HBHI country discussions. Following the HBHI initiation meetings, countries developed detailed activity plans to address challenges revealed during assessments. Mali and the United Republic of Tanzania are expected to have held their national consultation meeting by the end of the first quarter of 2020. The key HBHI response highlights in most countries in 2019 include launch or strengthening of social mobilization and advocacy movements through the launching of the campaign "Zero Malaria Starts With Me" (*26*) with support from the RBM Partnership; initiation of the process of developing national malaria data repositories and stratification for intervention mix analysis with support from WHO, in-country and international partners; and increased political accountability through work with parliamentarians and high level, multisectoral bodies.

In addition, to ensure greater flexibility in adoption and adaptation of WHO recommendations by countries, the GMP convened an informal consultation in

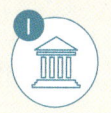

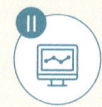

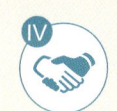

September 2019 to reconsider the formulation of malaria policy guidance. The outcome of this consultation was submitted to the Malaria Policy Advisory Committee (MPAC) during its meeting in October 2019 (27). The MPAC agreed with the conclusion of the informal consultation that intervention prioritization should not be driven solely by sequentially optimizing single interventions for maximal coverage; instead, intervention prioritization should be based on local evidence and aligned to the specific needs of different epidemiological strata or settings, as defined in the country's national strategic plan. The MPAC appreciated the concept of "universal coverage" in striving to save lives, reduce disease and ultimately eradicate malaria. The MPAC encouraged work towards universal coverage of the right mix of interventions, recognizing that the coverage of individual interventions will vary by setting.

This section summarizes the progress made in malaria burden, prevention, diagnosis and treatment for all HBHI countries. It ends with a discussion of trends in external and domestic direct funding (excluding estimated costs of patient care) in the HBHI countries.

**FIG. 4.1.**

**HBHI: a targeted malaria response to get countries back on target for the 2025 GTS milestones** *Source: WHO GMP and RBM Partnership.*

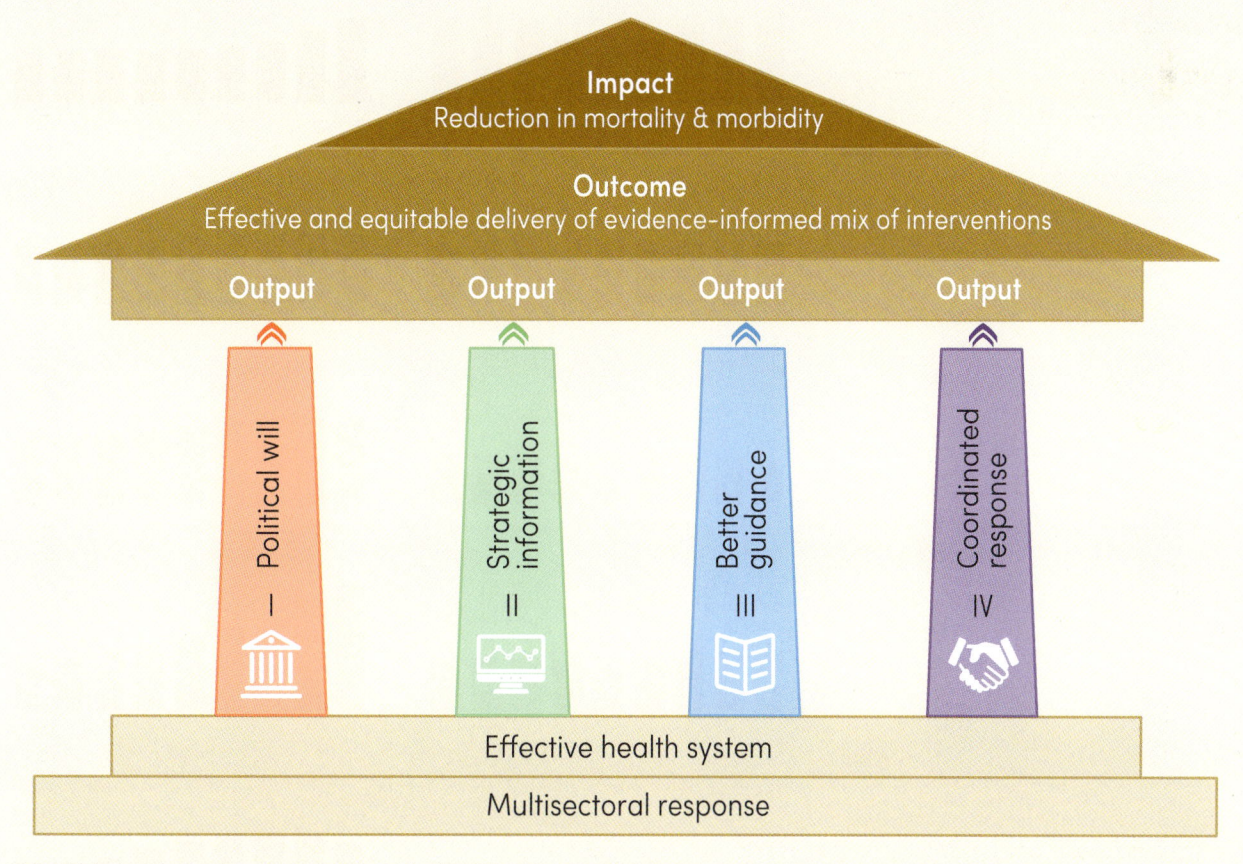

GMP: Global Malaria Programme; GTS: *Global technical strategy for malaria 2016–2030*; HBHI: high burden to high impact; RBM: Roll Back Malaria; WHO: World Health Organization.

# 4 High burden to high impact approach

## 4.2 BURDEN OF MALARIA CASES AND DEATHS

There were about 155 million estimated malaria cases in the 11 HBHI countries in 2018, compared with 177 million in 2010. The Democratic Republic of the Congo and Nigeria accounted for 84 million (54%) of total cases (**Fig. 4.2a**). Malaria deaths reduced from about 400 000 in 2010 to about 260 000 in 2018 (**Fig. 4.2a**).

**FIG. 4.2a.**

**Estimated malaria cases and deaths, 2010–2018** Countries are presented from highest to lowest number of estimated malaria cases in 2018. The estimated number of deaths for each country is shown in the right-hand column. *Source: WHO estimates.*

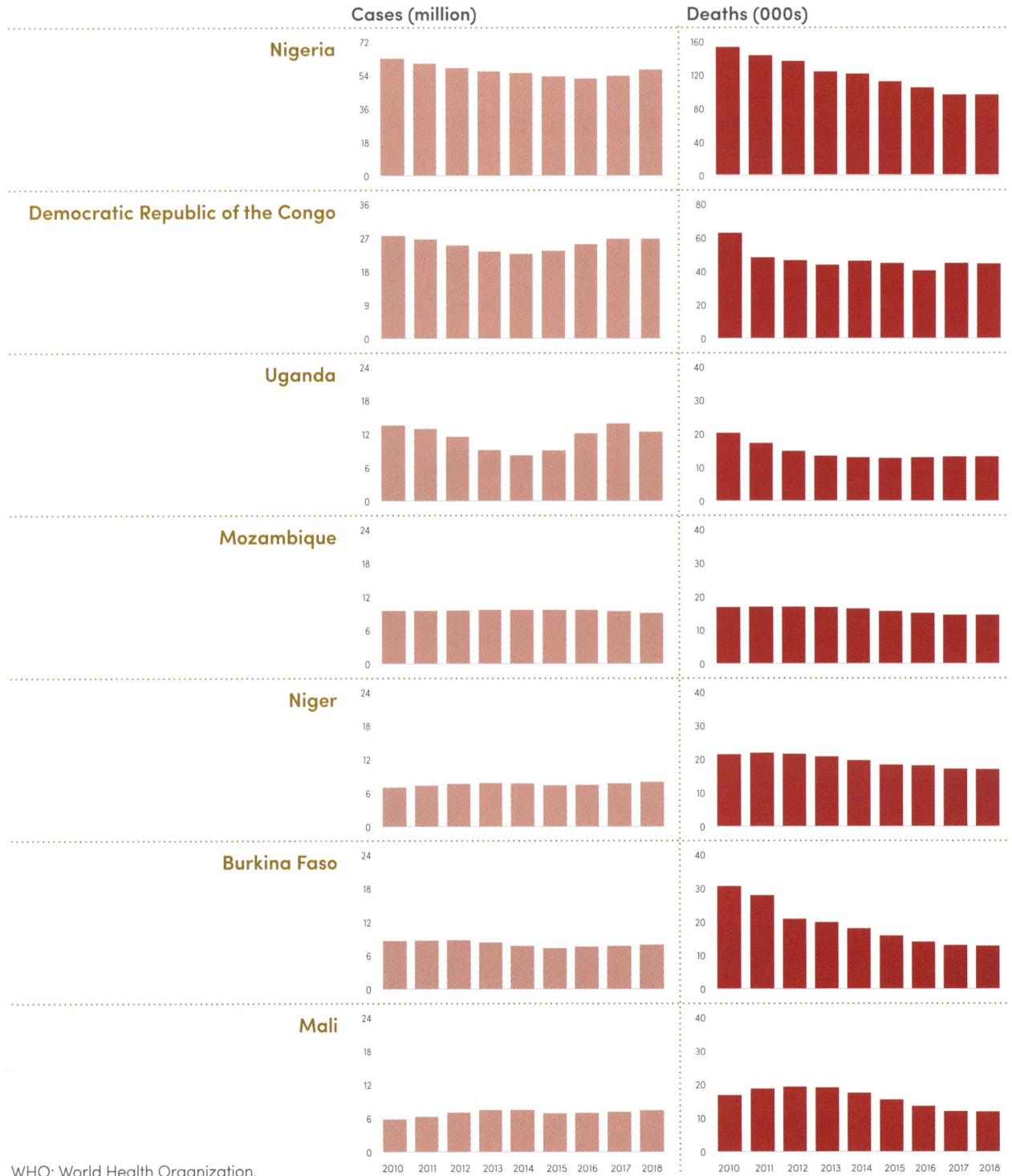

WHO: World Health Organization.

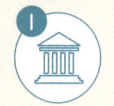

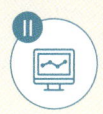

In India, only seven out of 36 states accounted for 90% of the estimated cases in 2018. In these seven states, there were large reductions in malaria cases in 2018 compared with 2010, from a total of 14.3 million cases to 5.7 million cases (**Fig. 4.2b**). For most other countries, however, the rates of reductions were generally slower in the past 3 years than in preceding years.

WHO: World Health Organization.

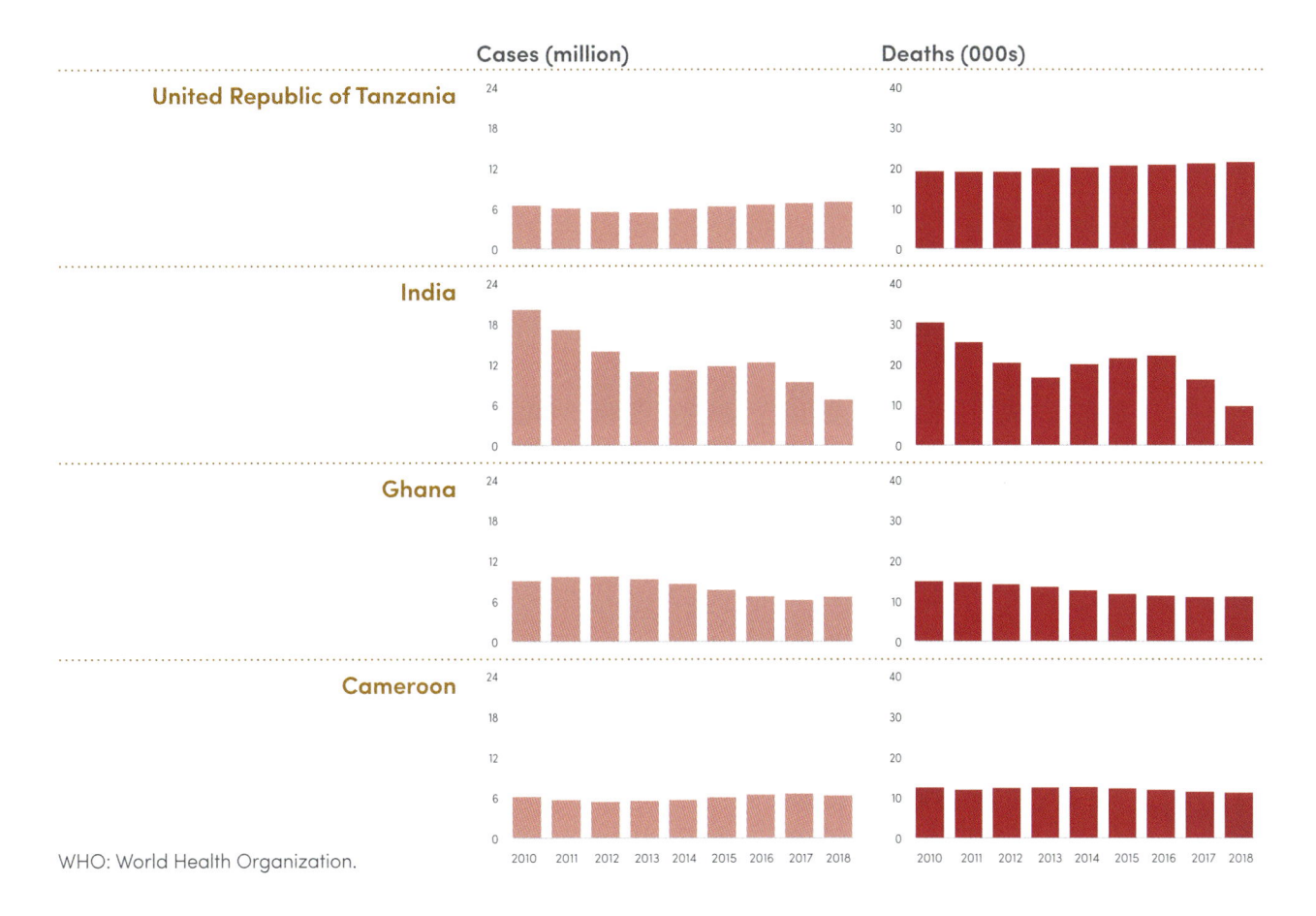

**FIG. 4.2b.**

**Estimated malaria cases in India, showing seven states that contributed a combined 90% of cases, 2010 versus 2018** *Source: WHO estimates.*

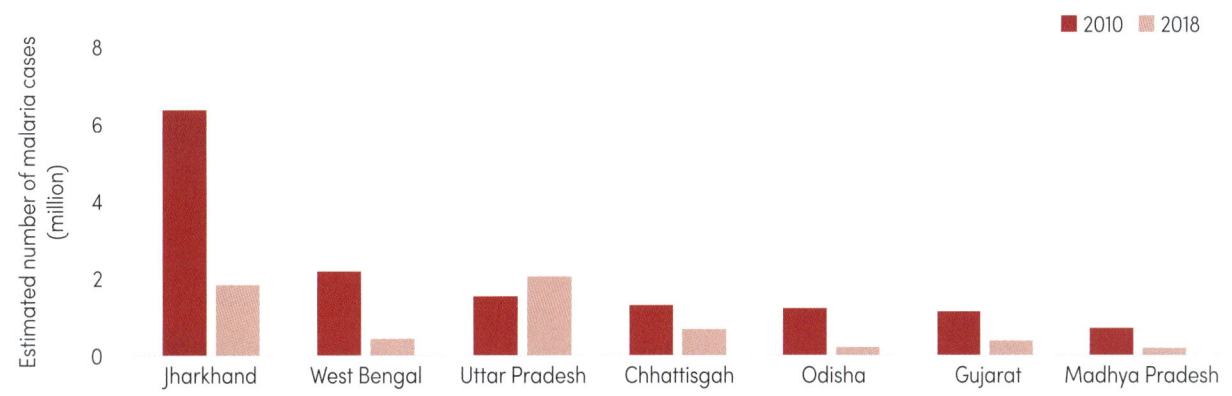

WHO: World Health Organization.

## 4 High burden to high impact approach

### 4.3 MALARIA PREVENTION

In the period 2016–2018, about 295 million long-lasting insecticidal nets (LLINs) were distributed in 11 HBHI countries, of which 116 million (39%) were distributed to communities in the Democratic Republic of the Congo and Nigeria (**Fig. 4.3a**). By 2018, access to LLINs was between 40% and 60% in Burkina Faso, Cameroon, Mozambique, Niger, Nigeria and the United Republic of Tanzania; between 60% and 70% in Mali; and between 70% and 80% in the Democratic Republic of the Congo, Ghana and Uganda (**Fig. 4.3b**). The percentage of the population sleeping under LLINs was highest in Uganda and lowest in Nigeria (**Fig. 4.3c**). The percentage of children sleeping under LLINs was about 50% in Burkina Faso and Nigeria, but above 70% in the

**FIG. 4.3.**
**Distribution and coverage of preventive interventions** *Source: NMP reports and WHO estimates.*

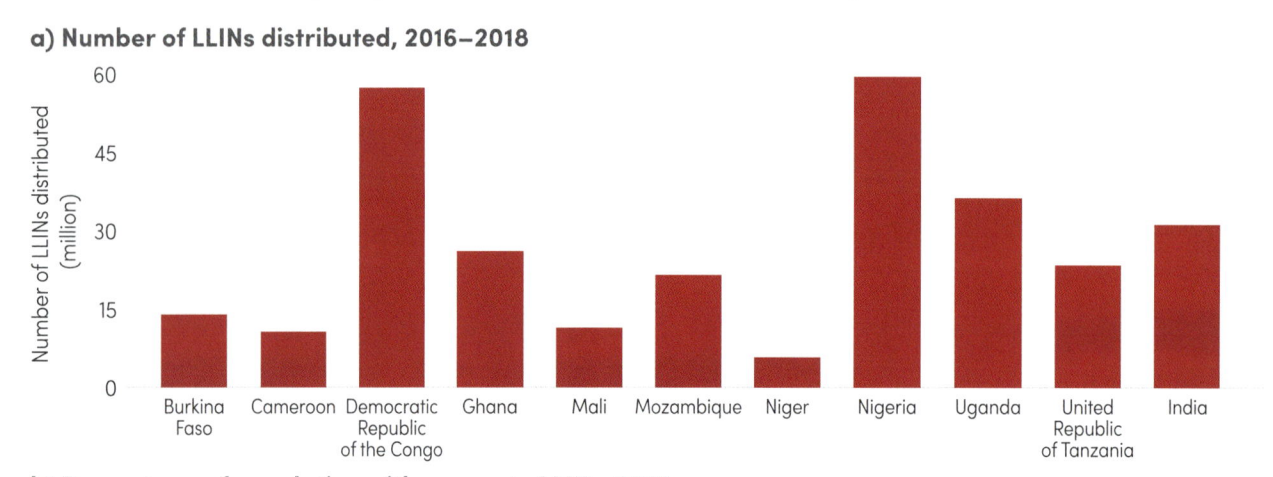

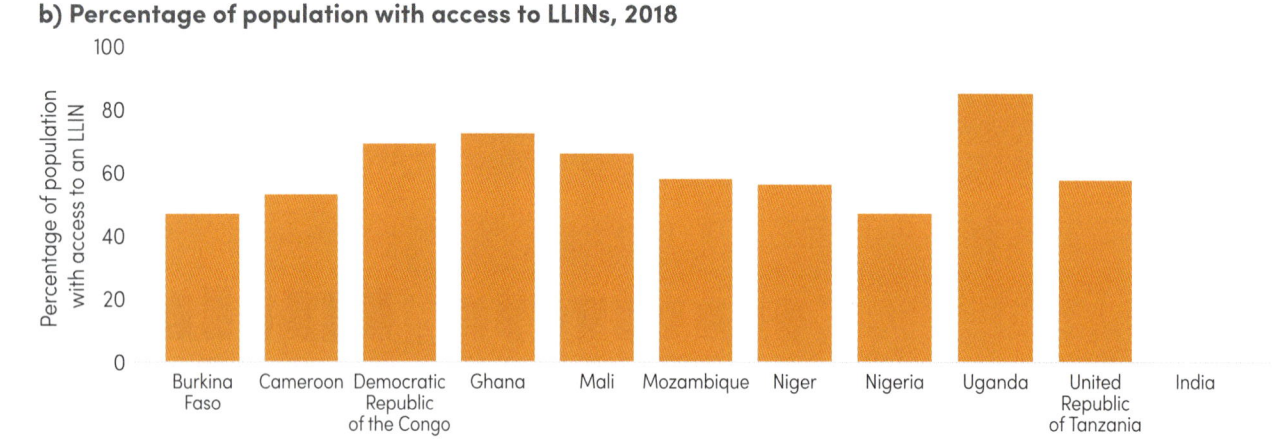

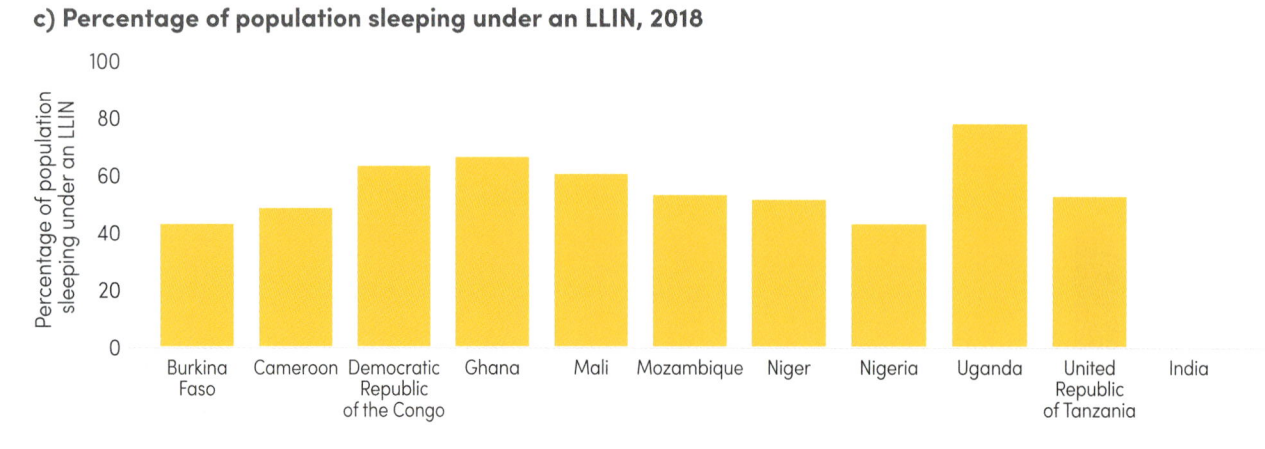

a) Number of LLINs distributed, 2016–2018

b) Percentage of population with access to LLINs, 2018

c) Percentage of population sleeping under an LLIN, 2018

LLIN: long-lasting insecticidal net; NMP: national malaria programme; WHO: World Health Organization

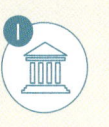

Democratic Republic of Congo, Ghana and Uganda (**Fig. 4.4d**). LLIN use by pregnant women was almost exactly the same as that of children aged under 5 years. Coverage of the recommended three doses of SP for IPTp (IPTp3) was low to moderate, with only Burkina Faso and the United Republic of Tanzania estimated as having more than half of pregnant women receiving IPTp3 in 2018. In Cameroon, Nigeria and Uganda, the estimated coverage was about 30% or less (**Fig. 4.3e**). Of the 10 HBHI countries in Africa, six countries within the sub-Sahelian ecological zone implemented SMC; by 2018, a mean total of 17 million children, out of the 26 million targeted, were treated per SMC cycle. The gap in treatment was greatest in Ghana and Nigeria (**Fig. 4.3f**).

**d) Percentage of children sleeping under an LLIN, 2018**

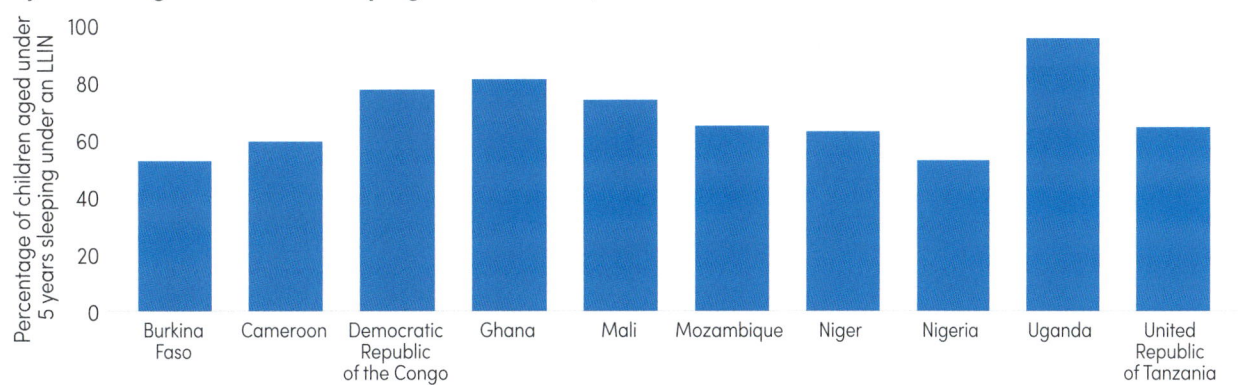

**e) Percentage of pregnant women who received IPTp3, 2018**

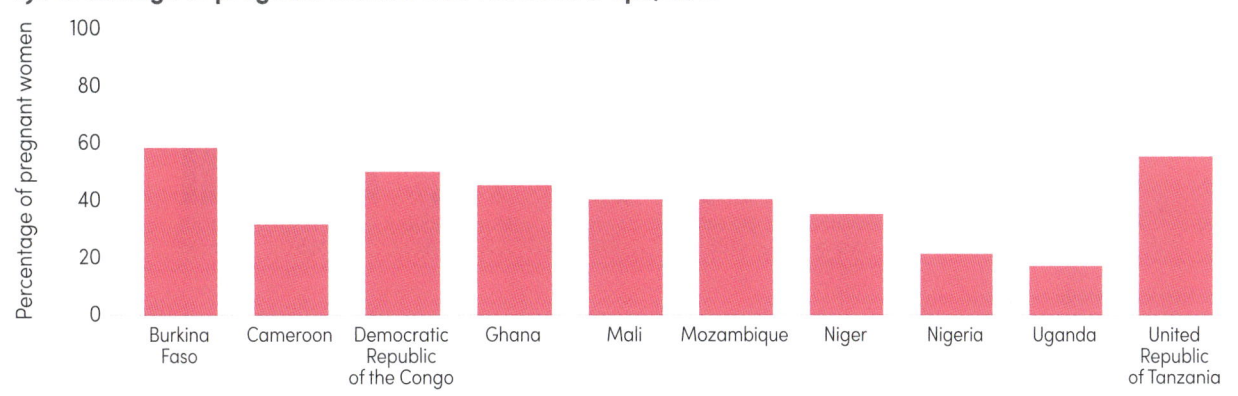

**f) SMC targeted children and mean treatments per cycle, 2018**

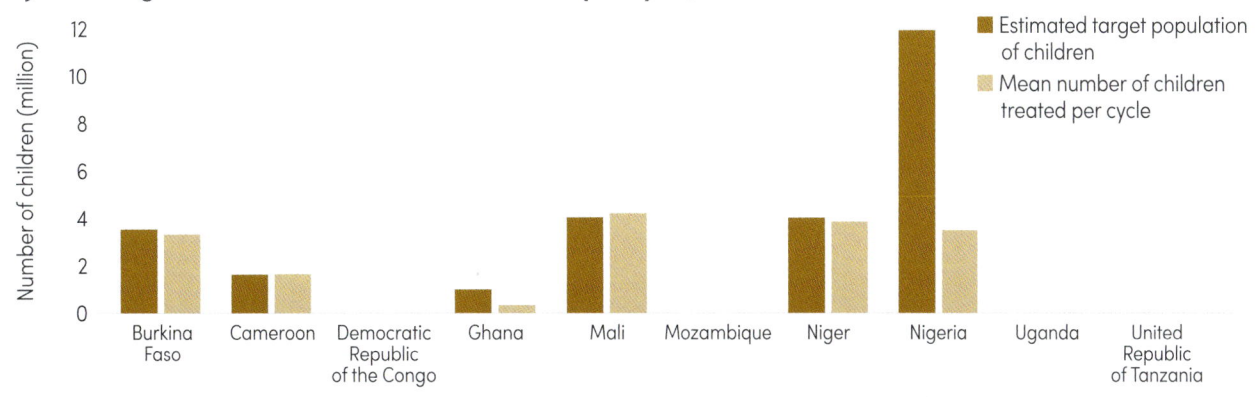

HBHI: high burden to high impact; IPTp3: third dose of intermittent preventive treatment in pregnancy; LLIN: long-lasting insecticidal net; SMC: seasonal malaria chemoprevention.
Note: population level coverage of malaria interventions not shown for India due to lack of household surveys. Out of 11 HBHI countries, only Burkina Faso, Cameroon, Ghana, Mali, Niger and Nigeria have areas eligible for SMC.

# 4 High burden to high impact approach

## 4.4 MALARIA DIAGNOSIS AND TREATMENT

The percentage of children aged under 5 years with fever (in the 2 weeks preceding the survey) varied by country, from 16% in Cameroon to 41% in Nigeria (**Fig. 4.4a**). Among these children, the proportion seeking treatment ranged from 58% in Mali to 82% in Uganda. Only in Burkina Faso and Mozambique were more than 50% of these children treated in the public health sector; in other countries, 37% or less of these children were treated in this sector. The use of the private sector was highest in Nigeria and Uganda (48%), and lowest in Burkina Faso and Mozambique (<4%) (**Fig. 4.4a**). Worryingly, a considerable number of children were not brought for care, and in the Democratic Republic of the Congo and Mali, this figure was more than 40%. Among children who were brought for care, the percentage who were tested for malaria was about 30% or less in Cameroon, the Democratic Republic of the Congo, Mali, Niger and Nigeria; and about 50% or more in Burkina Faso, Ghana, Mozambique, Uganda and the United Republic of Tanzania (**Fig. 4.4b**).

**FIG. 4.4.**

**Diagnosis and treatment of febrile children in HBHI African countries, (a) Treatment seeking for fevers in children aged under 5 years, and source of treatment by health sector, (b) Percentage of children aged under 5 years with fever who sought treatment and were diagnosed using a parasitological test** *Source: Household surveys.*

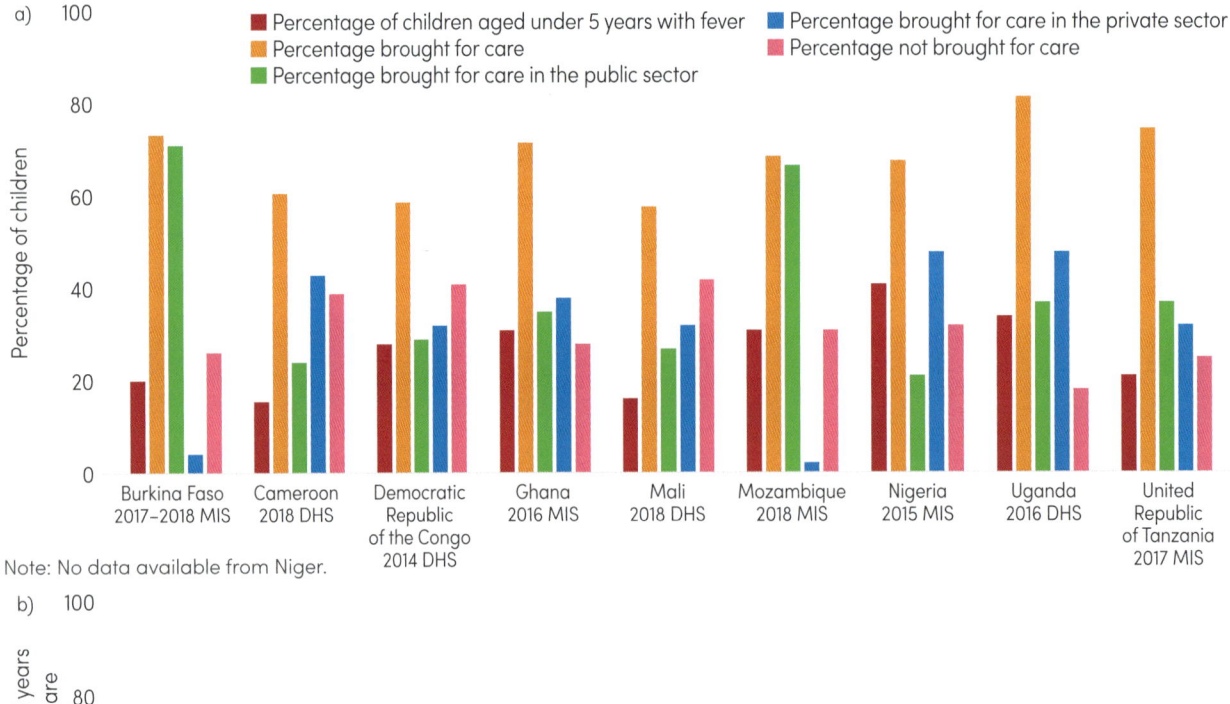

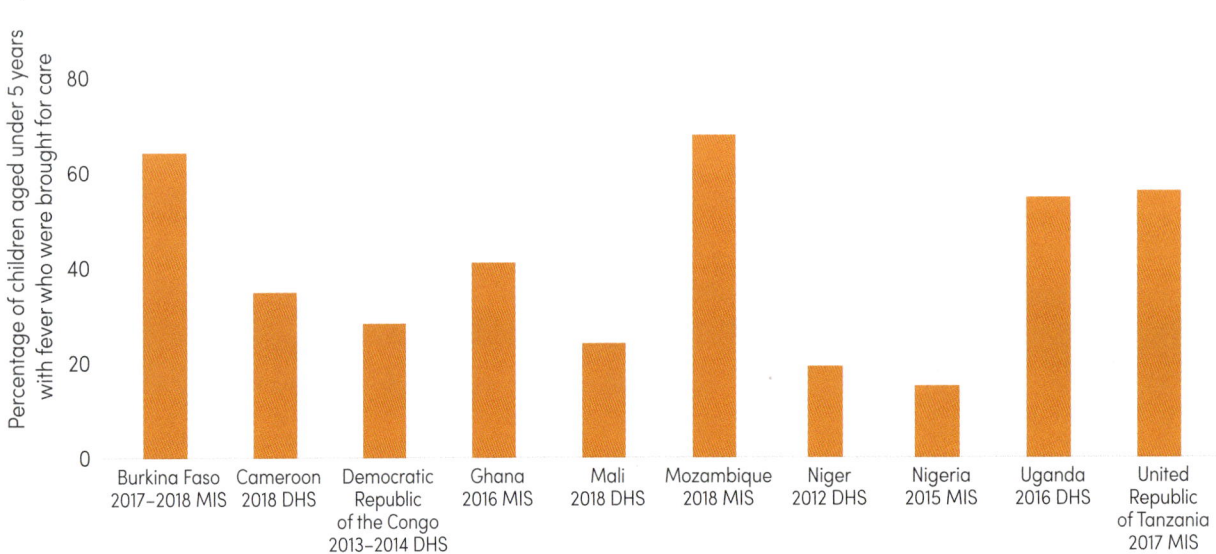

DHS: demographic and health surveys; HBHI: high burden to high impact; MIS: malaria indicator surveys.
Note: Data not available for the Democratic Republic of the Congo and Niger.

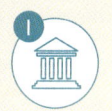

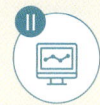

## 4.5 MALARIA FUNDING

An estimated US$ 9.4 billion in funding was directed at the 11 HBHI countries in the period 2010–2018. Of this, US$ 7.7 billion (82%) came from international sources. This funding represents direct budgetary investment in malaria control, but excludes the cost of health workers' time spent on treating patients. Over the 2010–2018 period, the Democratic Republic of the Congo and Nigeria received the largest amount of international funding (**Fig. 4.5a** and **Fig. 4.5b**). In the past 3 years (2016–2018), about US$ 3.5 billion of direct malaria funding was reported in the 11 HBHI countries, with about 31% of this funding being in the Democratic Republic of the Congo and Nigeria (**Fig. 4.5b**). Except for India, direct domestic investment remains very low in the HBHI countries.

### FIG. 4.5.

**Total international and domestic direct funding for malaria in the 11 HBHI countries, (a) 2010–2018 and (b) 2016–2018** Sources: ForeignAssistance.gov, United Kingdom Department for International Development, Global Fund, NMP reports, OECD creditor reporting system database, World Bank Data Bank and WHO estimates.

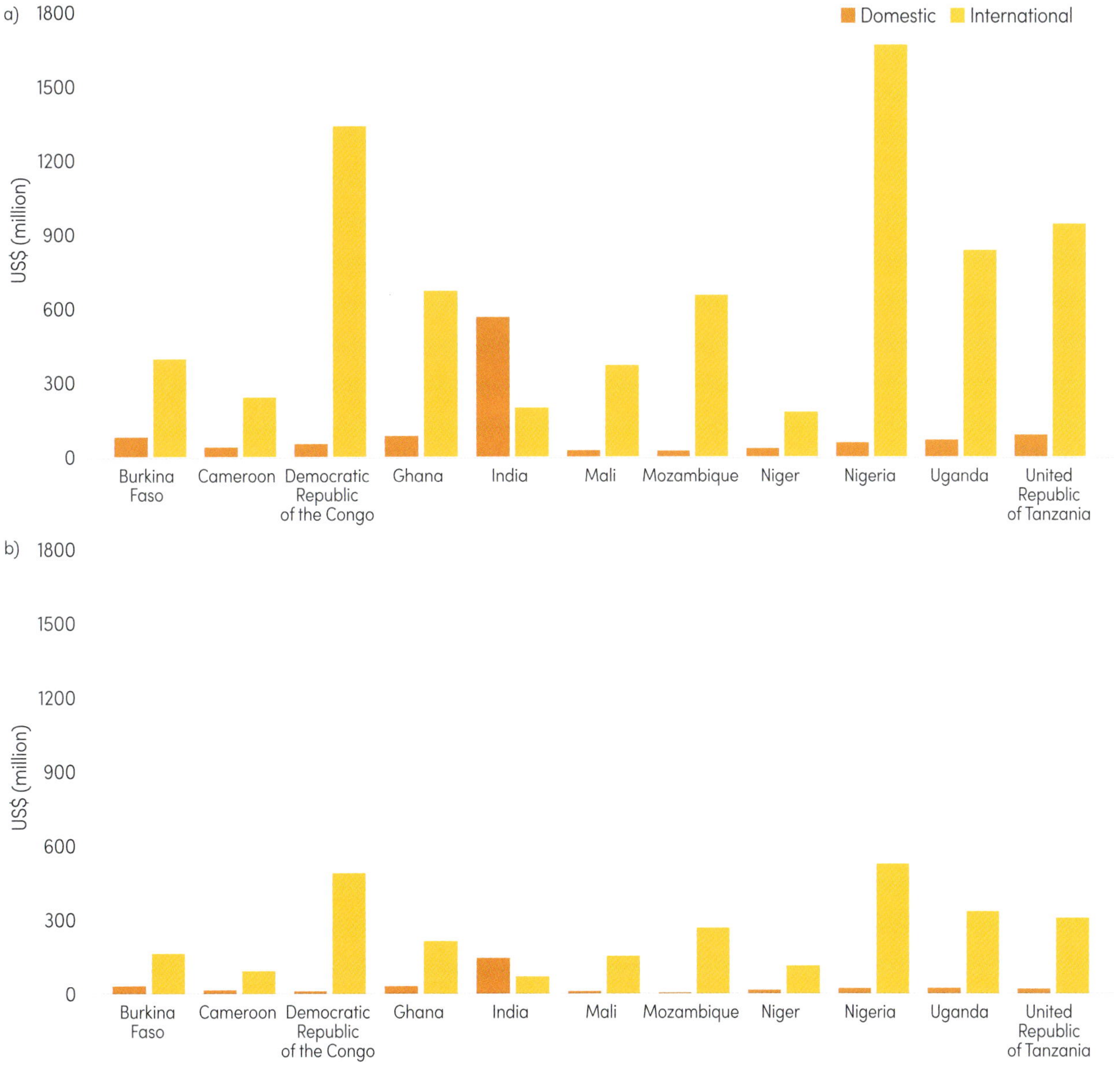

Global Fund: Global Fund to Fight AIDS, Tuberculosis and Malaria; NMP: national malaria programme; OECD: Organisation for Economic Co-operation and Development; WHO: World Health Organization.

# 5. Malaria elimination and prevention of re-establishment

An increasing number of countries are progressing towards elimination of malaria. Globally, the number of countries that were malaria endemic in 2000 and that reported fewer than 10 000 malaria cases increased from 40 in 2010 to 49 in 2018; in the same period, the number of countries with fewer than 100 indigenous cases increased from 17 to 27. Between 2017 and 2018, the number of countries with fewer than 10 indigenous cases increased from 19 to 24 (**Fig. 5.1**).

The GTS milestone for 2020 is to eliminate malaria from at least 10 countries that were malaria endemic in 2015 (*1*). Between 2000 and 2018, 19 countries attained zero indigenous cases for 3 years or more (**Table 5.1**); four countries that were malaria endemic in 2015 have since eliminated malaria. In 2018, no malaria endemic country reached zero indigenous malaria cases for the third consecutive year. However, several countries recorded zero indigenous cases for the first time in 2018, or for a second consecutive year (**Section 5.1**).

Certification of elimination by WHO is the official recognition of a country being free from indigenous malaria cases; this is based on an independent evaluation verifying the interruption of transmission and the country's ability to prevent re-establishment of transmission. Paraguay and Uzbekistan were awarded WHO certification of elimination in 2018, with Algeria and Argentina achieving certification in early 2019.

## 5.1 E-2020 INITIATIVE

In April 2016, WHO published an assessment of the likelihood of countries achieving malaria elimination by 2020. This assessment was based on the countries' trends in the number of indigenous malaria cases, their declared malaria elimination objectives and the informed opinions of WHO experts in the field (*28*). Twenty-one countries, across five WHO regions, were identified as being the most likely to reach zero indigenous cases by 2020. These countries were termed as the "eliminating countries for 2020" (E-2020), and they are the special focus of WHO efforts to accelerate national elimination efforts and monitor progress towards malaria free status (**Fig. 5.2**). An inaugural meeting of the national malaria programmes (NMPs) for the E-2020 countries, referred to as the Global Forum of Malaria-Eliminating Countries (Global Forum), was organized by WHO in March 2017 in Geneva, Switzerland; the Global Forum was held again in June 2018 in San José, Costa Rica, and in June 2019 in Wuxi, China.

In April 2018, WHO established the Malaria Elimination Oversight Committee (MEOC) to help countries to reach their elimination goals. The MEOC attended the 2018 and 2019 Global Forums and, in February 2019, met with a small group of countries on track to reach malaria elimination by 2020, to support those countries in their attempts to achieve malaria elimination. The MEOC has produced a series of recommendations to help countries accelerate towards this goal.

## TABLE 5.1.

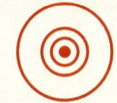

**Countries eliminating malaria since 2000** Countries are shown by the year that they attained 3 consecutive years of zero indigenous cases; countries that have been certified as free from malaria are shown in green (with the year of certification in parentheses). *Source: Country reports and WHO.*

|  | | | | |
|---|---|---|---|---|
| 2000 | Egypt | United Arab Emirates (2007) | | |
| 2001 | | | | |
| 2002 | | | | |
| 2003 | | | | |
| 2004 | Kazakhstan | | | |
| 2005 | | | | |
| 2006 | | | | |
| 2007 | Morocco (2010) | Syrian Arab Republic | Turkmenistan (2010) | |
| 2008 | Armenia (2011) | | | |
| 2009 | | | | |
| 2010 | | | | |
| 2011 | Iraq | | | |
| 2012 | Georgia | Turkey | | |
| 2013 | Argentina (2019) | Kyrgyzstan (2016) | Oman | Uzbekistan (2018) |
| 2014 | Paraguay (2018) | | | |
| 2015 | Azerbaijan | Sri Lanka (2016) | | |
| 2016 | Algeria (2019) | | | |
| 2017 | Tajikistan | | | |
| 2018 | | | | |

WHO: World Health Organization.

## FIG. 5.1.

**Number of countries that were malaria endemic in 2000, with fewer than 10, 100, 1000 and 10 000 indigenous malaria cases between 2010 and 2018** Sources: NMP reports and WHO estimates.

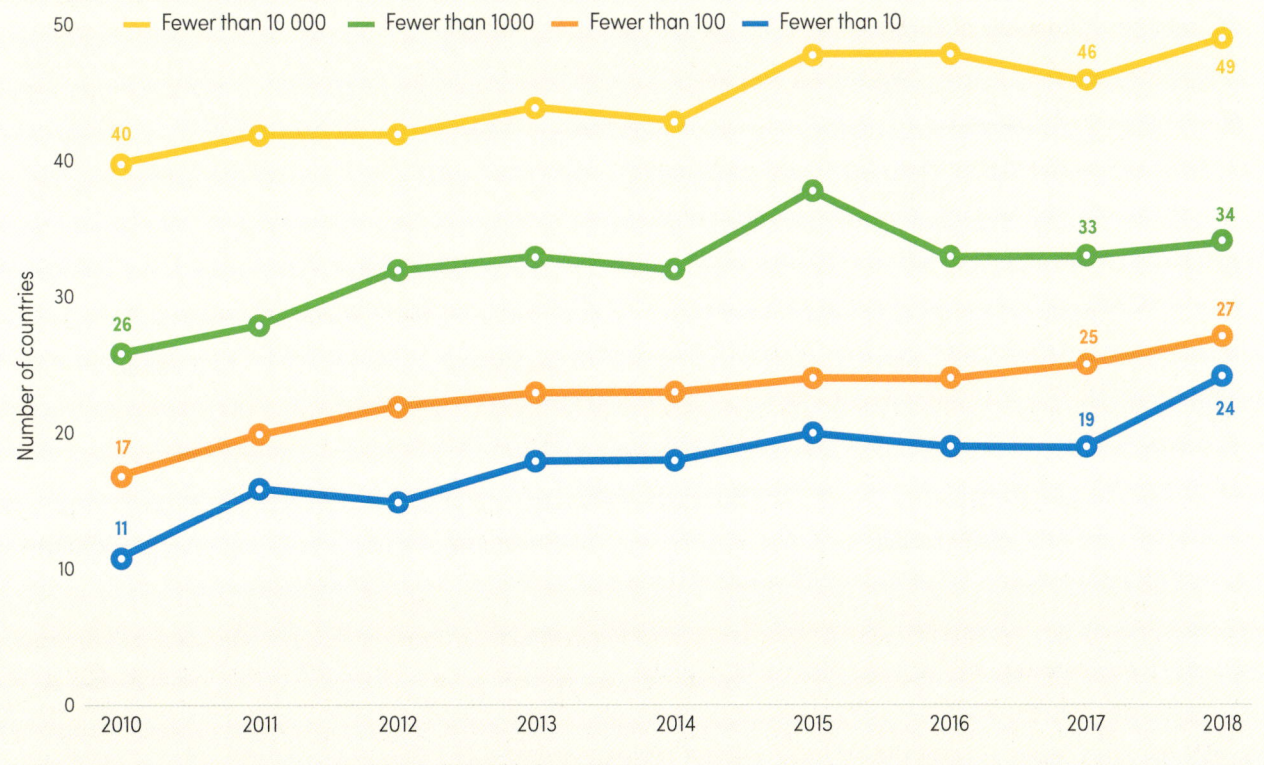

NMP: national malaria programme; WHO: World Health Organization.

In 2018, several countries reported significant progress towards elimination (**Fig. 5.2**). For the first time, Iran (Islamic Republic of), Malaysia and Timor-Leste reported zero indigenous cases, while China and El Salvador reported their second year of zero indigenous cases. Cabo Verde, Eswatini, Saudi Arabia and South Africa reported large reductions in the number of cases in 2018 compared with 2017. Comoros and Costa Rica, however, reported large increases in the number of cases.

## 5.2 GREATER MEKONG SUBREGION

The six countries of the Greater Mekong subregion (GMS) – Cambodia, China (Yunnan Province), Lao People's Democratic Republic, Myanmar, Thailand and Viet Nam – continue to make significant gains as

### FIG. 5.2.

**Trends in indigenous malaria cases in E-2020 countries, 2010–2018** Countries are presented from highest to lowest number of indigenous malaria cases at baseline year, 2010; the graphs show the number of indigenous malaria cases from 2010 to 2018. Years with zero indigenous malaria cases are represented by green dots. *Source: NMP reports.*

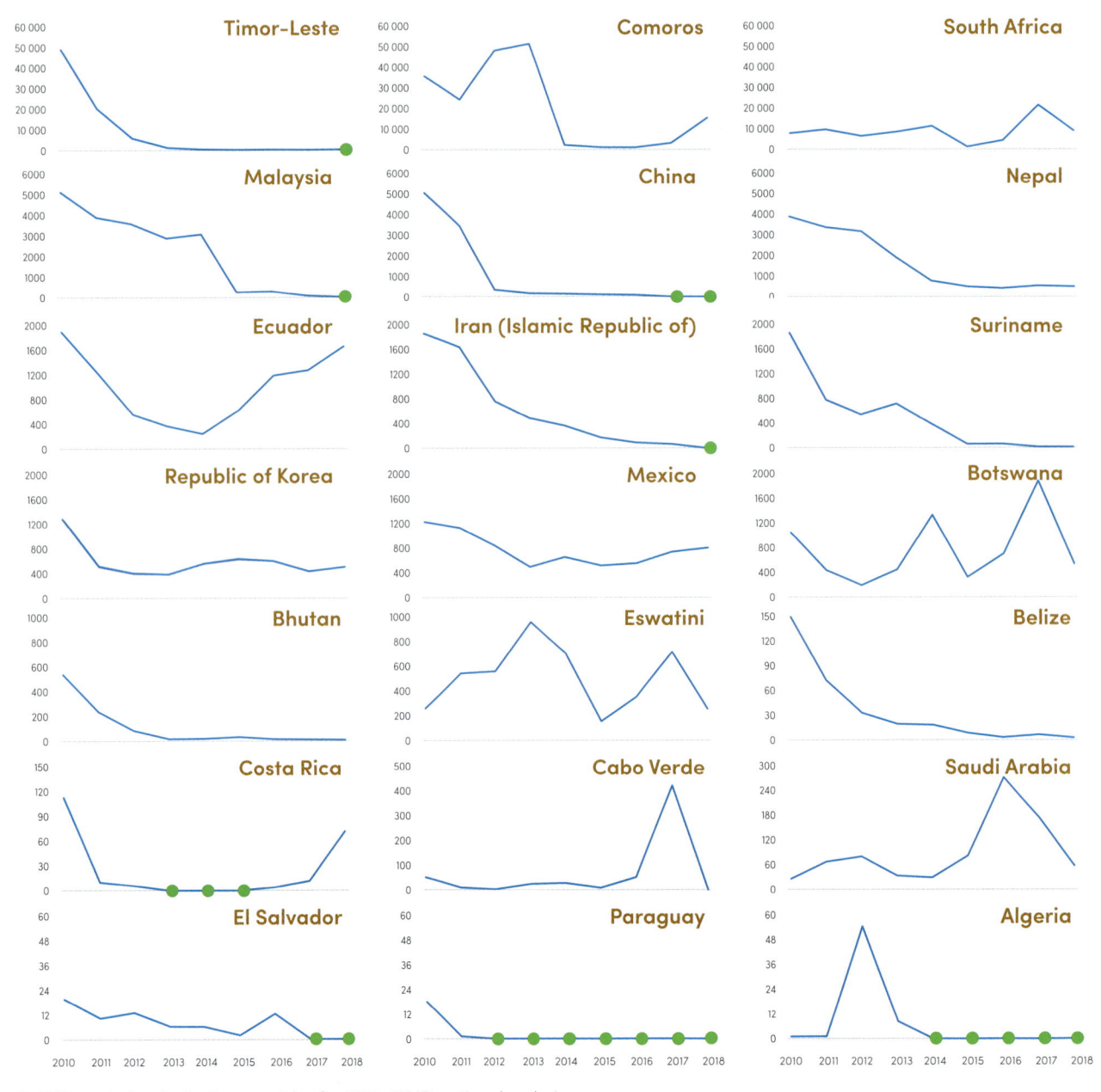

E-2020: malaria-eliminating countries for 2020; NMP: national malaria programme.

Note: Cases for Botswana, Nepal and Timor-Leste are derived from adjusting reported data for reporting and testing rates, and treatment seeking in different health sectors.

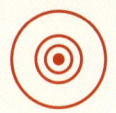

they aim for malaria elimination by 2030. Between 2010 and 2018, the reported number of malaria cases fell by 76% (**Fig. 5.3**); over the same period, malaria deaths fell by 95%. The GMS has reported a steep decline in *P. falciparum* cases: a decrease of 48% since 2010, and an 80% reduction in 2018 from the peak of 390 000 cases in 2012. This accelerated decrease in *P. falciparum* is especially critical because of drug resistance: in the GMS, *P. falciparum* parasites have developed partial resistance to artemisinin – the core compound of the best available antimalarial drugs.

In 2018, Cambodia reported no malaria-related deaths for the first time in the country's history. China also reported its second consecutive year of zero indigenous cases. Meanwhile, Thailand is nearing *P. falciparum* elimination, with a 38% decrease in *P. falciparum* cases between 2017 and 2018.

**FIG. 5.3.**

*P. falciparum* **cases in the GMS, 2010–2018** Source: NMP reports.

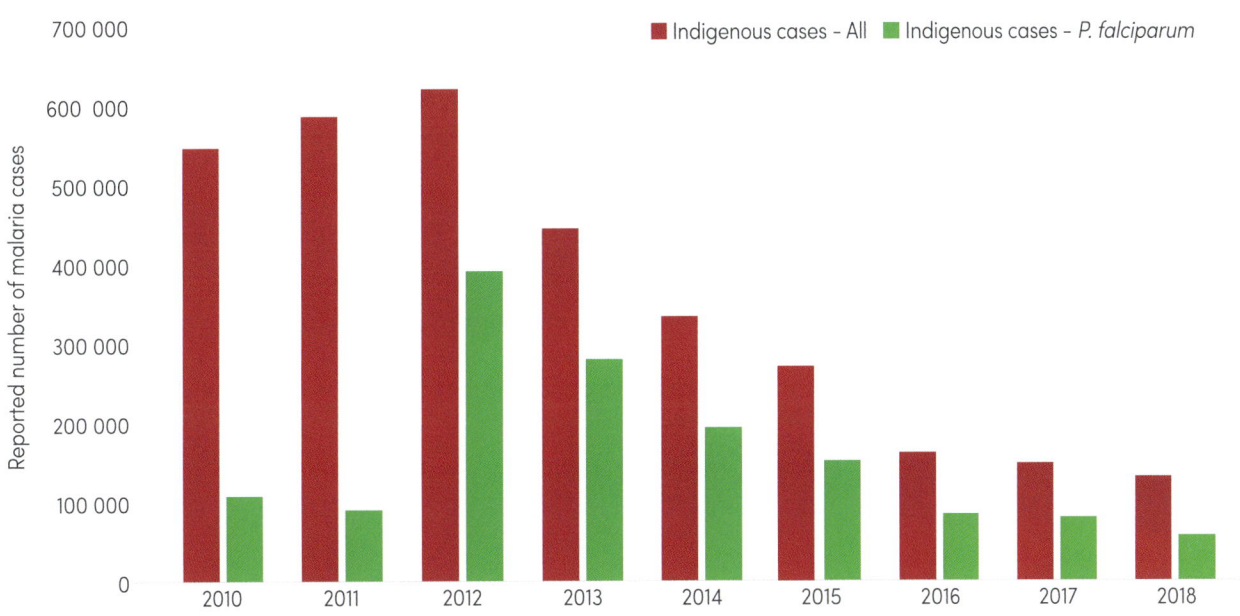

GMS: Greater Mekong subregion; NMP: national malaria programme; *P. falciparum*: *Plasmodium falciparum*.

**FIG. 5.4.**

**Regional map of malaria incidence in the GMS by area, 2018** Source: NMP reports.

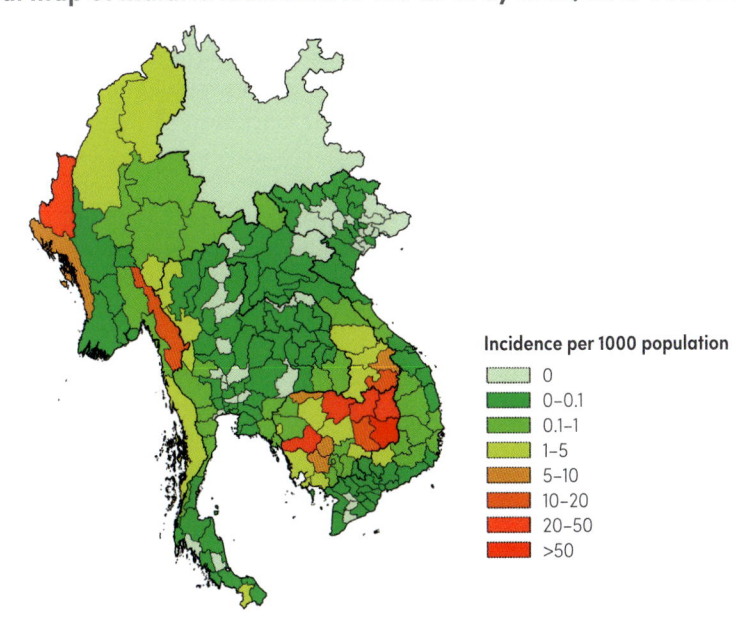

GMS: Greater Mekong subregion; NMP: national malaria programme.

# 6 Investments in malaria programmes and research

For 2020, the GTS milestones are a global reduction of at least 40% in malaria case incidence and mortality rates compared with 2015, elimination in at least 10 countries and prevention of re-establishment in all malaria free countries (*1*). Estimates of the funding required to achieve these milestones have been set out in the GTS. Total annual resources needed were estimated at US$ 4.1 billion in 2016, rising to US$ 6.8 billion in 2020. An additional US$ 0.72 billion is estimated to be required annually for global malaria research and development (*1*).

This section presents the most up-to-date funding trends for malaria control and elimination, by source and channel of funding for the period 2010–2018, both globally and for major country groupings. It then presents investments in malaria-related research and development (R&D) for the same period.

A large proportion of the investment in malaria is spent on scaling up malaria prevention, diagnosis and treatment. This section presents trends in the sales and in-country distribution of insecticide-treated mosquito nets (ITNs), artemisinin-based combination therapies (ACTs) and RDTs.

## 6.1 FUNDING FOR MALARIA CONTROL AND ELIMINATION

For the 91 countries analysed in this section, total funding for malaria control and elimination was estimated at US$ 2.7 billion in 2018, compared with US$ 3.2 billion in 2017. The amount invested in 2018 falls short of the US$ 5.0 billion estimated to be required globally to stay on track towards the GTS milestones (*1*). Moreover, the funding gap between the amount invested and the resources needed widened from US$ 1.3 billion in 2017 to US$ 2.3 billion in 2018.

Over the period 2010–2018, nearly 70% of the total funding for malaria control and elimination was provided by international sources (**Fig. 6.1**). However, the aggregated figures hide substantial variations in the relative share of funding from domestic and international sources across country groups, as noted later in this section.

Of the US$ 2.7 billion invested in 2018, US$ 1.8 billion came from international funders. The government of the United States of America (USA) contributed a total of US$ 1.0 billion through planned bilateral funding and contributions to multilateral funding agencies, followed by bilateral and multilateral disbursements from the United Kingdom of Great Britain and Northern Ireland (United Kingdom) of US$ 0.2 billion; France, Japan and Germany with contributions of about US$ 0.1 billion each; and other country members of the Development Assistance Committee and private sector contributors of about US$ 0.3 billion combined (**Fig. 6.2**).

Governments of malaria endemic countries continued to contribute about 30% of the total funding (**Fig. 6.1**), with investments reaching US$ 0.9 billion in 2018 (**Fig. 6.2**). Of this amount, US$ 0.6 billion was invested in malaria control activities, and US$ 0.3 billion was estimated to have been spent on malaria case management in the public sector.

**FIG. 6.1.**

**Funding for malaria control and elimination over the period 2010–2018 (% of total funding), by source of funds (constant 2018 US$)** *Sources: ForeignAssistance.gov, United Kingdom Department for International Development, Global Fund, NMP reports, OECD creditor reporting system database, the World Bank Data Bank and WHO estimates.*

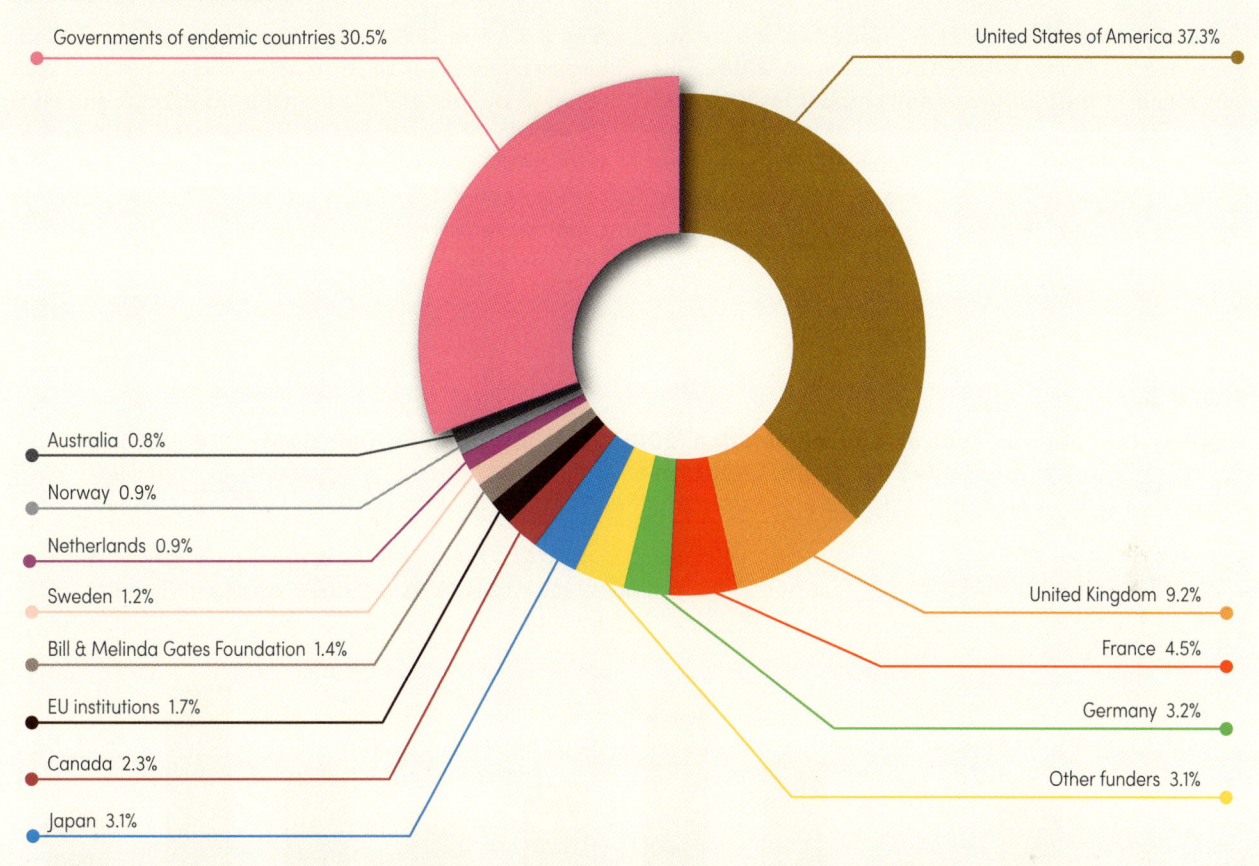

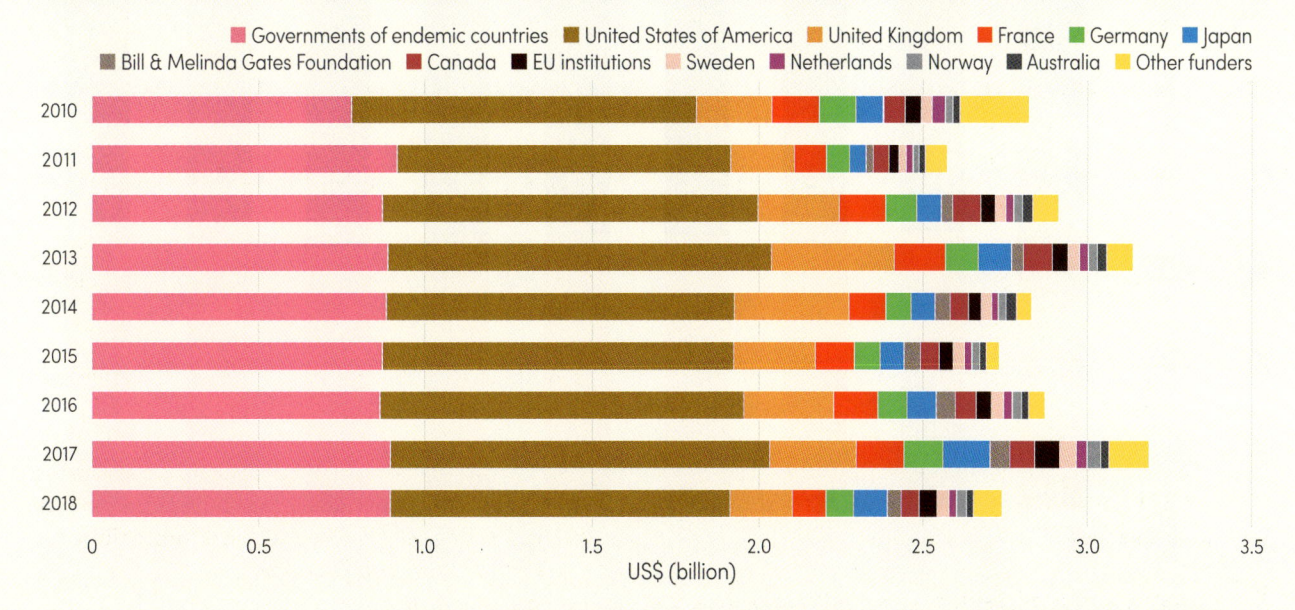

- Governments of endemic countries 30.5%
- United States of America 37.3%
- United Kingdom 9.2%
- France 4.5%
- Germany 3.2%
- Other funders 3.1%
- Japan 3.1%
- Canada 2.3%
- EU institutions 1.7%
- Bill & Melinda Gates Foundation 1.4%
- Sweden 1.2%
- Netherlands 0.9%
- Norway 0.9%
- Australia 0.8%

EU: European Union; Global Fund: Global Fund to Fight AIDS, Tuberculosis and Malaria; NMP: national malaria programme; OECD: Organisation for Economic Co-operation and Development; WHO: World Health Organization.

**FIG. 6.2.**

**Funding for malaria control and elimination 2010–2018, by source of funds (constant 2018 US$)** *Sources: ForeignAssistance.gov, United Kingdom Department for International Development, Global Fund, NMP reports, OECD creditor reporting system database, the World Bank Data Bank and WHO estimates.*

EU: European Union; Global Fund: Global Fund to Fight AIDS, Tuberculosis and Malaria; NMP: national malaria programme; OECD: Organisation for Economic Co-operation and Development; WHO: World Health Organization.

# 6 Investments in malaria programmes and research

Of the US$ 2.7 billion invested in 2018, nearly US$ 1.0 billion (35%) was channelled through the Global Fund to Fight AIDS, Tuberculosis and Malaria (Global Fund) (**Fig. 6.3**). Compared with 2017, the Global Fund's disbursements to malaria endemic countries decreased by about US$ 0.4 billion in 2018. This difference in the disbursement amount in 2018 and 2017 reflects the cyclical distribution of ITNs supported by the Global Fund, and an increase in disbursements in 2017, corresponding to the end of most malaria grants in that year (**Fig. 6.3**).

Planned bilateral funding from the government of the USA amounted to US$ 0.8 billion in 2018, which was slightly lower than in 2017, although above the levels of all other annual planned contributions since 2010 (**Fig. 6.3**). The United Kingdom remains the second-largest bilateral funder, with about US$ 0.1 billion in 2018, followed by contributions from the World Bank and other Development Assistance Committee members (**Fig. 6.3**). With US$ 0.9 billion invested in 2018, the total contribution from governments of malaria endemic countries remained the same as in 2017.

**FIG. 6.3.**
**Funding for malaria control and elimination 2010–2018, by channel (constant 2018 US$)** *Sources: ForeignAssistance.gov, United Kingdom Department for International Development, Global Fund, NMP reports, OECD creditor reporting system database, the World Bank Data Bank and WHO estimates.*

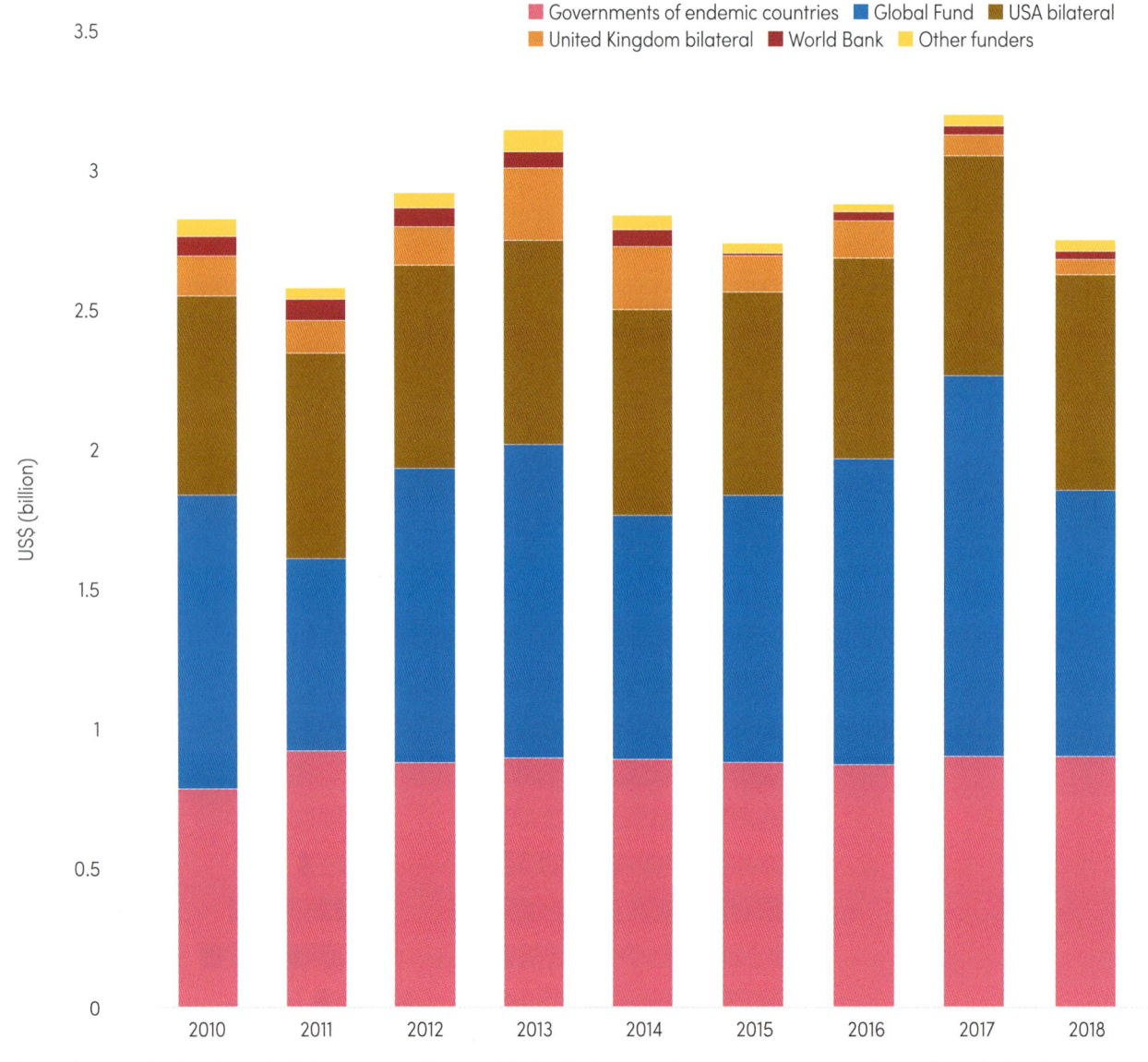

Global Fund: Global Fund to Fight AIDS, Tuberculosis and Malaria; NMP: national malaria programme; OECD: Organisation for Economic Co-operation and Development; USA: United States of America; WHO: World Health Organization.

**Fig. 6.4** shows the substantial variation across country income groups in the share of funding from domestic and international sources. The 29 low-income countries accounted for 47% of total funding for malaria in 2018 (and >90% of global malaria cases and deaths, respectively) with 85% of their funding coming from international sources. International funding also dominated in the group of 36 lower-middle-income countries (43% of total funding in 2018), accounting for 61% of the amount invested in these countries. In contrast, in the group of 23 upper-middle-income countries (11% of the total funding in 2018), 5% of their malaria funding came from international sources, and 95% came from domestic public funding.

Of the US$ 2.7 billion invested in 2018, nearly three quarters benefited the WHO African Region, followed by the WHO Region of the Americas (7%), WHO South-East Asia Region (6%), and WHO Eastern Mediterranean Region and WHO Western Pacific Region (5% each) (**Fig. 6.5**). Funding flows for which no geographical information on recipients was available represented 5% of the total funding in 2018 (**Fig. 6.5**).

## FIG. 6.4.

**Funding for malaria control and elimination 2010–2018, by World Bank 2018 income group and source of funding (constant 2018 US$)**[a] *Sources: ForeignAssistance.gov, United Kingdom Department for International Development, Global Fund, NMP reports, OECD creditor reporting system database, the World Bank Data Bank and WHO estimates.*

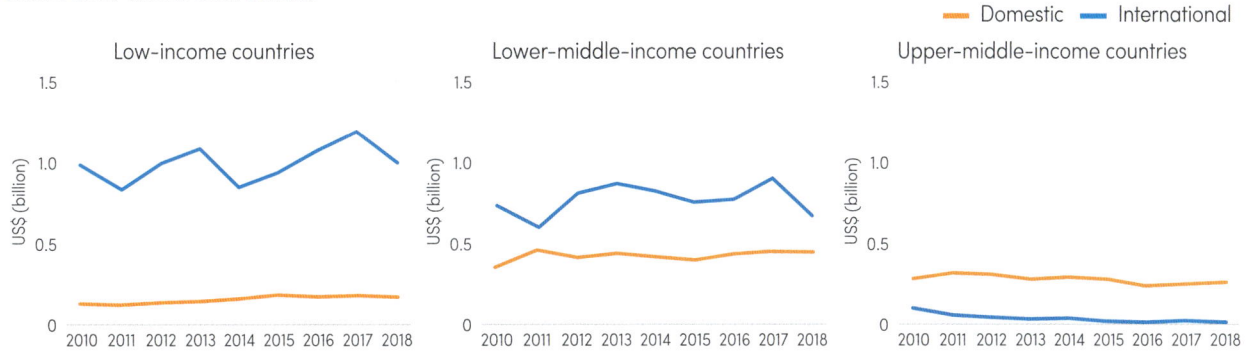

Global Fund: Global Fund to Fight AIDS, Tuberculosis and Malaria; NMP: national malaria programme; OECD: Organisation for Economic Co-operation and Development; WHO: World Health Organization.
[a] Domestic excludes out-of-pocket spending by households.

## FIG. 6.5.

**Funding for malaria control and elimination 2010–2018, by WHO region (constant 2018 US$)**[a] *Sources: ForeignAssistance.gov, United Kingdom Department for International Development, Global Fund, NMP reports, OECD creditor reporting system database, World Bank Data Bank and WHO estimates.*

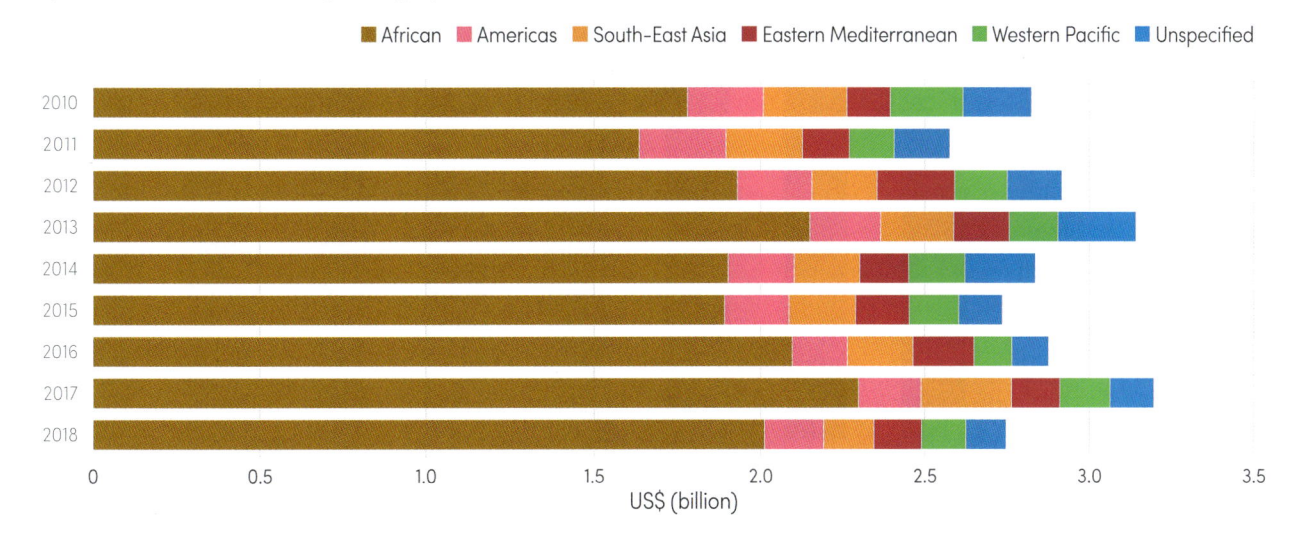

Global Fund: Global Fund to Fight AIDS, Tuberculosis and Malaria; NMP: national malaria programme; OECD: Organisation for Economic Co-operation and Development; WHO: World Health Organization.
[a] "Unspecified" category refers to funding flows, with no information on the geographical localization of their recipients.

# 6 Investments in malaria programmes and research

## 6.2 INVESTMENTS IN MALARIA R&D

Globally, a total funding of US$ 663 million was invested in basic research and product development for malaria in 2018. This was a modest increase from the previous year (an increase of US$ 18 million, or 2.8%), but marked the third consecutive year of increased funding, and the largest annual investment in malaria R&D since its peak of US$ 676 million in 2009.

Funding for drug R&D increased to the highest level ever recorded (from US$ 228 million in 2017 to US$ 252 million in 2018) (**Fig. 6.6**), driven by increased private sector industry investment in several Phase II trials of new chemical entities with the potential for single-exposure radical cure. Funding for basic research also increased (from US$ 143 million in 2017 to US$ 163 million in 2018) (**Fig. 6.6**), as did funding for vector control product R&D (from US$ 35 million in 2017 to US$ 56 million in 2018) (**Fig. 6.6**), although this latter change was due largely to the cyclical funding patterns of the Bill & Melinda Gates Foundation.

Funding for vaccine R&D decreased (from US$ 181 million in 2017 to US$ 156 million in 2018)

### FIG. 6.6.
**Funding for malaria-related R&D 2010–2018, by product type (constant 2018 US$)** *Sources: Policy Cures Research – G-FINDER 2019 report (in preparation).*

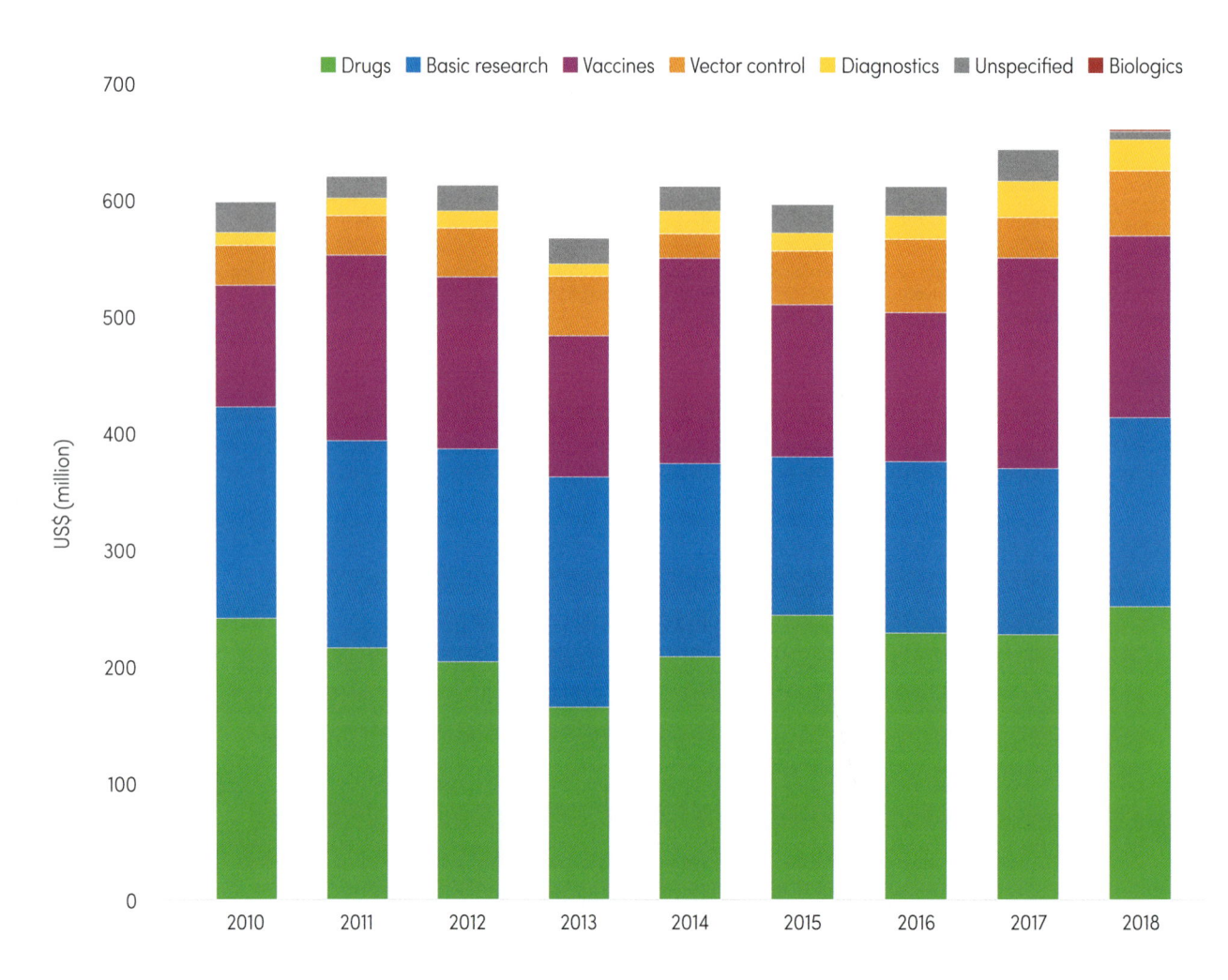

R&D: research and development.

(**Fig. 6.6**), owing to lower investment from private sector industry, which in turn reflects a pipeline that saw no new candidates advance from or enter into late-stage clinical trials, and pilot implementation studies for the vaccine RTS,S not commencing until 2019. Diagnostic R&D was the only other product area to receive lower funding in 2018, falling from US$ 31 million in 2017 to US$ 27 million in 2018 (**Fig. 6.6**).

Just over half (US$ 352 million, or 53%) of all malaria R&D funding in 2018 was for basic and early stage research; a further 27% (US$ 176 million) went to clinical development and post-registration studies. The remaining funding was not allocated to specific products or R&D stages, but mostly consisted of core funding to product development partnerships.

The public sector provided just over half (US$ 353 million, or 53%) of all malaria R&D funding in 2018 (**Fig. 6.7**), which was the same as in each of the previous 8 years. The remaining funding was split evenly between private sector industry (US$ 158 million, or 24%) and the philanthropic sector (US$ 152 million, or 23%) (**Fig. 6.7**). This was a record high investment by private sector industry, and marked the fourth consecutive year that its contribution equalled that of the philanthropic sector.

## FIG. 6.7.

**Malaria R&D funding in 2018, by sector (constant 2018 US$)** *Sources: Policy Cures Research – G-FINDER 2019 report (in preparation).*

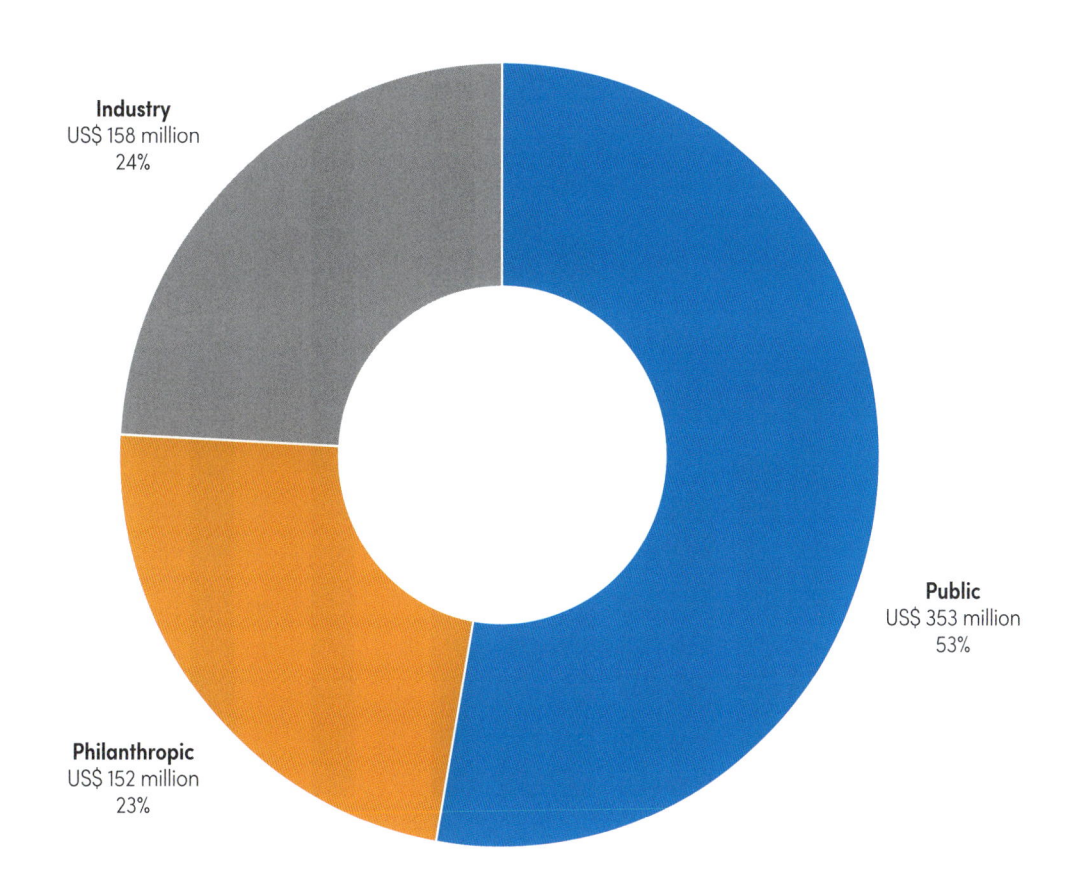

- Industry: US$ 158 million, 24%
- Philanthropic: US$ 152 million, 23%
- Public: US$ 353 million, 53%

R&D: research and development.

# 6 Investments in malaria programmes and research

## 6.3 PROCUREMENT AND DISTRIBUTIONS OF ITNs

The peak year for manufacturer deliveries of ITNs was 2017, when 251 million nets were reported as having been delivered globally. In 2018, about 197 million ITNs were delivered by manufacturers, of which more than 87% were delivered to countries in sub-Saharan Africa. This is fewer than in 2017, when 224 million nets were delivered worldwide (**Fig. 6.8**). Globally, the main channel of delivery was mass campaigns, while routine

**FIG. 6.8.**

**Number of ITNs delivered by manufacturers[a] and distributed[b] by NMPs, 2010–2018** *Sources: Milliner Global Associates and NMP reports.*

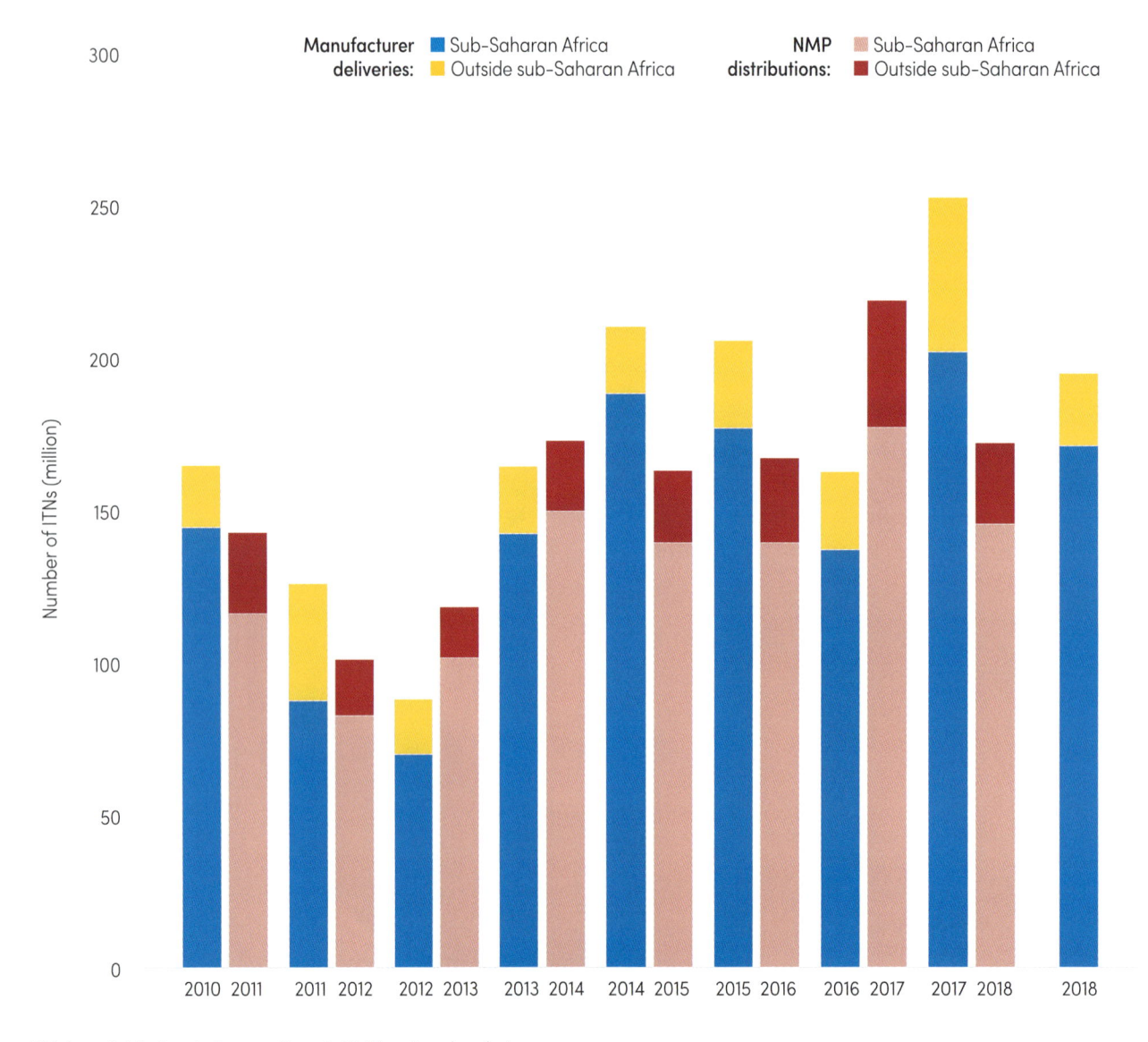

ITN: insecticide-treated mosquito net; NMP: national malaria programme.
[a] Deliveries by manufacturers in a given year are often not reflected in distributions by NMPs in that year; a lag of up to 1 year may occur.
[b] Distributions of ITNs reported by NMPs do not always reflect all the nets that have been distributed to communities, depending on completeness of recording.
Note: A lag between manufacturer deliveries to countries and NMP distributions of about 6–12 months is expected, which should be considered when interpreting the relationship between manufacturer deliveries, NMP distributions and likely population coverage. Additional considerations include nets that are in storage in country but have not yet been distributed by NMPs, and those sold through the private sector that are not reported by the programmes.

distributions through immunization programmes in ANC facilities continue to play an important role.

During the 3-year period 2016–2018, 578 million ITNs – most of which were LLINs – were distributed globally by NMPs in malaria endemic countries. Of these, about 90% were delivered to 29 countries (**Fig. 6.9**), with 50% going to Côte d'Ivoire, the Democratic Republic of the Congo, Ethiopia, Ghana, India, Nigeria, Uganda and the United Republic of Tanzania.

**FIG. 6.9.**
**Total LLINs distributed to communities by country in the period 2016–2018, in countries accounting for about 90% of global distributions by NMPs** Source: NMP reports.

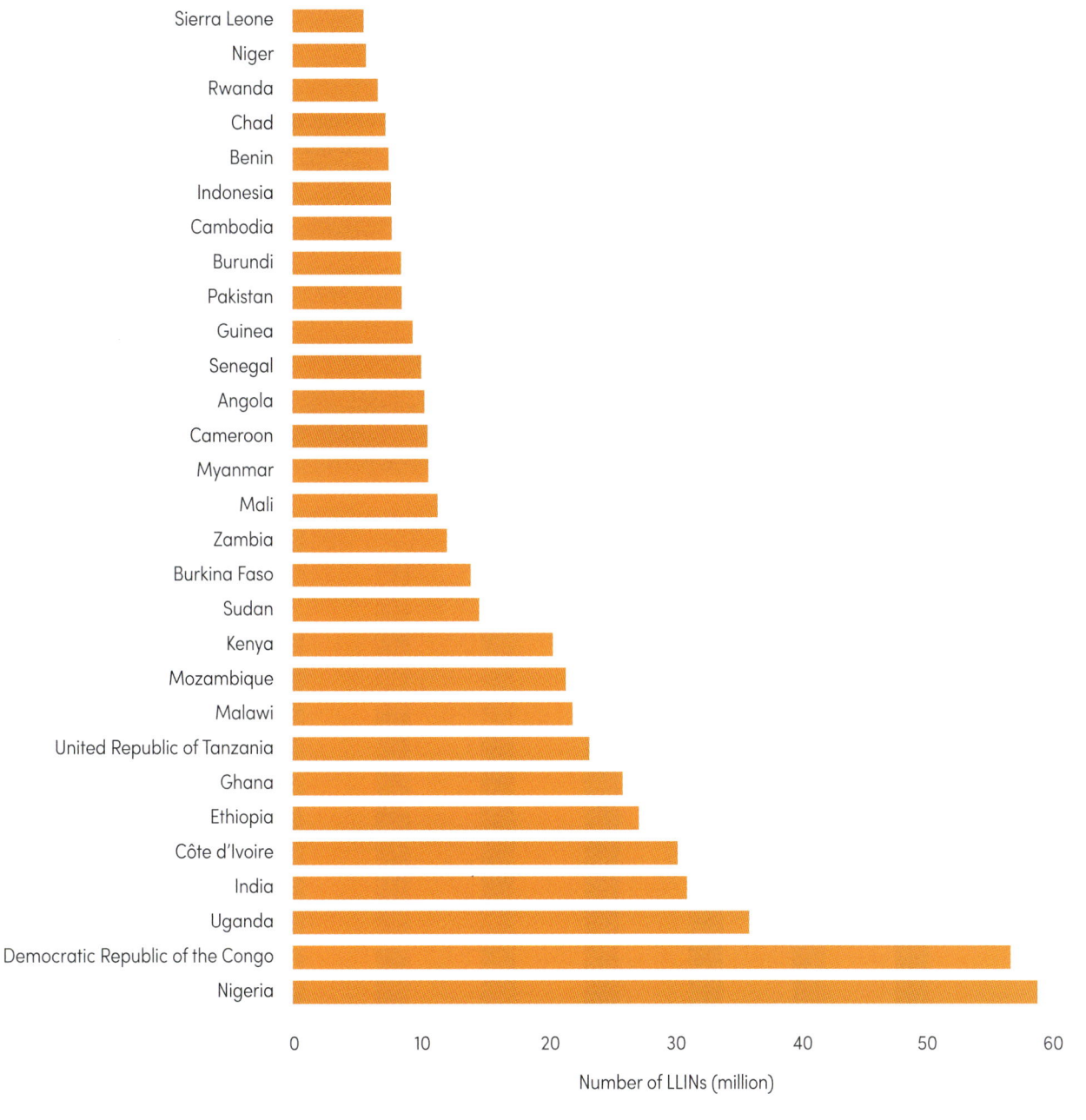

LLIN: long-lasting insecticidal net; NMP: national malaria programme.

# 6 Investments in malaria programmes and research

## 6.4 DELIVERIES OF RDTs

Globally, 2.3 billion RDTs for malaria were sold by manufacturers in the period 2010–2018, with nearly 80% of these sales to countries in sub-Saharan Africa. These were sales by manufacturers that were eligible for procurement according to the Malaria RDT Product Testing Programme and WHO Prequalification and NMP distributions of RDTs. In the same time period NMPs distributed 1.6 billion RDTs.

In 2018, 412 million RDTs were sold by manufacturers, compared with 276 million in 2017 (**Fig. 6.10**). However, NMPs distributed 259 million RDTs in 2018, compared with 245 million in 2017, with 80% of distributions also occurring in sub-Saharan Africa. Usually, differences between sales and distributions of RDTs can be attributed to one or more of the following causes: manufacturer data include both public and private health sector sales, whereas NMP-distributed RDTs represent tests in the public sector only; an initial high distribution may be followed by a lower one, as countries use commodities procured in the previous year; misreporting may occur, where RDTs in ministry of health central stores are not included in NMP distributions; and reporting systems may be weak or manufacturer data may represent recent orders that are yet to arrive in the country. Most of the RDTs sold globally (266 million), particularly in sub-Saharan Africa, were tests that detected only *P. falciparum*.

### FIG. 6.10.

**Number of RDTs sold by manufacturers and distributed by NMPs for use in testing suspected malaria cases,**[a] **2010–2018** *Sources: NMP reports and sales data from manufacturers eligible for WHO's Malaria RDT Product Testing Programme.*

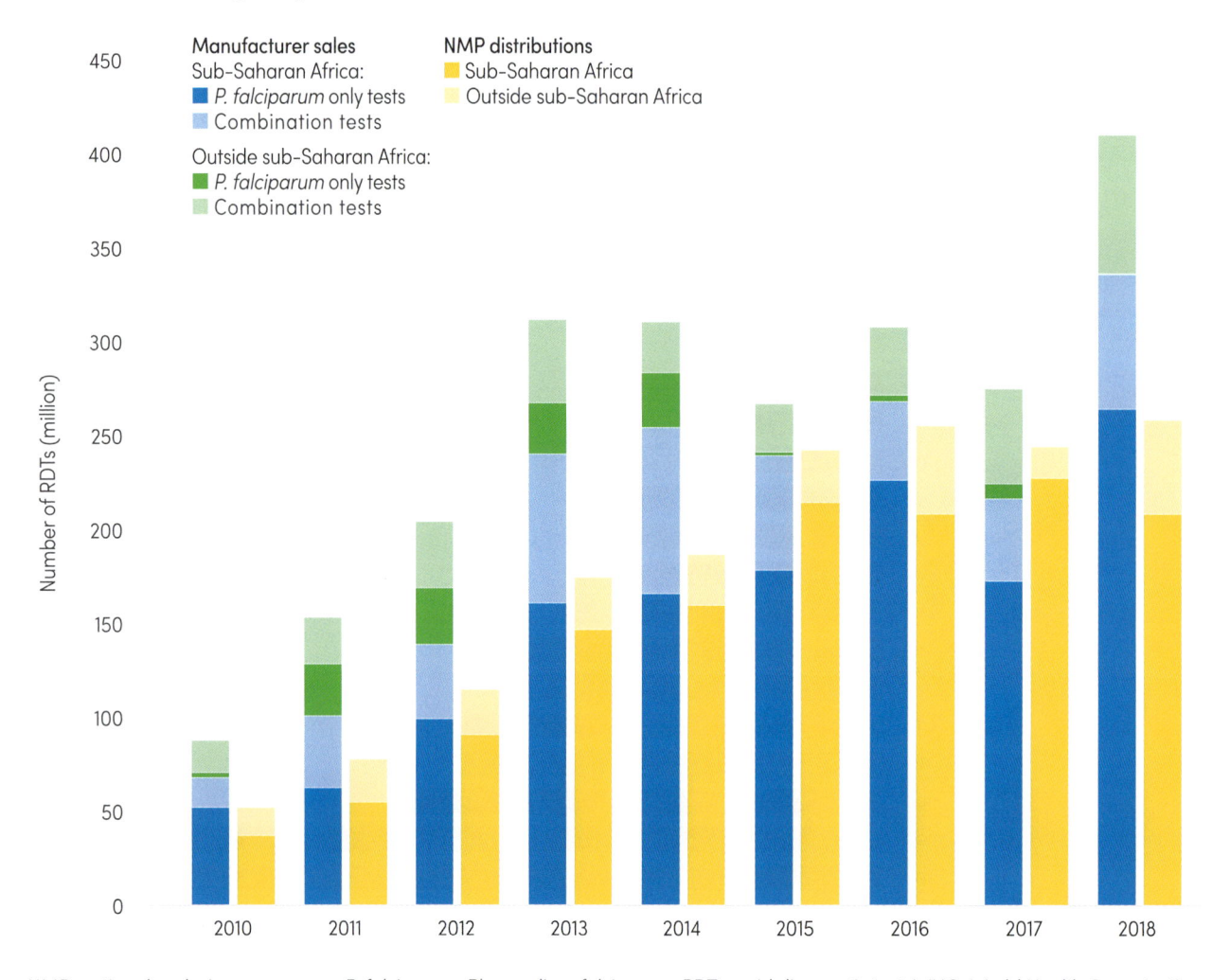

NMP: national malaria programme; *P. falciparum*: *Plasmodium falciparum*; RDT: rapid diagnostic test; WHO: World Health Organization.
[a] NMP distributions do not reflect those RDTs still in storage that have yet to be delivered to health facilities and community health workers.

## 6.5 DELIVERIES OF ACTs

More than 3 billion treatment courses of ACT were sold globally by manufacturers in the period 2010–2018 (**Fig. 6.11**). About 1.9 billion of these sales were to the public sector in malaria endemic countries, and the rest were sold through either public or private sector co-payments (or both), or sold exclusively through the private retail sector. National data reported by NMPs show that, in the same period, 1.7 billion ACTs were delivered to health facilities to treat malaria patients in the public health sector. The discrepancy between global sales and national distributions is, in part, due to the lack of reports from the private sector for most countries. However, with declines in co-payments from the Global Fund, the number of ACTs procured for the private sector has decreased substantially since 2016. In 2018, some 249 million ACTs were sold by manufacturers to the public health sector, and in the same year 214 million ACTs were distributed to this sector by NMPs, of which 98% were in sub-Saharan Africa.

### FIG. 6.11.

**Number of ACT treatment courses delivered by manufacturers and distributed by NMPs to patients, 2010–2018**[a,b] Sources: Companies eligible for procurement by WHO/UNICEF and NMP reports.

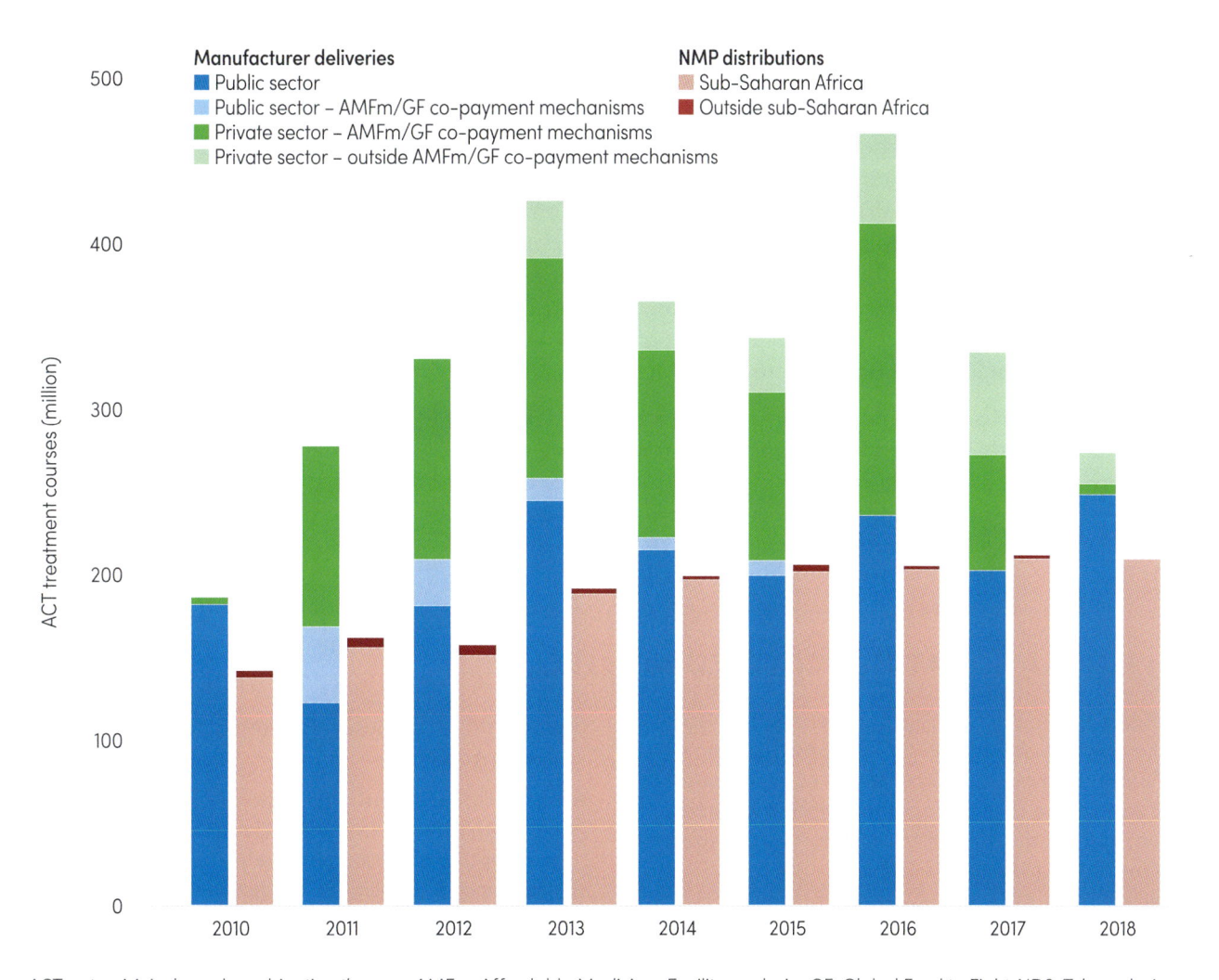

ACT: artemisinin-based combination therapy; AMFm: Affordable Medicines Facility–malaria; GF: Global Fund to Fight AIDS, Tuberculosis and Malaria; NMP: national malaria programme; UNICEF: United Nations Children's Fund; WHO: World Health Organization.
[a] NMP deliveries to patients reflect consumption reported in the public health sector.
[b] AMFm/GF indicates that the AMFm operated from 2010 to 2013, with the GF co-payment mechanism operating from 2014.

# 7 Preventing malaria

For the prevention of malaria, WHO recommends vector control (i.e. reducing the chances of mosquitoes biting human beings) or chemoprevention (i.e. providing drugs that suppress infections) in specific population subgroups (i.e. pregnant women, children and other high-risk groups) or in specific contexts (e.g. complex emergencies and elimination). The core interventions recommended by WHO to prevent mosquito bites are sleeping under an ITN and indoor residual spraying (IRS). In a few specific settings and circumstances, ITNs and IRS can be supplemented by larval source management or other environmental modifications (*29*).

With regard to chemoprevention, WHO recommends a number of context-specific interventions. In sub-Saharan Africa, IPTp with SP has been shown to reduce maternal anaemia, low birthweight and perinatal mortality (*30*). IPTi with SP provides protection against clinical malaria and anaemia (*31*). SMC with amodiaquine (AQ) plus SP (AQ+SP) for children aged 3–59 months reduces the incidence of clinical attacks and severe malaria by about 75%, and could avert millions of cases and thousands of deaths among children living in areas of highly seasonal malaria transmission (*32*). Since March 2012, WHO has recommended SMC for children aged 3–59 months living in areas of highly seasonal malaria transmission in the Sahel subregion of Africa. Mass drug administration is defined as the time-limited administration of antimalarial treatment to all age groups of a defined population or to every person living in a defined geographical area (except those for whom the medicine is contraindicated) at about the same time and at specific repeated intervals. It is recommended for malaria elimination settings in combination with high coverage of core interventions and as a means of rapidly reducing the malaria burden in epidemics and complex emergencies, as part of the rapid initial response (*33*).

This section discusses the population-level coverage of ITNs, IRS, IPTp and SMC. Analysis of coverage indicators for ITNs is limited to sub-Saharan Africa, where there are sufficient household survey data to measure progress. IPTp and SMC are also reported only for sub-Saharan Africa, where these interventions are applicable. The coverage of IPTi is not reported because, as for 2018, no country has adopted it. In 2019, Sierra Leone began national scale-up of IPTi.

## 7.1 POPULATION AT RISK COVERED WITH ITNs

Indicators of population-level coverage of ITNs were estimated for countries in sub-Saharan Africa in which ITNs are the main method of vector control. Household surveys were used, together with manufacturer deliveries and NMP distributions, to estimate the following main indicators (*34, 35*):

- net use (i.e. the percentage of a given population group that slept under an ITN the night before the survey);
- ITN ownership (i.e. the percentage of households that owned at least one ITN);
- percentage of households with at least one ITN for every two people;
- percentage of the population with access to an ITN within their household (i.e. the percentage of the population that could be protected by an ITN, assuming that each ITN in a household can be used by two people); and
- household ITN ownership gap, measured as the percentage of households with at least one ITN for every two people among households owning any ITN.

By 2018, 72% of households in sub-Saharan Africa had at least one ITN and about 57% of the population had access to an ITN, while 40% of the population lived in households with enough ITNs for all occupants. These indicators represented impressive progress from 2010, but no significant change since 2016 (**Fig. 7.1**).

Use of ITNs by household members, measured as the percentage of people who slept under an ITN the night before the survey, was 61% in 2018 compared with 36% in 2010 for both pregnant women and children aged under 5 years, and was 50% in 2018 compared with 29% in 2010 for the overall population (**Fig. 7.2**).

**FIG. 7.1.**

**Percentage of population at risk with access to an ITN, and percentage of households with at least one ITN and enough ITNs for all occupants, sub-Saharan Africa, 2010–2018** Source: ITN coverage model from MAP.[a]

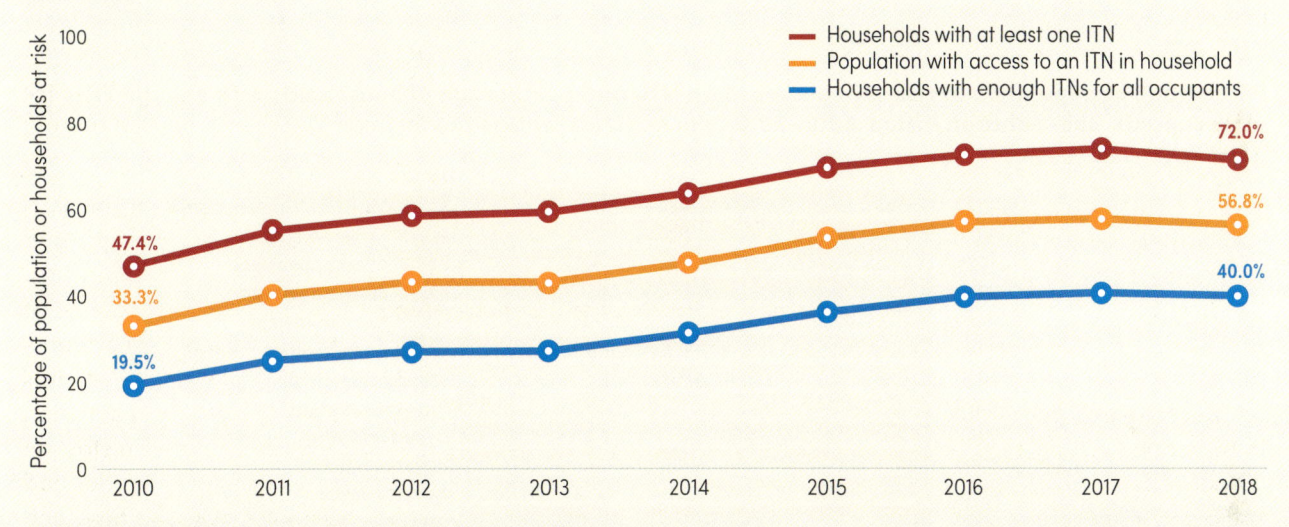

ITN: insecticide-treated mosquito net; MAP: Malaria Atlas Project.
[a] https://map.ox.ac.uk/

**FIG. 7.2.**

**Percentage of population at risk, pregnant women and children aged under 5 years[a] sleeping under an ITN, sub-Saharan Africa, 2010–2018** Source: ITN coverage model from MAP.[b]

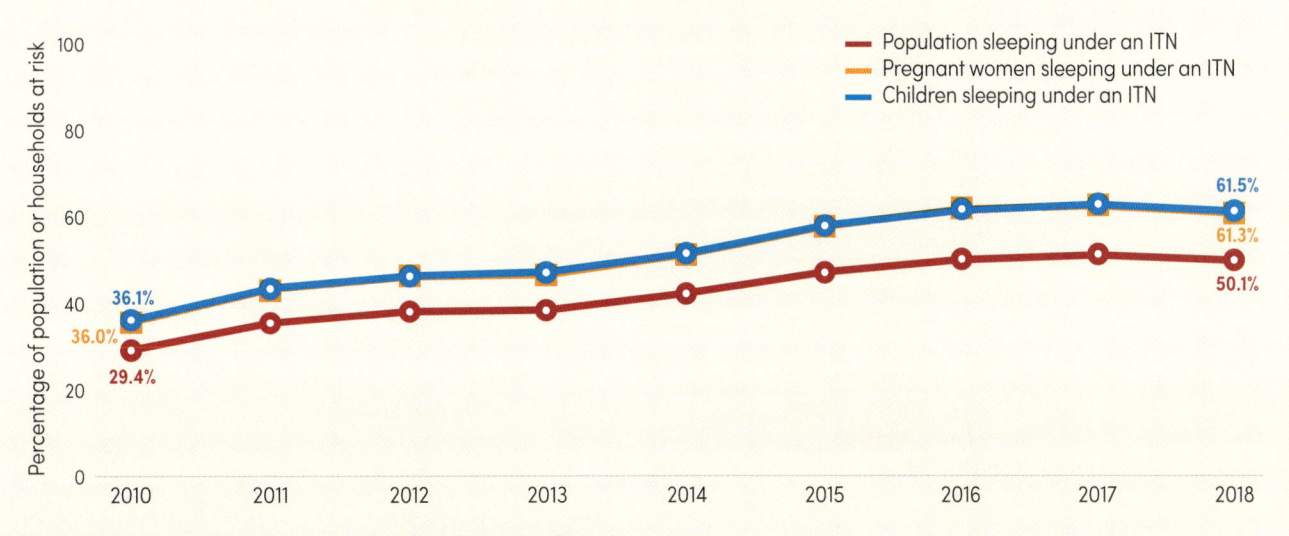

ITN: insecticide-treated mosquito net; MAP: Malaria Atlas Project.
[a] Estimates for children aged under 5 years and pregnant women highly overlap and show the same values in the trend since 2010.
[b] https://map.ox.ac.uk/

# 7 Preventing malaria

Results by country in sub-Saharan Africa on percentage of population with access to ITNs and proportion of households with enough ITNs for all occupants are shown in **Fig. 7.3**. These are countries where ITNs are the main vector control intervention. The analysis showed high levels of access (>70%) in 13 of 37 countries, moderate levels of access (50–70%) in an additional 13 countries, and access levels below 50% in 11 countries, including Burkina Faso and Nigeria, two very high burden countries. The percentage of households with at least one ITN for each two people was, as expected, highly correlated with, but consistently lower than, the percentage with access to ITN.

## 7.2 POPULATION AT RISK PROTECTED BY IRS

In most countries, IRS is targeted at a few focal areas, which may vary over time. Operational coverage of IRS is likely to be very high among the targeted populations. However, when interpreting the trends in IRS coverage presented here, the denominator of "population at risk" used is that of all populations

**FIG. 7.3.**

**Percentage of population at risk with access to an ITN, and percentage of households with enough ITNs for all occupants, sub-Saharan Africa, 2010–2018** *Source: ITN coverage model from MAP.*[a]

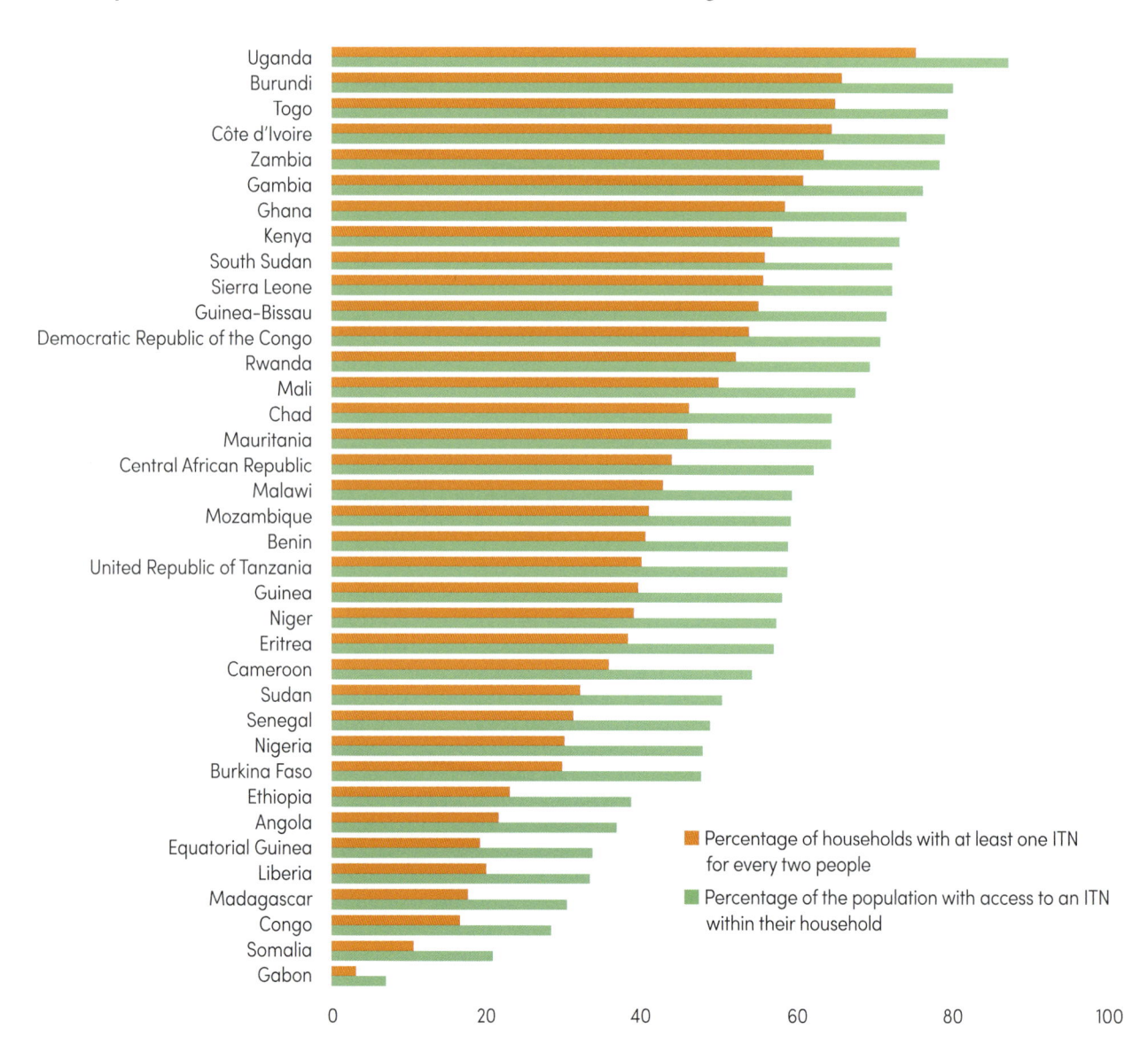

ITN: insecticide-treated mosquito net; MAP: Malaria Atlas Project.
[a] https://map.ox.ac.uk/

living in areas where there is ongoing malaria transmission, to allow for consistency in trend.

Globally, the percentage of the populations at risk protected by IRS declined from 5% in 2010 to 2% in 2018, with increases seen in 2018 compared with 2017 in the regions for which data were analysed: the WHO Region of the Americas and WHO Eastern Mediterranean Region (**Fig. 7.4**). The number of people protected in 2010 was 180 million globally, but by 2018 this number had reduced to about 93 million, with a decrease of 13 million compared with 2017.

Reasons for the declining global IRS coverage may include the switch from pyrethroids to more expensive insecticides in response to increasing pyrethroid resistance, or changes in operational strategies (e.g. decreasing at-risk populations in countries aiming for elimination of malaria). **Fig. 7.5** shows the main chemical class used for IRS across countries that have reported the implementation of this intervention. Most countries still rely on pyrethroids, although in 2018 about half of countries reported using other insecticides, mainly organophosphates (**Section 10.3**).

### FIG. 7.4.

**Percentage of the population at risk protected by IRS, by WHO region, 2010–2018** *Source: NMP reports and IVCC data.*

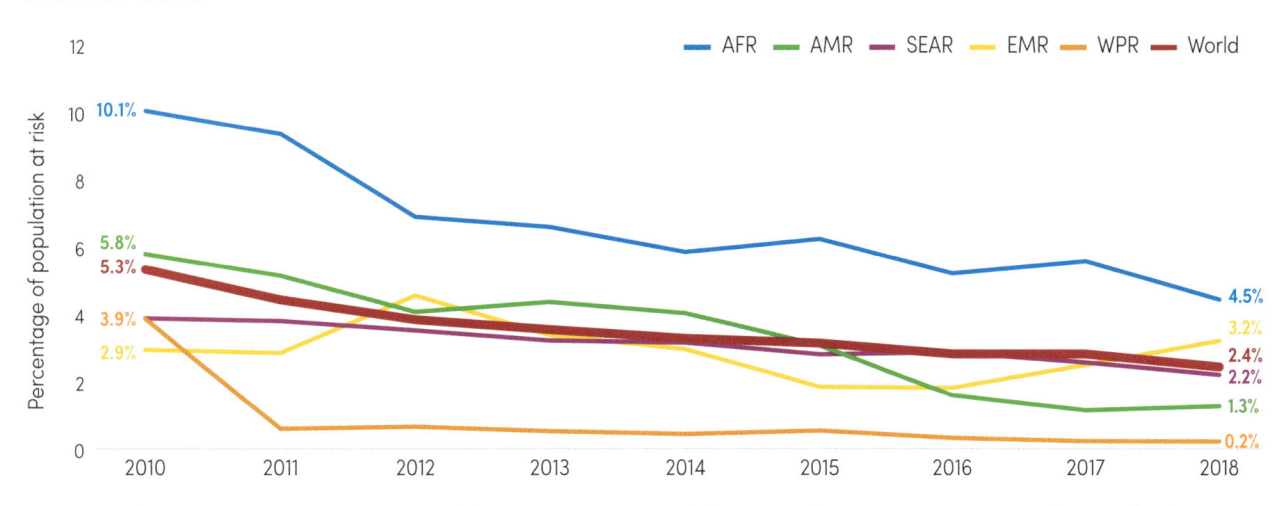

AFR: WHO African Region; AMR: WHO Region of the Americas; EMR: WHO Eastern Mediterranean Region; IRS: indoor residual spraying; IVCC: Innovative Vector Control Consortium; NMP: national malaria programme; SEAR: WHO South-East Asia Region; WHO: World Health Organization; WPR: WHO Western Pacific Region.

### FIG. 7.5.

**Main chemical classes used for IRS by national programmes globally, 2010–2018** *Source: NMP reports.*

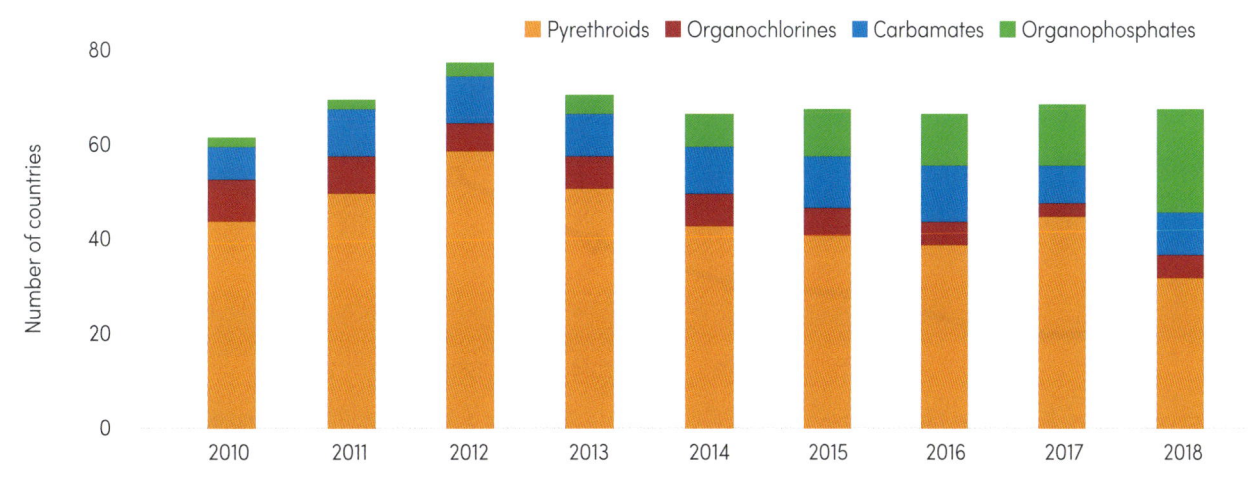

IRS: indoor residual spraying; NMP: national malaria programme.

# 7 Preventing malaria

## 7.3 PREGNANT WOMEN RECEIVING THREE OR MORE DOSES OF IPTp

WHO recommends that IPTp be given to all pregnant women at each ANC visit, starting as early as possible in the second trimester (i.e. not during the first trimester). Each SP dose should be given at least 1 month apart, with women receiving at least three SP doses (IPTp3) during each pregnancy (30). To date, 36 African countries have adopted this policy. These countries reported routine health facility data from the public sector on the number of women receiving the first, second, third and fourth doses of IPTp (i.e. IPTp1, IPTp2, IPTp3 and IPTp4). Using annual expected pregnancies, discounted for fetal loss and stillbirths, as the denominator, the percentage IPTp use by dose was computed. As of 2018, coverage rates of IPTp1, IPTp2 and IPTp3 were 60%, 49% and 31%, respectively (**Fig. 7.6**). The 2018 estimate of IPTp3 coverage, relative to the 22% in 2017, represents the highest single annual increase in this indicator, indicating

**FIG. 7.6.**
**Percentage of pregnant women attending ANC at least once and receiving IPTp, by dose, sub-Saharan Africa, 2010–2018** *Source: NMP reports, WHO and US Centers for Disease Control and Prevention estimates.*

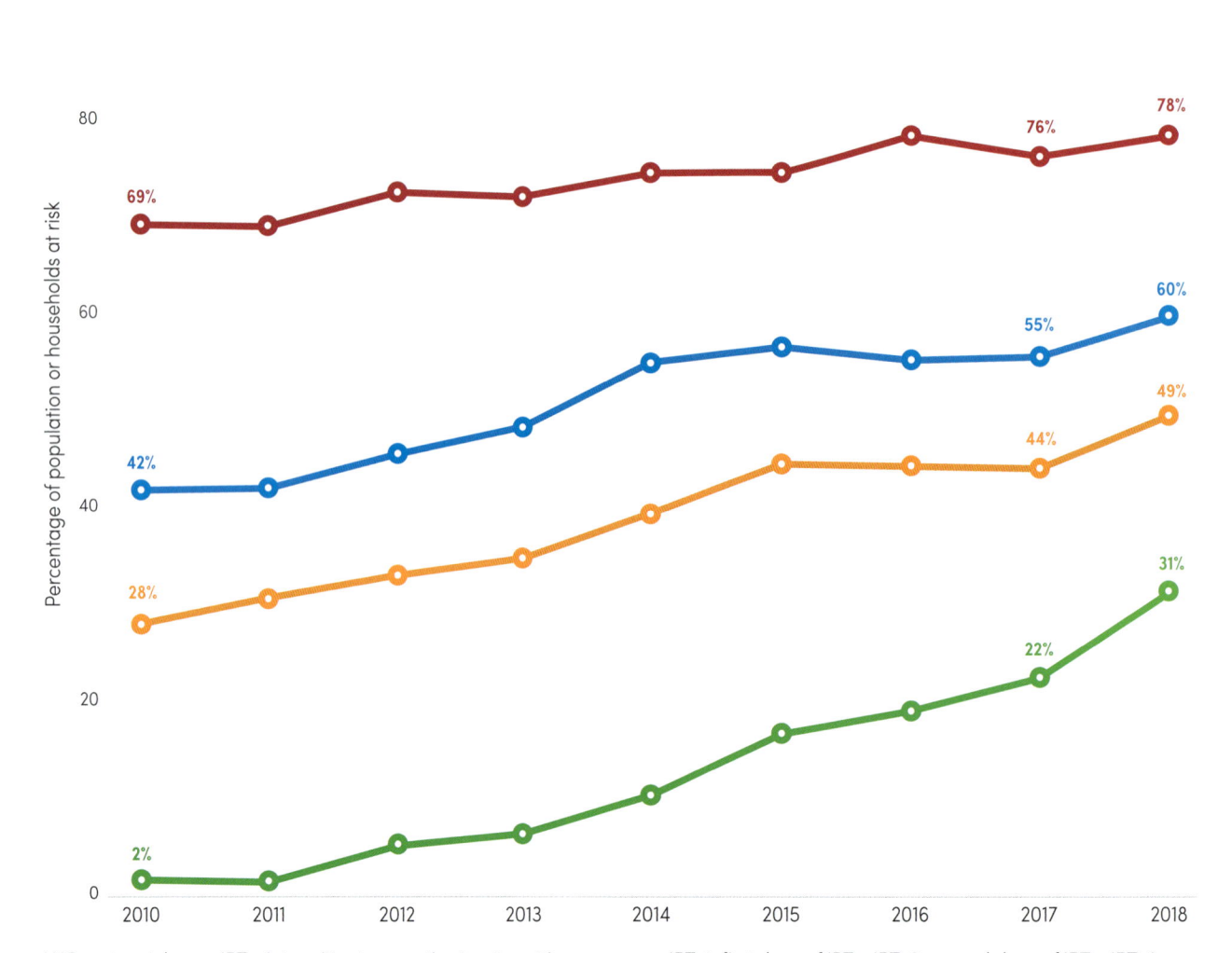

ANC: antenatal care; IPTp: intermittent preventive treatment in pregnancy; IPTp1: first dose of IPTp; IPTp2: second dose of IPTp; IPTp3: third dose of IPTp; NMP: national malaria programme; US: United States; WHO: World Health Organization.

considerable improvements in country uptake. The analysis suggests, however, that about 18% of women who use ANC services at least once do not receive any IPTp, representing a missed opportunity that, if harnessed, could considerably and rapidly improve IPTp coverage.

## 7.4 SEASONAL MALARIA CHEMOPREVENTION

In the 12 countries in the Sahel subregion that have scaled up SMC, 31 million children aged under 5 years were in SMC-eligible areas; of these, 19 million children (62%) were treated. The main gaps in treatment were in Nigeria (70%, 8.4 million), Chad (67%, 1.8 million), Ghana (66%, 0.7 million), Senegal (100%, 0.7 million) and Gambia (47%, 0.1 million). All targeted children received treatment in Cameroon, Guinea, Guinea-Bissau and Mali (**Fig. 7.7**).

### FIG. 7.7.
**Number of SMC treatments administered in scale-up countries in 2018** Source: London School of Hygiene & Tropical Medicine.

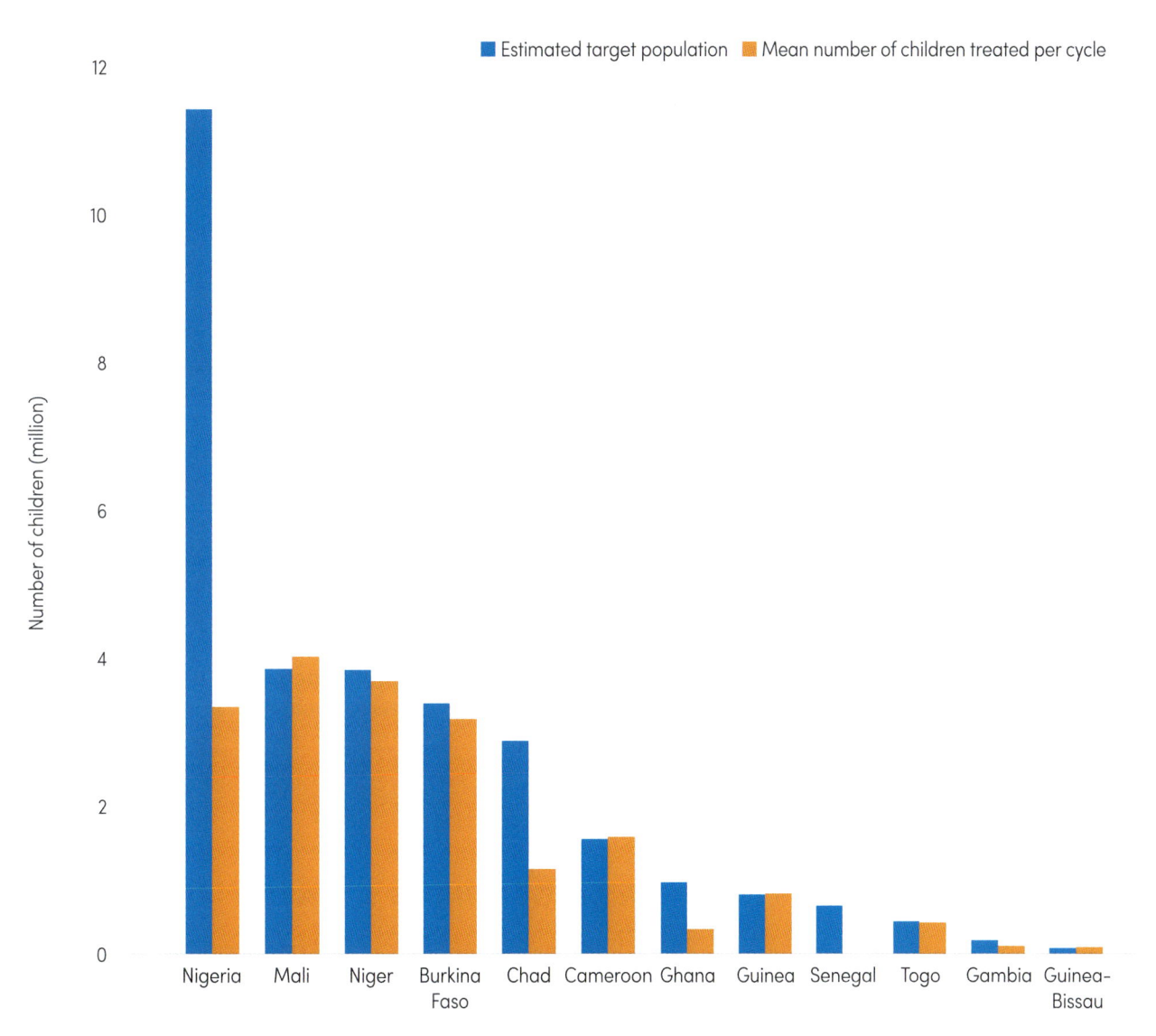

SMC: seasonal malaria chemoprevention.

# 8. Diagnostic testing and treatment

Diagnostic testing and treatment is a key component of malaria control and elimination strategies. In addition to the treatment of uncomplicated malaria illness, prompt and effective case management helps to prevent severe disease and probable death; it may also reduce the pool of individuals who contribute to malaria transmission. Diagnosing patients rather than treating them presumptively may help health service providers to further investigate other potential causes of febrile illnesses that have a negative parasitological result, reduce the unnecessary use of antimalarial drugs and associated side-effects, and contribute to reducing the spread of drug resistance (*36*).

The ability of health systems to provide quality malaria case management at high coverage is influenced by three indicators: the extent to which patients with suspected malaria seek treatment, receive a diagnostic test after seeking care, and (if that test is positive for malaria) receive appropriate treatment. These indicators are usually measured through household surveys, such as MIS and DHS. For reasons of data availability, the analysis in this section is largely confined to sub-Saharan Africa, the region that carries the highest share of the global malaria burden; it covers 4-year periods because most countries conduct household surveys once every 3–5 years. **Annex 1** discusses the countries included, the calculation methods, and the limitations of the use of DHS and MIS data.

The signs and symptoms of malaria are similar to those of many other febrile illnesses. In non-immune individuals, malaria typically presents with fever, sometimes accompanied by chills, sweats, headache or other symptoms that may resemble signs or symptoms of other febrile illnesses. Consequently, fever is the main basis for suspecting malaria and triggering diagnostic testing of the patient in most malaria endemic settings. A history of fever in children aged under 5 years and subsequent steps taken to seek treatment have been the basis of measuring access to malaria case management. However, some important limitations of these data are as follows: what constitutes a "fever" varies by cultural context, which means that making comparisons across cultural groups can be problematic; the percentage of fevers that are due to malaria varies according to the underlying transmission intensity and level of control; there is no conclusive evidence that the household-level and individual-level processes for making the decision to seek treatment for malaria fevers are the same as those for other fevers or across different ages; and a percentage of respondents may not recall the medication they received, resulting in misclassification of the drugs that were prescribed.

## 8.1 PREVALENCE OF FEVER IN CHILDREN AGED UNDER 5 YEARS

Based on 20 household surveys conducted in sub-Saharan Africa between 2015 and 2018, a median of 26% of children (interquartile range [IQR]: 19–35%) had a fever in the 2 weeks preceding the survey. Children aged 6 months to 3 years had a higher prevalence (around 30%) of fever than children aged under 6 months or over 3 years (**Fig. 8.1**). Prevalence of fever ranged from more than 40% in Malawi and Nigeria to less than 20% in Angola, Ethiopia, Madagascar, Mali and Zimbabwe (**Annex 3-Eb**). However, the data should be interpreted with caution because of potential bias in the season in which surveys are conducted.

## 8.2 NUMBERS OF CHILDREN WITH FEVER BROUGHT FOR CARE

Based on 20 nationally representative household surveys in sub-Saharan Africa conducted between 2015 and 2018, a median of 42% (IQR: 34–49%) of febrile children aged under 5 years were brought for care in the public sector compared with 10% (IQR: 8–22%) in the formal private sector and 3% (IQR: 2–7%) in the informal private sector (i.e. shops, markets, kiosks, itinerant drug sellers, traditional healers, friends and relatives, and other nonmedical health facilities). A considerable percentage of febrile children were not brought for care (median: 36%, IQR: 28–45%). When looking more closely at the subcategories of health sectors, visits to public health facilities and community health workers (CHWs) accounted for 37% (IQR: 31–48%) and 3% (IQR: 1–4%), respectively. Visits to the formal private sector were to the formal medical private sector, excluding pharmacies (median: 8%, IQR: 4–11%), and to pharmacies or accredited drug stores (median: 5%, IQR: 1–10%). Overall, a median of 58% (IQR: 47–70%) of febrile children brought for care were taken to a trained provider (i.e. to public sector health facilities, CHWs, formal private health facilities or pharmacies) (**Fig. 8.2**).

### FIG. 8.1.

**Median percentage of children who had a fever in the 2 weeks preceding the survey, overall and by age group, sub-Saharan Africa, 2015–2018 (latest survey)** *Sources: Nationally representative household survey data from DHS and MIS.*

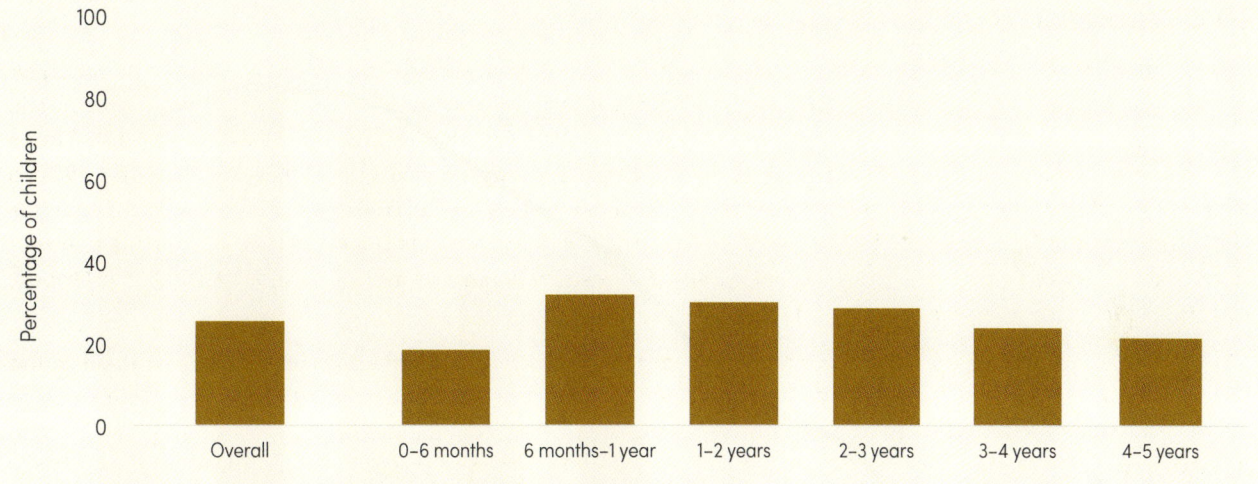

DHS: demographic and health surveys; MIS: malaria indicator surveys.

### FIG. 8.2.

**Median percentage of febrile children brought for care, by health sector, sub-Saharan Africa, 2015–2018 (latest survey)** *Sources: Nationally representative household survey data from DHS and MIS.*

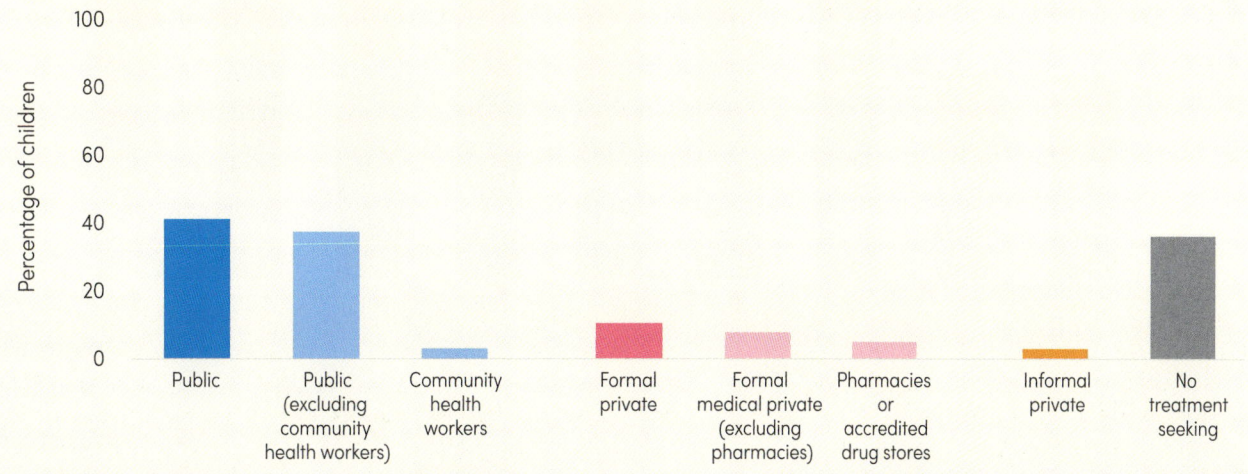

DHS: demographic and health surveys; MIS: malaria indicator surveys.

# 8 Diagnostic testing and treatment

Variation in care-seeking behaviour was substantial across countries. In Burkina Faso, Mozambique and Sierra Leone, most febrile children (>60%) were brought for care in the public sector, whereas in Nigeria and Uganda they were mainly taken to the private sector. In Benin, Ghana, Mali and Togo, more than 10% of febrile children attended the informal private sector. Also, in Benin, Ethiopia, Malawi, Mali, Senegal, Togo and Zimbabwe, most febrile children were not brought for care (**Annex 3-Eb**).

## 8.3 PARASITOLOGICAL TESTING OF FEBRILE CHILDREN

Data from NMP country reports show that, because of the increasing scale-up of diagnostics, the percentage of patients suspected of having malaria who are seen in public health facilities and tested with either an RDT

**FIG. 8.3.**
**Malaria patients examined using RDT and microscopy, and percentage of suspected cases tested in public health facilities, sub-Saharan Africa, 2010–2018** *Source: NMP reports.*

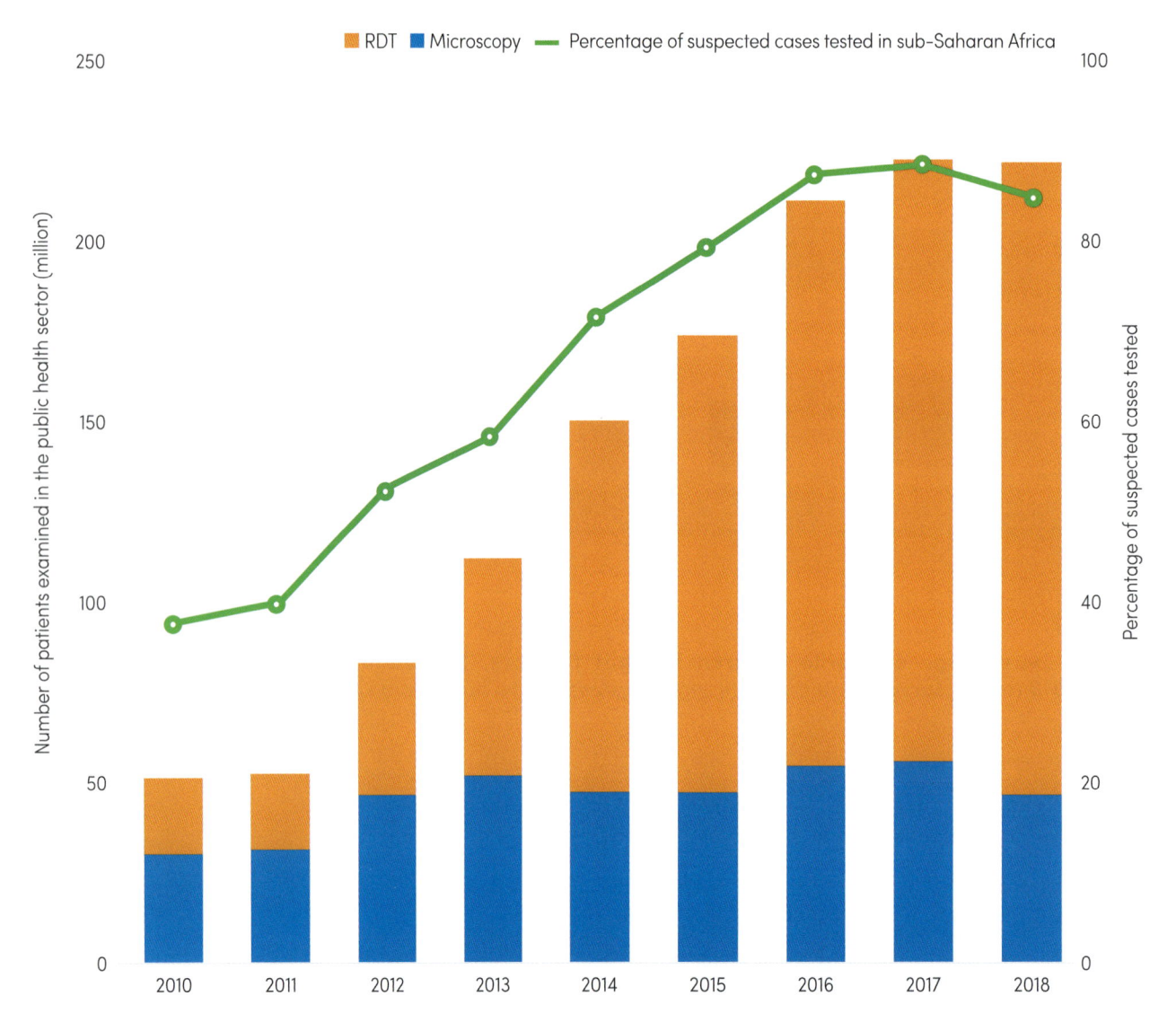

NMP: national malaria programme; RDT: rapid diagnostic test.

or microscopy, has risen from 38% in 2010 to 85% in 2018 (**Fig. 8.3**).

Data reported by NMPs from 38 moderate to high transmission countries in sub-Saharan Africa show a considerable increase between 2010 and 2018 in the number of suspected malaria cases tested with a parasitological test (**Fig. 8.4**). In 27 of these countries, the percentage of suspected cases tested was greater than 80% in 2018; however, in Congo, Gabon, Kenya and Mauritania, less than 50% of suspected cases in the public health sector were tested for malaria.

### FIG. 8.4.
**Percentage of suspected cases tested in public health facilities, sub-Saharan Africa, 2010–2018** *Source: NMP reports.*

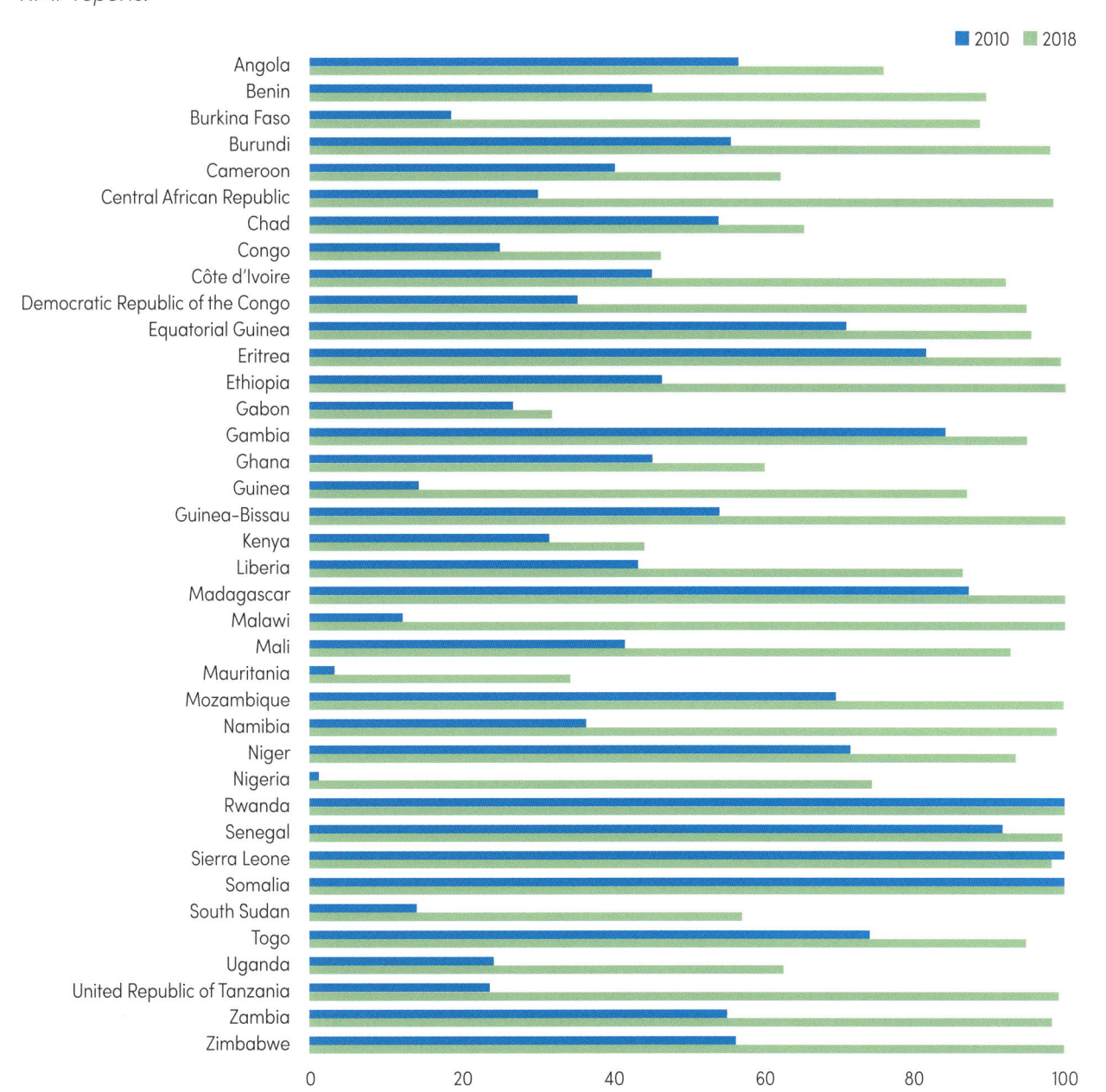

NMP: national malaria programme.

# 8 Diagnostic testing and treatment

At community level, based on 19 nationally representative household surveys conducted between 2015 and 2018 in sub-Saharan Africa, the median percentage of febrile children brought for care who received a finger or heel stick (suggesting that a malaria diagnostic test may have been performed) was greater in the public sector (median: 66%, IQR: 49–75%) than in the formal private sector (median: 40%, IQR: 16–46%) or the informal private sector (median: 9%, IQR: 5–22%). In the public sector, 66% of febrile children received a diagnostic test in public health facilities (IQR: 49–75%) and 58% when visiting a CHW (IQR: 39–75%). In the formal private sector, the percentage of those brought for care who had a blood test was 58% in the formal medical private sector, excluding pharmacies (IQR: 30–76%), compared with 13% in pharmacies (IQR: 9–22%). Overall, 57% of children brought to a trained provider for care received a diagnostic test (IQR: 36–68%) (**Fig. 8.5**). This percentage ranged from more than 70% in Burundi,

**FIG. 8.5.**
**Median percentage of febrile children who received a blood test, by health sector, sub-Saharan Africa, 2015–2018 (latest survey)** *Sources: Nationally representative household survey data from DHS and MIS.*

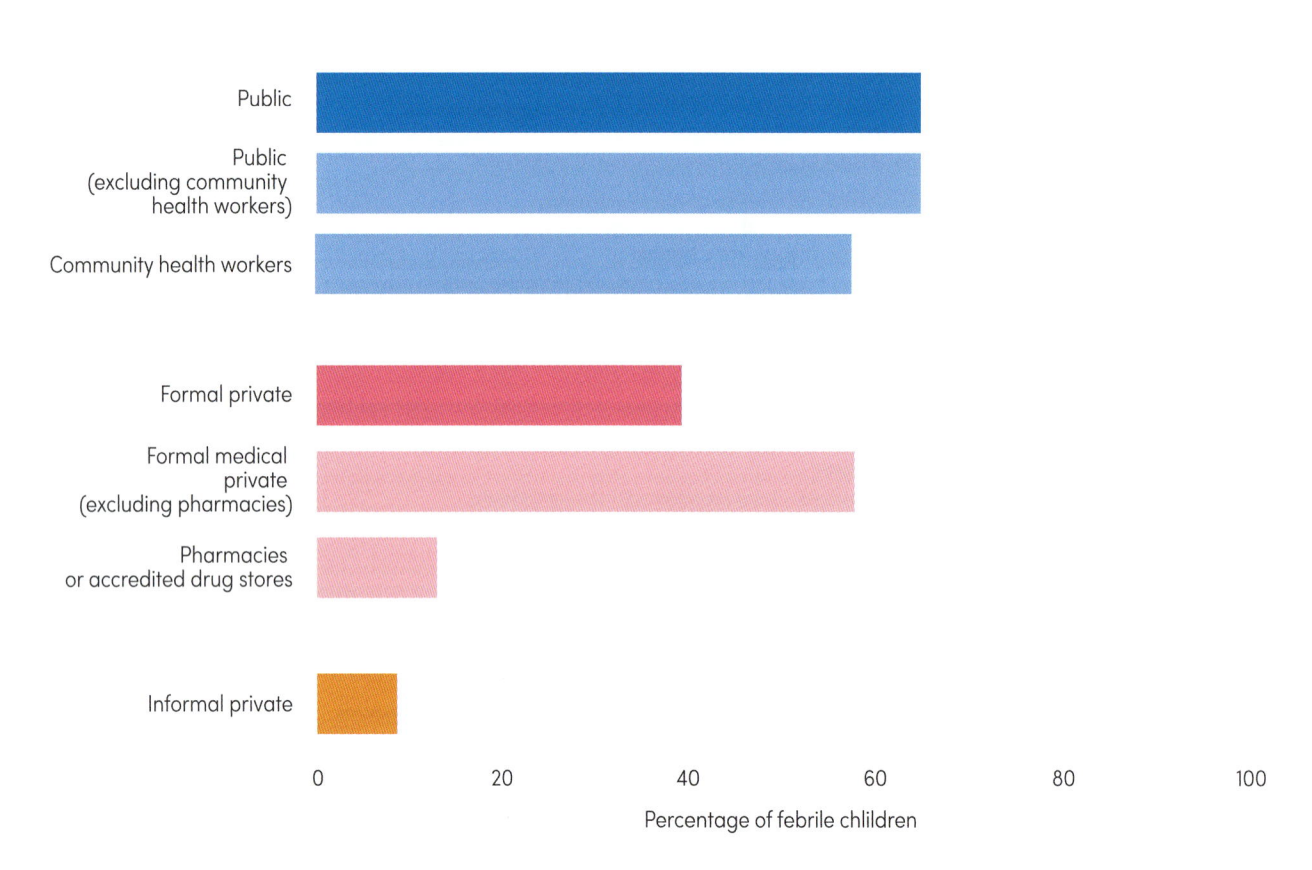

DHS: demographic and health surveys; MIS: malaria indicator surveys.

Malawi and Sierra Leone, to less than 20% in Nigeria (**Annex 3-Eb**).

Based on 61 surveys conducted in 29 sub-Saharan African countries between 2010 and 2018, the percentage of febrile children attending public health facilities who had a blood test before treatment increased from a median of 48% (IQR: 30–62%) in 2010–2013 to a median of 76% (IQR: 60–86%) in 2015–2018. In the formal private sector, this median percentage also increased, from 32% (IQR: 16–49%) in 2010–2013 to 45% (IQR: 34–62%) in 2015–2017 (**Fig. 8.6**). Although median percentages are relatively high, antimalarial treatment continues to be prescribed based on fever without laboratory confirmation. The availability of high-quality, inexpensive RDTs in the public sector has significantly improved and expanded, but RDTs are often unavailable in the formal private sector.

## FIG. 8.6.

**Trend in the median percentage of febrile children who received a blood test among those treated with an antimalarial drug, by health sector, sub-Saharan Africa, 2010–2018 (all surveys)** *Sources: Nationally representative household survey data from DHS and MIS.*

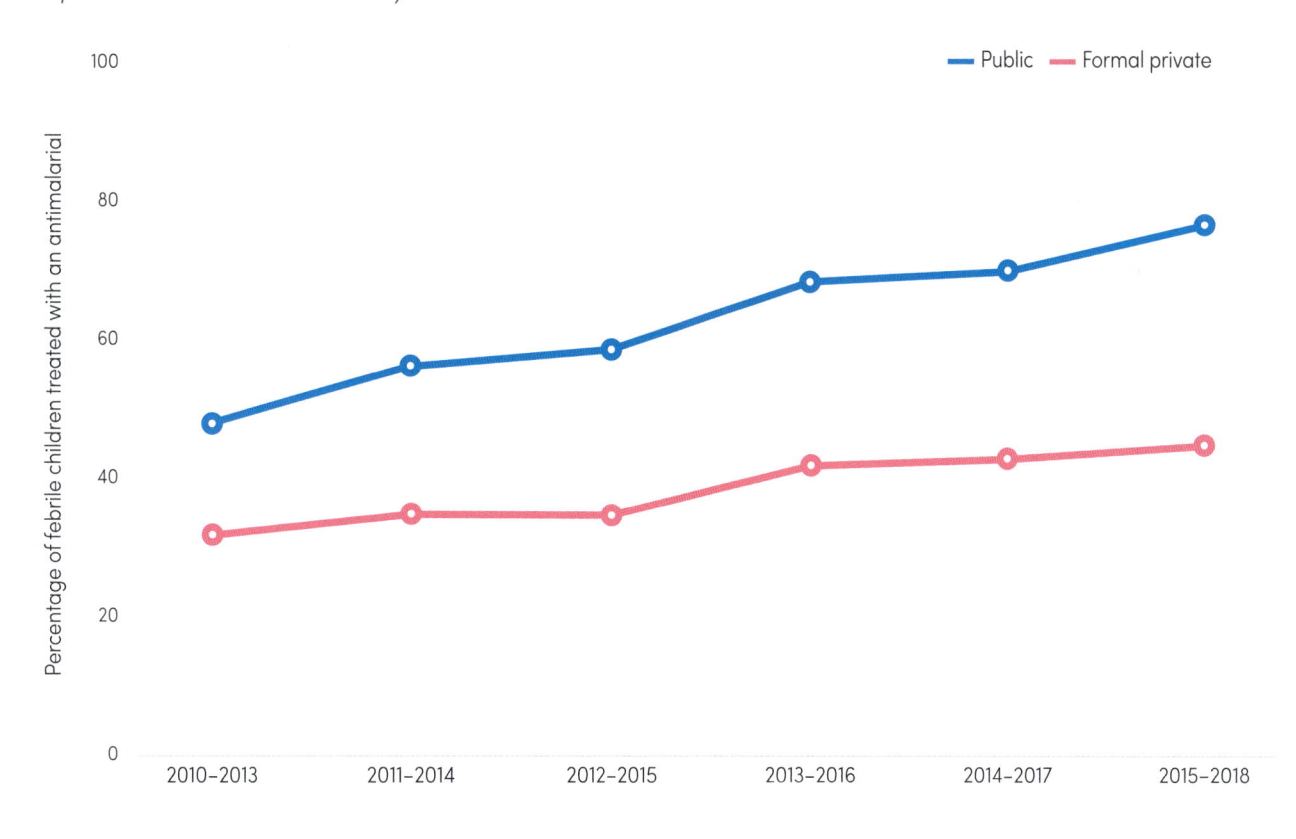

DHS: demographic and health surveys; MIS: malaria indicator surveys.

# 8 Diagnostic testing and treatment

## 8.4 TREATMENT OF FEBRILE CHILDREN WITH ANTIMALARIAL DRUGS

Based on 20 household surveys conducted in sub-Saharan Africa in 2015–2018, the median percentage of febrile children who were treated with any antimalarial drug was higher in the public sector (median: 48%, IQR: 30–69%) than in the formal private sector (median: 40%, IQR: 21–51%) or the informal private sector (median: 18%, IQR: 10–29%) (**Fig. 8.7**). This pattern was consistent across countries except in Angola, Ethiopia, Kenya, Nigeria and the United Republic of Tanzania, where febrile children mainly received antimalarial drugs through the formal private sector. In some countries (e.g. Ghana, Liberia and Uganda), antimalarial treatment coverage was high in the informal private sector, where there is a risk that non-recommended treatments and poor-quality products may be used (**Annex 3-Eb**). When analysed by subcategory of source of care, the median percentage of children receiving antimalarial drugs was 47% (IQR: 29–69%) among those attending public health facilities, and 59% (IQR: 53–84%) among those visiting a CHW. In the private sector, this percentage was 49% (IQR: 19–55%) among those attending the formal medical private sector (excluding pharmacies), and 41% among those visiting pharmacies (IQR: 23–56%). Overall, 48% (IQR: 31–66%) of febrile children received an antimalarial drug among those visiting a trained provider. Among febrile children not brought for care, 8% (IQR: 5–19%) received an antimalarial drug as part of self-treatment at home.

Although there is considerable variation among countries, the median percentage of febrile children

### FIG. 8.7.

**Median percentage of febrile children who were treated with an antimalarial drug, by health sector, sub-Saharan Africa, 2015–2018 (latest survey)** *Sources: Nationally representative household survey data from DHS and MIS.*

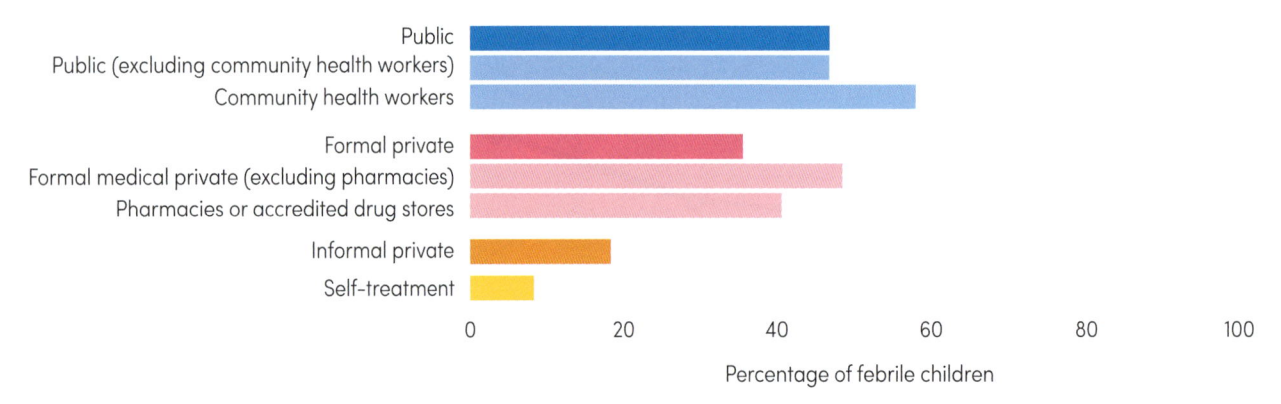

DHS: demographic and health surveys; MIS: malaria indicator surveys.

### FIG. 8.8.

**Trend in the median percentage of febrile children who were treated with an antimalarial drug, by health sector, sub-Saharan Africa, 2010–2018 (all surveys)** *Sources: Nationally representative household survey data from DHS and MIS.*

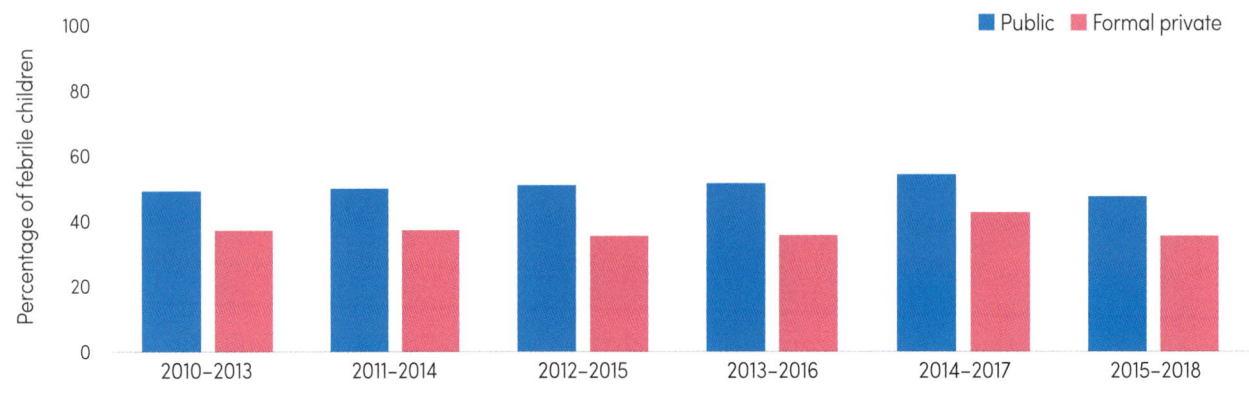

DHS: demographic and health surveys; MIS: malaria indicator surveys.

receiving antimalarial drugs has remained stable, both in the public sector (around 50%) and in the formal private sector (close to 40%) (**Fig. 8.8**). Interpretation of levels and trends in malaria treatment coverage among all febrile children is limited because fevers are not always the result of malaria infection. Even if a country achieves a reasonably high level of treatment of fevers with an antimalarial drug, this measure can be misleading because it includes inappropriate treatment of non-malarial fevers.

## 8.5 USE OF ACT FOR THE TREATMENT OF FEBRILE CHILDREN

Based on 19 surveys, ACT was the most commonly used drug-based therapy among febrile children who received antimalarial medicine (median: 80%, IQR: 45–94%). Antimalarial treatments were slightly more likely to be ACT if treatment was sought in the public sector (median: 80%, IQR: 45–94%) than in the formal private sector (median: 77%, IQR: 43–87%) or the informal private sector (median: 60%, IQR: 40–84%) (**Fig. 8.9**). However, those relatively high percentages do not guarantee that each ACT was a quality-assured ACT, especially in the private sector.

Based on 69 nationally representative household surveys conducted in 32 sub-Saharan African countries between 2010 and 2018, the percentage of febrile children receiving an ACT among those treated with antimalarial medicine in public health facilities increased from a median of 45% (IQR: 29–77%) in 2010–2013 to 82% (IQR: 44–95%) in 2015–2018 (**Fig. 8.10**).

### FIG. 8.9.

**Median percentage of febrile children who received an ACT among those treated with an antimalarial drug, by health sector, sub-Saharan Africa, 2015–2018 (latest survey)** *Sources: Nationally representative household survey data from DHS and MIS.*

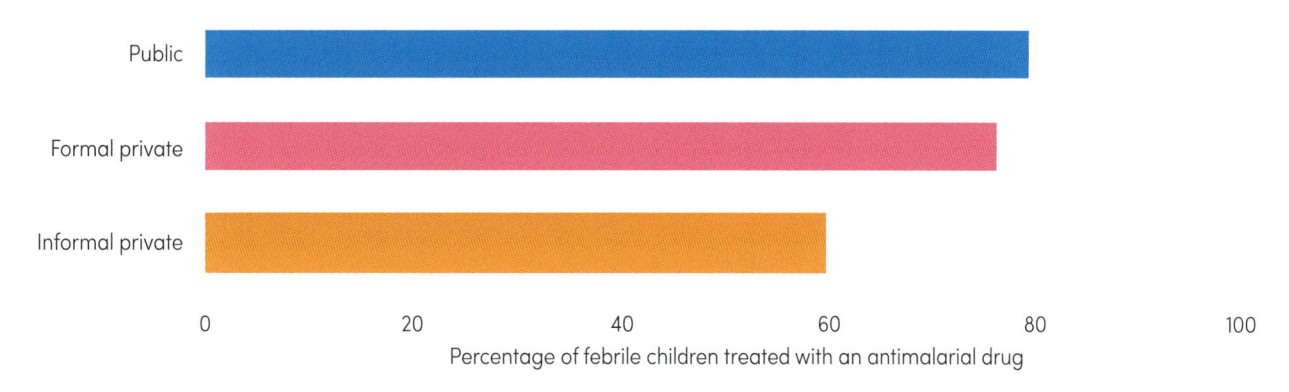

ACT: artemisinin-based combination therapy; DHS: demographic and health surveys; MIS: malaria indicator surveys.

### FIG. 8.10.

**Trend in the median percentage of febrile children who received an ACT among those treated with an antimalarial drug, by health sector, sub-Saharan Africa, 2010–2018 (all surveys)** *Sources: Nationally representative household survey data from DHS and MIS.*

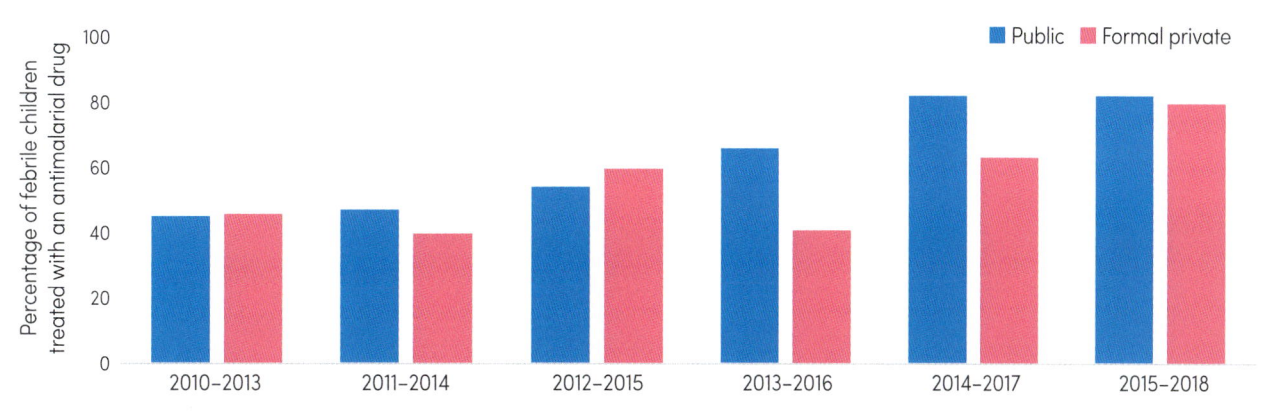

ACT: artemisinin-based combination therapy; DHS: demographic and health surveys; MIS: malaria indicator surveys.

# 8 Diagnostic testing and treatment

## 8.6 INTEGRATED COMMUNITY CASE MANAGEMENT

Nearly 40% of children with fever do not access care (**Fig. 8.2**). Integrated community case management (iCCM) is a proven strategy to deliver effective and simple life-saving interventions for major killers of children (i.e. malaria, pneumonia and diarrhoea) to hard-to-reach and under-served communities. iCCM involves using trained CHWs who may or may not be paid, to deliver health services to these communities. Thirty countries now implement iCCM at different levels, with only a few implementing nationally.

The Global Fund financed a thematic review report on iCCM across 18 countries through desk reviews and field visits with support from WHO and the United Nations Children's Fund (UNICEF). Released in September 2018, this report found that from 2014 to 2017 major donors and development partners increased their funding and technical support for iCCM implementation in all 18 countries. The report also found that many factors that contributed to iCCM success included establishment of national iCCM policies, strong leadership and partnership, and the presence of an existing competent pool of CHWs partnership support.[1]

In 2012, the Government of Canada awarded a grant to the WHO's GMP to support the scale-up of iCCM of pneumonia, diarrhoea and malaria among children aged under 5 in sub-Saharan Africa under the Rapid Access Expansion Programme (RAcE). The two main objectives of the programme were to contribute to the reduction of child mortality, and to document best practices to catalyse scale-up of iCCM. In 2019, WHO and implementing partners published the results of the implementation research on the impact of the RAcE programme, as well the best practices to improving coverage of iCCM in routine health systems (*37*).

To build on the lessons from these studies and experiences from country programmes that are implementing iCCM, in July 2019 UNICEF and WHO co-hosted in Addis Ababa, Ethiopia, a meeting on institutionalizing iCCM to end preventable child deaths. The technical consultation brought together technical experts and country teams to refine guiding principles and develop recommendations for iCCM, and priorities for national strategic plans to strengthen country programming and to identify needs and gaps for resource mobilization. Several challenges and possible solutions for achieving and maintaining an acceptable level of quality of care and coverage were identified during this meeting (**Box 8.1**).

---

[1] Desk review in the following 18 countries: Burundi, Ethiopia, Kenya, Rwanda, South Sudan and Uganda (East Africa); Malawi and Zambia (Southern Africa); and Benin, Burkina Faso, Cameroon, the Democratic Republic of the Congo, Ghana, Mali, Niger, Nigeria, Senegal and Sierra Leone (West and Central Africa). Field visits were conducted in Burkina Faso, Cameroon, Malawi, Nigeria, South Sudan and Zambia.

## BOX. 8.1.
### Challenges to and proposed solutions for the scale-up of iCCM
*Source: WHO-UNICEF*

### Challenges

- Weaknesses in sustainable financing and integration of iCCM into national health system
- In some countries it is not clear which institution is in charge of activities
- Only a few countries have institutionalized CHWs as part of the system. Most countries rely on unpaid or volunteer CHWs
- Poor supervision due to shortage of staff at health facilities, weak links between CHWs and health facilities
- Non-integrated supply chain, poor data on iCCM commodity consumption
- Inadequate funding for pneumonia and diarrhoea commodities in some countries limit scale-up of malaria interventions through iCCM
- Multiple parallel community information systems supported, lack of complete information on performance of CHWs

### Proposed solutions

- Planning for iCCM should take place under the umbrella of primary health care and overall health sector development
- National community health policies and strategies should be in place, containing clear, official guidelines for recruitment, job description and motivation of CHWs, as well as clear criteria for implementing iCCM with a focus on hardest to reach populations
- Domestic and external funding should be targeted at system strengthening, with an inclusive focus on malaria, pneumonia and diarrhoea as well as community and facility based provision of care
- iCCM should be included in the national costing exercise and the annual health sector budgeting processes, with specific budget lines
- To promote institutionalization and sustainability, donors should coordinate iCCM funding with the ministry of health and support the ministry's iCCM implementation plan, instead of funding disease-specific or site-specific projects
- iCCM commodities should be an integral part of health facility and district level quantification
- Supportive supervision of CHWs as part of the primary health care system is core to quality iCCM, and needs to be budgeted and included in district implementation plans
- iCCM requires continuum of care from community to first level health facility to referral facility, having the capacity to fully manage referred children
- Community engagement is key to institutionalization of iCCM: local communities are central for effective planning, implementation and uptake of quality ICCM services
- The training of CHWs should not be considered complete until demonstration of defined competencies, with post training follow-up (time to be fixed as per area context) as part of training programme

# 9. Malaria surveillance

Pillar 3 of the GTS (*1*) is to transform malaria surveillance into a core intervention. This requires surveillance systems that can accurately and reliably track the burden of malaria, the interventions to reduce it, and the impact achieved geographically and temporally. To understand whether malaria surveillance systems are fit for purpose, WHO recommends the regular monitoring and evaluation of surveillance systems (*38*). This involves assessment of the structure, core and support functions, and the quality of the data, across both passive and active case-detection systems. Such information is critical to the continuous improvement of surveillance systems.

This section provides a summary of WHO initiatives to work with NMPs and partners in developing surveillance standards and tools to support the strengthening of national systems. It also presents an example of a country surveillance system assessment, to demonstrate the type of information such assessments provide and their potential role in improving surveillance systems (**Box 9.1**).

## 9.1 STRENGTHENING NATIONAL SURVEILLANCE SYSTEMS

Over the past 3 years, GMP has embarked on an intensified process of improving national surveillance systems and the use of data for programmatic decision-making. This includes the development of the following information products and tools:

- the *WHO Malaria surveillance, monitoring and evaluation: a reference manual* (*38*), released in March 2018, which outlines the global standards and core features of malaria surveillance across the transmission continuum;
- malaria surveillance modules that are based on the above WHO surveillance reference manual and are built into the District Health Information Software 2 (DHIS2),[1] for burden reduction (aggregate data) and elimination (case-based data) settings, entomological surveillance and vector-control interventions;
- national malaria data repositories that consolidate routine surveillance and non-routine data sources as part of the support provided to the HBHI countries; and
- surveillance system assessments to evaluate the ability of the surveillance system to collect complete, timely and accurate data that can be used to inform decisions, stratification of transmission and deployment of interventions.

## 9.2 MALARIA MODULES

The DHIS2 malaria modules were developed, in collaboration with partners, as part of the Health Data Collaborative, which is coordinated by the WHO Integrated Services Department and includes

---

[1] https://www.dhis2.org/inaction

surveillance support activities across WHO departments dealing with health information systems; immunization; maternal, newborn and child health; tuberculosis; and HIV/AIDS. The modules comprise a standard set of data elements and indicators, validation rules and dashboards for visualization of core epidemiological and data quality indicators, as charts, tables and maps. Routine reports and data exports can be easily generated for rapid dissemination of information to decision-makers. The modules, which are configurable and can be used either separately or in conjunction with one another, are accompanied by a guidance document and a curriculum for facility-level data analysis,[1] to help programmes to understand the content and how the data can be used in practice.

### 9.2.1 Aggregate malaria module

In settings in which transmission remains relatively high and where the main aim of NMPs is to reduce the burden of morbidity and mortality, data are aggregated to provide an overall picture of where and when malaria occurs and who is most affected.[2] Surveillance data in high-transmission settings is used to monitor trends in the number of cases and deaths, over time and by geography; the characteristics of people infected or dying from malaria; and the seasonality of transmission. In high-transmission settings, surveillance data can also be used to stratify geographical units by their malaria prevalence or annual parasite incidence, to better target interventions and optimize resource allocation.

As of October 2019, 23 countries have installed the WHO aggregate malaria module and another six installations are planned over the next year (**Fig. 9.1**). Five countries have already developed and integrated their own malaria module into DHIS2.

### 9.2.2 Case-based malaria module

The case-based malaria module, due to be released soon, will support case investigations in elimination settings by allowing the collection of line-listed data for

---

[1] https://www.who.int/healthinfo/tools_data_analysis_routine_facility/en/
[2] https://www.who.int/malaria/areas/surveillance/support-tools/en/

**FIG. 9.1.**

**Status of malaria surveillance modules implemented in DHIS2, October 2019** *Source: NMPs and the African Leaders Malaria Alliance.*

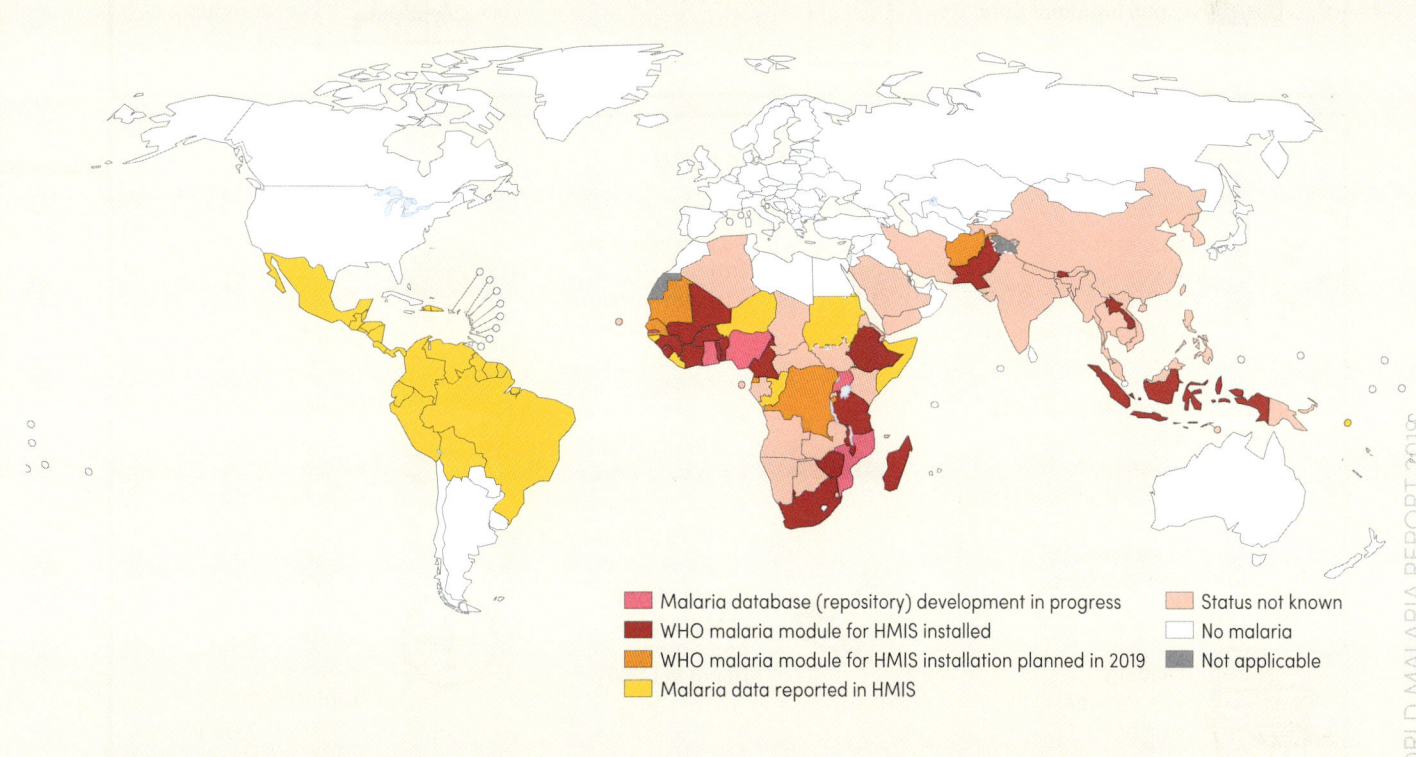

- Malaria database (repository) development in progress
- WHO malaria module for HMIS installed
- WHO malaria module for HMIS installation planned in 2019
- Malaria data reported in HMIS
- Status not known
- No malaria
- Not applicable

DHIS2: District Health Information Software 2; HMIS: health management information system; NMP: national malaria programme; WHO: World Health Organization.

# 9 Malaria surveillance

suspected cases (optional); diagnosis and treatment; treatment follow-up (optional); case investigation; and foci investigation, response and follow-up. Data will be aggregated and displayed on elimination dashboards for analysis and reporting. This work is being developed in partnership with the Clinton Health Access Initiative and the University of Oslo.

### 9.2.3 Entomology and vector control modules

These modules have been developed to facilitate the collection and use of entomology and vector-control data to inform decision-making at country level. The modules consist of electronic data collection forms, standard indicators and automatically generated dashboards that cover the following interventions areas: ITN mass campaign distribution, ITN bioefficacy monitoring, IRS campaigns, IRS residual efficacy monitoring, insecticide resistance monitoring, adult mosquito surveillance and identification, and monitoring of mosquito larval habitats. All modules have been designed based on WHO-recommended data collection protocols and standard indicators. As of November 2019, one country was already using the modules and implementation had started in another two countries. In the course of 2020, significant geographical scale-up across Africa is planned and a module for ITN durability monitoring will be developed.

### 9.2.4 National malaria data repositories

WHO has been working in coordination with national health management information systems (HMIS) departments of ministries of health, in particular the HBHI countries, to establish structured dynamic databases (**Fig. 9.2**) that support NMPs subnationally

**FIG. 9.2.**

**Proposed structure and examples of thematic areas for national malaria data repositories** *Source: WHO-GMP.*

### HMIS and LMIS data

- **Routine outpatient and inpatient data**
- **Routine interventions**
  - Case management
  - Routine LLINs
  - IPTp and IPTi
- **Stock**
  - Distribution and consumption
  - Stock-outs

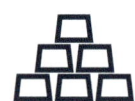

### Other data

- **Survey data**
  - Prevalence
  - Intervention coverage
  - Treatment seeking
- **Human resources/Training**
  - Health workforce
  - Training sessions
- **Climate**
  - Temperature
  - Rainfall
  - Transmission season
- **Entomological data**
  - Vector species and bionomics
  - Insecticide resistance
- **Partnership**
  - Type (local, international)
  - Areas of work
  - Type of activities
  - Funding source and budget
- **Document library**
  - Guidelines
  - SoPs
  - Operational plans
- **Drug efficacy and resistance**
- **Commodities procurement and supply (if not in LMIS)**
- Geocoded data
- Health facilities
- CHWs
- School
- Intervention micro planning
- Shapefiles, etc.
- **Funding**
  - Government
  - External

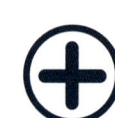

CHW: community health worker; GMP: Global Malaria Programme; HMIS: health management information system; IPTi: intermittent preventive treatment in infants; IPTp: intermittent preventive treatment in pregnancy; LLIN: long-lasting insecticidal net; LMIS: logistics management and information system; SoP: standard operating procedure; WHO: World Health Organization.

to implement targeted malaria activities informed by clear stratification, to monitor disease trends, to effectively respond to epidemics, to evaluate programme performance and to develop national strategic plans.

These national data repositories are developed either as part of WHO-supported national health observatories or as a direct service provided by the HMIS to disease programmes. GMP has developed an easily adaptable repository structure in DHIS2 with guidance on relevant data elements and indicators, their definitions and computation to cover key thematic areas (**Fig. 9.2**). So far, work to develop these databases has started in Gambia, Ghana, Mozambique, Nigeria, Uganda and the United Republic of Tanzania.

## 9.3 ASSESSMENT OF NATIONAL SURVEILLANCE SYSTEMS

Surveillance systems need to be assessed regularly to enable understanding of the quality of the data generated by the system, the use of the data to inform decision-making and the bottlenecks that impede the efficiency and effectiveness of the system. WHO recommends surveillance system assessments that monitor the following: structure, core functions, support functions and quality of surveillance (*38*).

A Mozambique case study is presented (**Box 9.1**) to illustrate the process of a surveillance assessment, the core findings and their contribution to strengthening the surveillance system.

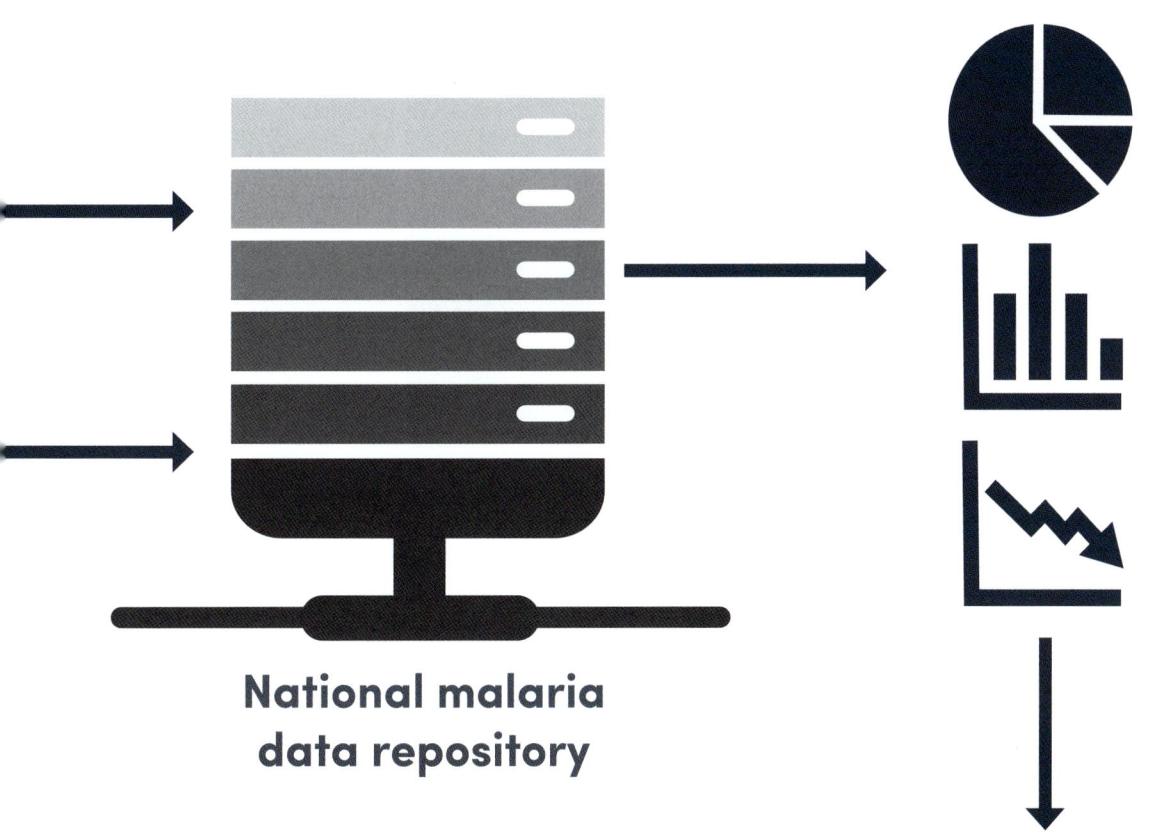

**National malaria data repository**

✓ Trigger actions sub-nationally
✓ Re-orient national malaria programme strategies
✓ Support monitoring and evaluation, malaria programme reviewers, etc.
✓ Support global reporting

# 9 Malaria surveillance

## BOX. 9.1.
## Assessing and strengthening malaria surveillance: an example from Mozambique

**Background:** In July 2017, Mozambique's national malaria programme (NMP) and partners developed a National Malaria Surveillance Roadmap that outlines the core component of a surveillance system required to support malaria elimination (**Fig. B.9.1**). To determine whether the current surveillance system was able to provide good-quality epidemiological and intervention data for timely stratification of transmission and subsequent deployment of targeted interventions, a comprehensive malaria surveillance system assessment was carried out in July 2018. The main objective of this assessment was to assess performance and to identify bottlenecks that may hinder the collection, transmission, analysis and use of data. The NMP implemented the assessment with Malaria Consortium as the lead partner. WHO provided technical support and the Bill & Melinda Gates Foundation provided funding.

**Fig. B.9.1. Surveillance components for evaluation during field assessment**

| HIS performance | HIS processes | Technical factors | Organizational factors | Behavioural factors |
|---|---|---|---|---|
| Data quality completeness | Data collection | Complexity of forms | Staff training | Self efficacy |
| Data quality timeliness | Data transmission | Availability of forms | Discussion on use of information | Promotion of a culture of information |
| Data quality completeness | Data processing /analysis | Software complexity | Promotion and use of information | Personal motivation |
| Report production | | | Supervision | |
| Display of information | | | Organizational factors | |

**Methods:** Adapted Performance Review Information System Management (PRISM) (*39*) tools were used to collect data from a sample of 80 health facilities and 58 CHW sites, in 15 randomly sampled districts across eight provinces (**Fig. B.9.2**). Technical, organizational and behavioural factors that influence key surveillance system processes and data quality were evaluated to assess the overall performance of MIS. The assessment focused on the public health sector.

**Results**: Reporting completeness was more than 90% across all administrative levels, and completeness of key data fields was more than 80% (**Fig. B.9.3**). There were challenges, however, with receiving timely reports from CHWs, and accuracy of data was poor at both health facility and CHW levels. Also, a significant number of patients who were tested with RDTs and confirmed cases treated with ACTs were not reported, which can result in stock-outs, poor commodity quantification and resource allocation. The main reason for inaccurate data was the lack of recording tools (e.g. registers and consultation books) (**Fig. B.9.4**).

**Fig. B.9.2. Map showing location of health facilities and community health worker sites from which data were collected**

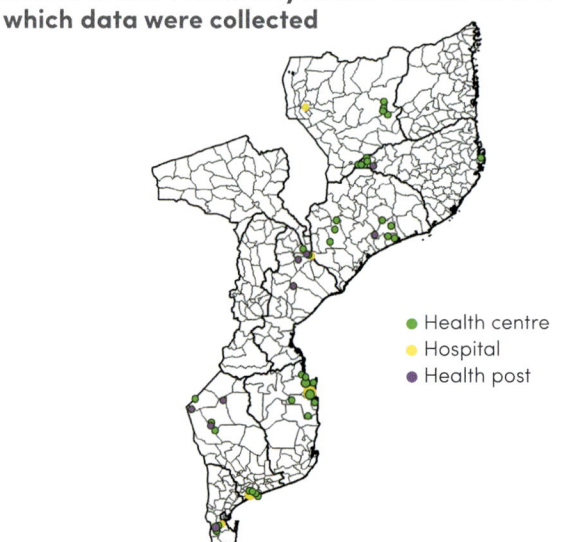

- ● Health centre
- ● Hospital
- ● Health post

With regard to data analysis and use, although the capacity to perform basic analysis and interpretation was greater than was self-perceived at both health facility (70% versus 56%) and district levels (89% versus 63%), there was a lack of regular production of analytical reports and bulletins, and the analysis carried out was limited, particularly at the health facility level. This was partly from lack of training and problems with computer and internet access. As a consequence, the district was found to be overburdened with data management responsibilities, resulting in low motivation.

**Conclusions:** Inaccurate and incomplete data have a direct impact on key epidemiological indicators that inform decision-making, strategic planning, and programmatic action at all levels. This assessment allowed the NMP of Mozambique to investigate and identify the reasons behind the suboptimal performance of MIS, and to define the activities and investments required to strengthen malaria surveillance. The key recommendations were to prioritize enforcement of data quality checks; nurture the use of information; and provide and enforce simple and clear technical guidelines for data management.

Following these recommendations, Mozambique's NMP and partners' support have initiated the following activities aimed at strengthening surveillance: capacity-building and training on quality of data to data management staff at all levels of government; initiation of integrated supportive supervision of CHWs, health facility and district malaria focal points; development of iMISS technical requirements; piloting of automated data visualization dashboards at different levels; development of standard operating procedures for routine data management activities and actions that should be undertaken in response to findings; and initiation of operational protocols for malaria case and foci investigations and responses in very low transmission settings. Lessons learned from these surveillance strengthening activities are being documented through an ongoing adaptive learning cycle, to inform improvements of surveillance system performance and guide further rollout of activities.

**Fig. B.9.3. Reporting completeness**

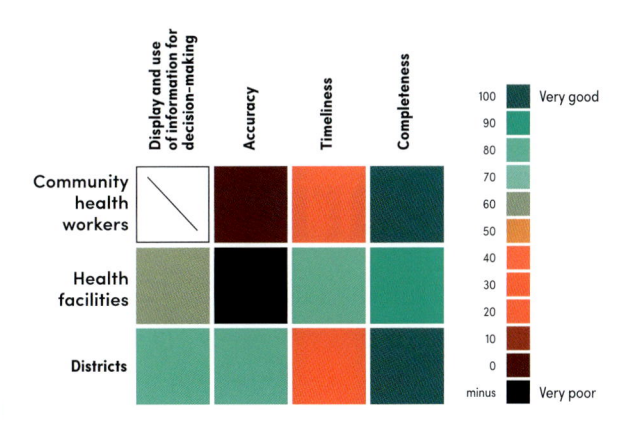

**Fig. B.9.4. Proportion of health facilities with data verification carried out in the past 3 months**

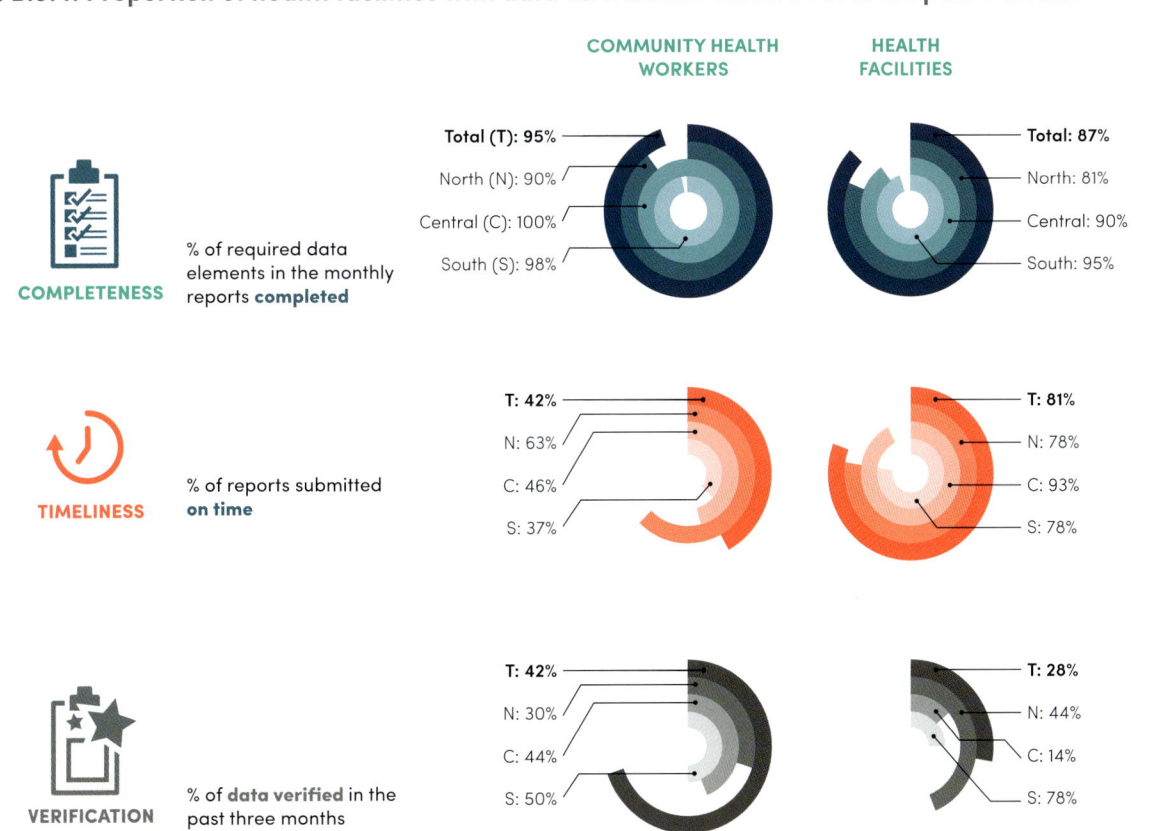

COMMUNITY HEALTH WORKERS | HEALTH FACILITIES

**COMPLETENESS** — % of required data elements in the monthly reports **completed**
- Community health workers: Total (T): 95%, North (N): 90%, Central (C): 100%, South (S): 98%
- Health facilities: Total: 87%, North: 81%, Central: 90%, South: 95%

**TIMELINESS** — % of reports submitted **on time**
- Community health workers: T: 42%, N: 63%, C: 46%, S: 37%
- Health facilities: T: 81%, N: 78%, C: 93%, S: 78%

**VERIFICATION** — % of **data verified** in the past three months
- Community health workers: T: 42%, N: 30%, C: 44%, S: 50%
- Health facilities: T: 28%, N: 44%, C: 14%, S: 78%

# 10 Responding to biological threats to the fight against malaria

The GTS (*1*) recognizes challenges in the fight against malaria, including the lack of robust, predictable and sustained international and domestic financing; the risks posed by conflict and other complex situations; the emergence of parasite resistance to antimalarial medicines and of mosquito resistance to insecticides; and the inadequate performance of health systems. One of WHO's major roles is to bring emerging challenges to the attention of the global community and to coordinate responses to address these challenges. This section of the report documents these challenges and proposed responses.

## 10.1 *PF-HRP2/3* GENE DELETIONS

HRP2 is the predominant target of the 412 million *P. falciparum*-detecting malaria RDTs sold annually. Parasites that no longer express HRP2 may not be detectable by HRP2-based RDTs, and those that no longer express HRP2 and HRP3 are completely invisible to these RDTs. Deletions in the *pfhrp2* and *pfhrp3* (*pfhrp2/3*) genes of clinical isolates were first identified in 2010 in the Peruvian Amazon basin by researchers characterizing blood samples that were negative by HRP2-RDTs but positive by microscopy. In recent years, *pfhrp2/3* deleted parasites have been documented outside of South America, including in East, Central, West and Southern Africa, in Asia and in the Middle East. Prevalence estimates vary widely both within and between countries. The examples of Eritrea and Peru, where the prevalence of dual *pfhrp2* and *pfhrp3* deletions among symptomatic patients reached as high as 80%, demonstrate that these parasites can become dominant in the population, posing a serious global threat to patients and the continued use of HRP2-based RDTs.

WHO has published guidance on investigating suspected *pfhrp2/3* deletions (*40*), and recommends that countries that have reports of *pfhrp2/3* deletions or that border countries with reports should conduct representative baseline surveys among suspected malaria cases, to determine whether the prevalence of *pfhrp2/3* deletions causing false negative RDT results has reached a threshold for RDT change (>5% *pfhrp2* deletions causing false negative RDT results). Alternative RDT options (e.g. based on detection of the parasite's lactate dehydrogenase [pLDH]) are limited; in particular, there is a lack of WHO-prequalified non-HRP2 combination tests that can detect and distinguish between *P. falciparum* and *P. vivax*.

WHO is tracking published reports of *pfhrp2/3* deletions using the Malaria Threat Map mapping tool,[1] and is encouraging a harmonized approach to mapping and reporting *pfhrp2/3* deletions through publicly available survey protocols. To date, 28 countries have reported *pfhrp2* deletions, but owing

---
[1] https://apps.who.int/malaria/maps/threats/

to variable methods in sample selection and laboratory analysis, the scale and scope of clinically significant *pfhrp2/3* deletions have not been fully elucidated. The WHO Global Response Plan for *pfhrp2/3* deletions outlines several areas for action beyond scaling up surveillance; the plan includes discovery of new biomarkers and improving the performance of non-HRP2 RDTs, as well as market forecasting and strengthened laboratory networks to support the demands of molecular characterization to rule in or rule out the presence of these gene deletions.

## 10.2 PARASITE RESISTANCE – STATUS OF ANTIMALARIAL DRUG EFFICACY (2010–2018)

*Plasmodium* resistance to antimalarial medicines is one of the key recurring challenges in the fight against malaria. Monitoring antimalarial drug efficacy supports early detection of changes in how well the recommended treatments work; this enables rapid action to mitigate any impact of resistance and prevent its spread. Therapeutic efficacy studies (TESs) provide a measure of clinical and parasitological patient outcomes, and are the main source of data on which the NMPs base their decisions regarding which treatment to recommend (*41*). In areas implementing malaria elimination activities, the routine surveillance system can track treatment and follow-up of all malaria cases, and use the data generated for integrated drug efficacy surveillance (iDES) (*38*). Information from TESs and iDES is supplemented by information on the prevalence and spread of molecular markers – genetic changes in the parasite – that are found to be associated with resistance. *PfKelch13* mutations have been identified as molecular markers of partial artemisinin resistance. *PfKelch13* mutations associated with artemisinin resistance are widespread in the GMS in South-East Asia, and have also been detected at a significant prevalence (over 5%) in Guyana, Papua New Guinea and Rwanda.

The WHO global database on antimalarial drug efficacy and resistance contains data from TESs conducted on *P. falciparum*, *P. vivax*, *P. knowlesi*, *P. malaria* and *P. ovale*, as well as molecular marker studies of *P. falciparum* drug resistance (*PfKelch13*, *PfPlasmepsin 2-3*, *Pfmdr1* and *Pfcrt* in Mesoamerica). Summary reports are regularly updated and are available on the WHO website (*42*). In addition, the Malaria Threats Maps provide a geographical representation of drug efficacy and resistance data.[1]

This section outlines the status of antimalarial drug efficacy in the WHO regions for 2010–2018.

### WHO African Region

The first-line treatments used in most African countries for *P. falciparum* are artemether-lumefantrine (AL) and artesunate-amodiaquine (AS-AQ), with some countries' treatment policies also allowing for the use of dihydroartemisinin-piperaquine (DHA-PPQ). Between 2010 and 2018, treatment efficacy data for AL were available from 28 countries, for AS-AQ from 26 and for DHA-PPQ from 14. The overall average efficacy rates of AL, AS-AQ and DHA-PPQ for *P. falciparum* were 98.0%, 98.5% and 99.3%, respectively. When the failure rates of all three treatments were analysed separately by year, it was found that their high efficacy has remained constant over time. Treatment failure rates above 10% detected in Gambia and Malawi in 2010 are likely to be statistical outliers; recent studies show that most treatment failure rates remain low. The high reported failure rate from two studies in Angola was probably due to methodological issues. For all other medicines, treatment failure rates remain below 10%.

In Africa, artemisinin partial resistance has not yet been confirmed. Surveys are detecting a number of different validated and unvalidated *PfKelch13* mutations at low prevalence, except in Rwanda, where clearance and efficacy of the first-line treatment AL does not seem to be affected. There have been unconvincing case reports of travellers returning from Africa with malaria and not responding as expected to treatment. These include a Vietnamese male returning in 2013 to Viet Nam from Angola, who developed malaria that did not respond to intravenous artesunate, clindamycin or DHA-PPQ (*43*). Another case was reported in a Chinese male, who developed malaria 8 weeks after returning from Equatorial Guinea in 2013. The patient responded to treatment with DHA-PPQ but had low-level parasitaemia on day 3 after the start of treatment, and the infection was identified as carrying the *PfKelch13* mutation M579I, previously only reported once in Myanmar (*44, 45*). Three recent surveys conducted in Equatorial Guinea did not identify M579 among a total of 721 samples.

Eleven cases of treatment failure were reported in European travellers returning from different locations in Africa and treated with DHA-PPQ or AL (*46–48*). The patients were infected with parasites not carrying *PfKelch13* mutations, and molecular markers or blood levels of the partner medicines could not confirm resistance. Combined, these cases do not provide convincing evidence for the presence of resistance to artemisinin or ACT partner drugs in Africa. Nevertheless, reporting on these cases is important because

---

[1] https://apps.who.int/malaria/maps/threats/

# 10 Responding to biological threats to the fight against malaria

resistance or treatment failures in travellers could be an early warning signal, supplementing the information collected in the endemic countries.

The *P. vivax* species is only endemic in a few countries in the WHO African Region. TESs with chloroquine (CQ) were conducted in Ethiopia, Madagascar and Mauritania. Ethiopia confirmed high rates of treatment failure for both CQ and AL. The high failure rate of AL without primaquine (PQ) is probably caused by the short half-life of artemisinin, which fails to prevent the first relapse. Madagascar monitored the efficacy of AS-AQ in 2012 and 2013, and Mauritania monitored CQ in 2012. The efficacy in these studies was found to be 100%.

## WHO Region of the Americas

The first-line treatments for *P. falciparum* in the Amazon region are AL and artesunate-mefloquine (AS-MQ). Treatment efficacy was high for both medicines. One treatment failure was detected in a TES of AL, conducted in Suriname, among 11 patients. In Guatemala, Haiti, Honduras and Nicaragua, where the first-line treatment is CQ, molecular marker studies of *Pfcrt* are conducted to supplement TESs. Between 2010 and 2018, a low prevalence of *Pfcrt* mutation was observed in Haiti, Honduras and Nicaragua. TESs almost always confirmed the high efficacy of CQ in these countries.

A retrospective study of Guyanese samples collected in 2010 identified the *PfKelch13* mutation C580Y in five out of 98 samples (5.1%). A larger survey done in 2016–2017 found C580Y in 14 out of 877 samples (1.6%). Genetic studies have confirmed that these parasites were not imported from South-East Asia; rather, the mutation emerged in parasites of South American origin.

The first-line treatment policy for *P. vivax* in all endemic countries in this region is CQ. Between 2010 and 2018, TESs of *P. vivax* were conducted in Bolivia (Plurinational State of), Brazil, Colombia, Peru and Venezuela (Bolivarian Republic of). All countries conducted studies for *P. vivax* with CQ alone or with CQ and PQ. One study conducted in the Plurinational State of Bolivia confirmed CQ resistance. Additionally, Brazil conducted studies of AS-AQ, AL+PQ and AS-MQ+PQ. None of these resulted in treatment failures above 10%.

## WHO South-East Asia Region

In Bhutan, Nepal and Timor-Leste, the first-line treatment policy for *P. falciparum* is AL. TESs conducted in these countries between 2010 and 2013 found high treatment efficacy, with less than 10% treatment failure.

Indonesia monitored DHA-PPQ efficacy between 2010 and 2017. All studies resulted in less than 10% treatment failures.

In Bangladesh, the first-line treatment policy includes AL, AS-AQ, AS-MQ and DHA-PPQ. Bangladesh monitored AL treatment failure between 2010 and 2018, and found rates above 10% in two studies, each with a small number of patients.

India's first-line treatment policy includes AL and AS-SP. India has extensively monitored the efficacy of AS-SP and found treatment failure rates ranging from 0% to 21.4%. Failure rates above 10% in north-eastern parts of India led to the treatment policy in this region changing to AL. All studies conducted for AL in India between 2011 and 2017 found treatment failure rates to be less than 10%.

Thailand's first-line treatment policy was AS-MQ until treatment failure rates began to progressively increase. The first-line treatment was changed to DHA-PPQ in 2015. Treatment failure for DHA-PPQ was monitored between 2014 and 2017, and treatment failure rates as high as 92.9% (13/14) were detected in 2017 in the north-eastern part of the country, probably from importation of malaria from Cambodia. As a result, the first-line treatment has since been changed to artesunate-pyronaridine (AS-PY) in eastern Thailand.

Myanmar's first-line treatment policy includes AL, AS-MQ and DHA-PPQ. Treatment failure rates were less than 10% despite the high prevalence of artemisinin partial resistance. In addition, Myanmar monitored AS-PY efficacy in four studies in 2017 and 2018, and found the treatment to be 100% efficacious.

The presence of molecular markers of artemisinin resistance has been reported in Bangladesh, India, Myanmar and Thailand. In Myanmar, seven different validated mutations have been reported, and the most frequently identified since 2010 is F446I. In Thailand, eight different validated mutations have been reported. In western Thailand, it is still possible to identify a range of different K13 mutations, whereas C580Y is becoming dominant in eastern Thailand. In Bangladesh, one C580Y mutation has been identified in a sample collected in 2018. Recently, two articles reported the emergence of artemisinin resistance in West Bengal, India based on the results from a TES with AS-SP done in the period 2014–2016 (*49*, *50*). Among the 226 patients in the study, 10.6% (24/226) were found to have parasite clearance half-lives of more than 5 hours, 5.8% (13/226) were found to carry the *PfKelch13* mutation G625R, and 0.9% (2/226) carried R539T. The treatment failure rate was 8% (18/226). These results should be interpreted with caution (*51*). The data contrast with other available data on drug efficacy from India, including from West Bengal. *PfKelch13* mutations are rare in India, and the G625R mutation has not yet been validated as an artemisinin resistance marker; further investigation is needed to examine the role of G625R in delayed parasite clearance. TESs are now being conducted in West Bengal, with an evaluation of parasite clearance times and analysis of *PfKelch13* mutations. Until appropriate validation and external quality control is completed, it is premature to claim that artemisinin resistance has emerged in India.

For *P. vivax*, CQ is the first-line treatment in Bangladesh, Bhutan, the Democratic People's Republic of Korea, India, Myanmar, Nepal, Sri Lanka and Thailand. DHA-PPQ is the first-line treatment in Indonesia, and AL in Timor-Leste. Although most studies demonstrated high efficacy of CQ, high failure rates of treatment with CQ were confirmed in Myanmar and Timor-Leste.

## WHO Eastern Mediterranean Region

Studies conducted in Somalia and Sudan between 2011 and 2015 detected high failure rates of treatment with AS-SP, ranging from 12.3% to 22.2%. The evidence prompted a decision to change the new first-line treatment policy to AL. Therefore, the first-line treatment for *P. falciparum* in Afghanistan, Djibouti, Pakistan, Somalia and Sudan is AL. The efficacy of AL has been monitored in each of these countries, except in Djibouti. All TESs show low rates of AL treatment failure (<5%).

For infection with *P. vivax*, the first-line treatment policy is AL in Somalia and Sudan, and CQ in Afghanistan, Djibouti, Iran (Islamic Republic of), Pakistan, Saudi Arabia and Yemen. TESs of AL were conducted in Afghanistan and Sudan, and TESs of CQ were conducted in Iran (Islamic Republic of) and Pakistan. All studies showed high treatment efficacy. A study conducted in Pakistan in 2013 for DHA-PPQ detected one treatment failure among 103 cases (1%).

## WHO Western Pacific Region

For *P. falciparum*, AL is the first-line treatment policy in countries outside the GMS as well as in Lao People's Democratic Republic. All studies conducted outside of the GMS resulted in failure rates of less than 10% for treatment with AL. In Lao People's Democratic Republic, treatment failure rates above 10% were found in three of nine studies between 2011 and 2017. However, the recommended samples sizes were not achieved.

In Cambodia, AS-MQ is the current first-line treatment. AS-MQ replaced DHA-PPQ after high rates of treatment failure were observed. Of the 17 studies conducted with AS-MQ since 2014, the treatment failure rate has been less than 2%. One study of AL found a treatment failure rate of 5% (3/60). The most recent studies with AS-PY in 2017 and 2018 showed efficacy of more than 95%. Treatment failure rates for AS-AQ ranged between 13.8% and 22.6%.

In Viet Nam, the first-line treatment policy is DHA-PPQ. Of the 42 TESs of DHA-PPQ conducted between 2010 and 2017, five studies detected treatment failure rates between 14.3% and 46.3%, all from 2015 to 2017. These studies were concentrated in the south, in the neighbouring provinces of Dak Nong and Binh Phuoc. Most recently, high failure rates for treatment with DHA-PPQ were observed in a third province, Dak Lak. Viet Nam has also monitored the efficacy of AL and AS-PY, with overall efficacies of 100% and 95.5%, respectively. Papua New Guinea monitored the efficacy of DHA-PPQ, and Malaysia monitored that of AS-MQ; both countries found 100% treatment efficacy for these medicines.

Artemisinin resistance has been confirmed in Cambodia, Lao People's Democratic Republic and Viet Nam through several studies conducted between 2001 and 2018. Between 2010 and 2018, eight *PfKelch13* mutations were identified in Cambodia and Lao People's Democratic Republic. C580Y was the most frequent, with about 71.7% of the genotypes carrying this mutation. In Viet Nam, six *PfKelch13* mutations were identified, and C580Y was also the most predominant, appearing on an average of 33.3% of the genotypes. The *PfKelch13* mutation C580Y has been identified twice in Papua New Guinea: in a survey in 2017 where 2.3% (3/132) of the samples carried the mutation (the percentage was higher in 2018) and in one traveller. No validated molecular markers of artemisinin resistance were found in studies conducted in Malaysia, the Philippines, Solomon Islands or Vanuatu.

The first-line treatment for *P. vivax* in Lao People's Democratic Republic, Malaysia, Papua New Guinea, Solomon Islands and Vanuatu is AL. High failure rates of treatment with AL were observed in Papua New Guinea (35% in 2011), Solomon Islands (31.6% in 2011), and Vanuatu (12.1% in 2013). These high rates in areas where early relapses occur are possibly explained by the short half-life of lumefantrine. In China, the Republic of Korea and Viet Nam, the first-line treatment for *P. vivax* is CQ. China and Viet Nam conducted TESs of CQ; only Viet Nam detected a treatment failure rate above 10% in 2015. In the Philippines, the recommended first-line treatments for *P. vivax* are AL and CQ. The nine studies in the Philippines conducted on CQ between 2010 and 2016 all showed treatment failure rates below 10%. In Cambodia, the first-line treatment for *P. vivax* is AS-MQ. Three recent TESs conducted in Cambodia showed 100% efficacy for AS-MQ. The efficacy of AS-MQ was also monitored in Lao People's Democratic Republic and Malaysia between 2012 and 2018. Both studies showed 100% efficacy. The efficacy of DHA-PPQ was monitored in Cambodia, Papua New Guinea and Viet Nam between 2010 and 2015. All studies found treatment failure rates below 10%.

# 10 Responding to biological threats to the fight against malaria

## 10.3 VECTOR RESISTANCE TO INSECTICIDES

Resistance of malaria vectors to insecticides commonly used for malaria vector control – namely, pyrethroids, organophosphates, carbamates and the occasionally used organochlorine dichlorodiphenyltrichloroethane (DDT) – threatens malaria control and elimination efforts.

From 2010 through 2018, some 81 countries reported data from a total of 3075 sites to WHO, 10% more sites than in the period 2010–2017. The extent and frequency of insecticide resistance monitoring continue to vary considerably between countries. Of these 81 countries, 63 reported insecticide resistance monitoring data at least once within the past 3 years and 18 did not. Only 59 out of the 81 countries reported on their insecticide resistance status consistently every year for the past 3 years. The number of sites per country for which resistance monitoring data were reported between 2010 and 2018 varied widely, from a single site to 271 sites.

A total of 73 countries confirmed resistance to at least one insecticide in one malaria vector species from one mosquito collection site within the period 2010–2018, an increase of five countries compared with the previous reporting period (2010–2017). The number of countries that reported insecticide resistance to all four main insecticide classes used to date in at least one malaria vector species increased from 22 to 26, and the number of countries that reported resistance to three of these four classes in at least one malaria vector species increased from 16 to 18. Of those countries that reported insecticide resistance monitoring data to WHO, the proportion of countries that confirmed resistance to each of these insecticide classes was 87.5% for pyrethroids, 81.5% for organochlorines, 68% for carbamates and 56% for organophosphates. Only eight of the countries that reported data did not confirm resistance to any insecticide class.

Resistance to the four insecticide classes mentioned above was detected in all WHO regions except for the WHO European Region. Globally, resistance to pyrethroids was detected in at least one malaria vector in 68% of the sites for which data were available, and resistance to organochlorines was detected in 63% of the sites. Resistance to carbamates and organophosphates was less prevalent, being detected in 31% and 26%, respectively, of the sites that reported monitoring data. However, the geographical extent of confirmed resistance to each insecticide class differed considerably across regions (**Fig. 10.1**).

Collection and reporting of data to guide deployment of recently prequalified vector control tools covered by WHO policy recommendations have significantly improved. Further enhancement will be needed to guide strategic deployment of tools currently undergoing WHO evaluation. Until 2018, a total of 17 countries had monitored the involvement of metabolic resistance mechanisms in pyrethroid resistance by means of piperonyl butoxide (PBO) pre-exposure bioassays. By 2018, the number of countries reporting data from these bioassays to WHO rose to 23, all of which detected partial or full involvement of metabolic resistance mechanisms in phenotypic resistance to pyrethroids in at least one monitoring site for at least one vector species and one pyrethroid insecticide. Of the 190 sites for which data were reported until 2018, 187 detected full or partial involvement of metabolic resistance mechanisms for at least one vector species and one pyrethroid insecticide.

Results of biochemical and molecular assays conducted to detect metabolic resistance mechanisms are available for 24 countries and 160 sites for the period 2010–2018. Mono-oxygenases were detected in 64% of the sites for which reports are available (84/160), glutathione-S-transferases were detected in 76% of the sites (83/160) and esterases in 77% of the sites (114/160). Results of assays conducted to detect target-site resistance mechanisms are now available for 43 countries and 628 sites. *Kdr L1014F* was detected in 76% of the sites (514/628) and *Kdr L1014S* in 42% of the sites (311/628).

Recently, WHO Member States and their implementing partners have started to explore procedures and dosages to monitor resistance to neonicotinoid and pyrrole insecticides. A formal WHO process to establish discriminating dosages and test procedures for these two insecticide classes is ongoing and will be completed in 2020. The data on mosquito mortality after exposure to neonicotinoid and pyrrole insecticides reported so far to WHO will be assessed against these discriminating dosages once they have been finalized. WHO test procedures for insecticide resistance monitoring will be updated in 2020 to incorporate the new discriminating dosages and potential changes to the test procedures.

All the standard insecticide resistance data reported to WHO are included in the WHO Global Insecticide Resistance Database and are available for exploration via the online mapping tool, Malaria Threats Map.[1] This tool was extended in 2019 to cover a fourth threat to malaria control and elimination: invasive mosquito vector species. At present, this new theme shows the geographical extent of reports on the detection of *Anopheles stephensi*; it may be further extended to other invasive vector species as reported to WHO.

---
[1] https://apps.who.int/malaria/maps/threats/

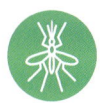

## 10.3.1 Mitigating and managing insecticide resistance

Among other considerations, the selection of effective vector-control interventions needs to be based on routine and representative data on the susceptibility of local vectors to insecticides recommended and prequalified by WHO. In addition, insecticide resistance data are crucial for assessing the potential impact that resistance may have on the effectiveness of malaria vector control, an area that continues to be poorly understood. To meet these data needs, countries and their partners are advised to conduct regular insecticide resistance monitoring following the WHO-recommended *Test procedures for insecticide resistance monitoring in malaria vector mosquitoes* (*52*), and to report and share results in a timely manner. To facilitate reporting, WHO has developed and supports the rollout of data-reporting templates and DHIS2 modules for use by its Member States and their implementing partners.

Ultimately, it is likely that insecticide resistance will reduce the efficacy of currently available interventions. Countries should therefore not delay the development and application of policies and practices for resistance prevention, mitigation and management. Two relatively

**FIG. 10.1.**

**Reported insecticide resistance status as a proportion of sites for which monitoring was conducted, by WHO region, 2010–2018, (a) Pyrethroids, (b) Organochlorines, (c) Carbamates, (d) Organophosphates** Status was based on mosquito mortality where <90% = confirmed resistance, 90–97% = possible resistance, and ≥98% = susceptibility. Where multiple insecticide classes or types, mosquito species or time points were tested at an individual site, the highest resistance status was considered. Numbers above bars indicate the total number of sites for which data were reported (n). *Sources: reports from NMPs and national health institutes, their implementation partners, research institutions and scientific publications.*

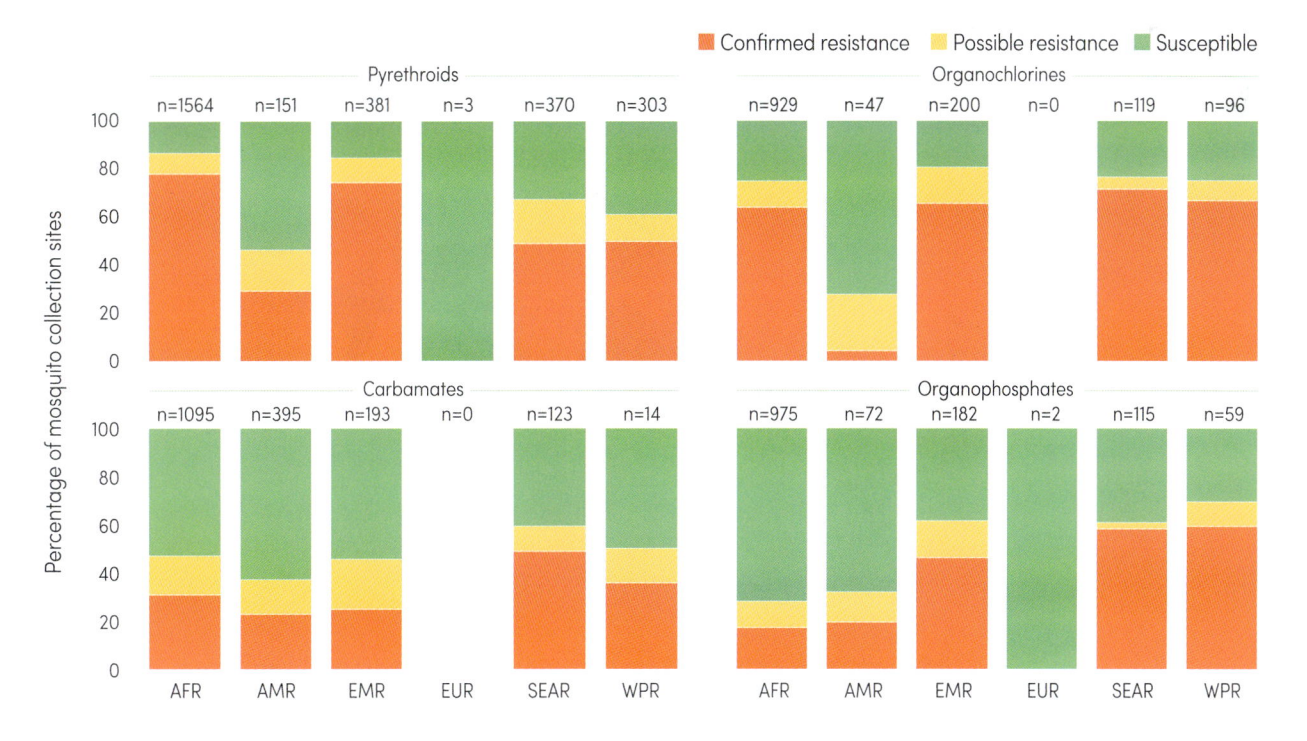

AFR: WHO African Region; AMR: WHO Region of the Americas; EMR: WHO Eastern Mediterranean Region; EUR: WHO European Region; n: number; NMP: national malaria programme; SEAR: WHO South-East Asia Region; WHO: World Health Organization; WPR: WHO Western Pacific Region.

# 10 Responding to biological threats to the fight against malaria

new vector control options that should be considered as part of a strategy to mitigate or manage insecticide resistance – pyrethroid-PBO nets and neonicotinoid insecticides for IRS – have been recommended by WHO in the past 2 years; a number of prequalified products are now available, as well as a high-level map to support in-country discussion on pyrethroid-PBO net deployment (**Fig. 10.2**). Additional vector-control interventions to provide options for insecticide resistance management or to address outdoor transmission are under development; a number of these are already under WHO evaluation, supported by the WHO Vector Control Advisory Group.

To guide resistance management, countries should develop and implement a national plan for insecticide-resistance monitoring and management, drawing on the WHO *Framework for a national plan for monitoring and management of insecticide resistance in malaria vectors* (*53*). Through 2018, some countries have made progress in developing such plans. By the end of 2018 a total of 45 countries had finalized plans for resistance monitoring and management, and 36 were developing them. Further effort and support will be required to ensure that every country has such a plan, updates it regularly and has the necessary resources to implement it.

**FIG. 10.2.**

**Status of monitoring WHO-recommended criteria for pyrethroid-PBO net deployment, 2010–2018** NMPs and their partners should consider the deployment of pyrethroid-PBO nets in areas where the main malaria vectors meet the criteria recommended by WHO in 2017 (*54*). Deployment of pyrethroid-PBO nets should be guided by whether geographical areas of operational relevance (e.g. districts or provinces) – rather than the whole country – meet the criteria specified by WHO and should be considered in the context of resource availability and potential for deployment of alternative malaria control interventions. *Sources: reports from NMPs and national health institutes, their implementation partners, research institutions and scientific publications.*

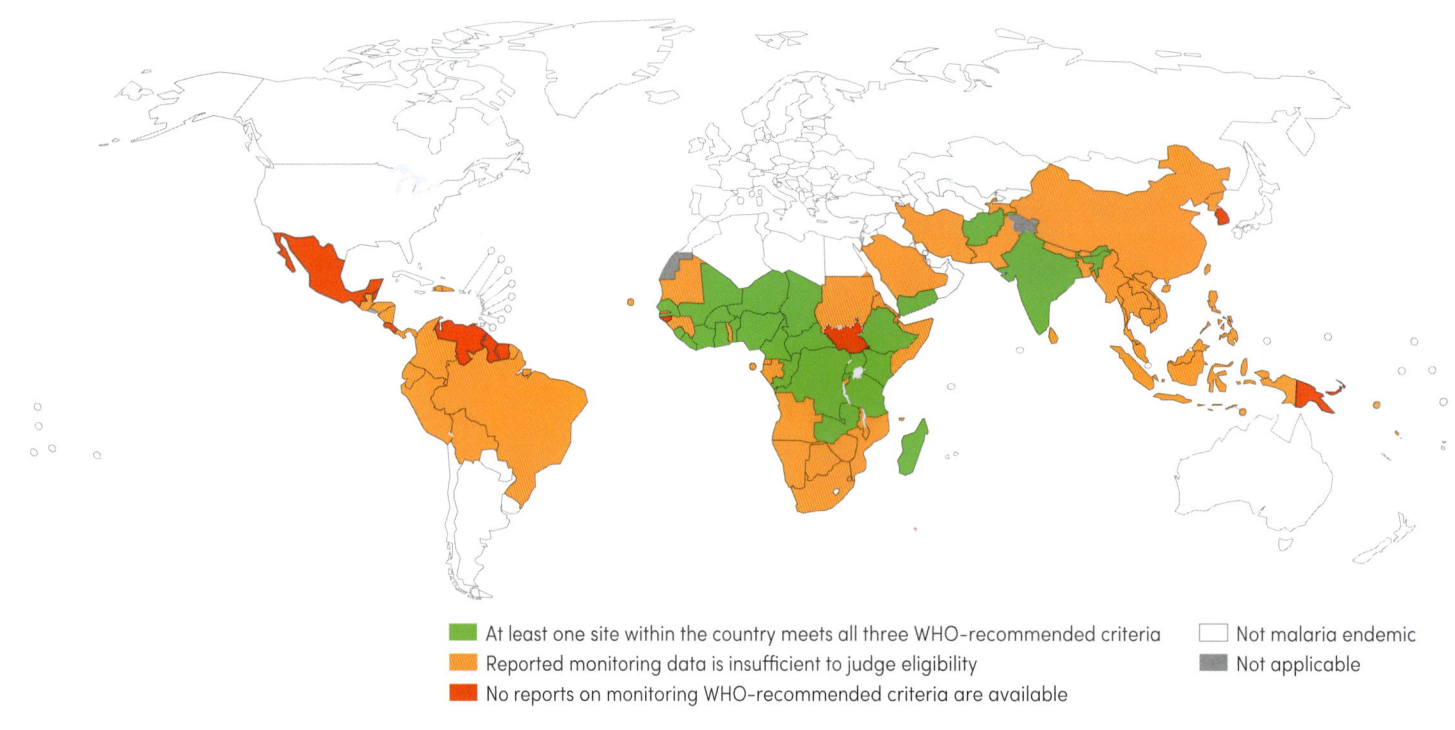

NMP: national malaria programme; PBO: piperonyl butoxide; WHO: World Health Organization.

# 11 Conclusion

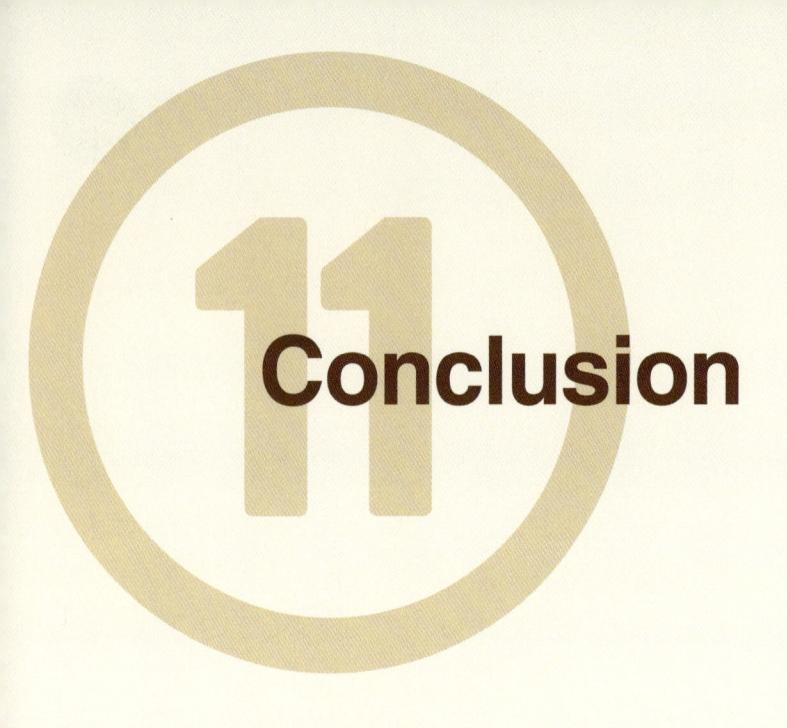

WHO's *World malaria report 2019* summarizes global progress in the fight against malaria up to the end of 2018. This is the fourth world malaria report since the launch of the GTS (*1*). From a baseline of 2015, the GTS aims to achieve, by 2020, a reduction of 40% of malaria morbidity incidence and mortality rate, elimination in at least 10 countries and prevention of reintroduction in all countries that achieved elimination (*1*). To this end, the analysis shows that in 2018 there were an estimated 228 million cases and 405 000 deaths globally, concentrated mainly in Africa and India. This represents about 3 million fewer cases and 11 000 fewer deaths compared with 2017.

On the one hand, the analysis shows that if malaria case incidence and mortality rate remained the same as those in 2000, globally there would be 320 million cases and nearly 1 million malaria deaths in 2018. Instead, there were an estimated 228 million malaria cases and 405 000 malaria deaths in 2018. These represent about 30% fewer cases and 60% fewer deaths in 2018 than would have been the case had levels of malaria incidence and malaria death remained similar to those in 2000. While the gains to date are impressive, the global malaria challenge remains enormous, and the rate of progress is slowing. For example, on the current trajectory, globally, the 2020 GTS milestones for morbidity will not be achieved, and unless there is accelerated change, the 2025 and 2030 milestones will not be achieved. A global malaria case incidence of 45 per 1000 population at risk in 2018 would have been required to get the world on target for the 2020 milestones, but current estimated incidence is 57 cases per 1000 population at risk. If the current trend in incidence is maintained, estimated malaria case incidence (per 1000 population at risk) would be 54 in 2020, 48 in 2025 and 42 in 2030, instead of the 35, 14 and 6 required to achieve the GTS milestones.

Progress towards the GTS elimination goals is on track. At least 10 countries that are part of the WHO E-2020 initiative are on track to reach the 2020 elimination milestone of our global malaria strategy. In 2015, all of these countries were malaria endemic; now they have either achieved zero malaria cases or are nearing the finish line. Across the six countries of the GMS – Cambodia, China (Yunnan Province), Lao People's Democratic Republic, Myanmar, Thailand and Viet Nam – there was a 76% reduction in malaria cases and a 95% reduction in deaths in the period 2010–2018. Notably, the report shows a steep decline in cases of *P. falciparum* malaria, the primary target in view of the ongoing threat of antimalarial drug resistance. In 2018, Cambodia reported zero malaria-related deaths for the first time in the country's history, China reported its second consecutive year of zero indigenous malaria cases and Thailand reported a 38% drop in *P. falciparum* cases compared with the previous year.

By November 2019, the HBHI approach had been initiated in nine high-burden countries in Africa. Countries have developed detailed activity plans to address the challenges revealed during the assessments. Two HBHI countries achieved significant reductions in malaria cases in 2018 compared with previous year – India (2.6 million fewer cases) and Uganda (1.5 million fewer cases). Notable increases were estimated in Ghana and Nigeria; however, overall, malaria case incidence and mortality rates continued to decline, but at a slower rate in recent years.

In 2018, total funding for malaria control and elimination reached an estimated US$ 2.7 billion, falling far short of the US$ 5 billion funding target of the GTS. Moreover, the funding gap widened between 2017 and 2018, from US $1.3 billion to US $2.3 billion. Over the period 2010–2018, nearly 70% of total malaria funding in 2018 was provided by international sources. Governments of malaria endemic countries contributed about 30% of total funding, with investments reaching US $0.9 billion in 2018. Of the US $2.7 billion invested in 2018, the government of the USA contributed about $1 billion; the United Kingdom contributed about $200 million; and France, Japan and Germany each contributed about $100 million. About US $1 billion in malaria funding was channelled through the Global Fund. Approximately three quarters of total funding benefited the WHO African Region, followed by the WHO Region of the Americas (7%), the WHO South-East Asia Region (6%), and the WHO Eastern Mediterranean Region and the WHO Western Pacific Region (5% each).

The scourge of malaria continues to strike hardest against pregnant women and children in Africa. The *World malaria report 2019* includes a special section focused on the burden and consequences of the disease among these two most-at-risk groups. In 2018, an estimated 11 million pregnant women in sub-Saharan Africa were infected with malaria, and 872 000 children were born with a low birthweight. About 24 million children in the region were estimated to be infected with the *P. falciparum* parasite in 2018; of these, 12 million had moderate anaemia and 1.8 million had severe anaemia. An estimated 70% of all malaria deaths globally, most of which were in sub-Saharan Africa, were of children aged under 5 years.

In 2018, 31% of pregnant women in 36 African countries received the recommended three or more doses of IPTp, up from 22% in 2017 and 0% in 2010. Notably, Burkina Faso and the United Republic of Tanzania reached IPTp coverage of more than 50% in 2018. Nearly 40% of pregnant women and children aged under 5 years did not sleep under an ITN in 2018. In the same year, two thirds of pregnant women also did not receive the recommended three or more doses of preventive therapy. In Africa's Sahel subregion, WHO recommends SMC during the peak transmission season. More than 60% of children living in SMC-eligible areas benefited from this preventive therapy in 2018. A high proportion of febrile children in sub-Saharan Africa (36%) do not receive any medical attention. Although impressive gains have been made in preventing and treating malaria in pregnant women and children, important gaps in access to care remain. Effective and equitable delivery of primary health care interventions is required to rapidly reduce the burden of malaria among these vulnerable groups.

# References

1. Global technical strategy for malaria 2016–2030. Geneva: World Health Organization; 2015 (https://www.who.int/malaria/areas/global_technical_strategy/en, accessed 20 October 2019).

2. Roll Back Malaria Partnership Secretariat. Action and investment to defeat malaria 2016–2030. For a malaria-free world. Geneva: World Health Organization; 2015 (https://endmalaria.org/sites/default/files/RBM_AIM_Report_0.pdf, accessed 20 October 2019).

3. Sustainable Development Goals: 17 goals to transform our world [website]. United Nations; 2015 (https://www.un.org/sustainabledevelopment/sustainable-development-goals, accessed 20 October 2019).

4. Thirteenth general programme of work 2019–2023 [website]. Geneva: World Health Organization; 2018 (https://www.who.int/about/what-we-do/gpw-thirteen-consultation/en/, accessed 20 October 2019).

5. Malaria and the UN Sustainable Development Goals (SDGs) 2030. Swiss Tropical and Public Health Institute (TPH) Swiss TPH for the Swiss Malaria Group; 2018 (https://www.swissmalariagroup.ch/fr/assets/uploads/files/New%20factsheet%20Malaria%20and%20the%20UN%20Sustainable%20Development%20Goals%20x.pdf, accessed 20 October 2019).

6. Country profiles [website]. Geneva: World Health Organization; (https:///www.who.int/malaria/publications/country-profiles/en/, accessed 20 October 2019).

7. Malaria in pregnant women. Geneva: World Health Organization; 2017 (https://www.who.int/malaria/areas/high_risk_groups/pregnancy/en/, accessed 20 October 2019).

8. Stevens GA, Finucame MM, De-Regil LM, Paciorek CJ, Flaxman SR, Branca F et al. Global, regional, and national trends in haemoglobin concentration and prevalence of total and severe anaemia in children and pregnant and non-pregnant women for 1995-2011: a systematic analysis of population-representative data. Lancet Glob Health. 2013 Jul;1(1):e16-25 (https://www.ncbi.nlm.nih.gov/pubmed/25103581, accessed 14 November 2019).

9. Guyatt HL, Snow RW. The epidemiology and burden of *Plasmodium falciparum*-related anemia among pregnant women in sub-Saharan Africa. Am J Trop Med Hyg. 2001 Jan-Feb;64(1-2 Suppl):36-44 (https://www.ncbi.nlm.nih.gov/pubmed/11425176, accessed 14 November 2019).

10. Guyatt HL, Snow RW. Impact of malaria during pregnancy on low birth weight in sub-Saharan Africa. Clin Microbiol Rev. 2004;17(4):760-9 (https://www.ncbi.nlm.nih.gov/pmc/articles/PMC523568/, accessed 20 October 2019).

11. Guyatt HL, Snow RW. Malaria in pregnancy as an indirect cause of infant mortality in sub-Saharan Africa. Trans R Soc Trop Med Hyg. 2001;95(6):569–76 (https://academic.oup.com/trstmh/article-abstract/95/6/569/1905057?redirectedFrom=fulltext, accessed 20 October 2019).

12. Menendez C. Malaria during pregnancy. Curr Mol Med. 2006 Mar;6(2):269-73.

13. Bardaji A, Martinez-Espinosa FE, Arevalo-Herrera M, Padilla N, Kochar S, Ome-Kaius M et al. Burden and impact of *Plasmodium vivax* in pregnancy: A multi-centre prospective observational study. PLoS Negl Trop Dis. 2017 Jun 12;11(6):e0005606.

14. WHA Global Nutrition Targets 2015: Anaeamia Policy Brief. Geneva: World Health Organization; 2014 (https://www.who.int/nutrition/topics/globaltargets_anaemia_policybrief.pdf, accessed 14 November 2019).

15. Crawley J. Reducing the burden of anemia in infants and young children in malaria-endemic countries of Africa: from evidence to action. Am J Trop Med Hyg. 2004;71(2_suppl):25–34 (https://www.ajtmh.org/content/journals/10.4269/ajtmh.2004.71.25, accessed 20 October 2019).

16. Walker PG, ter Kuile FO, Garske T, Menendez C, Ghani AC. Estimated risk of placental infection and low birthweight attributable to *Plasmodium falciparum* malaria in Africa in 2010: a modelling study. Lancet Glob Health. 2014;2(8):e460–e7.

17. Walker PGT, Griffin JT, Cairns M, Rogerson SJ, van Eijk AM; Ter Kuile F, Ghani AC. A model of parity-dependent immunity to placental malaria. Nat Commun. 2013;4:1609.

18. World Population Prospects. The 2019 Revision [website]. United Nations Population Division; 2019 (http://data.un.org/Data.aspx?d=PopDiv&f=variableID%3A54, accessed 14 November 2019).

19. Antimalarial drug efficacy and drug resistance (updated 27 April 2018) [website]. Geneva: World Health Organization; 2018 (https://www.who.int/malaria/areas/treatment/drug_efficacy/en/, accessed 15 October 2018).

20. UNICEF-WHO. Low birthweight estimates: Levels and trends 2000–2015. Geneva: World Health Organization; 2019 (https://www.unicef.org/media/53711/file/UNICEF-WHO%20Low%20birthweight%20estimates%202019%20.pdf, accessed 14 November 2019).

21. World health statistics overview 2019: monitoring health for the SDGs, sustainable development goals. Geneva: World Health Organization; 2019 (https://apps.who.int/iris/bitstream/handle/10665/311696/WHO-DAD-2019.1-eng.pdf, accessed 14 November 2019).

22. UNICEF Data: Monitoring the situation of children and women [website]. UNICEF; 2019 (https://data.unicef.org/topic/maternal-health/antenatal-care/, accessed 14 November 2019).

23. High burden to high impact: a targeted malaria response. Geneva: World Health Organization; 2019 (https://www.who.int/malaria/publications/atoz/high-impact-response/en/, accessed 22 October 2019).

24. World malaria report. Geneva: World Health Organization; 2017 (https://www.who.int/malaria/publications/world-malaria-report-2017/en/, accessed 20 October 2019).

25. World malaria report. Geneva: World Health Organization; 2018 (https://www.who.int/malaria/publications/world-malaria-report-2018/en/, accessed 20 October 2019).

26. Zero Malaria Starts with Me Toolkit. RBM Partnership to End Malaria African and the African Union Commission (https://endmalaria.org/sites/default/files/Zero%20Malaria%20Toolkit%20Final.pdf, accessed 15 November 2019).

27. WHO Malaria Policy Advisory Committee (MPAC): meeting report. Geneva: World Health Organization Global Malaria Programme; 2019 (https://www.who.int/publications-detail/malaria-policy-advisory-committee-meeting-report-october-2019, accessed 15 November 2019).

28. Malaria elimination: report from the inaugural global forum of countries with potential to eliminate malaria by 2020. Wkly Epidemiol Rec. 2017;92(39):578–86 (https://www.ncbi.nlm.nih.gov/pubmed/28960948, accessed 16 October 2018).

29. Guidelines for malaria vector control. Geneva: World Health Organization; 2019 (https://www.who.int/malaria/publications/atoz/9789241550499/en/, accessed 25 October 2019).

30. Intermittent preventive treatment in pregnancy (IPTp) (updated 21 June 2018) [website]. Geneva: World Health Organization; 2018 (https://www.who.int/malaria/areas/preventive_therapies/pregnancy/en/, accessed 15 October 2018).

31. Intermittent preventive treatment in infants (updated 1 May 2017) [website]. Geneva: World Health Organization; 2017 (https://www.who.int/malaria/areas/preventive_therapies/infants/en/, accessed 15 October 2018).

32. Seasonal malaria chemoprevention with sulfadoxine-pyrimethamine plus amodiaquine in children: a field guide. Geneva: World Health Organization; 2013 (https://apps.who.int/iris/bitstream/handle/10665/85726/9789241504737_eng.pdf?sequence=1, accessed 15 October 2018).

33. Mass drug administration for falciparum malaria: a practical field manual. Geneva: World Health Organization; 2017 (https://extranet.who.int/iris/restricted/handle/10665/259367, accessed 20 October 2019).

34. Acosta A, Obi E, Selby RA, Ugot I, Lynch M, Maire M et al. Design, implementation, and evaluation of a school insecticide-treated net distribution program in Cross River State, Nigeria. J Glob Health Sci. 2018;6(2):272–87.

35. Bhatt S, Weiss DJ, Cameron E, Bisanzio D, Mappin B, Dalrymple U et al. The effect of malaria control on *Plasmodium falciparum* in Africa between 2000 and 2015. Nature. 2015;526(7572):207–11.

36. Guidelines for the treatment of malaria, third edition. Geneva: World Health Organization; 2015 (https://apps.who.int/iris/bitstream/handle/10665/162441/9789241549127_eng.pdf;sequence=1, accessed 20 October 2010).

37. Sadruddin S, Pagnoni P, Baugh G. Lessons from the integrated community case management (iCCM) Rapid Access Expansion Program. JoGH 2019;9: 020101 (http://www.jogh.org/documents/issue201902/jogh-09-020101.pdf, accessed 15 November 2019).

# References

38. Malaria surveillance, monitoring & evaluation: a reference manual. Geneva: World Health Organization; 2018 (https://apps.who.int/iris/bitstream/handle/10665/272284/9789241565578-eng.pdf?ua=1, accessed 15 October 2018).

39. Adapted Performance Review Information System Management (PRISM) [website]. Measure Evaluation; (https://www.measureevaluation.org/resources/tools/health-information-systems/prism, accessed 21 October 2019).

40. False-negative RDT results and implications of new reports of *P. falciparum* histidine-rich protein 2/3 gene deletions World Health Organization; 2017 (https://apps.who.int/iris/bitstream/10665/258972/1/WHO-HTM-GMP-2017.18-eng.pdf, accessed 27 October 2017).

41. Methods for surveillance of antimalarial drug efficacy. Geneva: World Health Organization; 2009 (https://www.who.int/malaria/publications/atoz/9789241597531/en/, accessed 20 October 2019).

42. Global database on antimalaria drug efficacy and resistance (updated 27 April 2018). Geneva: World Health Organization; 2018 (https://www.who.int/malaria/areas/drug_resistance/drug_efficacy_database/en/, accessed 15 November 2019).

43. Van Hong N, Amambua-Ngwa A, Quang Tuan N, Duy Cuong D, Thi Huong Giang N, Van Dung N et al. Severe malaria not responsive to artemisinin derivatives in man returning from Angola to Vietnam. Emerg Infect Dis. 2014. 20(7):1199-202 (https://wwwnc.cdc.gov/eid/article/20/7/14-0155_article, accessed 15 November 2019).

44. Lu F, Culleton R, Zhang M, Ramaprasad A, von Seidlein L, Zhou H et al. Emergence of indigenous artemisinin-resistant *Plasmodium falciparum* in Africa. N Engl J Med. 2017 Mar 9;376(10):991-993 (https://www.nejm.org/doi/10.1056/NEJMc1612765, accessed 15 November 2019).

45. Rasmussen C, Nyunt MM, Ringwald P. Artemisinin-resistant *Plasmodium falciparum* in Africa. N Engl J Med. 2017 Jul 20;377(3):305-306 (https://www.nejm.org/doi/10.1056/NEJMc1705789, accessed 15 November 2019).

46. Russo G, L'Episcopia M, Menegon M, Souza SS, Dongho BGD, Vullo V et al. Dihydroartemisinin-piperaquine treatment failure in uncomplicated *Plasmodium falciparum* malaria case imported from Ethiopia. Infection. 2018 Dec;46(6):867-870 (https://link.springer.com/article/10.1007%2Fs15010-018-1174-9, accessed 15 November 2019).

47. Sonden K, Wyss K, Jovel I, Vieira da Silva A, Pohanka A, Asghar M et al. High rate of treatment failures in nonimmune travelers treated with artemether-lumefantrine for uncomplicated *Plasmodium falciparum* malaria in Sweden: retrospective comparative analysis of effectiveness and case series. Clin Infect Dis. 2017 Jan 15;64(2):199-206 (https://academic.oup.com/cid/article/64/2/199/2698880, accessed 15 November 2019).

48. Sutherland CJ, Lansdell P, Sanders M, Muwanguzi J, van Schalkwyk DA, Kaur H et al. Pfk13-independent treatment failure in four imported cases of *Plasmodium falciparum* malaria treated with artemether-lumefantrine in the United Kingdom. Antimicrob Agents Chemother. 2017 Feb 23;61(3): e02382-16 (https://www.ncbi.nlm.nih.gov/pmc/articles/PMC5328508/, accessed 15 November 2019).

49. Das S, Saha B, Hati AK, Roy S. Evidence of artemisinin-resistant *Plasmodium falciparum* malaria in Eastern India. N Engl J Med. 2018 Nov 15;379(20):1962-1964 (https://www.nejm.org/doi/10.1056/NEJMc1713777, accessed 15 November 2019).

50. Das S, Manna S, Saha B, Hati AK, Roy S. Novel pfkelch13 gene polymorphism associates with artemisinin resistance in Eastern India. Clin Infect Dis. 2019 Sep 13;69(7):1144-1152 (https://academic.oup.com/cid/article/69/7/1144/5236823, accessed 15 November 2019).

51. Rasmussen C, Valecha N, Ringwald P. Lack of convincing evidence of artemisinin resistance in India. Clin Infect Dis. 2019, 1461-1462 (https://academic.oup.com/cid/article-abstract/69/8/1461/5367393?redirectedFrom=fulltext, accessed 15 November 2019).

52. Test procedures for insecticide resistance monitoring in malaria vector mosquitoes (second edition). Geneva: World Health Organization; 2018 (https://apps.who.int/iris/bitstream/handle/10665/250677/9789241511575-eng.pdf, accessed 15 November 2019).

53. Framework for a national plan for monitoring and management of insecticide resistance in malaria vectors. Geneva: World Health Organization; 2017 (https://apps.who.int/iris/bitstream/handle/10665/254916/9789241512138-eng.pdf, accessed 15 November 2019).

54. Conditions for deployment of mosquito nets treated with a pyrethroid and piperonyl butoxide. Geneva: World Health Organization; 2017 (https://apps.who.int/iris/bitstream/handle/10665/258939/WHO-HTM-GMP-2017.17-eng.pdf, accessed 15 November 2019).

# Annexes

**Annex 1 – Data sources and methods**

**Annex 2 – Regional profiles**
- A. WHO African Region
    - a. West Africa
    - b. Central Africa
    - c. Countries with high transmission in East and Southern Africa
    - d. Countries with low transmission in East and Southern Africa
- B. WHO Region of the Americas
- C. WHO Eastern Mediterranean Region
- D. WHO South-East Asia Region
- E. WHO Western Pacific Region

**Annex 3 – Data tables**
- A. Policy adoption, 2018
- B. Antimalarial drug policy, 2018
- C. Funding for malaria control, 2016–2018
- D. Commodities distribution and coverage, 2016–2018
- Ea. Household survey results, 2015–2018, compiled through STATcompiler
- Eb. Household survey results, 2015–2018, compiled through WHO calculations
- F. Population at risk and estimated malaria cases and deaths, 2010–2018
- G. Population at risk and reported malaria cases by place of care, 2018
- H. Reported malaria cases by method of confirmation, 2010–2018
- I. Reported malaria cases by species, 2010–2018
- J. Reported malaria deaths, 2010–2018

# Annex 1 – Data sources and methods

### Fig. 1.1. Countries with indigenous cases in 2000 and their status by 2018

Data on the number of indigenous cases (an indicator of whether countries are endemic for malaria) were as reported to the World Health Organization (WHO) by national malaria programmes (NMPs). Countries with 3 consecutive years of zero indigenous cases are considered to have eliminated malaria.

### Table 1.1. GTS: global targets for 2030 and milestones for 2020 and 2025

Targets and milestones are as described in the *Global technical strategy for malaria 2016–2030* (GTS) (*1*) and *Action and investment to defeat malaria 2016–2030* (AIM) (*2*).

### Fig. 1.2. Malaria and the SDGs 2016–2030

This figure was adapted from a fact sheet on malaria and the Sustainable Development Goals (SDGs) (*3*) produced by the Swiss Tropical and Public Health Institute (a WHO Collaborating Centre) for the Swiss Malaria Group.

### Fig. 1.3. The WHO triple billion targets and the contribution of the fight against malaria

This figure is extracted from the document *Informal Member States Consultation GPW 13 WHO Impact Framework* (*4*).

### Table 2.1. Estimated malaria cases by WHO region, 2010–2018

The number of malaria cases was estimated by one of the following two methods:

#### Method 1

Method 1 was used for countries and areas outside Africa and for low-transmission countries and areas in Africa: Afghanistan, Bangladesh, Bolivia (Plurinational State of), Botswana, Brazil, Cambodia, Colombia, Dominican Republic, Eritrea, Ethiopia, French Guiana, Gambia, Guatemala, Guyana, Haiti, Honduras, India, Indonesia, Lao People's Democratic Republic, Madagascar, Mauritania, Myanmar, Namibia, Nepal, Nicaragua, Pakistan, Panama, Papua New Guinea, Peru, Philippines, Rwanda, Senegal, Solomon Islands, Timor-Leste, Vanuatu, Venezuela (Bolivarian Republic of), Viet Nam, Yemen and Zimbabwe.

Estimates were made by adjusting the number of reported malaria cases for completeness of reporting, the likelihood that cases were parasite positive, and the extent of health service use. The procedure, which is described in the *World malaria report 2008* (*5*), combines data reported by NMPs (reported cases, reporting completeness and likelihood that cases are parasite positive) with data obtained from nationally representative household surveys on health service use. Briefly:

$$T = (a + (c \times e))/d \times (1 + f/g + (1-g-f)/2/g)$$

where:

$a$ is malaria cases confirmed in public sector

$b$ is suspected cases tested

$c$ is presumed cases (not tested but treated as malaria)

$d$ is reporting completeness

$e$ is test positivity rate (malaria positive fraction) = $a/b$

$f$ is fraction seeking treatment in private sector

$g$ is fraction seeking treatment in public sector

No treatment seeking factor: $(1-g-f)$

Cases in public sector: $(a + (c \times e))/d$

Cases in private sector: $(a + (c \times e))/d \times f/g$

To estimate the uncertainty around the number of cases, the *test positivity rate* was assumed to have a normal distribution centred on the test positivity rate value and standard deviation, defined as $0.244 \times f^{0.5547}$, and truncated to be in the range 0, 1. *Reporting completeness* (*d*), when reported as a range or below 80%, was assumed to have one of three distributions, depending on the value reported by the NMP. If the value was greater than 80%, the distribution was assumed to be triangular, with limits of 0.8 and 1 and the peak at 0.8. If the value was greater than 50%, then the distribution was assumed to be rectangular, with limits of 0.5 and 0.8. Finally, if the value was lower than 50%, the distribution was assumed to be triangular, with limits of 0 and 0.5 and the peak at 0.5 (*6*). If the reporting completeness was reported as a value and was greater than 80%, a beta distribution was assumed with a mean value of the reported value (maximum of 95%) and confidence intervals (CIs) of 5% round the mean value. The fraction of children brought for care in the public sector and in the private sector were assumed to have a beta distribution, with the mean value being the estimated value in the survey and the standard deviation calculated from the range of the estimated 95% CIs divided by 4. The fraction of children not brought for care was assumed to have a rectangular distribution, with the lower limit being 0 and the upper limit calculated as 1 minus the proportion that were brought for care in the public and private sectors. The three distributions (fraction seeking treatment in public sector, fraction seeking treatment in private sector only and fraction not seeking treatment) were constrained to add up to 1.

Values for the fractions seeking care were linearly interpolated between the years that had a survey, and were extrapolated for the years before the first or after the last survey. Missing values for the distributions were imputed in a similar way or, if there was no value for any year in the country or area, a mixture of the distribution of the region for that year. CIs were obtained from 10 000 draws of the convoluted distributions. The data were analysed using the R statistical software (7).

For India, the values were obtained at subnational level using the same methodology, but adjusting the private sector for an additional factor due to the active case detection, estimated as the ratio of the test positivity rate in active case detection over the test positivity rate for passive case detection. This factor was assumed to have a normal distribution, with mean value and standard deviation calculated from the values reported in 2010.

No adjustment for private sector treatment seeking was made for the following countries and areas, because they report cases from the private and public sector together: Bangladesh, Bolivia (Plurinational State of), Botswana, Brazil, Colombia, Dominican Republic, French Guiana, Guatemala, Guyana, Haiti, Honduras, Myanmar (since 2013), Nicaragua, Panama, Peru, Rwanda, Senegal (70% of private sector reported together with public sector in 2018) and Venezuela (Bolivarian Republic of).

### Method 2

Method 2 was used for high-transmission countries in Africa and for some countries in the WHO Eastern Mediterranean Region in which the quality of surveillance data did not permit a robust estimate from the number of reported cases: Angola, Benin, Burkina Faso, Burundi, Cameroon, Central African Republic, Chad, Congo, Côte d'Ivoire, Democratic Republic of the Congo, Equatorial Guinea, Gabon, Ghana, Guinea, Guinea-Bissau, Kenya, Liberia, Malawi, Mali, Mozambique, Niger, Nigeria, Sierra Leone, Somalia, South Sudan, Sudan, Togo, Uganda, United Republic of Tanzania and Zambia. In this method, estimates of the number of malaria cases were derived from information on parasite prevalence obtained from household surveys.

First, data on parasite prevalence from nearly 60 000 survey records were assembled within a spatio-temporal Bayesian geostatistical model, along with environmental and sociodemographic covariates, and data distribution on interventions such as insecticide-treated mosquito net (ITNs), antimalarial drugs and indoor residual spraying (IRS). The geospatial model enabled predictions of *Plasmodium falciparum* prevalence in children aged 2–10 years, at a resolution of $5 \times 5$ km$^2$, throughout all malaria endemic African countries for each year from 2000 to 2018.[1] Second, an ensemble model was developed to predict malaria incidence as a function of parasite prevalence. The model was then applied to the estimated parasite prevalence in order to obtain estimates of the malaria case incidence at $5 \times 5$ km$^2$ resolution for each year from 2000 to 2018.[1] Data for each $5 \times 5$ km$^2$ area were then aggregated within country and regional boundaries, to obtain both national and regional estimates of malaria cases (8).

### Other methods

For most of the elimination countries and countries in prevention of reintroduction, the number of indigenous cases registered by the NMPs are reported without further adjustments. The countries in this category were Algeria, Argentina, Armenia, Azerbaijan, Belize, Bhutan, Cabo Verde, China, Comoros, Costa Rica, Democratic People's Republic of Korea, Djibouti, Ecuador, Egypt, El Salvador, Eswatini, Georgia, Iran (Islamic Republic of), Iraq, Kazakhstan, Kyrgyzstan, Malaysia, Mexico, Morocco, Oman, Paraguay, Republic of Korea, Sao Tome and Principe, Saudi Arabia, South Africa, Sri Lanka, Suriname, Syrian Arab Republic, Tajikistan, Thailand, Turkey, Turkmenistan, United Arab Emirates and Uzbekistan.

For some years, information was not always available or was not of sufficient quality to be used. For those countries, the number of cases was imputed from other years where the quality of the data was better, adjusting for population growth, as follows: for Ethiopia, the values were taken from a mixed distribution between values from Method 1 and Method 2 (50% from each method); for Gambia, 2010 values were imputed from 2011 to 2013 values; for Haiti, 2010 values were imputed from 2006 to 2008 values; for Namibia, 2012 values were imputed from 2010 and 2013 values; and for Papua New Guinea, 2012 values were imputed from 2009 to 2011 values. Estimated rates from 2017 were extrapolated to 2018 for Angola, Burundi, Central African Republic and Sudan. For Djibouti, 2011 and 2012 values were extrapolated from cases reported in 2009 and 2013. For Kenya, Mali, Niger and Somalia, the estimated series up to 2017 in the *World malaria report 2018* was used and extrapolated to 2018. To follow the current trends in reported cases in the public sector, modelled cases were adjusted for a factor of 1.1 in Uganda in 2018.

The number of malaria cases caused by *P. vivax* in each country was estimated by multiplying the country's reported proportion of *P. vivax* cases, computed as 1 − *P. falciparum*, by the total number of estimated cases for the country. For countries where the estimated proportion was not 0 or 1, the proportion of *P. falciparum* cases was assumed to have a beta distribution estimated from the proportion of *P. falciparum* cases reported by NMPs.

To transform malaria cases into incidence, a population at risk estimate was used. The proportion of the population at high, low or no risk of malaria was provided by NMPs. This was applied to United Nations (UN) population estimates, to compute the number of people at risk of malaria.

---

[1] For methods on the development of maps by the Malaria Atlas Project, see https://www.map.ox.ac.uk/making-maps/.

# Annex 1 – Data sources and methods

**Table 2.2. Estimated *P. vivax* malaria cases by WHO region, 2018**

See methods notes for **Table 2.1**.

**Fig. 2.1. Estimated country share of (a) total malaria cases and (b) *P. vivax* malaria cases, 2018**

See methods notes for **Table 2.1**.

**Fig. 2.2. Trends in malaria case incidence rate (cases per 1000 population at risk) globally and by WHO region, 2010–2018**

See methods notes for **Table 2.1**.

**Fig. 2.3. Map of malaria case incidence rate (cases per 1000 population at risk) by country, 2018**

See methods notes for **Table 2.1**.

**Fig. 2.4. Trends in malaria mortality rate (deaths per 100 000 population at risk), globally and in the WHO African Region, 2010–2018**

See methods notes for **Table 2.3**.

**Fig. 2.5. Trends in malaria mortality rate (deaths per 100 000 population at risk) in WHO regions, 2010–2018**

See methods notes for **Table 2.3**.

**Table 2.3. Estimated number of malaria deaths by WHO region, 2010–2018**

Numbers of malaria deaths were estimated using methods from Category 1, 2 or 3, as outlined below.

**Category 1 method**

A Category 1 method was used for low-transmission countries and areas outside Africa and for low-transmission countries and areas in Africa: Afghanistan, Bangladesh, Bolivia (Plurinational State of), Botswana, Cambodia, Comoros, Dominican Republic, Eritrea, Eswatini, Ethiopia, French Guiana, Guatemala, Guyana, Haiti, Honduras, India, Indonesia, Lao People's Democratic Republic, Madagascar, Myanmar, Namibia, Nepal, Nicaragua, Pakistan, Papua New Guinea, Philippines, Solomon Islands, Somalia, Sudan, Timor-Leste, Vanuatu, Venezuela (Bolivarian Republic of), Viet Nam, Yemen and Zimbabwe.

A case fatality rate of 0.256% was applied to the estimated number of *P. falciparum* cases, which represents the average of case fatality rates reported in the literature (*9-11*) and rates from unpublished data from Indonesia, 2004–2009.[1] The proportion of deaths then follows a categorical distribution of 0.01%, 0.19%, 0.30%, 0.38% and 0.40%, each one with equal probability. A case fatality rate of 0.0375% was applied to the estimated number of *P. vivax* cases, representing the midpoint of the range of case fatality rates reported in a study by Douglas et al. (*12*), following a rectangular distribution between 0.012% and 0.063%. Following the nonlinear association explained for the Category 2 method below, the proportion of deaths in children aged under 5 years was estimated as:

Proportion of deaths$_{under\ 5}$ = −0.2288 × Mortality$_{overall}^2$ + 0.823 × Mortality$_{overall}$ + 0.2239

where the Mortality$_{overall}$ is the number of estimated deaths over the estimated population at risk per 1000 (see **Annex 3.F** for national estimates of population at risk).

**Category 2 method**

A Category 2 method was used for countries in Africa with a high proportion of deaths due to malaria: Angola, Benin, Burkina Faso, Burundi, Cameroon, Central African Republic, Chad, Congo, Côte d'Ivoire, Democratic Republic of the Congo, Equatorial Guinea, Gabon, Gambia, Ghana, Guinea, Guinea-Bissau, Kenya, Liberia, Malawi, Mali, Mauritania, Mozambique, Niger, Nigeria, Rwanda, Senegal, Sierra Leone, South Sudan, Togo, Uganda, United Republic of Tanzania and Zambia.

In this method, child malaria deaths were estimated using a verbal autopsy multicause model that was developed by the WHO Maternal and Child Health Epidemiology Estimation Group (MCEE) to estimate causes of death in children aged 1–59 months (*13*). Mortality estimates (and 95% CI) were derived for seven causes of post-neonatal death (pneumonia, diarrhoea, malaria, meningitis, injuries, pertussis and other disorders), four causes arising in the neonatal period (prematurity, birth asphyxia and trauma, sepsis, and other conditions of the neonate), and other causes (e.g. malnutrition). Deaths due to measles, unknown causes and HIV/AIDS were estimated separately. The resulting cause-specific estimates were adjusted, country by country, to fit the estimated mortality envelope of 1–59 months (excluding HIV/AIDS and measles deaths) for corresponding years. Estimated prevalence of malaria parasites (see methods notes for **Table 2.1**) was used as a covariate within the model. It was assumed that the number of deaths follows a rectangular distribution, with limits being the estimated 95% CI. The malaria mortality rate in children aged under 5 years estimated with this method was then used to infer malaria-specific mortality in those aged over 5 years, using the relationship between levels of malaria mortality in a series of age groups and the intensity of malaria transmission (*14*), and assuming a nonlinear association between under-5-years mortality and over-5-years mortality, as follows:

---

[1] Dr Ric Price, Menzies School of Health Research, Australia, personal communication (November 2014).

Proportion of deaths$_{over 5}$ = −0.293 × Mortality$_{under 5}^2$ + 0.8918 × Mortality$_{under 5}$ + 0.2896

where Mortality$_{under 5}$ is estimated from the number of deaths from the MCEE model over the population at risk per 1000.

#### Category 3 method

For the Category 3 method, the number of indigenous malaria deaths registered by the NMPs is reported without further adjustments. This category includes the following countries: Algeria, Argentina, Armenia, Azerbaijan, Belize, Bhutan, Brazil, Cabo Verde, China, Colombia, Costa Rica, Democratic People's Republic of Korea, Djibouti, Ecuador, Egypt, El Salvador, Georgia, Iran (Islamic Republic of), Iraq, Kazakhstan, Kyrgyzstan, Malaysia, Mexico, Morocco, Oman, Panama, Paraguay, Peru, Republic of Korea, Sao Tome and Principe, Saudi Arabia, South Africa, Sri Lanka, Suriname, Syrian Arab Republic, Tajikistan, Thailand, Turkey, Turkmenistan, United Arab Emirates and Uzbekistan.

### Fig. 2.6. Percentage of estimated malaria deaths attributable to the 21 countries with nearly 85% of malaria deaths globally in 2018

See methods notes for **Table 2.3**.

### Fig. 2.7. Comparison of current estimated malaria cases with expected cases had malaria incidence remained at 2000 levels globally

Number of malaria cases by year was estimated using methods described for **Table 2.1**. Expected malaria cases if case incidence remained the same as the year 2000 were estimated using the 2000 incidence per 1000 population to estimated population at risk each year.

### Fig. 2.8. Comparison of current estimated malaria deaths with expected deaths had malaria incidence remained at 2000 levels globally

Number of malaria deaths by year was estimated using methods described for **Table 2.3**. Expected malaria deaths if mortality rate remained the same as the year 2000 were estimated using the 2000 rate per 100 000 population to estimated population at risk each year.

### Fig. 2.9. Comparison of progress in malaria case incidence considering three scenarios: current trajectory maintained (blue), GTS targets achieved (green) and worst case scenario, that is a return to mean peak past incidence in the period 2000–2007 (red)

GTS target 90% reduction of malaria incidence and mortality rate by 2030 with milestones of 40% and 75% reductions in both indicator for the years 2020 and 2025 respective (1). A curve based on a quadratic fit is used for the malaria incidence milestones. For projection of malaria incidence under current estimated trend, the same year on year trend observed from latest years (2016–2018) is forecast up to 2030. For the regress scenario, the trend in mean peak incidence of the 'pre-intervention scale-up' years (2000–2007) is projected forward to 2030.

### Fig. 3.1. Estimated prevalence of exposure to malaria infection during pregnancy overall and by subregion in 2018 in moderate to high transmission sub-Saharan Africa

Estimates of malaria-exposed pregnancies and preventable malaria-attributable low birthweight (LBW) deliveries in the absence of pregnancy-specific malaria prevention (i.e. LLIN delivery based on intermittent preventive treatment in pregnancy [IPTp] or antenatal care [ANC]) were obtained using a model of the relationship between these outcomes with slide microscopy prevalence in the general population and age- and gravidity-specific fertility patterns. This model was developed by fitting an established model of the relationship between malaria transmission and malaria infection by age (15) to patterns of infection in placental histology (16) and attributable LBW risk by gravidity in the absence of IPTp or other effective chemoprevention (17). The model was run across a 0.2 degree (5 km$^2$) longitude/latitude grid for 100 realisations of the MAP joint posterior estimated slide prevalence in 2-10 year olds in 2018 (8). Country-specific age-specific or gravidity-specific fertility rates, stratified by urban rural status, were obtained from demographic health surveys (DHS) and malaria indicator surveys (MIS) where such surveys had been carried out since 2014 and were available from the DHS program website (18). Countries where surveys were not available were allocated fertility patterns from a survey from a different country matched on the basis of total fertility rate (19) and geography. Fertility patterns of individual women within simulations at each grid-point were simulated according to the proportion of women estimated to be living in urban or rural locations. Urban/rural attribution at a 1 km$^2$ was conducted based upon WorldPop 1 km$^2$ 2018 population estimates (20) and an urban/rural threshold of 386/km$^2$ (21) which were then aggregated to the 0.2 degree (5 km$^2$) resolution of the MAP surfaces. This provided a risk of malaria infection and malaria-attributable LBW in the absence of prevention, along with a modelled per capita pregnancy rate for each grid-point, which was aggregated to country level, using WorldPop population estimates, to provide a per pregnancy risk of malaria infection and per livebirth estimate of malaria-attributable LBW in the absence of prevention. These were then multiplied by [X data source] country-level estimates of pregnancies and [Y data source] estimates of LBW in 2018.

# Annex 1 – Data sources and methods

**Table 3.1. Estimates of pregnancies, livebirths, low birthweights, exposure to malaria infection in pregnancy and malaria-attributable low birthweights in 2018 in moderate to high transmission sub-Saharan Africa**

Methods for estimating malaria infection in pregnancy and malaria-attributable LBWs are described in Walker et al. (*17*). Number of pregnancies and infection rates were estimated from latest UN population estimates and total fertility rates, while the underlying *P. falciparum* parasite prevalence estimates were the updated MAP series, methods described in Bhatt et al. (2015) (*8*).

**Fig. 3.2. Estimated maternal anaemia versus exposure to malaria infection in pregnancy in 2018 in moderate to high transmission countries in sub-Saharan Africa**

Malaria-related maternal anaemia prevalence estimates were derived from WHO, Global Health Observatory Data Repository/World Health Statistics.[1] The estimates have not been updated since 2016 and, for the purpose of this analysis, these estimates were maintained. For the methods used to compute malaria infection during pregnancy, see methods for **Table 3.1**.

**Fig. 3.3. Estimated low birthweights due to exposure to malaria infection during pregnancy overall and by subregion in 2018 in moderate to high transmission sub-Saharan Africa**

Overall LBW prevalence was obtained from a United Nations Children's Fund (UNICEF)–WHO publication (*22*). These rates have not been updated since 2015 and, for the purpose of the analysis, were applied to the number of livebirths in 2018 based on UN estimates of pregnancies and livebirths. For methods on low birthweights attributable to malaria infection during pregnancy, see methods for **Table 3.2**.

**Fig. 3.4. Prevalence of severe anaemia (<7 g/dL), moderate anaemia (7–9.9 g/dL) and mild anaemia (10–10.9 g/dL) in children aged under 5 years in sub-Saharan Africa, 2015–2018, by age and malaria infection status**

Estimates were derived from 16 nationally representative household surveys – demographic health surveys (DHS) and malaria indicator surveys (MIS) – conducted between 2015 and 2017 in Angola, Burundi, Ghana, Kenya, Liberia, Madagascar, Malawi, Mali, Mozambique, Nigeria, Rwanda, Senegal, Sierra Leone, Togo, Uganda and United Republic of Tanzania.

The numerator is the number of children in each category: not anaemic (Hb >11 g/dL), mild anaemia (Hb 10–10.9 g/dL), moderate anaemia (Hb 7–9.9 g/dL) and severe anaemia (Hb <7 g/dL). The denominator is the number of children aged under 5 years. Please refer to the methods for **Section 8** for more details about the limitations related to the use of DHS and MIS data.

**Fig. 3.5. Prevalence of severe anaemia (<7 g/dL), moderate anaemia (7–9.9 g/dL) and mild anaemia (10–10.9 g/dL) in children aged under 5 years in sub-Saharan Africa, 2015–2018, by country**

See methods notes for **Fig. 3.4**.

**Table 3.2. Estimated number of children aged 1–59 months infected with *P. falciparum* parasites in 2018 by subregion and overall in sub-Saharan Africa**

These were estimated from geospatial models of *P. falciparum* infection prevalence by age (*8*). These models use a combination of household parasite survey data, climatic and malaria intervention covariates, and information on age-specific patterns of parasite prevalence in diverse transmission settings (*23*). Prevalence estimates were applied to age-structured UN population estimates for 38 moderate to high malaria transmission countries in sub-Saharan Africa. Data were aggregated to the WHO African Region.

**Fig. 3.6. Country comparison of coverage of ANC4 and IPTp3 in moderate and high transmission sub Saharan Africa, 2018**

Estimates of at least four visits to ANC (ANC4) coverage were obtained from the UNICEF data on antenatal care coverage. This data are posted on https://data.unicef.org/topic/maternal-health/antenatal-care/ and contain a measure of ANC coverage by visit from household surveys. IPTp3 coverage was estimated using methods described for **Figure 7.6**.

**Fig. 4.1. HBHI: a targeted malaria response to get countries back on target for the 2025 GTS milestones**

This was taken from a recent WHO publication (*24*).

**Fig. 4.2a. Estimated malaria cases and deaths, 2010–2018**

See methods notes for **Table 2.1** and **Table 2.3**.

**Fig. 4.2b. Estimated malaria cases in India, showing seven states that contributed a combined 90% of cases, 2010 versus 2018**

See methods notes for **Table 2.1**.

---

[1] https://apps.who.int/gho/data/node.main.1?lang=en

**Fig. 4.3. Distribution and coverage of preventive interventions: (a) Number of LLINs distributed, 2016–2018, (b) Percentage of population with access to LLINs, 2018, (c) Percentage of population sleeping under an LLIN, 2018, (d) Percentage of children sleeping under an LLIN, 2018; (e) Percentage of pregnant women who received IPTp3, 2018; (f) SMC targeted children and mean treatments per cycle, 2018**

See methods notes for **Fig. 6.8**, **Fig. 7.1**, **Fig. 7.2**, **Fig. 7.6** and **Fig. 7.7**, respectively.

**Fig. 4.4. Diagnosis and treatment of febrile children in HBHI African countries: (a) Treatment seeking for fevers in children aged under 5 years, and source of treatment by health sector, (b) Percentage of children aged under 5 years with fever who sought treatment and were diagnosed with a parasitological test**

Data obtained from household surveys such as DHS, MIS and multiple indicator cluster surveys (MICS).

**Fig. 4.5. Total international and domestic direct funding for malaria in the 11 HBHI countries, (a) 2010–2018 and (b) 2016–2018**

See methods notes for **Fig. 6.3**.

**Table 5.1. Countries eliminating malaria since 2000**

Countries are shown by the year in which they attained zero indigenous cases for 3 consecutive years, according to reports submitted by NMPs.

**Fig. 5.1. Number of countries that were malaria endemic in 2000 with fewer than 10, 100, 1000 and 10 000 indigenous malaria cases between 2010 and 2018**

For the 16 countries that attained zero indigenous cases for 3 consecutive years between 2000 and 2018, the number of NMP-reported indigenous cases was tabulated according to the number of years preceding the attainment of zero cases. Data from years before the peak number of cases were excluded. Thus, if a country had experienced zero cases and malaria returned, cases were only included from the year in which they peaked. This inclusion criterion generates a slope that is steeper than it would be if cases from all years were included (because some increases are excluded). In some earlier years where data on indigenous cases were not available, the total number of reported cases was used (i.e. for country-years with larger numbers of cases, in which the proportion of imported cases is expected to be low).

**Fig. 5.2. Trends in indigenous malaria cases in E-2020 countries, 2010–2018**

Data were derived from NMP reports.

**Fig. 5.3. *P. falciparum* cases in the GMS, 2010–2018**

Data were derived from NMP reports to the Greater Mekong subregion (GMS) Malaria Elimination Database (MEDB).

**Fig. 5.4. Regional map of malaria incidence in the GMS by area, 2018**

Data were derived from NMP reports to the GMS MEDB.

**Fig. 6.1. Funding for malaria control and elimination over the period 2010–2018 (% of total funding), by source of funds (constant 2018 US$)**

Total funding for malaria control and elimination over the period 2010–2018 was estimated using data obtained from several sources.

Contributions from governments of endemic countries were estimated as the sum of government contributions reported by NMPs for the world malaria report of the relevant year plus the estimated costs of patient care delivery services at public health facilities. If NMP contributions were missing for 2018, data reported from previous years were used after conversion in constant 2018 US$. The number of reported malaria cases attending public health facilities was sourced from NMP reports, adjusted for diagnosis and reporting completeness. Between 1% and 3% of uncomplicated reported malaria cases were assumed to have moved to the severe stage of disease, and 50–80% of these severe cases were assumed to have been hospitalized. Costs of outpatient visits and inpatient bed-stays were estimated from the perspective of the public health care provider, using unit cost estimates[1] from WHO-CHOosing Interventions that are Cost-Effective (WHO-CHOICE). For each country, WHO-CHOICE 2010 unit cost estimates expressed in national currency were estimated for the period 2011–2018 using the gross domestic product (GDP) annual price deflator published by the World Bank[2] on 28 August 2019 and converted in base year 2010. Country-specific unit cost estimates were then converted from national currency to constant 2018 US$ for each year during 2010–2018. For each country, the number of adjusted reported malaria cases attending public health facilities was then multiplied by the estimated unit costs. In the absence of information on the level of care at which

---

[1] https://www.who.int/choice/en/
[2] https://data.worldbank.org/indicator

# Annex 1 – Data sources and methods

malaria patients attend public facilities, uncertainty around unit cost estimates was handled through probabilistic uncertainty analysis. The mean total cost of patient care service delivery was calculated from 1000 estimations.

International bilateral funding data were obtained from several sources. Data on planned funding from the government of the United States of America (USA) were sourced from the US government Foreign Assistance website,[1] with the technical assistance of the Kaiser Family Foundation. Country-level planned funding data were available for the United States Agency for International Development (USAID) for the period 2010–2018. Country-specific planned funding data from other agencies, such as the US Centers for Disease Control and Prevention (CDC) and the US Department of Defense, were not available; therefore, data on total annual planned funding from each of these two agencies were used for the period 2010–2018. For the government of the United Kingdom of Great Britain and Northern Ireland (United Kingdom), funding data towards malaria control for 2017 and 2018 were sourced from the Statistics on International Development: Final UK Aid Spend 2018[2] (UK Aid Spend) with the technical assistance of the United Kingdom Department for International Development. UK Aid Spend data do not capture all spending from the United Kingdom that may impact on malaria outcomes. The United Kingdom supports malaria control and elimination through a broad range of interventions; for example, via support to overall health systems in malaria endemic countries and research and development, which are not included in these data.

For the period 2010–2016, United Kingdom spending data were sourced from the Organisation for Economic Co-operation and Development (OECD) creditor reporting system (CRS) database on aid activity.[3] For all other donors, disbursement data were also obtained from the OECD CRS database on aid activity for the period 2010–2018. For each year and each funder, the country-level and regional-level project-type interventions and other technical assistance were extracted. All data were converted to constant 2018 US$.

Malaria-related annual funding from donors through multilateral agencies was estimated from data on (i) donors' contributions published by the Global Fund to Fight AIDS, Tuberculosis and Malaria (Global Fund)[4] and annual disbursements by the Global Fund to malaria endemic countries between 2010 and 2018 as reported by the Global Fund; and (ii) donors' disbursements to malaria endemic countries published in the OECD CRS and in the OECD Development Assistance Committee members' total use of the multilateral system.[5] All funding flows were converted to constant 2018 US$.

For (i), the amount of funding contributed by each donor was estimated as the proportion of funding paid by each donor out of the total amount received by the Global Fund in a given year, multiplied by the total amount disbursed by the Global Fund in the same year. Equal contributions were assumed every year by each donor over the 3-year periods for which data were available.

For (ii), contributions from donors to multilateral channels were estimated by calculating the proportion of the core contributions received by a multilateral agency each year by each donor, then multiplying that amount by the multilateral agency's estimated investment in malaria control in the same year.

Contributions from malaria endemic countries to multilateral agencies were allocated to governments of endemic countries under the "funding source" category. Contributions from non-DAC countries and other sources to multilateral agencies were not available and were, therefore, not included.

Annual estimated investments were summed up to estimate the total amount each funder contributed to malaria control and elimination over the period 2010–2018, and the relative percentage of the total spending contributed by each funder calculated for the period 2010–2018.

**Fig. 6.1** excludes household spending on malaria prevention and treatment in malaria endemic countries.

### Fig. 6.2. Funding for malaria control and elimination 2010–2018, by source of funds (constant 2018 US$)

See methods notes for **Fig. 6.1** for sources of information on total funding for malaria control and elimination from governments of malaria endemic countries and on international funding flows. **Fig. 6.2** excludes household spending on malaria prevention and treatment in malaria endemic countries.

### Fig. 6.3. Funding for malaria control and elimination 2010–2018, by channel (constant 2018 US$)

See methods notes for **Fig. 6.1** for sources of information on total funding for malaria control and elimination from governments of malaria endemic countries and on international funding flows. **Fig. 6.3** excludes household spending on malaria prevention and treatment in malaria endemic countries.

---

[1] https://foreignassistance.gov/
[2] https://www.gov.uk/government/statistics/statistics-on-international-development-final-uk-aid-spend-2018 (purpose code 12262)
[3] https://stats.oecd.org/Index.aspx?DataSetCode=CRS1
[4] https://www.theglobalfund.org/en/financials/
[5] https://stats.oecd.org/Index.aspx?DataSetCode=CRS1

### Fig. 6.4. Funding for malaria control and elimination 2010–2018, by World Bank 2018 income group and source of funding (constant 2018 US$)

See methods notes for **Fig. 6.1** for sources of information on total funding for malaria control and elimination from governments of malaria endemic countries and on international funding flows. Data on income group classification for 2018 were sourced from the World Bank.[1] **Fig. 6.4** excludes household spending on malaria prevention and treatment in malaria endemic countries.

### Fig. 6.5. Funding for malaria control and elimination 2010–2018, by WHO region (constant 2018 US$)

See methods notes for **Fig. 6.1** for sources of information on total funding for malaria control and elimination from governments of malaria endemic countries and on international funding flows. The "Unspecified" category includes all funding data for which there was no geographical information on the recipient. **Fig. 6.5** excludes household spending on malaria prevention and treatment in malaria endemic countries.

### Fig. 6.6. Funding for malaria-related R&D 2010–2018, by product type (constant 2018 US$)

Data on funding for malaria-related research and development for 2010–2018 were sourced directly from Policy Cures Research as advance preview of the forthcoming 2019 G-FINDER report.[2]

### Fig. 6.7. Malaria R&D funding in 2018, by sector (constant 2018 US$)

See methods notes for **Fig. 6.6**.

### Fig. 6.8. Number of ITNs delivered by manufacturers and distributed by NMPs, 2010–2018

Data on the number of ITNs delivered by manufacturers to countries were provided to WHO by Milliner Global Associates. Data from NMP reports were used for the number of ITNs distributed within countries.

### Fig. 6.9. Total LLINs distributed to communities by country in the period 2016–2018, in countries accounting for about 90% of global distributions by NMPs

Data on long-lasting insecticidal nets (LLINs) were derived from NMP reports.

### Fig. 6.10. Number of RDTs sold by manufacturers and distributed by NMPs for use in testing suspected malaria cases, 2010–2018

The numbers of rapid diagnostic tests (RDTs) distributed by WHO region are the annual totals reported as having been distributed by NMPs. Numbers of RDT sales were reported by 41 manufacturers that participated in RDT product testing by WHO, the Foundation for Innovative New Diagnostics (FIND), the CDC, and the Special Programme for Research and Training in Tropical Diseases. The number of RDTs reported by manufacturers represents total sales to the public and private sectors worldwide.

### Fig. 6.11. Number of ACT treatment courses delivered by manufacturers and distributed by NMPs to patients, 2010–2018

Data on artemisinin-based combination therapy (ACT) sales were provided by eight manufacturers eligible for procurement by WHO or UNICEF. ACT sales were categorized as being to either the public sector or the private sector. Data on ACTs distributed within countries through the public sector were taken from NMP reports.

### Fig. 7.1. Percentage of population at risk with access to an ITN, and percentage of households with at least one ITN and enough ITNs for all occupants, sub-Saharan Africa, 2010–2018

Estimates of ITN coverage were derived from a model developed by MAP,[3] using a two-stage process. First, a mechanism was designed for estimating net crop (i.e. the total number of ITNs in households in a country at a given time), taking into account inputs to the system (e.g. deliveries of ITNs to a country) and outputs (e.g. loss of ITNs from households). Second, empirical modelling was used to translate estimated net crops into resulting levels of coverage (e.g. access within households, use in all ages and use among children aged under 5 years).

The model incorporates data from three sources:

- the number of ITNs delivered by manufacturers to countries, as provided to WHO by Milliner Global Associates;
- the number of ITNs distributed within countries, as reported to WHO by NMPs; and
- data from nationally representative household surveys from 39 countries in sub-Saharan Africa, from 2001 to 2018.

---

[1] https://datahelpdesk.worldbank.org/knowledgebase/articles/906519-world-bank-country-and-lending-groups, accessed 1 October 2019
[2] https://www.policycuresresearch.org/, forthcoming
[3] https://www.map.ox.ac.uk/

# Annex 1 – Data sources and methods

**Countries for analysis**

The main analysis covered 40 of the 47 malaria endemic countries or areas of sub-Saharan Africa. The islands of Mayotte (for which no ITN delivery or distribution data were available) and Cabo Verde (which does not distribute ITNs) were excluded, as were the low-transmission countries of Eswatini, Namibia, Sao Tome and Principe, and South Africa, for which ITNs comprise a small proportion of vector control. Analyses were limited to populations categorized by NMPs as being at risk.

**Estimating national net crops through time**

As described by Flaxman et al. (25), national ITN systems were represented using a discrete-time stock-and-flow model. Nets delivered to a country by manufacturers were modelled as first entering a "country stock" compartment (i.e. stored in-country but not yet distributed to households). Nets were then available from this stock for distribution to households by the NMP or other distribution channels. To accommodate uncertainty in net distribution, the number of nets distributed in a given year was specified as a range, with all available country stock (i.e. the maximum number of nets that could be delivered) as the upper end of the range and the NMP-reported value (i.e. the assumed minimum distribution) as the lower end. The total household net crop comprised new nets reaching households plus older nets remaining from earlier times, with the duration of net retention by households governed by a loss function. Rather than the loss function being fitted to a small external dataset, as was done by Flaxman et al. (25), the loss function was fitted directly to the distribution and net crop data within the stock-and-flow model itself. Loss functions were fitted on a country-by-country basis, were allowed to vary through time, and were defined separately for conventional ITNs (cITNs) and LLINs. The fitted loss functions were compared to existing assumptions about rates of net loss from households. The stock-and-flow model was fitted using Bayesian inference and Markov chain Monte Carlo methods, which provided time-series estimates of national household net crop for cITNs and LLINs in each country, and an evaluation of under-distribution, all with posterior credible intervals.

**Estimating indicators of national ITN access and use from the net crop**

Rates of ITN access within households depend not only on the total number of ITNs in a country (i.e. the net crop), but also on how those nets are distributed among households. One factor that is known to strongly influence the relationship between net crop and net distribution patterns among households is the size of households, which varies among countries, particularly across sub-Saharan Africa.

Many recent national surveys report the number of ITNs observed in each household surveyed. Hence, it is possible not only to estimate net crop, but also to generate a histogram that summarizes the household net ownership pattern (i.e. the proportion of households with zero nets, one net, two nets and so on). In this way, the size of the net crop was linked to distribution patterns among households while accounting for household size, in order to generate ownership distributions for each stratum of household size. The bivariate histogram of net crop to distribution of nets among households by household size made it possible to calculate the proportion of households with at least one ITN. Also, because the number of both ITNs and people in each household was available, it was possible to directly calculate two additional indicators: the proportion of households with at least one ITN for every two people, and the proportion of the population with access to an ITN within their household. For the final ITN indicator – the proportion of the population who slept under an ITN the previous night – the relationship between ITN use and access was defined using 62 surveys in which both these indicators were available (ITN use$_{all\ ages}$ = 0.8133 × ITN access$_{all\ ages}$ + 0.0026, $R^2$ = 0.773). This relationship was applied to the MAP's country–year estimates of household access in order to obtain ITN use among all ages. The same method was used to obtain the country–year estimates of ITN use in children aged under 5 years (ITN use$_{children\ under\ 5}$ = 0.9327 × ITN access$_{children\ under\ 5}$ + 0.0282, $R^2$ = 0.754).

**Fig. 7.2. Percentage of population at risk, pregnant women and children aged under 5 years sleeping under an ITN, sub-Saharan Africa, 2010–2018**

See methods notes for **Fig. 7.1**.

**Fig. 7.3. Percentage of population at risk with access to an ITN, and percentage of households with enough ITNs for all occupants, sub-Saharan Africa, 2010–2018**

See methods notes for **Fig. 7.1**.

**Fig. 7.4. Percentage of the population at risk protected by IRS, by WHO region, 2010–2018**

The number of persons protected by IRS was reported to WHO by NMPs. The total population of each country was taken from the 2017 revision of the *World population prospects* (19), and the proportion at risk of malaria was derived from NMP reports.

**Fig. 7.5. Main chemical classes used for IRS by national programmes globally, 2010–2018**

Data on the type of insecticide used for IRS were reported to WHO by NMPs. Insecticides were classified into pyrethroids or other classes (carbamates, organochlorines or organophosphates). If data were not reported for a particular year, data from the most recent year were used. For the period 2010–2018, this method of imputation was used for an average of 19 countries each year.

### Fig. 7.6. Percentage of pregnant women attending ANC at least once and receiving IPTp, by dose, sub-Saharan Africa, 2010–2018

The total number of pregnant women eligible for intermittent preventive treatment in pregnancy (IPTp) was calculated by adding total live births calculated from UN population data and spontaneous pregnancy loss (specifically, miscarriages and stillbirths) after the first trimester. Spontaneous pregnancy loss has previously been calculated by Dellicour et al. (26). Country-specific estimates of IPTp coverage were calculated as the ratio of pregnant women receiving IPTp at antenatal care (ANC) clinics to the estimated number of pregnant women eligible for IPTp in a given year. ANC attendance rates were derived in the same way, using the number of initial ANC visits reported through routine information systems. Local linear interpolation or information for national representative surveys was used to compute missing values. Annual aggregate estimates exclude countries for which a report or interpolation was not available for the specific year. Among 38 countries with IPTp policy, dose coverage could be calculated for 34.

### Fig. 7.7. Number of SMC treatments administered in scale-up countries in 2018

Data were provided by the Seasonal Malaria Chemoprevention (SMC) Working Group.

## Diagnostic testing and treatment

The first step was to select for inclusion all nationally representative household surveys (DHS and MIS) conducted between 2015 and 2018 (and released before 4 October 2019), for which data on malaria case management were available. Sub-Saharan Africa is the region that carries the highest share of the global malaria burden, and more surveys were available from there than from other regions; hence, only surveys conducted in that region were included in the analyses. Data were only available for children aged under 5 years because DHS and MIS focus on the most vulnerable population groups. Interviewers ask caregivers whether the child has had fever in the 2 weeks preceding the interview and, if so, where care was sought; whether the child received a finger or heel stick as part of the care; what treatment was received for the fever and when; and, in particular, whether the child received an ACT or other antimalarial medicine. In addition to self-reported data, DHS and MIS also include biomarker testing for malaria, using RDTs that detect *P. falciparum* histidine-rich protein 2 (HRP2). Percentages were calculated for each country each year. Median values and interquartile ranges (IQRs) were calculated using country percentages over a 4-year period. For cross-sectional analysis over the period 2015–2018, in cases where more than one dataset were available for a country, the most recent survey was used. For trend analysis from 2010–2013 to 2015–2018, data were calculated over 4-year overlapping intervals and all surveys in all countries for all years were included.

The use of household survey data has several limitations. One issue is that, because of difficulty recalling past events, respondents may not provide reliable information, especially on episodes of fever and the identity of prescribed medicines, resulting in a misclassification of drugs. Also, because respondents can choose more than one source of care for one episode of fever, and because the diagnostic test and treatment question is asked broadly and is, therefore, not linked to any specific source of care, it has been assumed that the diagnostic test and treatment were received in all the selected sources of care. However, only a low percentage (<5%) of febrile children were brought for care in more than one source of care. Data may also be biased by the seasonality of survey data collection because DHS are carried out at various times during the year and MIS are usually timed to correspond with the high malaria transmission season. Another limitation, when undertaking trend analysis, is that DHS and MIS are done intermittently, or not at all in some countries, resulting in a relatively small number of countries for the region of sub-Saharan Africa or for any one 4-year period. Countries are also not the same across each 4-year period. In addition, depending on the sample size of the survey, the denominator for some indicators can be small – countries where the number of children in the denominator was less than 30 were excluded from the calculation.

### Fig. 8.1. Median percentage of children who had a fever in the 2 weeks preceding the survey, overall and by age group, sub-Saharan Africa, 2015–2018 (latest survey)

Estimates were derived from 20 nationally representative household surveys (DHS and MIS) conducted between 2015 and 2018 in Angola, Benin, Burkina Faso, Burundi, Ethiopia, Ghana, Kenya, Liberia, Madagascar, Malawi, Mali, Mozambique, Nigeria, Rwanda, Senegal, Sierra Leone, Togo, Uganda, United Republic of Tanzania and Zimbabwe. For each age group, the numerator was the number of children who had a fever in the 2 weeks preceding the survey, and the denominator was the number of children.

### Fig. 8.2. Median percentage of febrile children brought for care, by health sector, sub-Saharan Africa, 2015–2018 (latest survey)

Estimates were derived from 20 nationally representative household surveys (DHS and MIS) conducted between 2015 and 2018 in Angola, Benin, Burkina Faso, Burundi, Ethiopia, Ghana, Kenya, Liberia, Madagascar, Malawi,

# Annex 1 – Data sources and methods

Mali, Mozambique, Nigeria, Rwanda, Senegal, Sierra Leone, Togo, Uganda, United Republic of Tanzania and Zimbabwe. The numerator was the number of febrile children brought for care in each health sector, and the denominator was the number of febrile children aged under 5 years. Note that respondents could choose more than one source of care for one episode of fever. Community health worker data were based on 12 countries: Burkina Faso, Burundi, Madagascar, Malawi, Mali, Mozambique, Nigeria, Rwanda, Senegal, Togo, Uganda and Zimbabwe.

### Fig. 8.3. Malaria patients examined using RDT and microscopy, and percentage of suspected cases tested in health facilities, sub-Saharan Africa, 2010–2018

Data reported by NMPs on the number of tests (RDTs and microscopy) from the public health sector were combined to calculate the number of patients examined in this sector. The number of suspected cases was computed as the number of tests plus number of presumed cases. Percentage of suspected cases who were tested was computed as percentage of number of cases examined divided by number of suspected cases.

### Fig. 8.4. Percentage of suspected cases tested in health facilities, sub-Saharan Africa, 2010–2018

See methods notes for **Fig. 8.3**.

### Fig. 8.5. Median percentage of febrile children who received a blood test, by health sector, sub-Saharan Africa, 2015–2018 (latest survey)

Estimates were derived from 19 nationally representative household surveys (DHS and MIS) conducted between 2015 and 2018 in Angola, Benin, Burkina Faso, Burundi, Ghana, Kenya, Liberia, Madagascar, Malawi, Mali, Mozambique, Nigeria, Rwanda, Senegal, Sierra Leone, Togo, Uganda, United Republic of Tanzania and Zimbabwe. For each health sector, the numerator was the number of febrile children who received a blood test and the denominator was the number of febrile children aged under 5 years. Community health worker data were based on seven countries: Burundi, Madagascar, Mali, Mozambique, Rwanda, Togo and Uganda.

### Fig. 8.6. Trend in the median percentage of febrile children who received a blood test among those treated with an antimalarial drug, by health sector, sub-Saharan Africa, 2010–2018 (all surveys)

Estimates were derived from 61 nationally representative household surveys (DHS and MIS) conducted between 2010 and 2018 in 29 countries: Angola, Benin, Burkina Faso, Burundi, Chad, Comoros, Congo, Côte d'Ivoire, Democratic Republic of the Congo, Gabon, Gambia, Ghana, Guinea, Kenya, Liberia, Madagascar, Malawi, Mali, Mozambique, Namibia, Niger, Nigeria, Rwanda, Senegal, Sierra Leone, Togo, Uganda, United Republic of Tanzania and Zambia. For each health sector, the numerator was the number of febrile children who received a blood test, and the denominator was the number of febrile children aged under 5 years who were treated with an antimalarial drug.

### Fig. 8.7. Median percentage of febrile children who were treated with an antimalarial drug, by health sector, sub-Saharan Africa, 2015–2018 (latest survey)

Estimates were derived from 20 nationally representative household surveys (DHS and MIS) conducted between 2015 and 2017 in Angola, Benin, Burkina Faso, Burundi, Ethiopia, Ghana, Kenya, Liberia, Madagascar, Malawi, Mali, Mozambique, Nigeria, Rwanda, Senegal, Sierra Leone, Togo, Uganda, United Republic of Tanzania and Zimbabwe. For each health sector, the numerator was the number of febrile children who received an antimalarial drug, and the denominator was the number of febrile children aged under 5 years. Community health worker data were based on eight countries: Burundi, Madagascar, Mali, Mozambique, Nigeria, Rwanda, Togo and Uganda.

### Fig. 8.8. Trend in the median percentage of febrile children who were treated with an antimalarial drug, by health sector, sub-Saharan Africa, 2010–2018 (all surveys)

Estimates were derived from 71 nationally representative household surveys (DHS and MIS) conducted between 2010 and 2018 in 32 countries: Angola, Benin, Burkina Faso, Burundi, Cameroon, Chad, Comoros, Congo, Côte d'Ivoire, Democratic Republic of the Congo, Ethiopia, Gabon, Gambia, Ghana, Guinea, Kenya, Liberia, Madagascar, Malawi, Mali, Mozambique, Namibia, Niger, Nigeria, Rwanda, Senegal, Sierra Leone, Togo, Uganda, United Republic of Tanzania, Zambia and Zimbabwe. For each health sector, the numerator was the number of febrile children who received an antimalarial drug, and the denominator was the number of febrile children aged under 5 years.

### Fig. 8.9. Median percentage of febrile children who received an ACT among those treated with an antimalarial drug, by health sector, sub-Saharan Africa, 2015–2018 (latest survey)

Estimates were derived from 19 nationally representative household surveys (DHS and MIS) conducted between 2015 and 2018 in Angola, Benin, Burkina Faso, Burundi, Ethiopia, Ghana, Kenya, Liberia, Madagascar, Malawi,

Mali, Mozambique, Nigeria, Rwanda, Senegal, Sierra Leone, Togo, Uganda and United Republic of Tanzania. The numerator was the number of febrile children who received an ACT, and the denominator was the number of febrile children aged under 5 years who were treated with an antimalarial drug.

### Fig. 8.10. Trend in the median percentage of febrile children who received an ACT among those treated with an antimalarial drug, by health sector, sub-Saharan Africa, 2010–2018 (all surveys)

Estimates were derived from 70 nationally representative household surveys (DHS and MIS) conducted between 2010 and 2018 in 32 countries: Angola, Benin, Burkina Faso, Burundi, Cameroon, Chad, Comoros, Congo, Côte d'Ivoire, Democratic Republic of the Congo, Ethiopia, Gabon, Gambia, Ghana, Guinea, Kenya, Liberia, Madagascar, Malawi, Mali, Mozambique, Namibia, Niger, Nigeria, Rwanda, Senegal, Sierra Leone, Togo, Uganda, United Republic of Tanzania, Zambia and Zimbabwe. The numerator was the number of febrile children who received an ACT, and the denominator was the number of febrile children aged under 5 years who were treated with an antimalarial drug.

### Fig. 9.1. Status of malaria surveillance modules implemented in DHIS2, October 2019

Data on the implementation of District Health Information Software 2 (DHIS2) were obtained from communications with NMPs and WHO GMP project reports.

### Fig. 9.2. Proposed structure and examples of thematic areas for national malaria data repositories

The aim of national malaria data repositories is to assemble, in a structured way with ability for dynamic update, existing malaria-related databases in a malaria endemic country. These databases will be installed centrally and sub nationally by HMIS to allow for effective intervention against malaria. This figure illustrates the structure and some of the proposed content of such a database.

### Fig. 10.1. Reported insecticide resistance status as a proportion of sites for which monitoring was conducted, by WHO region, 2010–2018, (a) Pyrethroids, (b) Organochlorines, (c) Carbamates, and (d) Organophosphates

Insecticide resistance monitoring results were collated from data submissions to WHO by NMPs, the African Network for Vector Resistance, national public health institutes, universities and research centers, MAP and the US President's Malaria Initiative, and extracted from scientific publications. Only data from standard WHO tube tests or CDC bottle bioassays with discriminating concentrations of insecticides were considered. Where multiple insecticide classes or types, mosquito species or time points were tested at an individual site, the highest resistance status was considered.

### Fig. 10.2. Status of monitoring of the WHO-recommended criteria for pyrethroid-PBO net deployment, 2010–2018

The status of each country was judged based on whether their monitoring sites fulfill the following criteria, namely 1) resistance to pyrethroids was confirmed in at least one key malaria vector, 2) resistance was of moderate intensity and 3) it was conferred (at least in part) by monooxygenase-based resistance mechanism. Monitoring data was reported to WHO by NMPs, the US President's Malaria Initiative and extracted from scientific publications.

# References for Annex 1

1. Global technical strategy for malaria 2016–2030. Geneva: World Health Organization; 2015 (https://www.who.int/malaria/areas/global_technical_strategy/en, accessed 20 October 2019).

2. Roll Back Malaria Partnership Secretariat. Action and investment to defeat malaria 2016–2030. For a malaria-free world. Geneva: World Health Organization; 2015 (https://endmalaria.org/sites/default/files/RBM_AIM_Report_0.pdf, accessed 20 October 2019).

3. Malaria and the UN Sustainable Development Goals (SDGs) 2030. Swiss Tropical and Public Health Institute (TPH) Swiss TPH for the Swiss Malaria Group; 2018 (https://www.swissmalariagroup.ch/fr/assets/uploads/files/New%20factsheet%20Malaria%20and%20the%20UN%20Sustainable%20Development%20Goals%20x.pdf, accessed 20 October 2019).

4. Informal Member States Consultation GPW 13 WHO Impact Framework. Geneva: World Health Organization; 2019.

5. World malaria report 2008. Geneva: World Health Organization; 2008 (https://www.who.int/malaria/publications/atoz/9789241563697/en, accessed 15 October 2013).

6. Cibulskis RE, Aregawi M, Williams R, Otten M, Dye C. Worldwide incidence of malaria in 2009: estimates, time trends, and a critique of methods. PLoS Med. 2011;8(12):e1001142.

7. The R Core Team. R: A language and environment for statistical computing: reference index. Vienna, Austria: R Foundation for Statistical Computing.

8. Bhatt S, Weiss DJ, Cameron E, Bisanzio D, Mappin B, Dalrymple U et al. The effect of malaria control on *Plasmodium falciparum* in Africa between 2000 and 2015. Nature. 2015;526(7572):207–11.

9. Alles HK, Mendis KN, Carter R. Malaria mortality rates in South Asia and in Africa: implications for malaria control. Parasitol Today. 1998;14(9):369–75.

10. Luxemburger C, Ricci F, Nosten F, Raimond D, Bathet S, White NJ. The epidemiology of severe malaria in an area of low transmission in Thailand. Trans R Soc Trop Med Hyg. 1997;91(3):256–62.

11. Meek SR. Epidemiology of malaria in displaced Khmers on the Thai-Kampuchean border. SE Asian J Trop Med. 1988;19(2):243–52.

12. Douglas NM, Pontororing GJ, Lampah DA, Yeo TW, Kenangalem E, Poespoprodjo JR et al. Mortality attributable to *Plasmodium vivax* malaria: a clinical audit from Papua, Indonesia. BMC Medicine. 2014;12(1):217.

13. Liu L, Oza S, Hogan D, Perin J, Rudan I, Lawn JE et al. Global, regional, and national causes of child mortality in 2000–13, with projections to inform post-2015 priorities: an updated systematic analysis. Lancet. 2015;385(9966):430–40.

14. Ross A, Maire N, Molineaux L, Smith T. An epidemiologic model of severe morbidity and mortality caused by *Plasmodium falciparum*. Am J Trop Med Hyg. 2006;75(2 Suppl):63–73.

15. Griffin QJ, Ferguson NM, Ghani AC. Estimates of the changing age-burden of *Plasmodium falciparum* malaria disease in sub-Saharan Africa. Nat Commun. 2014;5:3136.

16. Walker PGT, Griffin JT, Cairns M, Rogerson SJ, van Eijk AM, Ter Kuile F, Ghani AC. A model of parity-dependent immunity to placental malaria. Nat Commun. 2013;4:1609.

17. Walker PGT, Ter Kuile FO, Garske T, Menendez C, Ghani AC. Estimated risk of placental infection and low birthweight attributable to *Plasmodium falciparum* malaria in Africa in 2010: a modelling study. Lancet Glob Health. 2014;2(8):e460–e7.

18. The DHS Program: Demographic and Health Surveys [website]. (httpp://dhsprogram.com/, accessed 22 October 2019).

19. World population prospects [website]. United Nations; 2017 (https://population.un.org/wpp/, accessed 24 October 2018).

20. WorldPop [website]. (https://www.worldpop.org/, accessed 22 October 2019).

21. Cairns M, Roca-Felter A, Garske T, Wilson AL, Diallo D, Milligan PJ et al. Estimating the potential public health impact of seasonal malaria chemoprevention in African children. Nat Commun. 2012;3:881.

22. UNICEF-WHO. Low birthweight estimates: levels and trends 2000–2015. Geneva: World Health Organization; 2015 (https://www.who.int/nutrition/publications/UNICEF-WHO-lowbirthweight-estimates-2019/en/, accessed 22 October 2019).

23. Cameron E, Battle KE, Bhatt S, Weiss DJ, Bisanzio D, Mappin B et al. Defining the relationship between infection prevalence and clinical incidence of *Plasmodium falciparum* malaria. Nat Commun. 2015;6:8170.

24. High burden to high impact: a targeted malaria response. Geneva: World Health Organization; 2019 (https://www.who.int/malaria/publications/atoz/high-impact-response/en/, accessed 22 October 2019).

25. Flaxman AD, Fullman N, Otten MW, Menon M, Cibulskis RE, Ng M et al. Rapid scaling up of insecticide-treated bed net coverage in Africa and its relationship with development assistance for health: a systematic synthesis of supply, distribution, and household survey data. PLoS Med. 2010;7(8):e1000328.

26. Dellicour S, Tatem AJ, Guerra CA, Snow RW, ter Kuile FO. Quantifying the number of pregnancies at risk of malaria in 2007: a demographic study. PLoS Med. 2010;7(1):e1000221.

# Annex 2 – A. WHO African Region, a. West Africa

## EPIDEMIOLOGY
**Population at risk:** 381 million
**Parasites:** P. falciparum (almost 100%)
**Vectors:** An. arabiensis, An. coluzzii, An. funestus s.l., An. gambiae s.l., An. hispaniola, An. labranchiae, An. melas, An. moucheti, An. multicolor, An. nili s.l., An. pharoensis and An. sergentii s.l.

## FUNDING (US$), 2010–2018
547.6 million (2010), 558.9 million (2015), 675.6 million (2017); increase 2010–2018: 23%
**Proportion of domestic source* in 2018:** 9%
**Regional funding mechanisms:** Senegal River Basin Development Organization (OMVS): Guinea, Mali, Mauritania and Senegal
* Domestic source excludes patient service delivery costs and out-of-pocket expenditure.

## INTERVENTIONS, 2018
**Countries with ≥80% coverage with either LLIN or IRS in 2018:** Côte d'Ivoire and Togo
**Countries with ≥50% coverage with either LLIN or IRS in 2018:** Benin, Gambia, Ghana, Guinea, Guinea-Bissau, Liberia, Mali, Mauritania, Niger, Nigeria, Senegal and Sierra Leone

**Countries implemented IPTp in 2018:** Benin, Burkina Faso, Côte d'Ivoire, Gambia, Ghana, Guinea, Guinea-Bissau, Mali, Mauritania, Niger, Nigeria, Senegal, Sierra Leone and Togo
**Countries with >30% IPTp3+ in 2018:** Burkina Faso, Côte d'Ivoire, Gambia, Ghana, Guinea, Guinea-Bissau, Mali, Niger, Senegal, Sierra Leone and Togo

**Percentage of suspected cases tested (reported):** 44% (2010), 71% (2015), 81% (2018)
**Number of ACT courses distributed:** 32.2 million (2010), 47.4 million (2015), 75.8 million (2018)
**Number of any antimalarial treatment courses (incl. ACT) distributed:** 32.2 million (2010), 49.3 million (2015), 75.8 million (2018)

## REPORTED CASES AND DEATHS IN PUBLIC SECTOR, 2010–2018
**Total (presumed and confirmed) cases:** 29.4 million (2010), 52.3 million (2015), 61.1 million (2018)
**Confirmed cases:** 7.1 million (2010), 33.3 million (2015), 46.5 million (2018)
**Percentage of total cases confirmed:** 24.3% (2010), 63.6% (2015), 76.2% (2018)
**Deaths*:** 39 000 (2010), 21 600 (2015), 19 600 (2018)
* No data reported for Nigeria

**Children aged under 5 years, presumed and confirmed cases:** 11.9 million (2010), 21.0 million (2015), 24.6 million (2018)
**Children aged under 5 years, percentage of total cases:** 40.6% (2010), 40.2% (2015), 40.2% (2018)
**Children aged under 5 years, deaths:** 214 100 (2010), 22 100 (2015), 27 700 (2018)

## ESTIMATED CASES AND DEATHS, 2010–2018
**Cases:** 118.9 million (2010), 107.6 million (2015), 111.1 million (2018); decrease 2010–2018: 7%
**Deaths:** 304 000 (2010), 220 000 (2015), 194 000 (2018); decrease 2010–2018: 36%

## ACCELERATION TO ELIMINATION
**Countries with nationwide elimination programme:** Cabo Verde
**Zero indigenous cases for 3 consecutive years (2016, 2017 and 2018):** Algeria
**Certified as malaria free since 2010:** Algeria (2019)

## THERAPEUTIC EFFICACY TESTS (CLINICAL AND PARASITOLOGICAL FAILURE, %)

| Medicine | Study years | No. of studies | Min. | Median | Max. | Percentile 25 | Percentile 75 |
|---|---|---|---|---|---|---|---|
| AL | 2010–2017 | 69 | 0.0 | 0.0 | 11.9 | 0.0 | 2.6 |
| AS-AQ | 2010–2017 | 59 | 0.0 | 0.0 | 6.6 | 0.0 | 1.7 |
| AS-PY | 2011–2014 | 6 | 0.0 | 0.5 | 0.6 | 0.0 | 0.6 |
| DHA-PPQ | 2010–2016 | 12 | 0.0 | 0.0 | 1.9 | 0.0 | 0.2 |

AL: artemether-lumefantrine; AS-AQ: artesunate-amodiaquine; AS-PY: artesunate-pyronaridine; DHA-PPQ: dihydroartemisinin-piperaquine.

## STATUS OF INSECTICIDE RESISTANCE[a] PER INSECTICIDE CLASS (2010–2018) AND USE OF EACH CLASS FOR MALARIA VECTOR CONTROL (2018)

|  | Pyrethroids | Organochlorines | Carbamates | Organophosphates |
|---|---|---|---|---|
| LLIN:[b] | 16 | – | – | – |
| IRS:[b] | 0 | 0 | 0 | 4 |

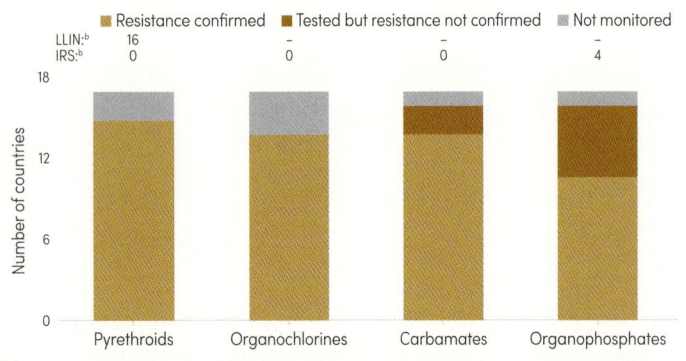

[a] Resistance is considered confirmed when it was detected to one insecticide in the class, in at least one malaria vector from one collection site.
[b] Number of countries that reported using the insecticide class for malaria vector control (2018).

### A. P. falciparum parasite prevalence (Pf PP), 2018

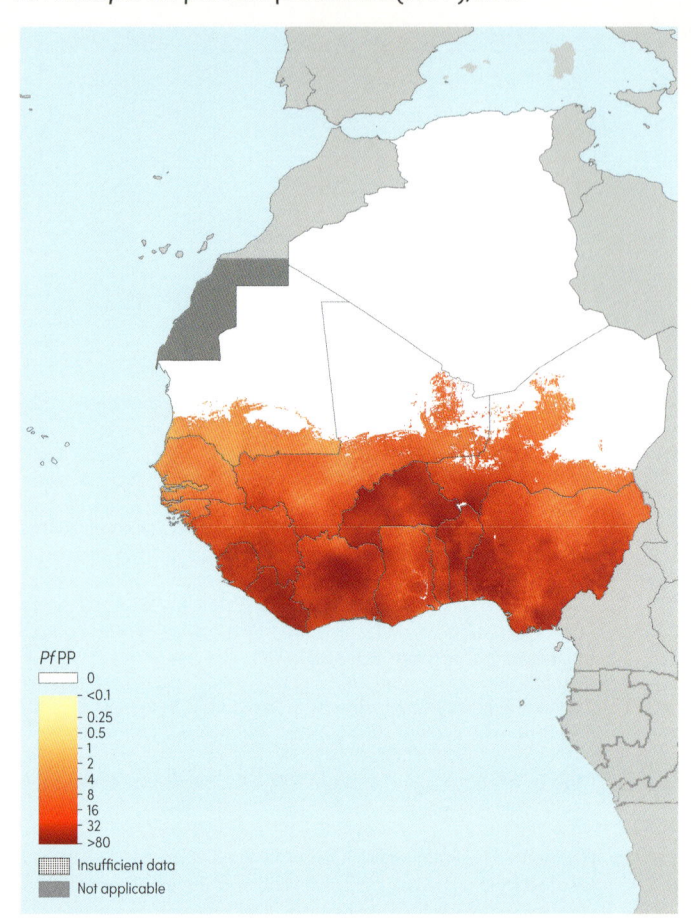

PfPP scale: 0, <0.1, 0.25, 0.5, 1, 2, 4, 8, 16, 32, >80; Insufficient data; Not applicable

### B. Malaria funding* by source, 2010–2018

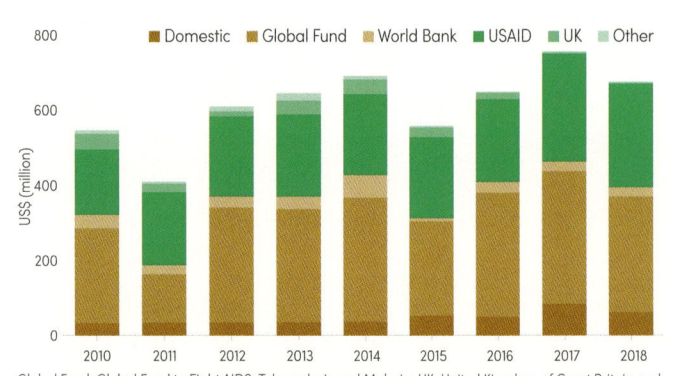

Legend: Domestic, Global Fund, World Bank, USAID, UK, Other

Global Fund: Global Fund to Fight AIDS, Tuberculosis and Malaria; UK: United Kingdom of Great Britain and Northern Ireland; USAID: United States Agency for International Development.
* Excludes patient service delivery costs and out-of-pocket expenditure.

### C. Malaria funding* per person at risk, average 2016–2018

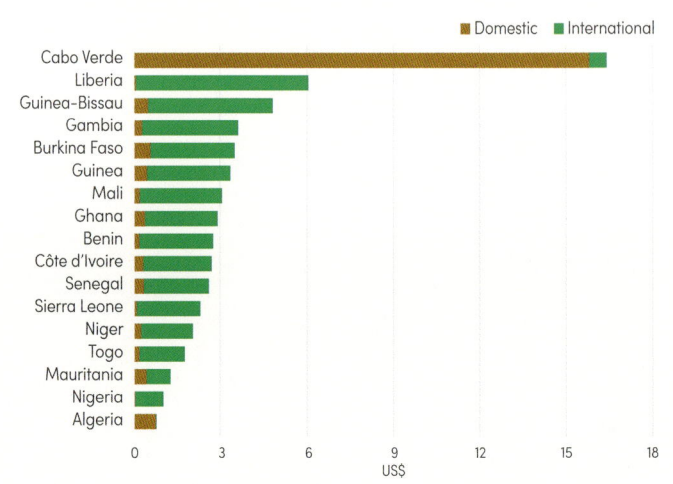

Legend: Domestic, International

Countries (top to bottom): Cabo Verde, Liberia, Guinea-Bissau, Gambia, Burkina Faso, Guinea, Mali, Ghana, Benin, Côte d'Ivoire, Senegal, Sierra Leone, Niger, Togo, Mauritania, Nigeria, Algeria

* Excludes costs related to health staff, costs at subnational level and out-of-pocket expenditure.

### D. Share of estimated malaria cases, 2018

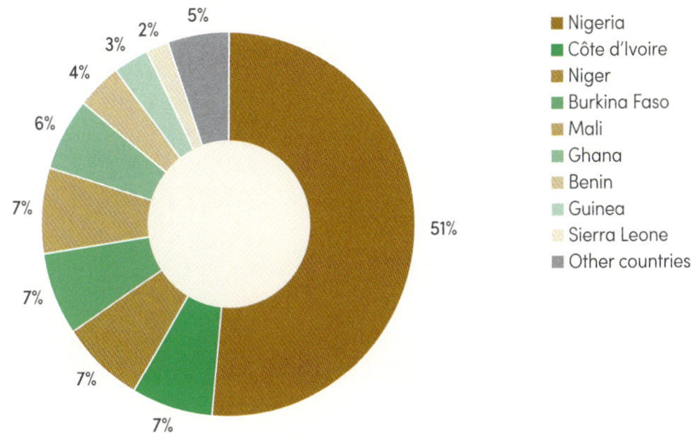

- Nigeria — 51%
- Côte d'Ivoire — 7%
- Niger — 7%
- Burkina Faso — 7%
- Mali — 7%
- Ghana — 6%
- Benin — 4%
- Guinea — 3%
- Sierra Leone — 2%
- Other countries — 5%

### E. Percentage of population with access to either LLINs or IRS, 2018
*Source: ITN coverage model from MAP*

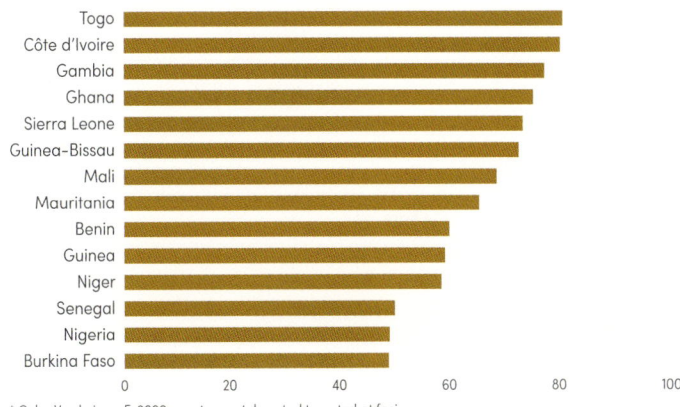

Countries (top to bottom): Togo, Côte d'Ivoire, Gambia, Ghana, Sierra Leone, Guinea-Bissau, Mali, Mauritania, Benin, Guinea, Niger, Senegal, Nigeria, Burkina Faso.

* Cabo Verde is an E-2020 country, vector control targeted at foci.

IRS: indoor residual spraying; ITN: insecticide-treated mosquito net; LLIN: long-lasting insecticidal net; MAP: Malaria Atlas Project.

### F. Countries on track to reduce case incidence by ≥40% by 2020
Algeria, Cabo Verde, Mauritania, Gambia, Togo. Baseline (2015). 2010–2018.

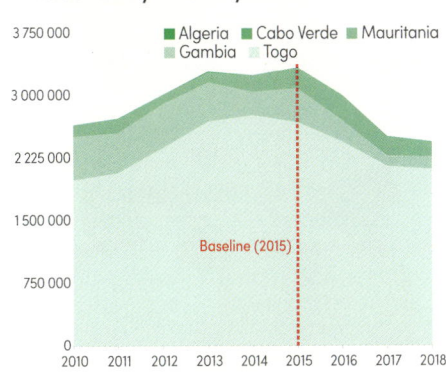

### G. Countries likely to reduce case incidence by <40% by 2020
Senegal, Sierra Leone, Benin, Guinea, Mali, Niger, Burkina Faso, Ghana, Nigeria. Baseline (2015). 2010–2018.

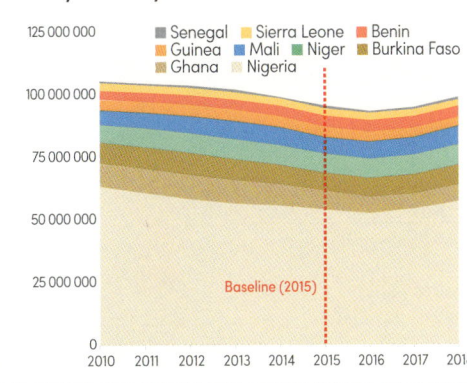

### H. Countries with an increase in case incidence, 2015–2018
Guinea-Bissau, Liberia, Côte d'Ivoire. Baseline (2015). 2010–2018.

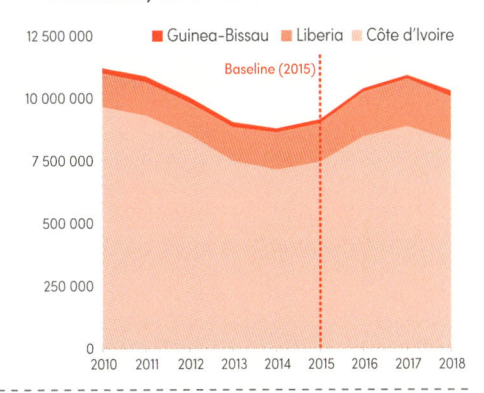

### I. Change in estimated malaria incidence and mortality rates, 2015–2018
Incidence, Mortality. 2020 milestone: −40%.

Countries (top to bottom): Cabo Verde, Gambia, Mauritania, Mali, Togo, Niger, Sierra Leone, Guinea, Ghana, Benin, Senegal, Nigeria, Burkina Faso, Côte d'Ivoire, Liberia, Guinea-Bissau.

### J. Incidence in 2018 compared to baseline (2015–2017)
75th percentile (2015–2017), 2018. 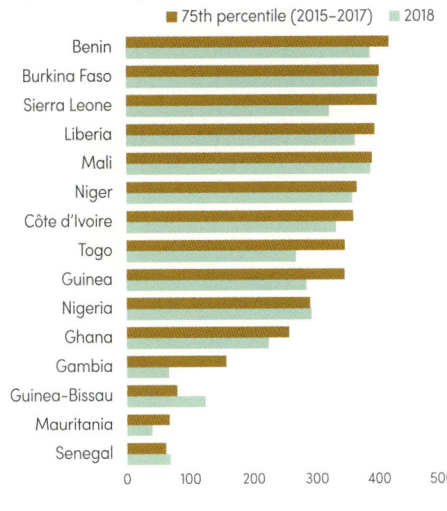

Countries (top to bottom): Benin, Burkina Faso, Sierra Leone, Liberia, Mali, Niger, Côte d'Ivoire, Togo, Guinea, Nigeria, Ghana, Gambia, Guinea-Bissau, Mauritania, Senegal.

### K. Reported indigenous cases in countries with national elimination activities, 2015 versus 2018
- Cabo Verde: 2015 = 7, 2018 = 2

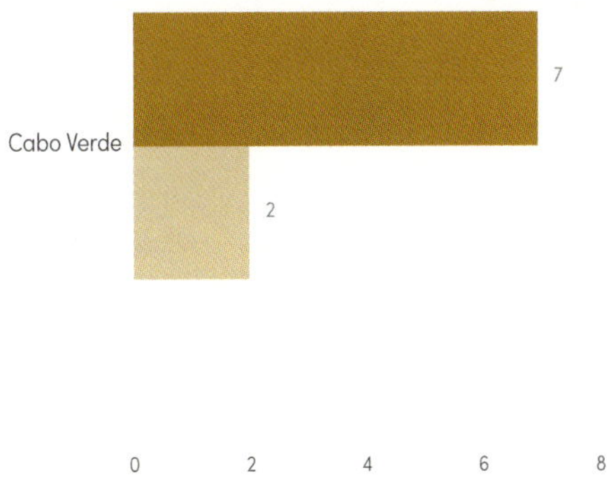

* Zero cases and deaths in Algeria since 2015.

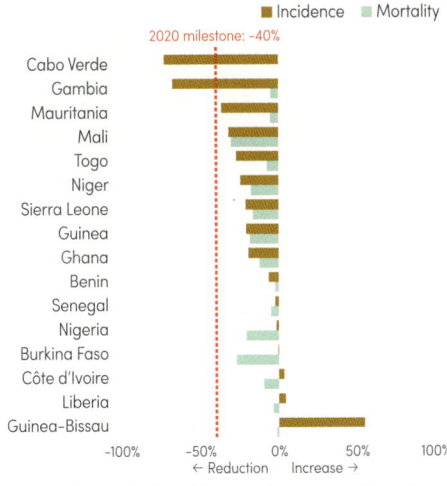

* Cabo Verde already achieved the 40% reduction in mortality rate in 2015; since then there has been no change.
** Zero cases and deaths in Algeria since 2015.

## KEY MESSAGES

- About 381 million people living in the 17 countries of West Africa are at high risk. Algeria was certified malaria free in May 2019, following 3 consecutive years with zero indigenous cases. In the rest of the countries in the subregion, malaria transmission is year-round and almost exclusively due to *P. falciparum* in most of the countries, with strong seasonality in the Sahelian countries.

- The subregion had more than 111 million estimated cases and about 194 000 estimated deaths, representing a 7% and 36% decrease compared with 2010, respectively. Six countries accounted for over 80% of the estimated cases: Nigeria (51%), Côte d'Ivoire (7%), Burkina Faso (7%), Mali and Niger (each 7%) and Ghana (6%). In the public health sector, about 61 million cases were reported, of which 40.2% were in children aged under 5 years and 46.5 million (76.2%) were confirmed. The proportion of total cases that were confirmed improved substantially over time, from only 24.3% in 2010. A total of 27 700 malaria deaths were reported in children aged under 5 years; this figure exceeded the total malaria deaths, indicating that there are challenges in the surveillance of malaria mortality in some countries.

- In 12 of the 15 countries in which routine distribution of LLINs or use of IRS is still applicable, at least 50% of the population had access to these interventions. Seven countries are on track to meet the GTS target by reducing case incidence by at least 40% by 2020 compared with 2015: Algeria (already certified malaria free), Cabo Verde, Gambia, Mali, Mauritania, Niger and Togo. Nine countries showed progress towards meeting the target but need efforts to be accelerated to achieve the 40% reduction: Benin, Burkina Faso, Ghana, Guinea, Mali, Niger, Nigeria, Senegal and Sierra Leone. Despite Senegal's progress in malaria reduction in recent years, the country saw an increase in 2017 and 2018. In Côte d'Ivoire, Guinea-Bissau and Liberia, incidence increased in 2018 compared with 2015. Following a large increase in indigenous cases in Cabo Verde between 2016 and 2017, the country reported only two indigenous cases in 2018, similar to 2015. In addition to Algeria and Cabo Verde, only Burkina Faso and Mali are on track to reduce malaria mortality rates by at least 40%.

- In line with the Nouakchott Declaration and the Sahel Malaria Elimination Initiative (SaME), eight ministers of the Sahelian countries (Burkina Faso, Cabo Verde, Chad, Gambia, Mali, Mauritania, Niger and Senegal) committed on 31 August 2018 to accelerate implementation, with the aim of eliminating malaria by 2030. In addition to Cabo Verde as an eliminating country, Gambia, Mauritania, Niger and Senegal are reorienting their programmes towards malaria subnational elimination.

- Vector resistance to pyrethroids was confirmed in most of the countries, and resistance to organochlorines and carbamates was confirmed in more than half of the countries. Guinea-Bissau has not reported standard resistance monitoring to any of the four insecticide classes.

- Challenges include inadequate political commitment and leadership, weak malaria programme management, insufficient prioritization and sustainability of interventions, inappropriate application of larviciding, inadequate domestic financing and weak surveillance systems, including a lack of well-functioning vital registration systems.

# Annex 2 - A. WHO African Region, b. Central Africa

### EPIDEMIOLOGY
**Population at risk:** 180 million
**Parasites:** P. falciparum (100%)
**Vectors:** An. arabiensis, An. funestus s.l., An. gambiae s.l., An. melas, An. moucheti, An. nili s.l. and An. pharoensis.

### FUNDING (US$), 2010–2018
246.2 million (2010), 370.0 million (2015), 318.7 million (2018); increase 2010–2018: 29%
**Proportion of domestic source* in 2018:** 20%
**Regional funding mechanisms:** none
* Domestic source excludes patient service delivery costs and out-of-pocket expenditure.

### INTERVENTIONS, 2018
**Countries with ≥80% coverage with either LLIN or IRS in 2018:** Burundi and Sao Tome and Principe
**Countries with ≥50% coverage with either LLIN or IRS in 2018:** Cameroon, Central African Republic, Chad and Democratic Republic of the Congo
**Countries implemented IPTp in 2018:** Angola, Burundi, Cameroon, Central African Republic, Chad, Congo, Democratic Republic of the Congo, Equatorial Guinea and Gabon
**Countries with >30% IPTp3+ in 2018:** Burundi, Cameroon, Central African Republic, Chad and Democratic Republic of the Congo
**Percentage of suspected cases tested (reported):** 41% (2010), 92% (2015), 92% (2018)
**Number of ACT courses distributed:** 18.2 million (2010), 22.4 million (2015), 26.8 million (2018)
**Number of any antimalarial treatment courses (incl. ACT) distributed:** 19.0 million (2010), 22.4 million (2015), 26.9 million (2018)

### REPORTED CASES AND DEATHS IN PUBLIC SECTOR, 2010–2018
**Total (presumed and confirmed) cases:** 20.4 million (2010), 24.6 million (2015), 35.1 million (2018)
**Confirmed cases:** 6.6 million (2010), 22.2 million (2015), 30.9 million (2018)
**Percentage of total cases confirmed:** 32.6% (2010), 90.1% (2015), 88.2% (2018)
**Deaths:** 40 400 (2010), 58 200 (2015), 39 500 (2018)
**Children aged under 5 years, presumed and confirmed cases:** 9.1 million (2010), 11.3 million (2015), 16.3 million (2018)
**Children aged under 5 years, percentage of total cases:** 44.9% (2010), 46.1% (2015), 46.4% (2018)
**Children aged under 5 years, deaths:** 26 000 (2010), 37 100 (2015), 25 100 (2018)

### ESTIMATED CASES AND DEATHS, 2010–2018
**Cases:** 46.0 million (2010), 42.8 million (2015), 49.2 million (2018); increase 2010–2018: 7%
**Deaths:** 118 400 (2010), 92 000 (2015), 89 900 (2018); decrease 2010–2018: 24%

### ACCELERATION TO ELIMINATION
**Countries with subnational/territorial elimination programme:** Sao Tome and Principe

### THERAPEUTIC EFFICACY TESTS (CLINICAL AND PARASITOLOGICAL FAILURE, %)

| Medicine | Study years | No. of studies | Min. | Median | Max. | Percentile 25 | Percentile 75 |
|---|---|---|---|---|---|---|---|
| AL | 2010–2018 | 27 | 0.0 | 2.1 | 13.6 | 0.0 | 3.6 |
| AS-AQ | 2010–2018 | 28 | 0.0 | 1.4 | 7.7 | 0.0 | 3.9 |

AL: artemether-lumefantrine; AS-AQ: artesunate-amodiaquine.

### STATUS OF INSECTICIDE RESISTANCE[a] PER INSECTICIDE CLASS (2010–2018) AND USE OF EACH CLASS FOR MALARIA VECTOR CONTROL (2018)

| | Pyrethroids | Organochlorines | Carbamates | Organophosphates |
|---|---|---|---|---|
| LLIN:[b] | 10 | – | – | – |
| IRS:[b] | 1 | 0 | 3 | 2 |

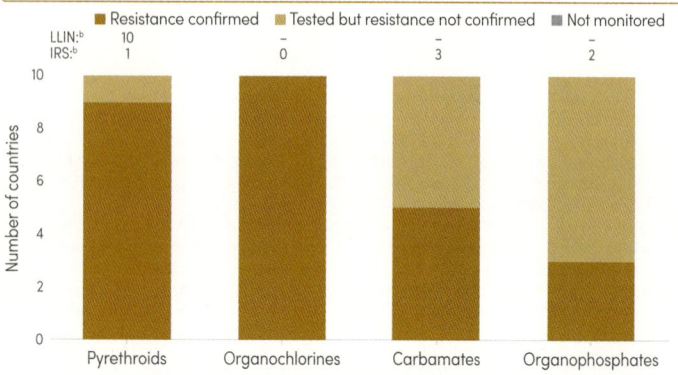

[a] Resistance is considered confirmed when it was detected to one insecticide in the class, in at least one malaria vector from one collection site.
[b] Number of countries that reported using the insecticide class for malaria vector control (2018).

## A. P. falciparum parasite prevalence (Pf PP), 2018

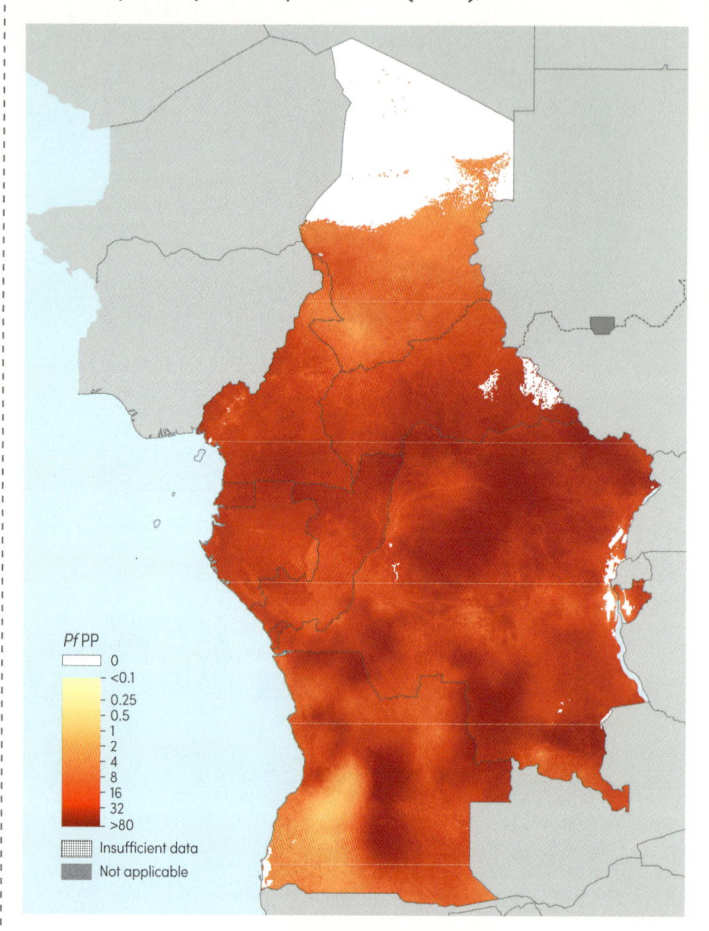

## B. Malaria funding* by source, 2010–2018

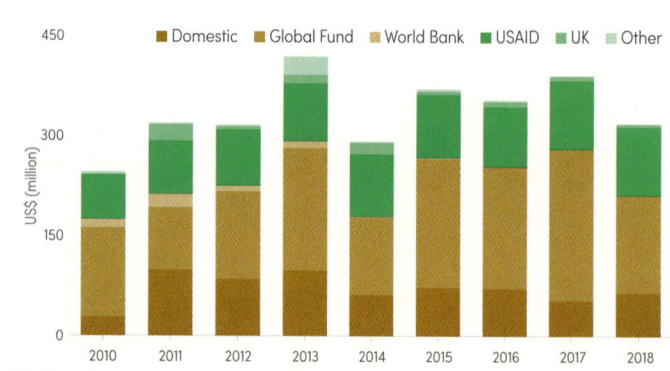

Global Fund: Global Fund to Fight AIDS, Tuberculosis and Malaria; UK: United Kingdom of Great Britain and Northern Ireland; USAID: United States Agency for International Development.
* Excludes patient service delivery costs and out-of-pocket expenditure.

## C. Malaria funding* per person at risk, average 2016–2018

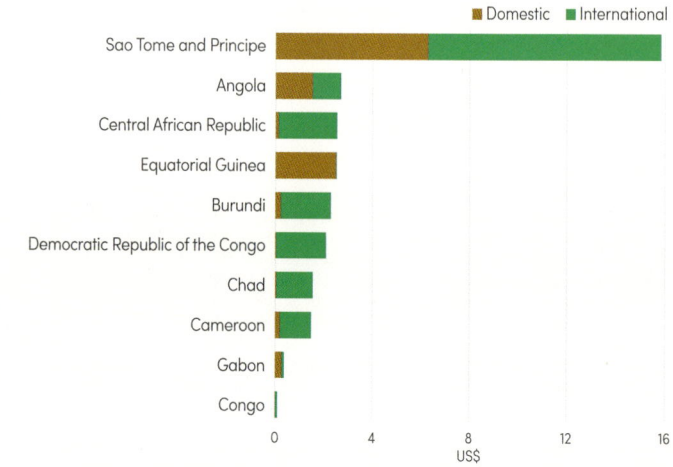

* Excludes costs related to health staff, costs at subnational level and out-of-pocket expenditure.

**D. Share of estimated malaria cases, 2018**

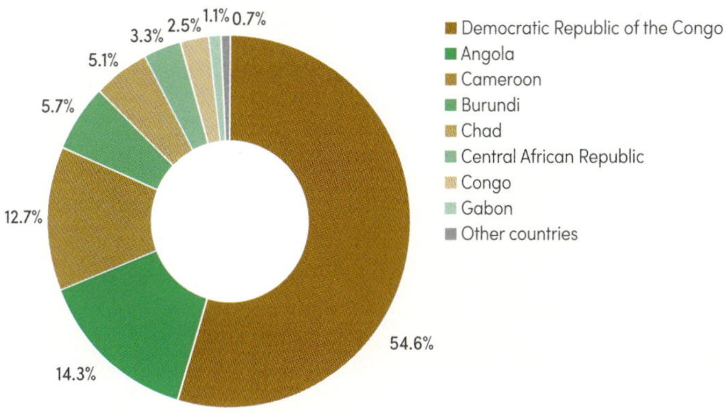

- Democratic Republic of the Congo: 54.6%
- Angola: 14.3%
- Cameroon: 12.7%
- Burundi: 5.7%
- Chad: 5.1%
- Central African Republic: 3.3%
- Congo: 2.5%
- Gabon: 1.1%
- Other countries: 0.7%

**E. Percentage of population with access to either LLINs or IRS, 2018**
*Source: ITN coverage model from MAP*

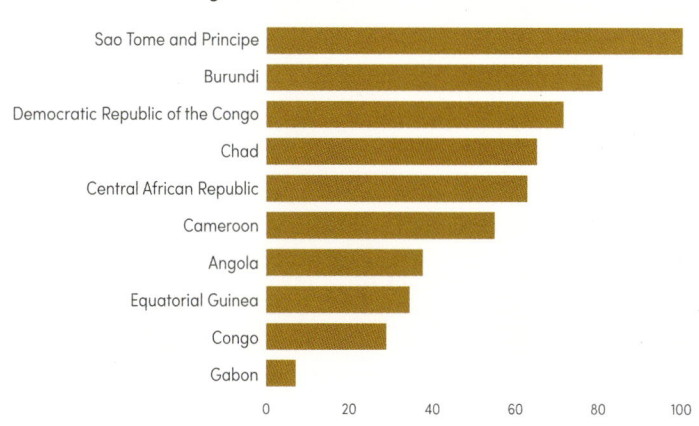

Ranking (approximate):
- Sao Tome and Principe: ~100
- Burundi: ~80
- Democratic Republic of the Congo: ~70
- Chad: ~65
- Central African Republic: ~60
- Cameroon: ~55
- Angola: ~40
- Equatorial Guinea: ~35
- Congo: ~30
- Gabon: ~10

IRS: indoor residual spraying; ITN: insecticide-treated mosquito net; LLIN: long-lasting insecticidal net; MAP: Malaria Atlas Project.

**F. Countries likely to reduce case incidence by <40% by 2020**

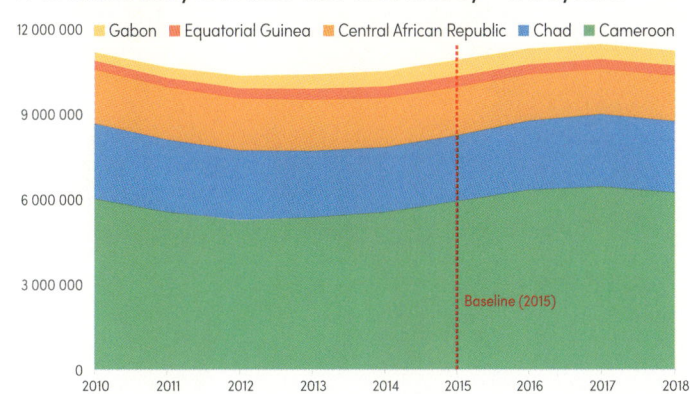

Legend: Gabon, Equatorial Guinea, Central African Republic, Chad, Cameroon. Baseline (2015). Years 2010–2018.

**G. Countries with an increase in case incidence, 2015–2018**

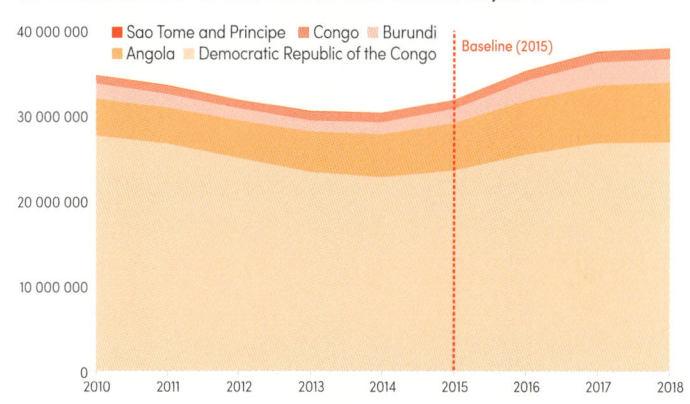

Legend: Sao Tome and Principe, Congo, Burundi, Angola, Democratic Republic of the Congo. Baseline (2015). Years 2010–2018.

**H. Change in estimated malaria incidence and mortality rates, 2015–2018**

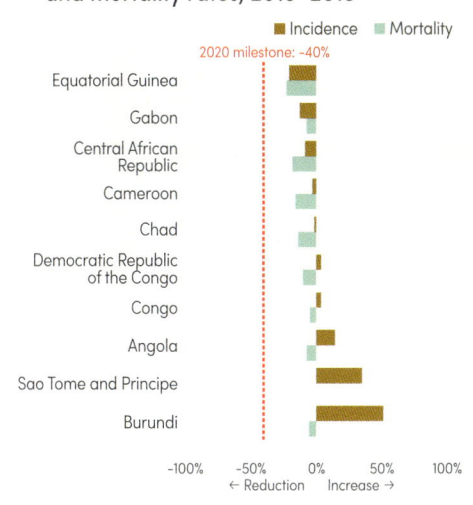

Legend: Incidence, Mortality. 2020 milestone: −40%.

Countries (top to bottom): Equatorial Guinea, Gabon, Central African Republic, Cameroon, Chad, Democratic Republic of the Congo, Congo, Angola, Sao Tome and Principe, Burundi.

← Reduction    Increase →

**I. Incidence in 2018 compared to baseline (2015–2017)**

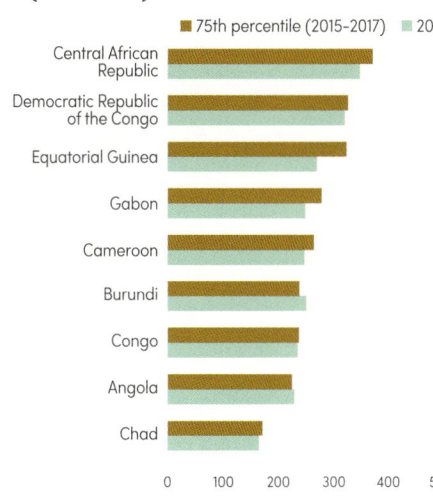

Legend: 75th percentile (2015–2017), 2018.

Countries: Central African Republic, Democratic Republic of the Congo, Equatorial Guinea, Gabon, Cameroon, Burundi, Congo, Angola, Chad.

**J. Reported indigenous cases in countries with national elimination activities, 2015 versus 2018**

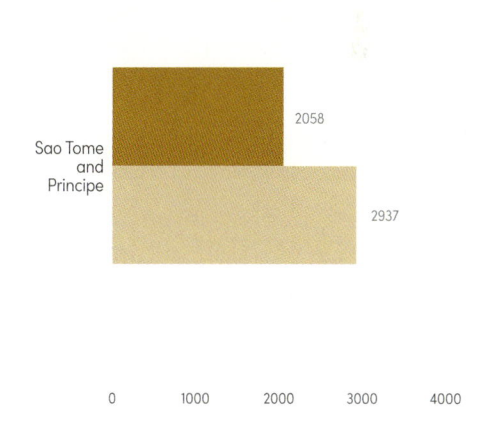

Legend: 2015, 2018.

Sao Tome and Principe: 2058 (2015), 2937 (2018)

* Sao Tome and Principe already achieved the 40% reduction in mortality rate in 2015; since then there has been no change.

# KEY MESSAGES

- About 180 million people living in the 10 countries of Central Africa are at high risk. Malaria transmission, almost exclusively due to *P. falciparum*, occurs throughout the year, except in Burundi, the highlands of eastern Cameroon, northern Chad and Congo.
- In 2018, the subregion had about 49 million estimated cases and almost 90 000 estimated deaths, representing a 7% increase and a 24% decrease compared with 2010, respectively. The Democratic Republic of the Congo accounted for 55% of estimated cases, followed by Angola (14%), Cameroon (13%), Burundi (6%) and Chad (5%). In the public health sector, about 35 million cases were reported, of which 46% were in children aged under 5 years and 30.9 million (87.7%) were confirmed. The proportion of total cases that were confirmed improved substantially over time from only 32.6% in 2010. There were 39 500 reported malaria deaths, of which 63% were in children aged under 5 years.
- Progress has been made towards achieving the GTS target of a 40% reduction in incidence by 2020 in Cameroon, Central African Republic, Chad, Equatorial Guinea and Gabon, but greater efforts are needed to ensure that these countries meet the target. Five countries saw an increase in cases between 2015 and 2018, with Burundi having the largest increase (51%). Although Sao Tome and Principe also saw a slight increase in reported cases, zero deaths were reported in 2018. In Cameroon, Central African Republic, Chad and the Democratic Republic of the Congo, 50% of the population had access to LLINs or IRS. Burundi and Sao Tome and Principe had more than 80% coverage, which is indicative of a rapid and efficient response to the increasing cases in the countries. In 2018, Angola, Central African Republic, Equatorial Guinea and Sao Tome and Principe conducted LLIN mass campaigns.
- Vector resistance to organochlorines was confirmed in all countries, and to pyrethroids in all countries except Sao Tome and Principe. All countries had standardized monitoring of carbamates and organophosphates, for which resistance is still lower.
- Challenges include weak health systems, insufficient domestic and international funding, and frequent malaria outbreaks. Equatorial Guinea and Gabon are no longer eligible for support from the Global Fund but domestic investments have increased to bridge the funding gap.

# Annex 2 – A. WHO African Region, c. Countries with high transmission in East and Southern Africa

## EPIDEMIOLOGY
**Population at risk:** 351 million
**Parasites:** *P. falciparum* (76%) and *P. vivax* (24%)
**Vectors:** An. arabiensis, An. funestus s.l., An. gambiae s.l., An. gambiae s.s., An. leesoni, An. nili, An. pharoensis, An. rivulorum, An. stephensi s.l.* and An. vaneedeni.

* A potential vector identified.

## FUNDING (US$), 2010–2018
745.6 million (2010), 721.1 million (2015), 698.1 million (2018); decrease 2010–2018: 6%
**Proportion of domestic source* in 2018:** 11%
**Regional funding mechanisms:** none

* Domestic source excludes patient service delivery costs and out-of-pocket expenditure.

## INTERVENTIONS, 2018
**Countries with ≥80% coverage with either LLIN or IRS in 2018:** Uganda
**Countries with ≥50% coverage with either LLIN or IRS in 2018:** Kenya, Malawi, Mozambique, Rwanda, South Sudan, United Republic of Tanzania and Zambia

**Countries implemented IPTp in 2018:** Kenya, Madagascar, Malawi, Mozambique, South Sudan, Uganda, United Republic of Tanzania, Zambia and Zimbabwe
**Countries with >30% IPTp3+ in 2018:** Mozambique, United Republic of Tanzania, Zambia and Zimbabwe

**Percentage of suspected cases tested (reported):** 30% (2010), 80% (2015), 89% (2018)
**Number of ACT courses distributed:** 84.5 million (2010), 108.2 million (2015), 108.3 million (2018)
**Number of any antimalarial treatment courses (incl. ACT) distributed:** 84.7 million (2010), 109.9 million (2015), 108.8 million (2018)

## REPORTED CASES AND DEATHS IN PUBLIC SECTOR, 2010–2018
**Total (presumed and confirmed) cases:** 53.2 million (2010), 54.3 million (2015), 56.7 million (2018)
**Confirmed cases:** 19.9 million (2010), 40.2 million (2015), 47.6 million (2018)
**Percentage of total cases confirmed:** 37.5% (2010), 74.1% (2015), 83.9% (2018)
**Deaths:** 70 700 (2010), 38 300 (2015), 14 000 (2018)

**Children aged under 5 years, presumed and confirmed cases:** 21.6 million (2010), 17.6 million (2015), 11.0 million (2018)
**Percentage of total cases under 5:** 40.5% (2010), 32.5% (2015), 19.4% (2018)
**Children aged under 5 years, deaths:** 25 300 (2010), 10 400 (2015), 6500 (2018)

## ESTIMATED CASES AND DEATHS, 2010–2018
**Cases*:** 53.5 million (2010), 48.7 million (2015), 52.2 million (2018); decrease 2010–2018: 2%
**Deaths:** 12 400 (2010), 5350 (2015), 6500 (2018); decrease 2010–2018: 48%

* Estimated cases are derived from the *Pf/Pr*-to-incidence model, which means that estimated cases are lower than reported by the country.

## ACCELERATION TO ELIMINATION
**Countries with subnational/territorial elimination programme:** United Republic of Tanzania

## THERAPEUTIC EFFICACY TESTS (CLINICAL AND PARASITOLOGICAL FAILURE, %)

| Medicine | Study years | No. of studies | Min. | Median | Max. | Percentile 25 | Percentile 75 |
|---|---|---|---|---|---|---|---|
| AL | 2010–2016 | 68 | 0.0 | 1.8 | 19.5 | 0.0 | 3.6 |
| AS-AQ | 2011–2016 | 14 | 0.0 | 0.0 | 2.0 | 0.0 | 1.2 |

AL: artemether-lumefantrine; AS-AQ: artesunate-amodiaquine.

## STATUS OF INSECTICIDE RESISTANCE[a] PER INSECTICIDE CLASS (2010–2018) AND USE OF EACH CLASS FOR MALARIA VECTOR CONTROL (2018)

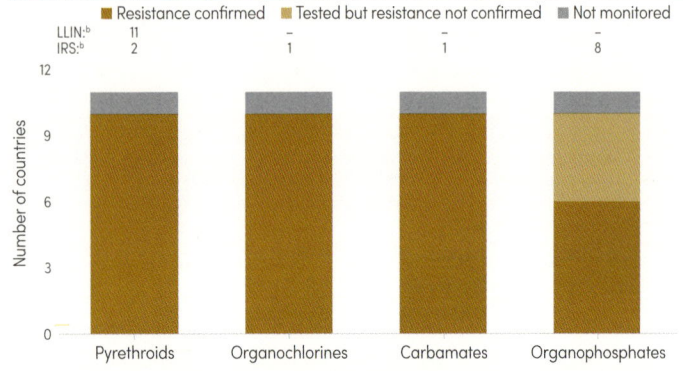

[a] Resistance is considered confirmed when it was detected to one insecticide in the class, in at least one malaria vector from one collection site.
[b] Number of countries that reported using the insecticide class for malaria vector control (2018).

## A. *P. falciparum* parasite prevalence (*Pf* PP), 2018

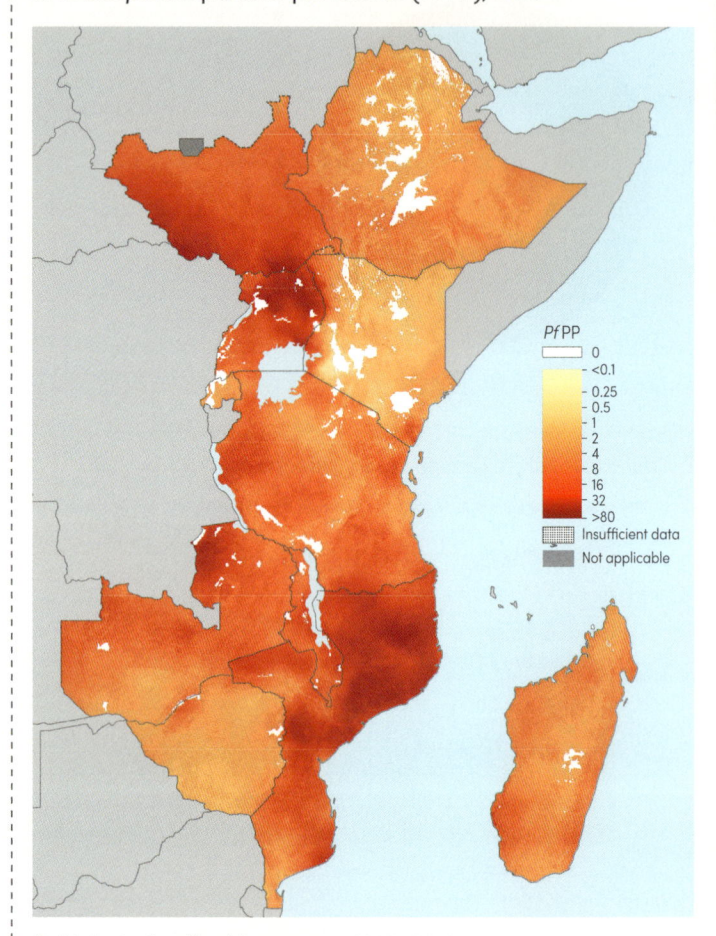

## B. Malaria funding* by source, 2010–2018

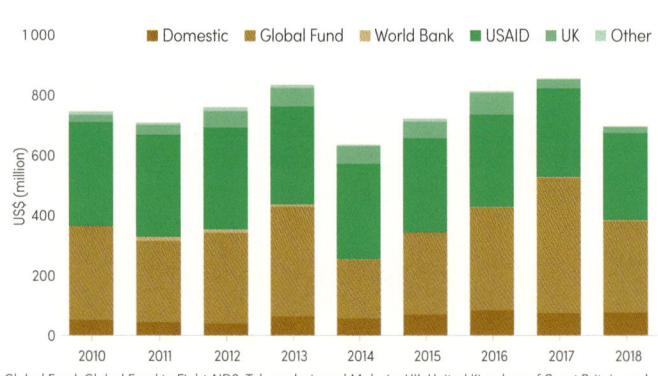

Global Fund: Global Fund to Fight AIDS, Tuberculosis and Malaria; UK: United Kingdom of Great Britain and Northern Ireland; USAID: United States Agency for International Development.
* Excludes patient service delivery costs and out-of-pocket expenditure.

## C. Malaria funding* per person at risk, average 2016–2018

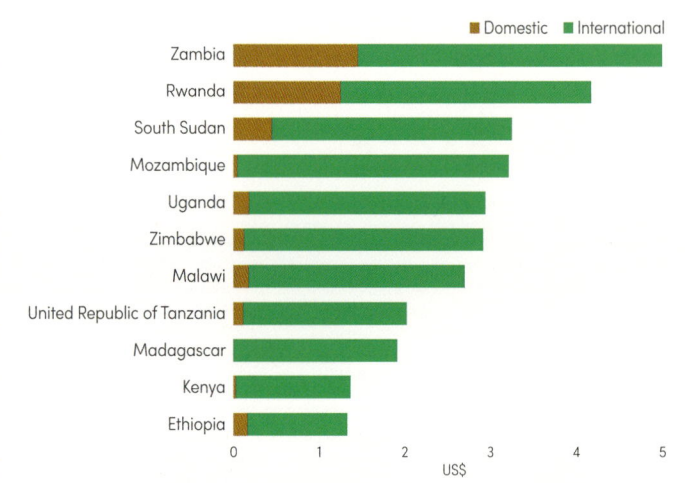

* Excludes costs related to health staff, costs at subnational level and out-of-pocket expenditure.

### D. Share of estimated malaria cases, 2018

- Uganda: 23.7%
- Mozambique: 17.2%
- United Republic of Tanzania: 13.4%
- Rwanda: 11.5%
- Malawi: 7.4%
- Kenya: 6.9%
- Zambia: 5.2%
- South Sudan: 5.0%
- Ethiopia: 4.5%
- Madagascar: 4.1%
- Zimbabwe: 1.1%

### E. Percentage of population with access to either LLINs or IRS, 2018
*Source: ITN coverage model from MAP*

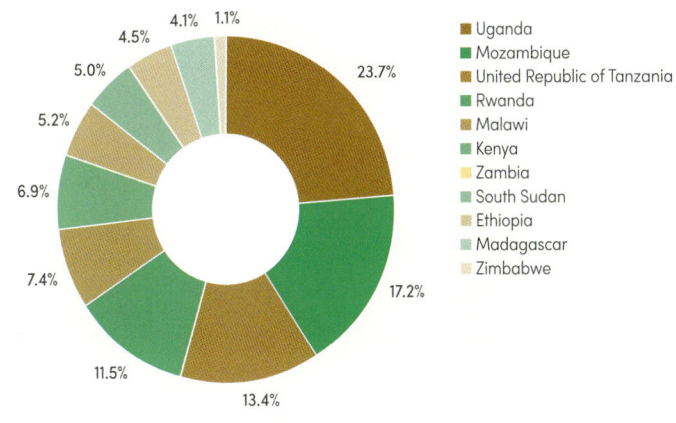

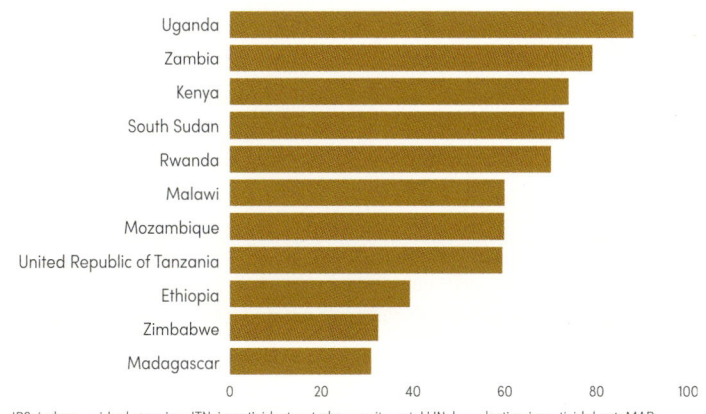

IRS: indoor residual spraying; ITN: insecticide-treated mosquito net; LLIN: long-lasting insecticidal net; MAP: Malaria Atlas Project.

### F. Countries on track to reduce case incidence by ≥40% by 2020
Zimbabwe, Zambia, Ethiopia

### G. Countries likely to reduce case incidence by <40% by 2020
Madagascar, South Sudan, Kenya, Malawi, Mozambique

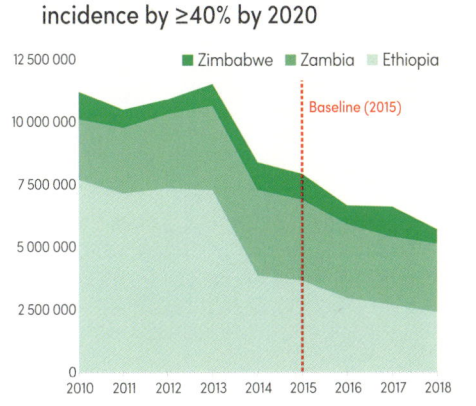

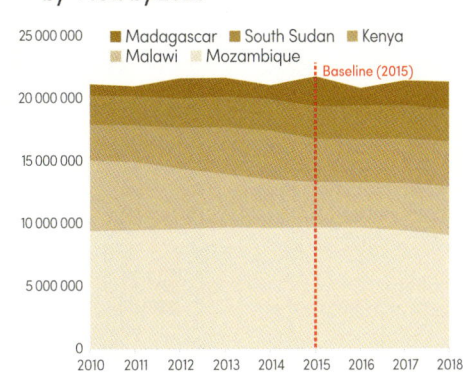

### H. Countries with an increase in case incidence, 2015–2018
Rwanda, United Republic of Tanzania, Uganda

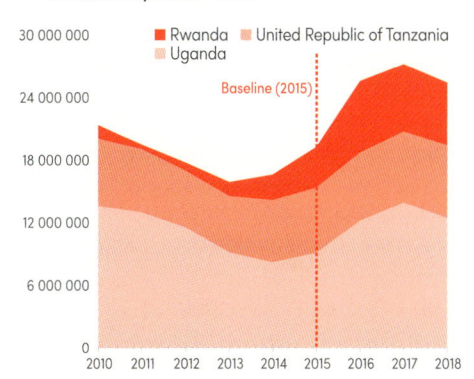

### I. Change in estimated malaria incidence and mortality rates, 2015–2018

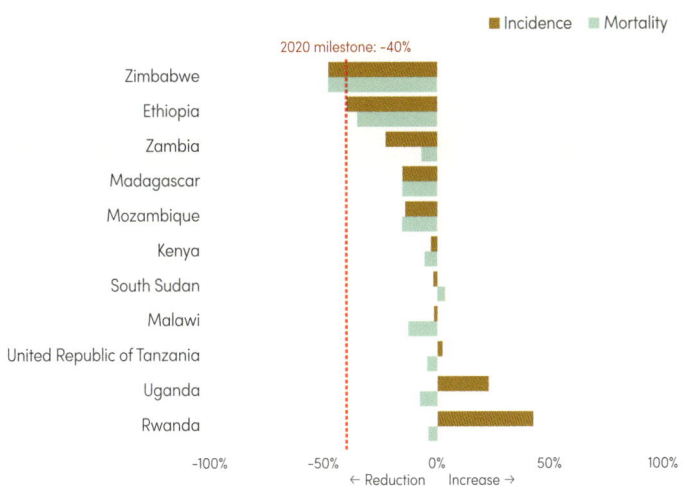

### J. Incidence in 2018 compared to 75th percentile of 2015–2017

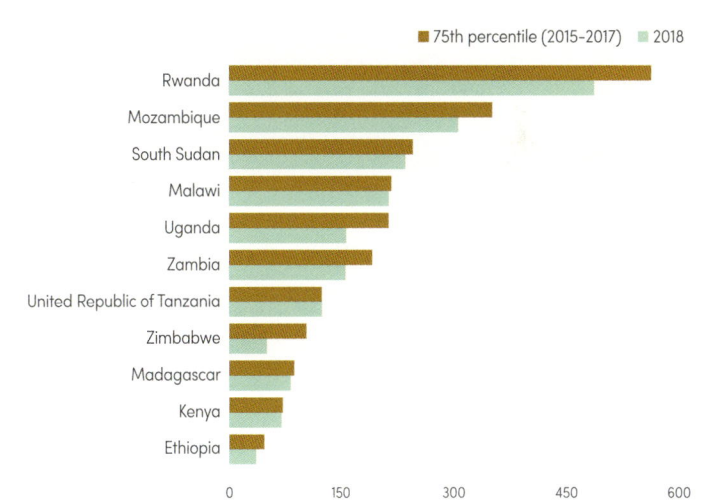

## KEY MESSAGES

- About 351 million people in the 11 countries of East and Southern Africa are at high risk. Malaria transmission is almost exclusively due to *P. falciparum* (except in Ethiopia), and is highly seasonal in Ethiopia, Madagascar and Zimbabwe, and in coastal and highland areas of Kenya. Malaria transmission is stable in most of Malawi, Mozambique, South Sudan, Uganda, the United Republic of Tanzania and Zambia.

- The subregion had 52 million estimated cases and about 6500 estimated deaths, representing a 2% and 48% decrease compared with 2010, respectively. Three countries accounted for over 60% of the estimated cases: Uganda (24%), Mozambique (17%) and the United Republic of Tanzania (13%). In the public health sector more than 55 million cases were reported, of which 19.4% were in children aged under 5 years and 47 million (83.9%) were confirmed. The proportion of total cases that were confirmed improved substantially over time, from only 37.5% in 2010. A significantly lower number of malaria deaths were reported in 2018 (14 000) compared with 2010 (70 700) and 2015 (38 300).

- Ethiopia, Rwanda, Zambia and Zimbabwe are all on track for a 40% reduction in incidence by 2020; all other countries either reported small reductions in incidence, or increases (Rwanda, Uganda and the United Republic of Tanzania). Only Ethiopia and Zambia are on track to reduce malaria mortality rates by at least 40%. In more than half of the countries, 50% or more of the population had access to LLINs or IRS in 2018, and Uganda had coverage of more than 80%.

- Reported cases in Rwanda increased from 2.5 million in 2015 to 4.2 million in 2018, an increase of 68%. Madagascar and Mozambique also reported increases of 30% and 20%, respectively, during the period 2015–2018. Causes of such increases can include inadequate vector control; climatic factors and improved reporting. Uganda saw a 51% decrease in 2018 compared with 2017, which may be as a result of a successful rapid public health response to the almost 25% increase in cases that was reported between 2016 and 2017. Zanzibar (United Republic of Tanzania) also reported a 54% decrease in cases (from 3349 to 1532) between 2017 and 2018.

- Vector resistance to pyrethroids, organochlorines and carbamates was confirmed in all countries except South Sudan, which did not report resistance monitoring. Resistance to organophosphates was confirmed in half of the countries.

- Challenges include frequent epidemics, emergencies and inadequate response (South Sudan), inadequate funding and weak surveillance systems in a number of the countries.

# Annex 2 – A. WHO African Region, d. Countries with low transmission in East and Southern Africa

## EPIDEMIOLOGY

**Population at risk:** 14 million
**Parasites:** *P. falciparum* (98%) and *P. vivax* (2%)
**Vectors:** *An. arabiensis, An. funestus s.l., An. funestus s.s., An. gambiae s.l.* and *An. gambiae s.s.*

## FUNDING (US$), 2010–2018

67.7 million (2010), 25.5 million (2015), 42.3 million (2018); decrease 2010–2018: 37%
**Proportion of domestic source in 2018:** 75%
**Regional funding mechanisms:** Southern Africa Malaria Elimination Eight Initiative

\* Domestic source excludes patient service delivery costs and out-of-pocket expenditure.

## INTERVENTIONS, 2018

**Countries with ≥80% coverage of at-risk population with either LLIN or IRS in 2018:** None
**Countries with ≥80% coverage of high risk population with either LLIN or IRS in 2018:** Botswana

**Countries with >30% IPTp3+ in 2018:** Comoros

**Percentage of suspected cases tested (reported):** 79% (2010), 98% (2015), 99% (2018)
**Number of ACT courses distributed:** 575 000 (2010), 366 000 (2015), 357 000 (2018)
**Number of any antimalarial treatment courses (incl. ACT) distributed:** 575 000 (2010), 366 000 (2015), 391 000 (2018)

## REPORTED CASES AND DEATHS IN PUBLIC SECTOR, 2010–2018

**Total (presumed and confirmed) cases:** 205 300 (2010), 47 800 (2015), 99 800 (2018)
**Confirmed cases:** 82 400 (2010), 33 900 (2015), 79 500 (2018)
**Percentage of total cases confirmed:** 40.2% (2010), 70.8% (2015), 79.7% (2018)
**Deaths:** 242 (2010), 178 (2015), 175 (2018)

**Children aged under 5 years, presumed and confirmed cases:** 56 400 (2010), 7300 (2015), 11 500 (2018)
**Children aged under 5 years, percentage of total cases:** 27.5% (2010), 15.2% (2015), 11.5% (2018)
**Children aged under 5 years, deaths:** 37 (2010), 16 (2015), 33 (2018)

## ESTIMATED CASES AND DEATHS, 2010–2018

**Cases:** 133 200 (2010), 87 300 (2015), 177 900 (2018); increase 2010–2018: 34%
**Deaths:** 344 (2010), 293 (2015), 438 (2018); increase 2010–2018: 27%

## ACCELERATION TO ELIMINATION

**Countries with nationwide elimination programme:** Botswana, Comoros, Eswatini, Namibia and South Africa

## THERAPEUTIC EFFICACY TESTS (CLINICAL AND PARASITOLOGICAL FAILURE, %)

| Medicine | Study years | No. of studies | Min. | Median | Max. | Percentile 25 | Percentile 75 |
|---|---|---|---|---|---|---|---|
| AL | 2011–2017 | 18 | 0.0 | 0.0 | 2.5 | 0.0 | 0.0 |
| AS-AQ | 2010–2016 | 18 | 0.0 | 2.4 | 7.9 | 0.0 | 5.2 |

AL: artemether-lumefantrine; AS-AQ: artesunate-amodiaquine.

## STATUS OF INSECTICIDE RESISTANCE[a] PER INSECTICIDE CLASS (2010–2018) AND USE OF EACH CLASS FOR MALARIA VECTOR CONTROL (2018)

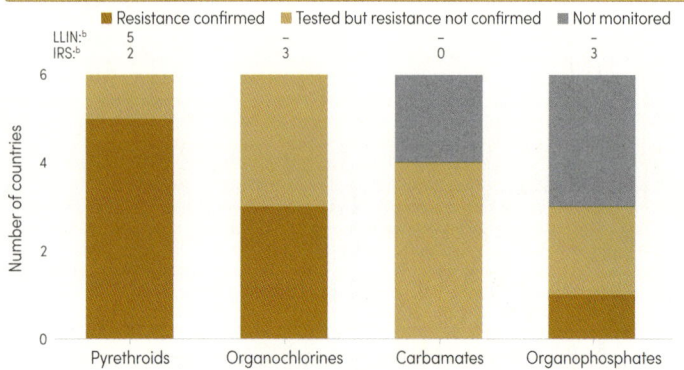

[a] Resistance is considered confirmed when it was detected to one insecticide in the class, in at least one malaria vector from one collection site.
[b] Number of countries that reported using the insecticide class for malaria vector control (2018).

### A. Confirmed malaria cases per 1000 population, 2018

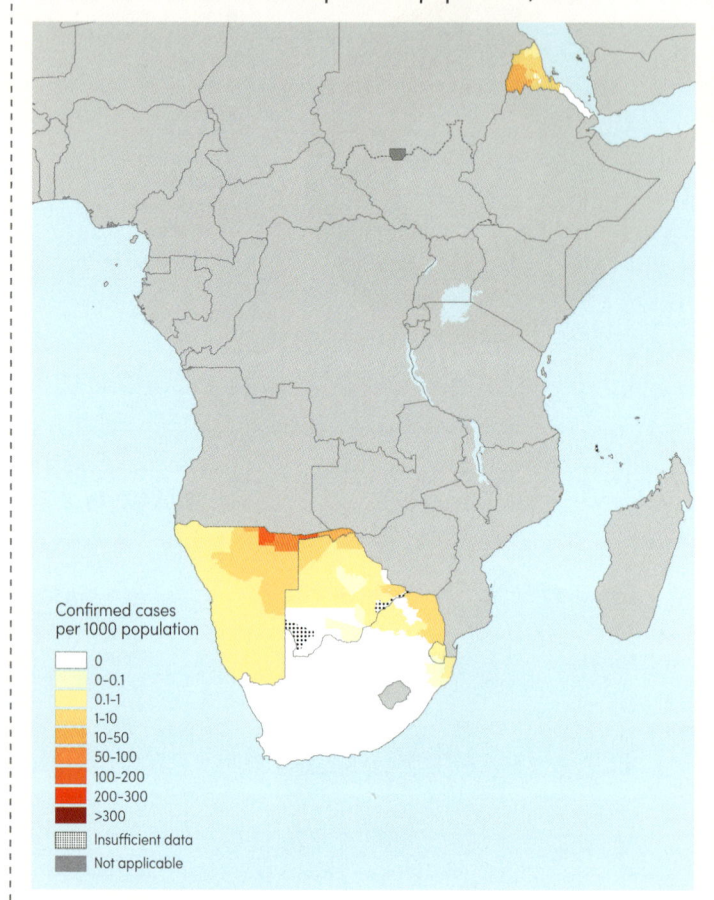

### B. Malaria funding* by source, 2010–2018

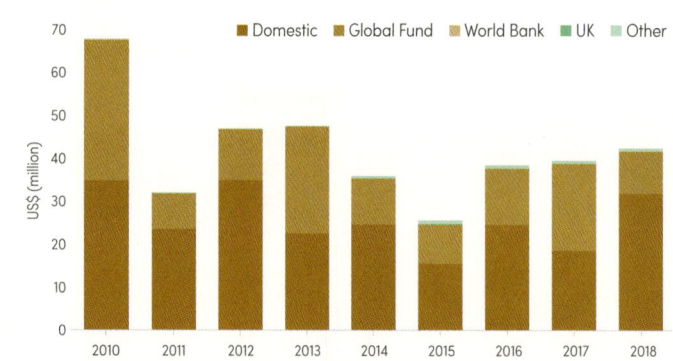

Global Fund: Global Fund to Fight AIDS, Tuberculosis and Malaria; UK: United Kingdom of Great Britain and Northern Ireland.
\* Excludes patient service delivery costs and out-of-pocket expenditure.

### C. Malaria funding* per person at risk, average 2016–2018

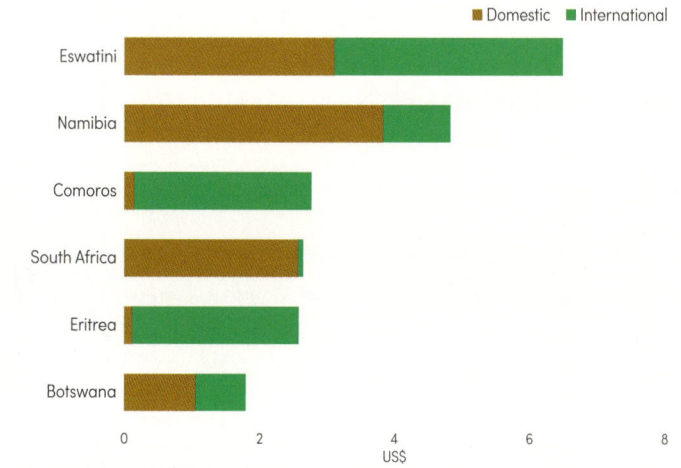

\* Excludes costs related to health staff, costs at subnational level and out-of-pocket expenditure.

### D. Share of estimated malaria cases, 2018

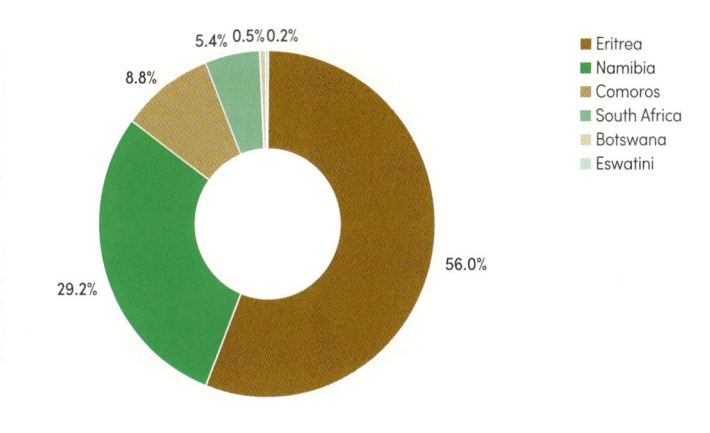

- Eritrea: 56.0%
- Namibia: 29.2%
- Comoros: 8.8%
- South Africa: 5.4%
- Botswana: 0.5%
- Eswatini: 0.2%

### E. Percentage of population with access to either LLINs or IRS, 2018
*Source: ITN coverage model from MAP*

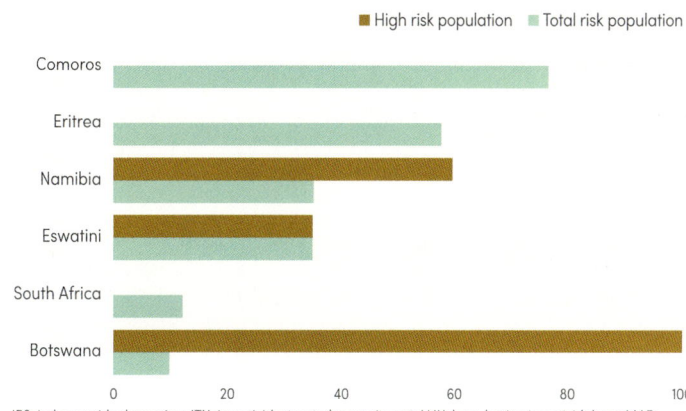

Legend: High risk population, Total risk population

(Bar chart showing Comoros, Eritrea, Namibia, Eswatini, South Africa, Botswana)

IRS: indoor residual spraying; ITN: insecticide-treated mosquito net; LLIN: long-lasting insecticidal net; MAP: Malaria Atlas Project.
* Comoros and Eritrea have ITN coverage estimated by a model from MAP.
** Namibia and South Africa LLIN and IRS coverage is combined because there is no overlap in the areas where they are used.
*** South Africa has no data for high risk population.

### F. Countries with an increase in case incidence, 2015–2018

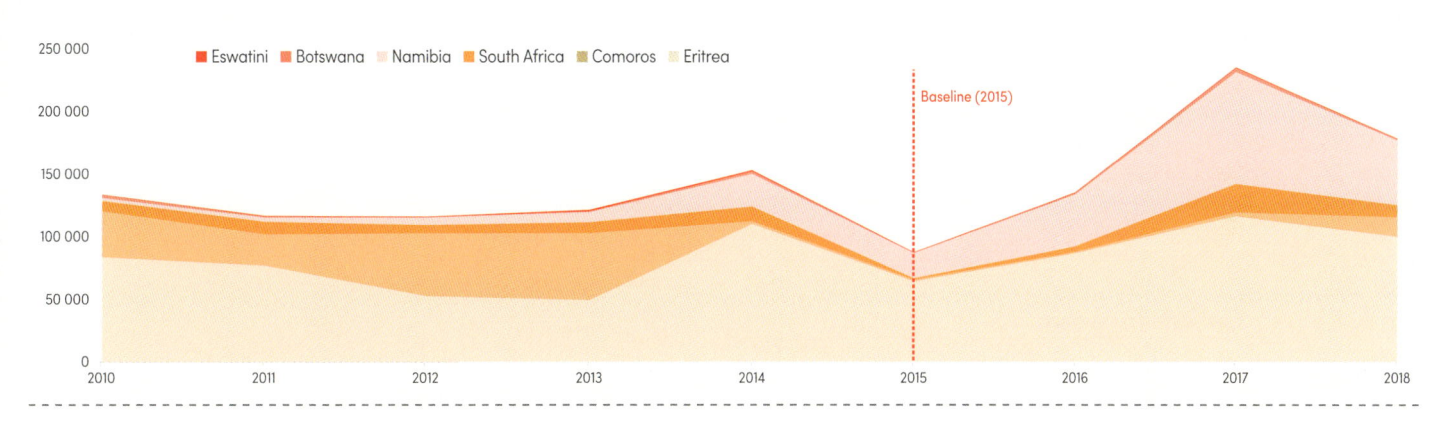

(Stacked area chart 2010–2018 for Eswatini, Botswana, Namibia, South Africa, Comoros, Eritrea; Baseline (2015) marked)

### G. Change in estimated malaria incidence and mortality rates, 2015–2018

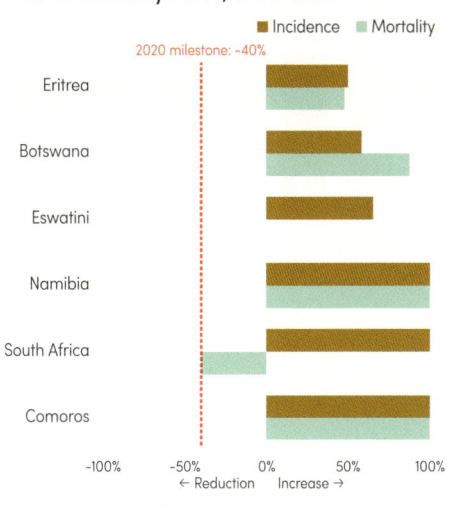

Legend: Incidence, Mortality; 2020 milestone: –40%

Countries: Eritrea, Botswana, Eswatini, Namibia, South Africa, Comoros

* Eswatini already achieved the 40% reduction in mortality rate in 2015; since then there has been no change

### H. Percentage of total confirmed cases investigated, 2018

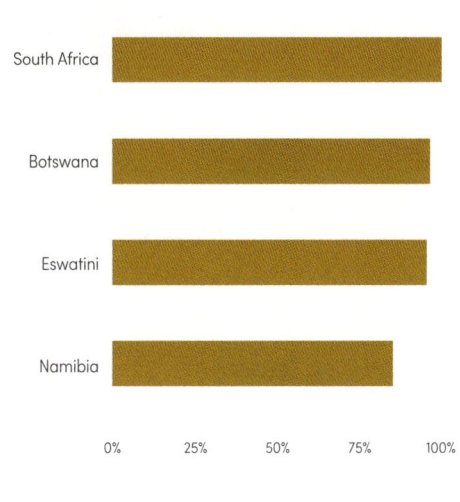

Countries: South Africa, Botswana, Eswatini, Namibia

### I. Reported indigenous cases in countries with national elimination activities, 2015 versus 2018

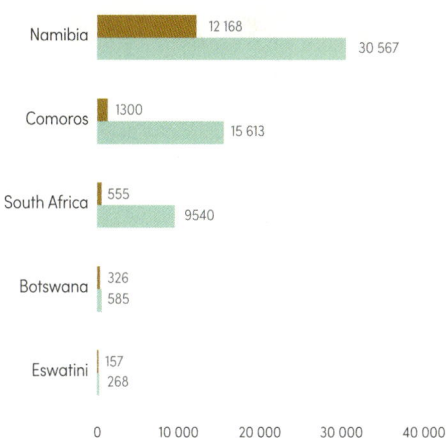

| Country | 2015 | 2018 |
|---|---|---|
| Namibia | 12 168 | 30 567 |
| Comoros | 1300 | 15 613 |
| South Africa | 555 | 9540 |
| Botswana | 326 | 585 |
| Eswatini | 157 | 268 |

## KEY MESSAGES

- About 14 million people in the six countries with low transmission in East and Southern Africa are at high risk of malaria. Malaria transmission is focal, highly seasonal and almost exclusively due to *P. falciparum* (except in Eritrea).
- The subregion had nearly 178 000 estimated malaria cases and about 440 estimated deaths, representing a 34% and 27% increase compared with 2010, respectively. The four frontline countries of the Elimination-8 (E8) initiative in Southern Africa (Botswana, Eswatini, Namibia and South Africa) accounted for almost 50% of cases and Eritrea accounted for almost 40%. In the public health sector almost 103 000 cases were reported, of which 11% were in children aged under 5 years and 79 500 (79.7%) were confirmed. The proportion of total cases that were confirmed improved substantially over time from only 40.2% in 2010.
- Despite previous decreases in case incidence between 2010 and 2015, all of the countries had an increase between 2015 and 2018, which means that currently none are on track to achieve the GTS target of at least a 40% reduction in incidence by 2020. Estimated cases in Namibia increased significantly, from only 2590 cases in 2010 to 89 155 in 2017, and only declined moderately (to 51 898) in 2018. South Africa is the only country on track for reducing the mortality rate by 40%. The proportion of cases investigated was high in all countries except Namibia, possibly because of a lack of resources as a result of the recent resurgence in cases.
- During 2016 and 2017 alone, the number of reported cases in South Africa increased more than fivefold (4323 to 22 061), but decreased to 9540 cases in 2018 (a reduction of 57%). Botswana and Eswatini also saw reductions in reported cases between 2017 and 2018, by 69% and 62%, respectively. Comoros, however, saw a huge increase of reported cases from 2274 in 2017 to 15 613 in 2018; an increase of 587%. There are multiple reasons for the increase in cases: improved diagnosis and reporting, inadequate vector control and climatic factors.
- Vector resistance to pyrethroids was confirmed in more than half of the countries. There are significant gaps in standard resistance monitoring for carbamates and organophosphates.
- Challenges include inadequate coverage of vector control, importation of cases from neighbouring countries and resurgence during the past 3 years.

# Annex 2 – B. WHO Region of the Americas

## EPIDEMIOLOGY
**Population at risk:** 138 million
**Parasites:** P. vivax (79.5%), P. falciparum and mixed (20.5%), and other (<1%)
**Vectors:** An. albimanus, An. albitarsis, An. aquasalis, An. argyritarsis, An. braziliensis, An. cruzii, An. darlingi, An. neivai, An. nuneztovari, An. pseudopunctipennis and An. punctimacula.

## FUNDING (US$), 2010–2018
218.5 million (2010), 195.6 million (2015), 168.0 million (2018); decrease 2010–2018: 23%
**Proportion of domestic source* in 2018:** 84%
**Regional funding mechanisms:** Regional Malaria Elimination Initiative

* Domestic source excludes patient service delivery costs and out-of-pocket expenditure.

## INTERVENTIONS, 2018
**Number of people protected by IRS:** 2.78 million (2010), 2.81 million (2015), 1.72 million (2018)
**Total LLINs distributed:** 363 000 (2010), 875 000 (2015), 957 000 (2018)
**Number of RDTs distributed:** 83 700 (2010), 534 000 (2015), 899 000 (2018)
**Number of ACT courses distributed:** 148 400 (2010), 209 400 (2015), 220 900 (2018)
**Number of any first-line antimalarial treatment courses (incl. ACT) distributed:** 1.25 million (2010), 669 000 (2015), 1.26 million (2018)

## REPORTED CASES AND DEATHS IN PUBLIC SECTOR*, 2010–2018
**Total (presumed and confirmed) cases:** 677 100 (2010), 434 000 (2015), 753 700 (2018)
**Confirmed cases:** 677 100 (2010), 434 000 (2015), 753 700 (2018)
**Percentage of total cases confirmed:** 100% (2010), 100% (2015), 100% (2018)
**Deaths:** 190 (2010), 98 (2015), 338 (2018)

* In Belize, Brazil, Colombia, Costa Rica, Ecuador, Haiti, Suriname and Venezuela (Bolivarian Republic of), cases from the private sector and/or community are included in 2018.

## ESTIMATED CASES AND DEATHS, 2010–2018
**Cases:** 814 000 (2010), 566 000 (2015), 929 000 (2018); increase 2010–2018: 14%
**Deaths:** 460 (2010), 320 (2015), 580 (2018); increase 2010–2018: 26%

## ACCELERATION TO ELIMINATION
**Countries with nationwide elimination programme:** Argentina, Belize, Costa Rica, Ecuador, El Salvador, Mexico and Suriname
**Zero indigenous cases for 3 consecutive years (2016, 2017 and 2018):** Argentina
**Zero indigenous cases in 2018:** Argentina and El Salvador
**Certified as malaria free since 2010:** Argentina (2019) and Paraguay (2018)

## THERAPEUTIC EFFICACY TESTS (CLINICAL AND PARASITOLOGICAL FAILURE, %)

| Medicine | Study years | No. of studies | Min. | Median | Max. | Percentile 25 | Percentile 75 |
|---|---|---|---|---|---|---|---|
| AL | 2011–2016 | 5 | 0.0 | 0.0 | 9.0 | 0.0 | 4.5 |
| AS-MQ | 2010–2017 | 6 | 0.0 | 0.0 | 0.0 | 0.0 | 0.0 |

AL: artemether-lumefantrine; AS-MQ: artesunate-mefloquine.

## STATUS OF INSECTICIDE RESISTANCE[a] PER INSECTICIDE CLASS (2010–2018) AND USE OF EACH CLASS FOR MALARIA VECTOR CONTROL (2018)

LLIN:[b] 18, 0, 3, 2
IRS:[b] 11

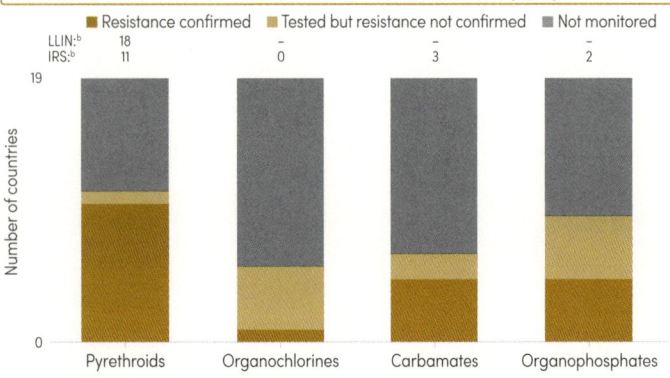

[a] Resistance is considered confirmed when it was detected to one insecticide in the class, in at least one malaria vector from one collection site.
[b] Number of countries that reported using the insecticide class for malaria vector control (2018).

### A. Confirmed malaria cases per 1000 population, 2018

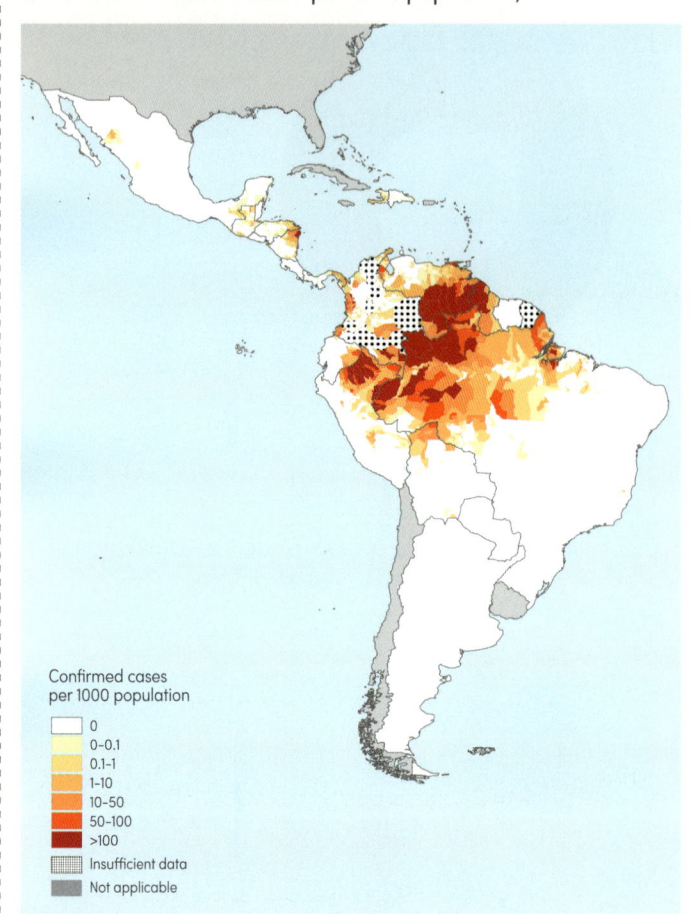

Confirmed cases per 1000 population: 0; 0–0.1; 0.1–1; 1–10; 10–50; 50–100; >100; Insufficient data; Not applicable

### B. Malaria funding* by source, 2010–2018

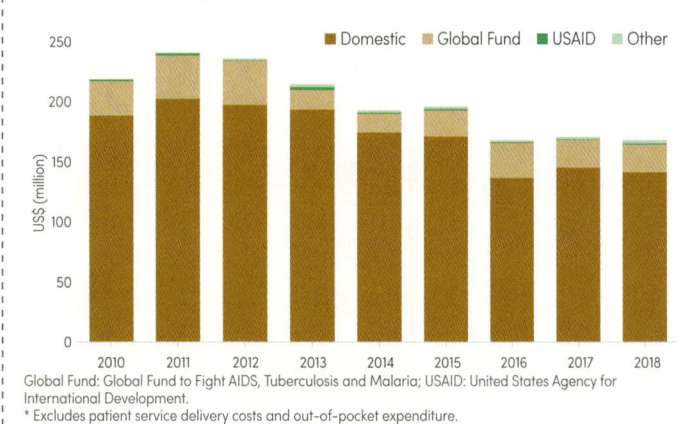

Domestic, Global Fund, USAID, Other

Global Fund: Global Fund to Fight AIDS, Tuberculosis and Malaria; USAID: United States Agency for International Development.
* Excludes patient service delivery costs and out-of-pocket expenditure.

### C. Malaria funding* per person at risk, average 2016–2018

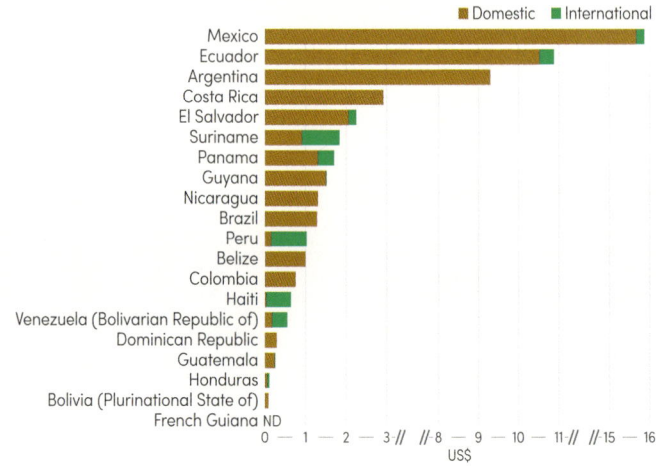

Domestic, International

Mexico, Ecuador, Argentina, Costa Rica, El Salvador, Suriname, Panama, Guyana, Nicaragua, Brazil, Peru, Belize, Colombia, Haiti, Venezuela (Bolivarian Republic of), Dominican Republic, Guatemala, Honduras, Bolivia (Plurinational State of), French Guiana ND

ND: No data.
* Excludes costs related to health staff, costs at subnational level and out-of-pocket expenditure.

### D. Share of estimated malaria cases, 2018

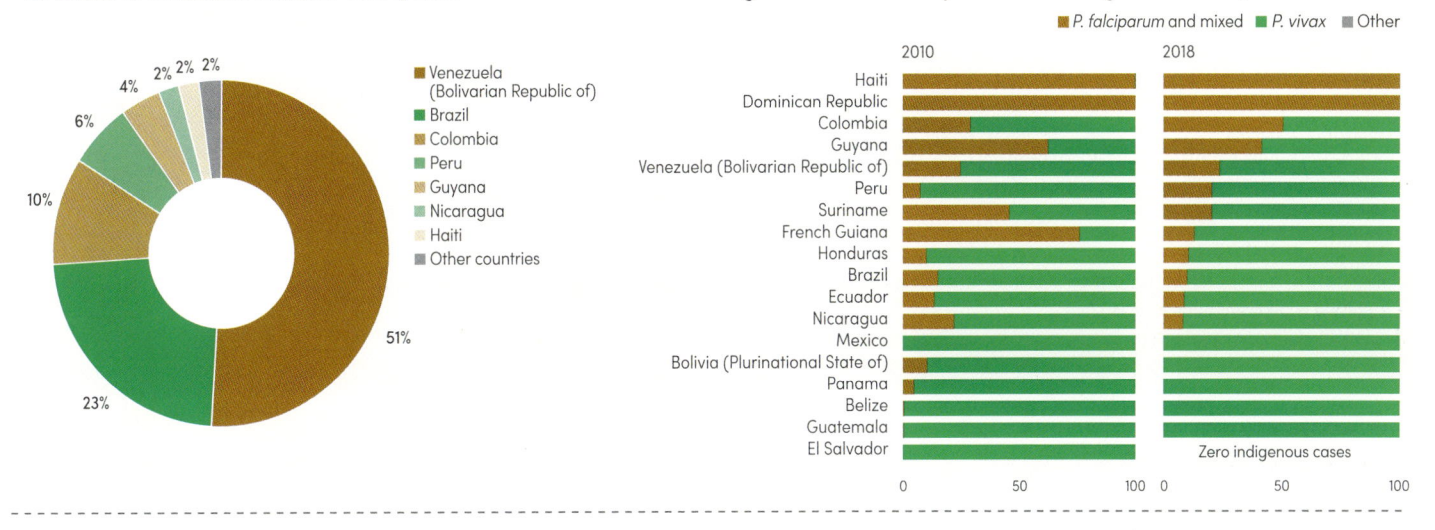

- Venezuela (Bolivarian Republic of): 51%
- Brazil: 23%
- Colombia: 10%
- Peru: 6%
- Guyana: 4%
- Nicaragua: 2%
- Haiti: 2%
- Other countries: 2%

### E. Percentage of *Plasmodium* species from indigenous cases, 2010 and 2018

■ *P. falciparum* and mixed  ■ *P. vivax*  ■ Other

(Countries listed: Haiti, Dominican Republic, Colombia, Guyana, Venezuela (Bolivarian Republic of), Peru, Suriname, French Guiana, Honduras, Brazil, Ecuador, Nicaragua, Mexico, Bolivia (Plurinational State of), Panama, Belize, Guatemala, El Salvador — Zero indigenous cases in 2018)

### F. Countries on track to reduce case incidence by ≥40% by 2020

(El Salvador, Belize, Suriname, Guatemala, Honduras, Bolivia (Plurinational State of), Peru, Haiti; Baseline 2015)

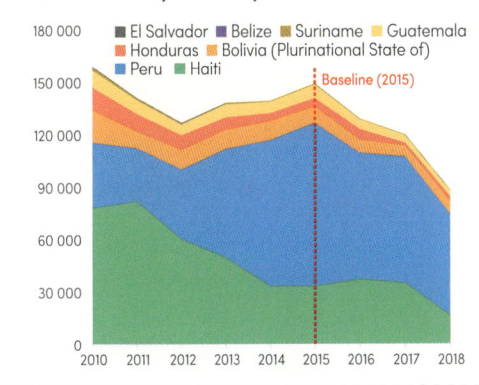

### G. Countries and areas likely to reduce case incidence by <40% by 2020

(French Guiana, Dominican Republic; Baseline 2015)

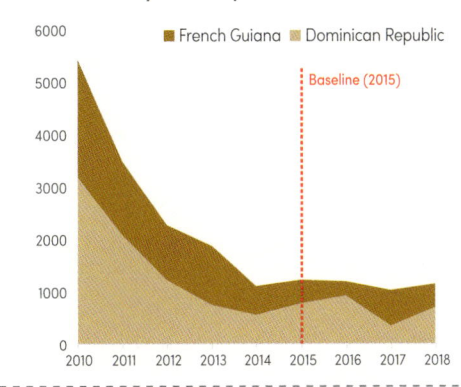

### H. Countries with an increase in case incidence, 2015–2018

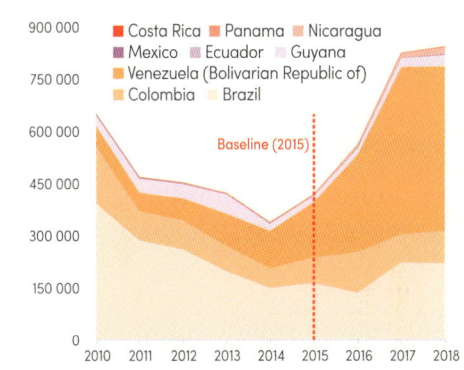

(Costa Rica, Panama, Nicaragua, Mexico, Ecuador, Guyana, Venezuela (Bolivarian Republic of), Colombia, Brazil; Baseline 2015)

### I. Change in estimated malaria incidence and mortality rates, 2015–2018

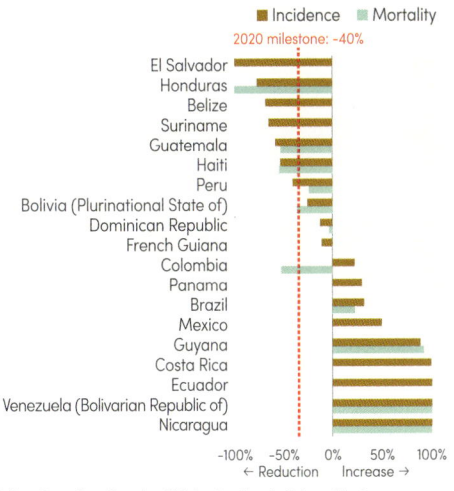

■ Incidence  ■ Mortality  — 2020 milestone: −40%

(Countries: El Salvador, Honduras, Belize, Suriname, Guatemala, Haiti, Peru, Bolivia (Plurinational State of), Dominican Republic, French Guiana, Colombia, Panama, Brazil, Mexico, Guyana, Costa Rica, Ecuador, Venezuela (Bolivarian Republic of), Nicaragua)

\* Belize, Costa Rica, Ecuador, El Salvador, French Guiana, Mexico, Panama and Suriname already achieved the 40% reduction in mortality rate in 2015; since then there has been no change.

### J. Percentage of total confirmed cases investigated, 2018

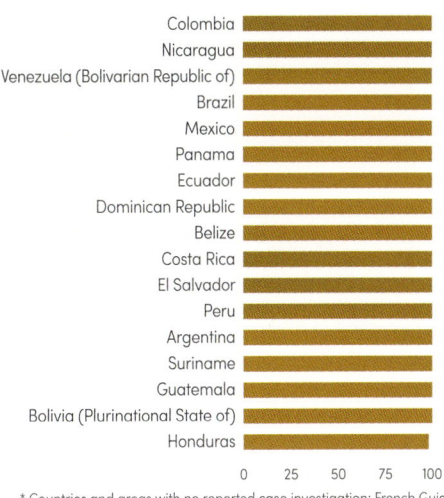

(Colombia, Nicaragua, Venezuela (Bolivarian Republic of), Brazil, Mexico, Panama, Ecuador, Dominican Republic, Belize, Costa Rica, El Salvador, Peru, Argentina, Suriname, Guatemala, Bolivia (Plurinational State of), Honduras)

\* Countries and areas with no reported case investigation: French Guiana, Guyana and Haiti.

### K. Number of reported indigenous cases in countries with national elimination activities, 2015 versus 2018

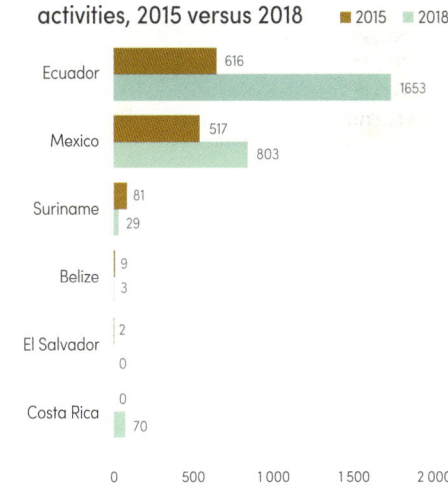

■ 2015  ■ 2018

| Country | 2015 | 2018 |
|---|---|---|
| Ecuador | 616 | 1653 |
| Mexico | 517 | 803 |
| Suriname | 81 | 29 |
| Belize | 9 | 3 |
| El Salvador | 2 | 0 |
| Costa Rica | 0 | 70 |

## KEY MESSAGES

- About 138 million people in 19 countries and areas are at risk of malaria, of which almost 80% is caused by *P. vivax*. In 2018, the region had almost 1 million estimated malaria cases and about 600 estimated deaths; increases of 14% and 26%, respectively, compared with 2010. Three countries – Brazil, Colombia and Venezuela (Bolivarian Republic of) – account for 80% of all estimated cases. In the public health sector, about 750 000 cases were reported, all of which were confirmed. Reported deaths due to malaria were few, at about 300 deaths.
- Eight out of the 19 malaria endemic countries and areas are on target to achieve a more than 40% reduction in case incidence by 2020, while Dominican Republic and French Guiana are on target to achieve a 20–40% reduction. Nine countries (Brazil, Colombia, Costa Rica, Ecuador, Guyana, Mexico, Nicaragua, Panama and Venezuela [Bolivarian Republic of]) saw increases in incidence in 2018 compared with 2015.
- The number of cases in French Guiana has fluctuated, largely because of variable detection efforts in the hinterland, whereas there have been large increases in Nicaragua (572%) and Venezuela (Bolivarian Republic of) (209%).
- Nevertheless, transmission in countries is focal, being particularly high in Choco in Colombia, Loreto in Peru and Bolivar in Venezuela (Bolivarian Republic of). More than one third of all cases in the region in 2018 were from five municipalities. Increases in other countries in 2018 are attributed to improved surveillance and focal outbreaks. El Salvador has reported zero indigenous cases for the past 2 years. Mexico and Bolivia have reported no local *P. falciparum* cases for more than 3 years, and Belize reported one case in 2018 and only two cases of *P. vivax*. The reported cases due to *P. falciparum* were below 10% in Brazil, Ecuador, Guatemala, Mexico, Nicaragua and Panama. LLIN distribution increased by 9% in 2018 compared with 2015, while the number of people protected by IRS decreased by 39%.
- Paraguay and Argentina were awarded malaria free certification by WHO in 2018 and 2019, respectively. Nine countries in Central America and Hispaniola are taking part in the subregional initiative to eliminate malaria by 2020. Despite Costa Rica reporting zero indigenous cases between 2013 and 2015, there has been a resurgence in cases in recent years, with eight cases being reported in 2016 and 70 cases in 2018, largely related to increased importation of cases from neighbouring countries and consequent re-establishment of transmission. Efforts are underway to enhance access to diagnosis and treatment, investigation of cases and adequate response.
- Vector resistance to pyrethroids was confirmed in more than half of the countries. There are significant gaps in standard resistance monitoring for all the five insecticide classes commonly used for vector control.

# Annex 2 – C. WHO Eastern Mediterranean Region

### EPIDEMIOLOGY
**Population at risk:** 317 million
**Parasites:** *P. falciparum* and mixed (75%), *P. vivax* (25%) and other (<1%)
**Vectors:** *An. annularis, An. arabiensis, An. culicifacies s.l., An. d'thali, An. fluviatilis, An. funestus s.l., An. gambiae s.s., An. maculipennis s.s., An. pulcherrimus, An. sacharovi, An. sergentii, An. stephensi* and *An. superpictus*.

### FUNDING (US$), 2010–2018
127.9 million (2010), 158.2 million (2015), 140.0 million (2018); increase 2010–2018: 9%
**Proportion of domestic source\* in 2017:** 52%
**Regional funding mechanisms:** none
\* Domestic source excludes patient service delivery costs and out-of-pocket expenditure.

### INTERVENTIONS, 2018
**Number of people protected by IRS:** 10.5 million (2010), 27.8 million (2015), 10.2 million (2018)
**Total LLINs distributed:** 2.8 million (2010), 5.7 million (2015), 10.4 million (2018)
**Number of RDTs distributed:** 2.0 million (2010), 6.1 million (2015), 8.3 million (2018)
**Number of ACT courses distributed:** 2.6 million (2010), 3.2 million (2015), 4.7 million (2018)
**Number of any first-line antimalarial treatment courses (incl. ACT) distributed:** 2.6 million (2010), 4.0 million (2015), 5.9 million (2018)

### REPORTED CASES AND DEATHS IN PUBLIC SECTOR\*, 2010–2018
**Total (presumed and confirmed) cases:** 6.4 million (2010), 5.4 million (2015), 5.2 million (2018)
**Confirmed cases:** 1.2 million (2010), 999 000 (2015), 2.4 million (2018)
**Percentage of total cases confirmed:** 18.3% (2010), 18.5% (2015), 46.4% (2018)
**Deaths:** 1140 (2010), 1020 (2015), 3320 (2018)
\* In Djibouti, Pakistan and Sudan, cases from the private sector are included in 2018.

### ESTIMATED CASES AND DEATHS, 2010–2018
**Cases:** 4.3 million (2010), 3.8 million (2015), 4.9 million (2018); increase 2010–2018: 12%
**Deaths:** 8300 (2010), 7120 (2015), 9330 (2018); increase 2010–2018: 13%
\* In Iran (Islamic Republic of) and Saudi Arabia, reported malaria cases were used.

### ACCELERATION TO ELIMINATION
**Countries with nationwide elimination programme:** Iran (Islamic Republic of) and Saudi Arabia
**Zero indigenous cases in 2018:** Iran (Islamic Republic of)
**Certified as malaria free since 2010:** Morocco (2010)

### THERAPEUTIC EFFICACY TESTS (CLINICAL AND PARASITOLOGICAL FAILURE, %)

| Medicine | Study years | No. of studies | Min. | Median | Max. | Percentile 25 | Percentile 75 |
|---|---|---|---|---|---|---|---|
| AL | 2010–2018 | 27 | 0.0 | 0.0 | 3.3 | 0.0 | 1.5 |
| AS-SP | 2010–2017 | 41 | 0.0 | 1.0 | 22.2 | 0.0 | 4.4 |
| DHA-PPQ | 2013–2016 | 6 | 0.0 | 0.5 | 2.5 | 0.0 | 2.2 |

AL: artemether-lumefantrine; AS-SP: artesunate-sulfadoxine-pyrimethamine; DHA-PPQ: dihydroartemisinin-piperaquine.

### STATUS OF INSECTICIDE RESISTANCE[a] PER INSECTICIDE CLASS (2010–2018) AND USE OF EACH CLASS FOR MALARIA VECTOR CONTROL (2018)

| | Pyrethroids | Organochlorines | Carbamates | Organophosphates |
|---|---|---|---|---|
| LLIN:[b] | 8 | – | – | – |
| IRS:[b] | 4 | 0 | 2 | 0 |

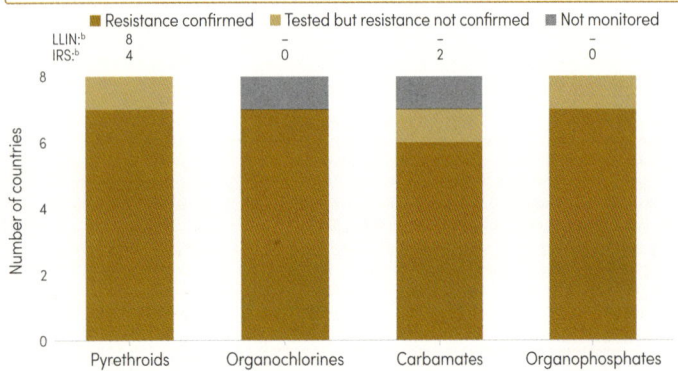

[a] Resistance is considered confirmed when it was detected to one insecticide in the class, in at least one malaria vector from one collection site.
[b] Number of countries that reported using the insecticide class for malaria vector control (2018).

### A. *P. falciparum* parasite prevalence (*Pf* PP)/confirmed malaria cases per 1000 population, 2018

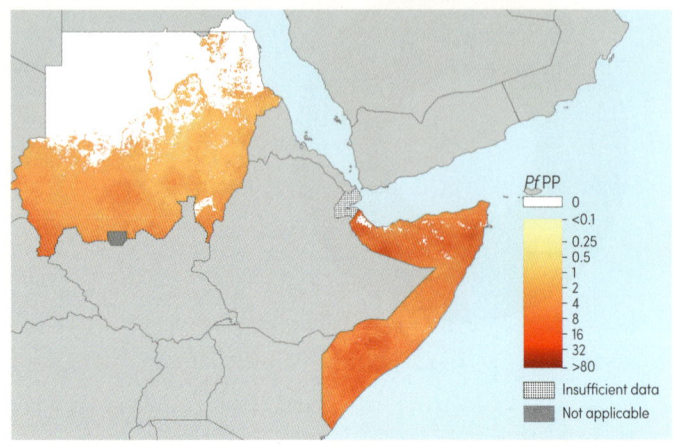

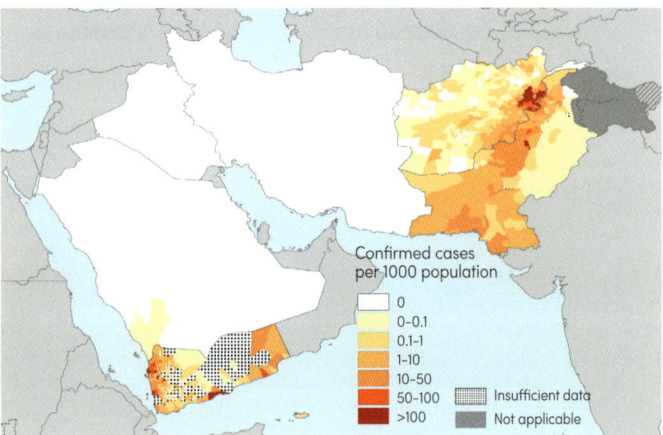

### B. Malaria funding\* by source, 2010–2018

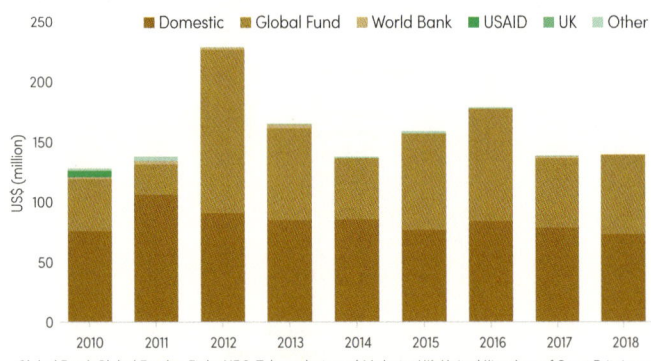

Global Fund: Global Fund to Fight AIDS, Tuberculosis and Malaria; UK: United Kingdom of Great Britain and Northern Ireland; USAID: United States Agency for International Development.
\* Excludes patient service delivery costs and out-of-pocket expenditure.

### C. Malaria funding\* per person at risk, average 2016–2018

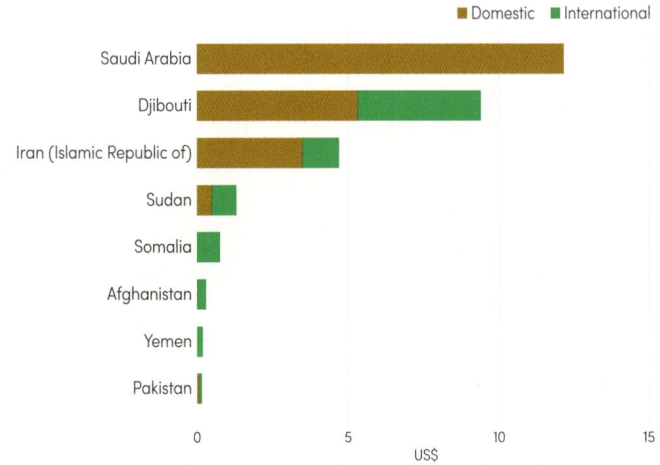

\* Excludes costs related to health staff, costs at subnational level and out-of-pocket expenditure.

D. Share of estimated malaria cases, 2018

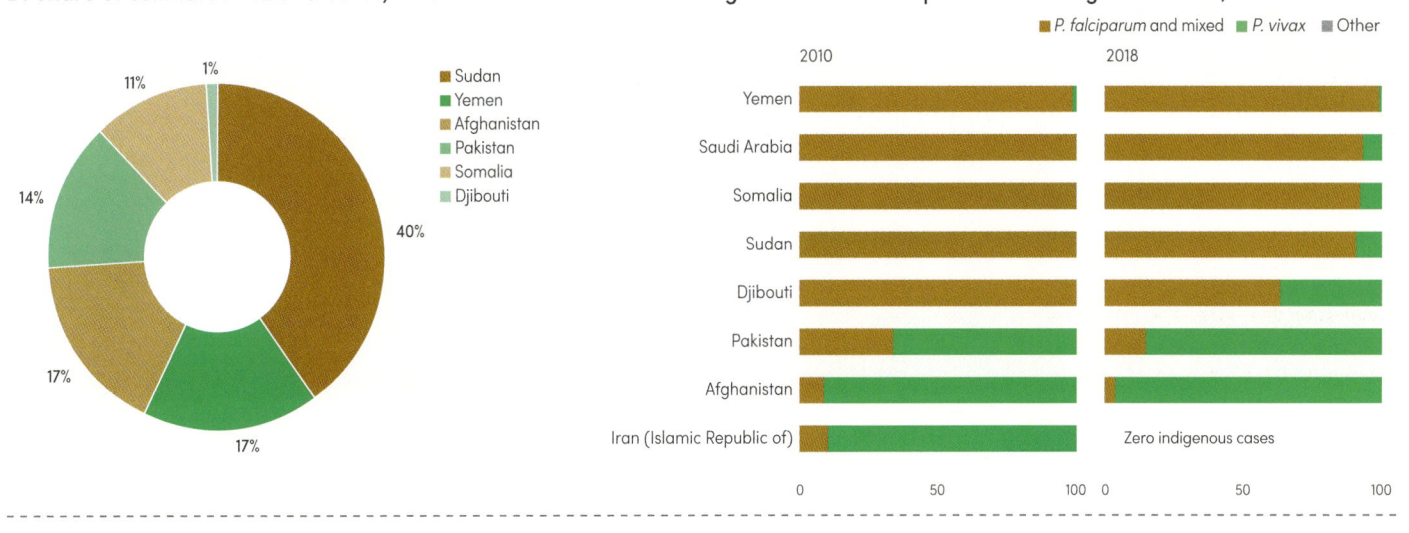

- Sudan: 40%
- Yemen: 17%
- Afghanistan: 17%
- Pakistan: 14%
- Somalia: 11%
- Djibouti: 1%

E. Percentage of *Plasmodium* species from indigenous cases, 2010 and 2018

*P. falciparum* and mixed | *P. vivax* | Other

2010 / 2018 by country: Yemen, Saudi Arabia, Somalia, Sudan, Djibouti, Pakistan, Afghanistan, Iran (Islamic Republic of) — 2018: Iran shows "Zero indigenous cases"

F. Countries with an increase in reported cases, 2015–2018

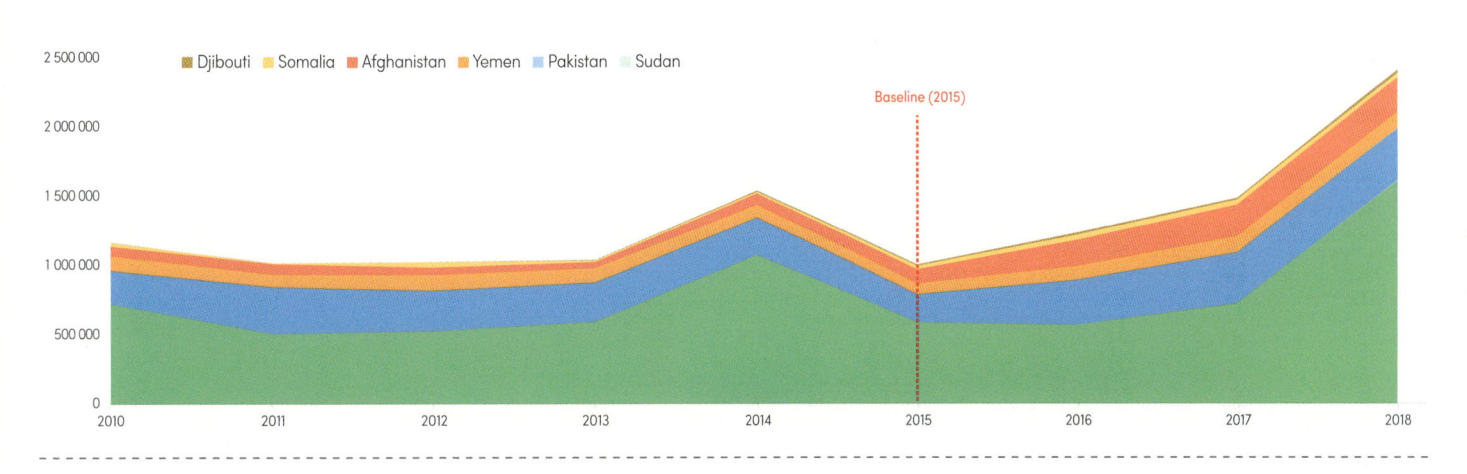

Djibouti | Somalia | Afghanistan | Yemen | Pakistan | Sudan

Baseline (2015)

G. Change in estimated malaria incidence and mortality rates, 2015–2018*

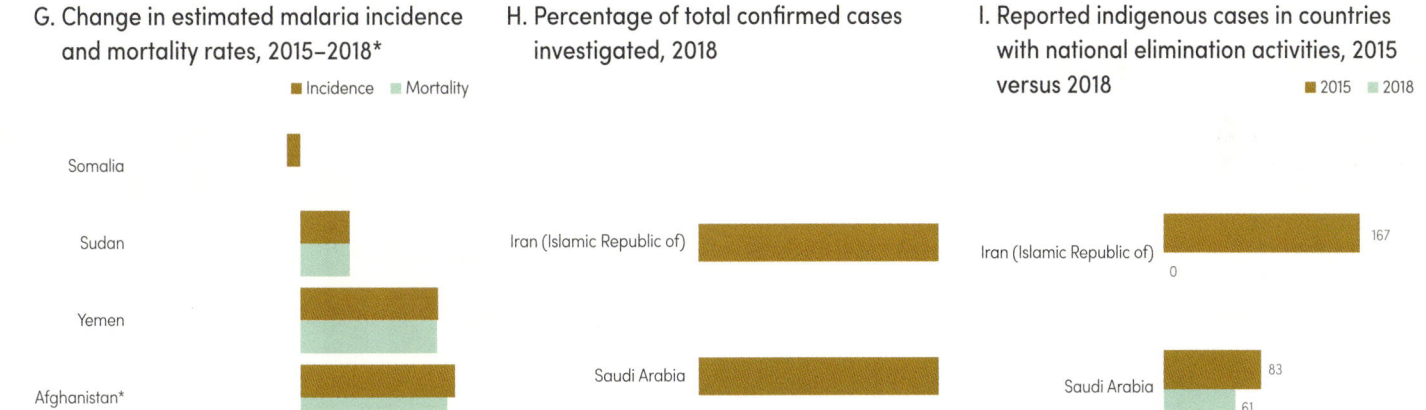

Incidence | Mortality

Somalia, Sudan, Yemen, Afghanistan*, Djibouti**

← Reduction −100% / −50% / 0% / 50% / 100% Increase →

H. Percentage of total confirmed cases investigated, 2018

Iran (Islamic Republic of), Saudi Arabia

I. Reported indigenous cases in countries with national elimination activities, 2015 versus 2018

■ 2015  ■ 2018

Iran (Islamic Republic of): 167 / 0
Saudi Arabia: 83 / 61

\* Estimates of change in Afghanistan may be exaggerated due to uncertainties in adjustments; estimates for Pakistan were excluded due to high uncertainties.

\*\* Reported confirmed cases are used for Djibouti (as opposed to estimated cases). No mortality data was reported for Djibouti for 2017 or 2018.

## KEY MESSAGES

- Fourteen countries in the WHO Eastern Mediterranean Region are free of indigenous malaria and are at the stage of prevention of re-establishment. There are eight malaria endemic countries in the region, and *P. falciparum* is responsible for 75% of all detected infections. Estimated malaria incidence in the region declined between 2010 and 2015, but increased over the past 3 years. Estimated malaria deaths also increased by 13% since 2010. Sudan accounted for 40% of reported cases. In 2018, the region reported 5.2 million cases (presumed and confirmed), of which only 2.4 million (46%) were confirmed. The proportion of confirmed cases was 18% in 2010 but has improved since then. The reported number of deaths increased from 1140 in 2010 to just over 3300 in 2018.
- The Islamic Republic of Iran and Saudi Arabia are both targeting elimination by 2020. The Islamic Republic of Iran reported zero indigenous cases for the first time in 2018, and 20 introduced cases. In Saudi Arabia, the number of indigenous malaria cases declined from 272 in 2016 to 61 in 2018. Both the Islamic Republic of Iran and Saudi Arabia have reported zero indigenous deaths over the past 3 years. These countries undertake continued vigilance for malaria in the general health service, and provide free-of-charge diagnosis and treatment to all imported cases.
- Vector resistance to pyrethroids and organochlorines was confirmed in all countries except for Saudi Arabia. Resistance to organophosphates and carbamates was confirmed in most of the countries of the region.
- Challenges include low coverage of essential interventions (below universal target) in most malaria endemic countries, inadequate funding and dependence on external resources, difficult operational environments and population displacements, a shortage of skilled technical staff (particularly at subnational level), and weak surveillance and health information systems. These challenges may have led to an overall increase in cases during the period 2015–2018 in some countries of the region.

# Annex 2 - D. WHO South-East Asia Region

## EPIDEMIOLOGY

**Population at risk:** 1.61 billion
**Parasites:** *P. falciparum* and mixed (52%), *P. vivax* (48%) and other (<1%)
**Vectors:** *An. albimanus, An. annularis, An. balabacensis, An. barbirostris, An. culicifacies s.l., An. dirus s.l., An. farauti s.l., An. fluviatilis, An. leteri, An. maculatus s.l., An. minimus s.l., An. peditaeniatus, An. philippinensis, An. pseudowillmori, An. punctulatus s.l., An. sinensis s.l., An. stephensi s.l., An. subpictus s.l., An. sundaicus s.l., An. tessellatus, An. vagus, An. varuna* and *An. yatsushiroensis*.

## FUNDING (US$), 2010–2018

246.6 million (2010), 198.4 million (2015), 151.0 million (2018); decrease 2010–2018: 39%
**Proportion of domestic source* in 2018:** 59%
**Regional funding mechanisms:** Malaria Elimination in the Greater Mekong Region (MME): Myanmar and Thailand
* Domestic source excludes patient service delivery costs and out-of-pocket expenditure.

## INTERVENTIONS, 2018

**Number of people protected by IRS:** 76.4 million (2010), 57.2 million (2015), 35.4 million (2018)
**Total LLINs distributed:** 7.4 million (2010), 7.3 million (2015), 2.9 million (2018)
**Number of RDTs distributed:** 11.4 million (2010), 23.5 million (2015), 14.0 million (2018)
**Number of ACT courses distributed:** 3.5 million (2010), 2.8 million (2015), 1.8 million (2018)
**Number of any first-line antimalarial treatment courses (incl. ACT) distributed:** 2.9 million (2010), 2.9 million (2015), 2.2 million (2018)

## REPORTED CASES AND DEATHS IN PUBLIC SECTOR*, 2010–2018

**Total (presumed and confirmed) cases:** 3.1 million (2010), 1.6 million (2015), 744 000 (2018)
**Confirmed cases:** 2.6 million (2010), 1.6 million (2015), 707 000 (2018)
**Percentage of total cases confirmed:** 84.8% (2010), 98.4% (2015), 95% (2018)
**Deaths:** 2421 (2010), 620 (2015), 165 (2018)
* In Bhutan, India, Indonesia, Myanmar, Thailand and Timor-Leste, cases from the private sector and/or community are included in 2018.

## ESTIMATED CASES AND DEATHS, 2010–2018

**Cases:** 25.1 million (2010), 13.6 million (2015), 7.9 million (2018); decrease 2010–2018: 69%
**Deaths:** 39 100 (2010), 24 500 (2015), 11 600 (2018); decrease 2010–2018: 70%

## ACCELERATION TO ELIMINATION

**Countries with subnational/territorial elimination programme:** Bangladesh, India, Indonesia, Myanmar and Thailand
**Countries with nationwide elimination programme:** Bhutan, Democratic People's Republic of Korea, Nepal and Timor-Leste
**Zero indigenous cases in 2018:** Timor-Leste
**Certified as malaria free since 2010:** Maldives (2015) and Sri Lanka (2016)

## THERAPEUTIC EFFICACY TESTS (CLINICAL AND PARASITOLOGICAL FAILURE, %)

| Medicine | Study years | No. of studies | Min. | Median | Max. | Percentile 25 | Percentile 75 |
|---|---|---|---|---|---|---|---|
| AL | 2010–2018 | 72 | 0.0 | 0.0 | 14.3 | 0.0 | 2.0 |
| AS-SP | 2010–2017 | 55 | 0.0 | 0.0 | 21.4 | 0.0 | 1.5 |
| AS-MQ | 2010–2016 | 22 | 0.0 | 1.8 | 49.1 | 0.0 | 17.3 |
| DHA-PPQ | 2010–2017 | 29 | 0.0 | 0.0 | 92.9 | 0.0 | 2.2 |

AL: artemether-lumefantrine; AS-MQ: artesunate-mefloquine; AS-SP: artesunate-sulfadoxine-pyrimethamine; DHA-PPQ: dihydroartemisinin-piperaquine.

## STATUS OF INSECTICIDE RESISTANCE[a] PER INSECTICIDE CLASS (2010–2018) AND USE OF EACH CLASS FOR MALARIA VECTOR CONTROL (2018)

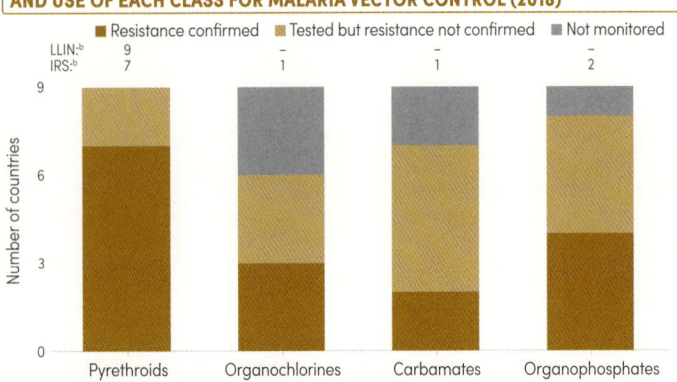

[a] Resistance is considered confirmed when it was detected to one insecticide in the class, in at least one malaria vector from one collection site.
[b] Number of countries that reported using the insecticide class for malaria vector control (2018).

## A. Confirmed malaria cases per 1000 population, 2018

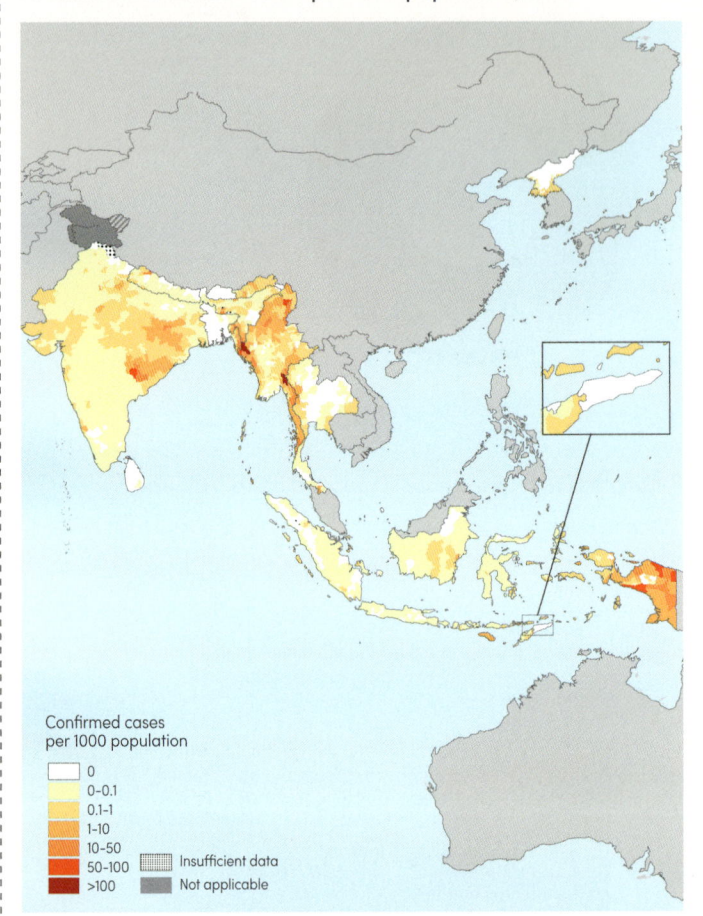

## B. Malaria funding* by source, 2010–2018

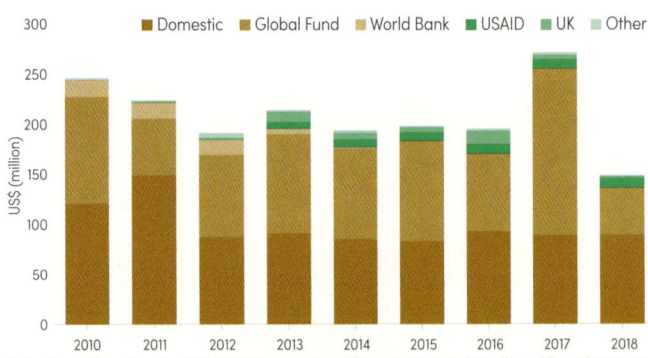

Global Fund: Global Fund to Fight AIDS, Tuberculosis and Malaria; UK: United Kingdom of Great Britain and Northern Ireland; USAID: United States Agency for International Development.
* Excludes patient service delivery costs and out-of-pocket expenditure.

## C. Malaria funding* per person at risk, 2016–2018

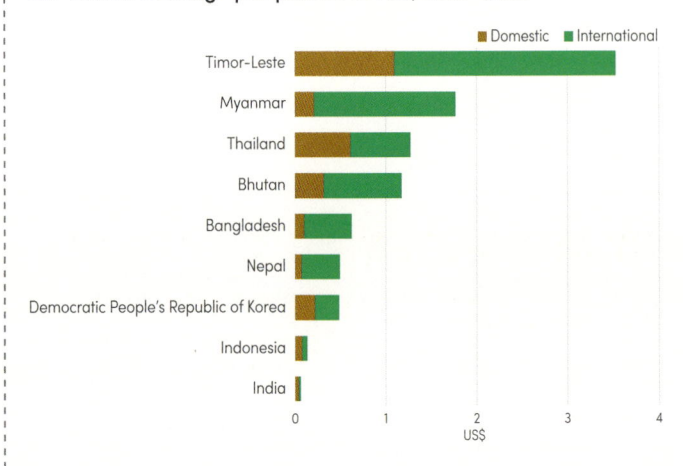

* Excludes costs related to health staff, costs at sub-national level and out-of-pocket expenditure.

**D. Share of estimated malaria cases, 2018**

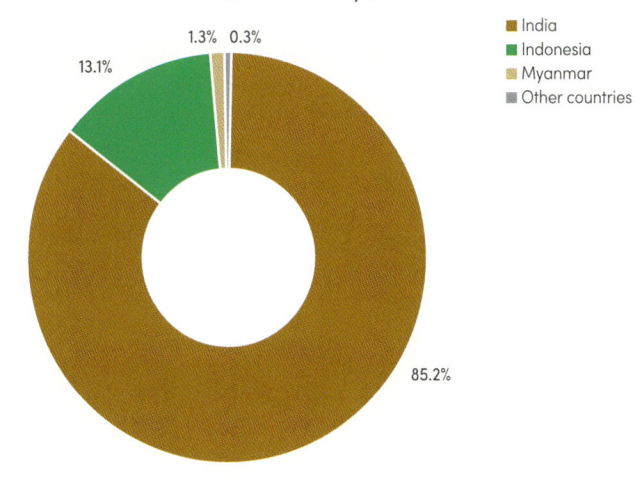

- India: 85.2%
- Indonesia: 13.1%
- Myanmar: 1.3%
- Other countries: 0.3%

**E. Percentage of *Plasmodium* species from indigenous cases, 2010 and 2018**

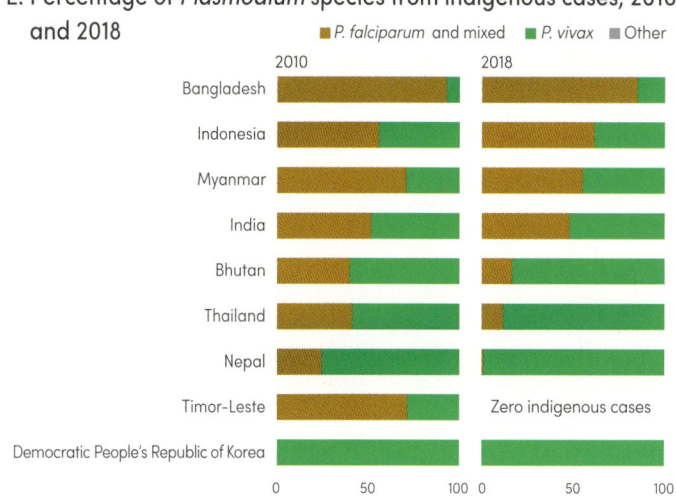

Legend: *P. falciparum* and mixed | *P. vivax* | Other

Countries (2010 and 2018): Bangladesh, Indonesia, Myanmar, India, Bhutan, Thailand, Nepal, Timor-Leste (Zero indigenous cases in 2018), Democratic People's Republic of Korea

**F. Countries on track to reduce case incidence by ≥40% by 2020**

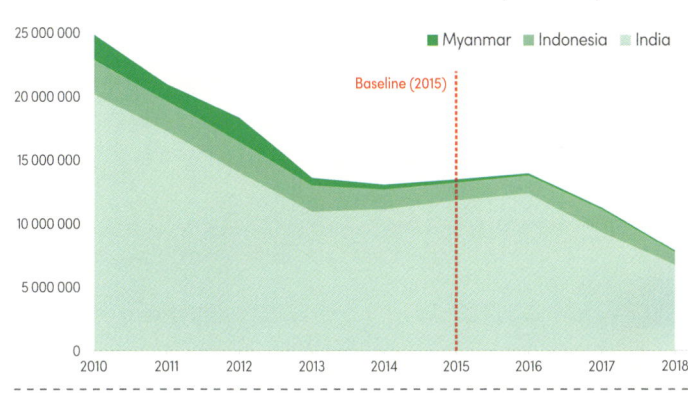

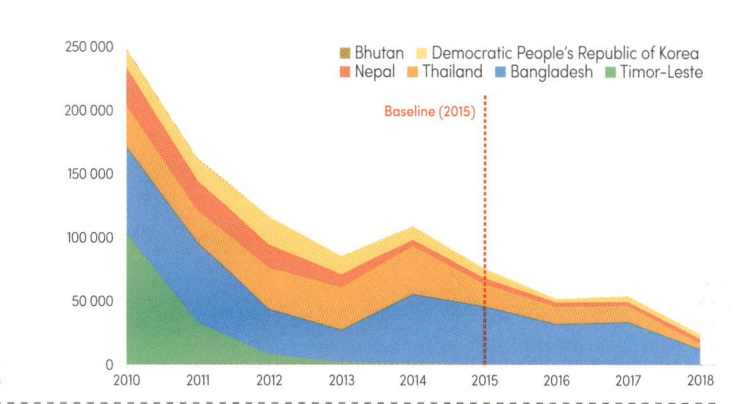

Left chart (Myanmar, Indonesia, India, 2010–2018), Baseline (2015)

Right chart (Bhutan, Democratic People's Republic of Korea, Nepal, Thailand, Bangladesh, Timor-Leste, 2010–2018), Baseline (2015)

**G. Change in estimated malaria incidence and mortality rates, 2015–2018**

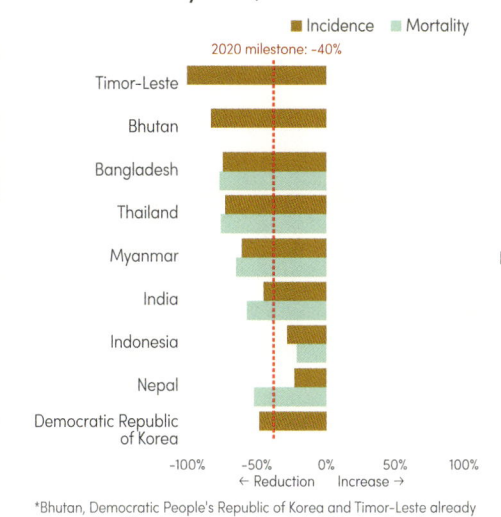

Legend: Incidence | Mortality
2020 milestone: -40%

Countries: Timor-Leste, Bhutan, Bangladesh, Thailand, Myanmar, India, Indonesia, Nepal, Democratic Republic of Korea

*Bhutan, Democratic People's Republic of Korea and Timor-Leste already achieved the 40% reduction in mortality rate in 2015; since then there has been no change.

** Reported confirmed cases are used for Bhutan and Democratic People's Republic of Korea (as opposed to estimated cases).

**H. Percentage of total confirmed cases investigated, 2018**

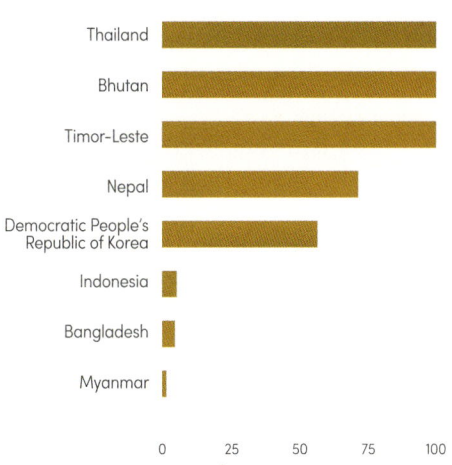

Thailand, Bhutan, Timor-Leste, Nepal, Democratic People's Republic of Korea, Indonesia, Bangladesh, Myanmar

* Countries with no reported case investigation: India.

**I. Reported indigenous cases in countries with national elimination activities, 2015 versus 2018**

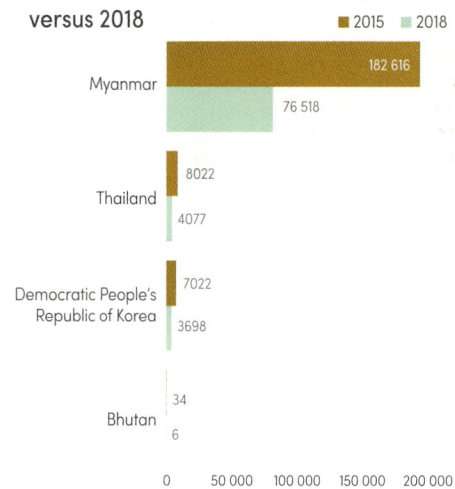

- Myanmar: 182 616 (2015); 76 518 (2018)
- Thailand: 8022 (2015); 4077 (2018)
- Democratic People's Republic of Korea: 7022 (2015); 3698 (2018)
- Bhutan: 34 (2015); 6 (2018)

# KEY MESSAGES

- An estimated 1.61 billion people in the WHO South-East Asia Region are at risk of malaria. The disease is endemic in 9 out of 11 countries of the region, accounting for 50% of the burden outside the WHO African Region. In 2018, the region had almost 8 million estimated cases and about 11 600 estimated deaths – reductions of 69% and 70%, respectively, compared with 2010 – representing the largest decline among all regions. All countries are on target to achieve a more than 40% reduction in case incidence by 2020, and all have strategic plans that aim for malaria elimination by 2030 at the latest.

- Three countries accounted for 98% of the total reported cases in the region, the main contributor being India (58%), followed by Indonesia (30%) and Myanmar (10%). Despite being the highest burden country of the region, India showed a reduction in reported cases of 51% compared with 2017 and of 60% compared with 2016. Although cases continue to decrease in the public sector, estimates indicate that there are still gaps in reporting from the private sector and in treatment seeking in the three countries (estimated versus reported: India 6.7 million versus 400 000, Indonesia 1 million versus 200 000, Myanmar 100 000 versus 76 500). Two other countries in the region reported substantial decline in total reported cases between 2017 and 2018: by 62% in Bangladesh and by 21% in Thailand.

- Timor-Leste had no indigenous malaria cases in a year for the first time, while Bhutan had only six indigenous (and 14 introduced) cases. Maldives and Sri Lanka, certified as malaria free in 2015 and 2016, respectively, continue to maintain their malaria free status.

- Continuing the declining trend, reported malaria deaths in the region dropped to 165 in 2018, reductions of 93% and 45 compared with 2010 and 2017, respectively. India, Indonesia and Myanmar accounted for 58%, 21% and 12% of the total reported deaths in the region, respectively. Bhutan, Democratic People's Republic of Korea and Timor-Leste continue to record zero indigenous deaths.

- Vector resistance to pyrethroids was confirmed in one third of the countries. Resistance to organophosphates was confirmed in almost half of the countries, and resistance to organochlorines and carbamates was confirmed in less than one third of them. There are still significant gaps in standard resistance monitoring for these three classes of vector control agents.

- Challenges include decreased funding, multiple ACT treatment failures in the countries of the GMS and vector resistance to pyrethroids. Efforts are underway to strengthen surveillance and to enhance reporting from private sector and nongovernmental organizations (where relevant), and case-based surveillance and response to accelerate towards elimination.

# Annex 2 - E. WHO Western Pacific Region

## EPIDEMIOLOGY
**Population at risk:** 762 million
**Parasites:** *P. falciparum* and mixed (66%), *P. vivax* (33%) and other (<1%)
**Vectors:** An. anthropophagus, An. balabacensis, An. barbirostris s.l., An. dirus s.l., An. donaldi, An. epirotivulus, An. farauti s.l., An. flavirostris, An. jeyporiensis, An. koliensis, An. litoralis, An. maculatus s.l., An. mangyanus, An. minimus s.l., An. punctulatus s.l., An. sinensis s.l. and An. sundaicus s.l.

## FUNDING (US$), 2010-2018
213.7 million (2010), 145.4 million (2015), 129.4 million (2018); decrease 2010-2018: 39%
**Proportion of domestic source* in 2018:** 60%
**Regional funding mechanisms:** Mekong Malaria Elimination (MME) Initiative in the Greater Mekong Subregion: Cambodia, China (Yunnan), Lao People's Democratic Republic and Viet Nam (supported by RAI2e Global Fund)
* Domestic source excludes patient service delivery costs and out-of-pocket expenditure.

## INTERVENTIONS, 2018
**Number of people protected by IRS:** 27.9 million (2010), 3.3 million (2015), 1.5 million (2018)
**Total LLINs distributed:** 3.4 million (2010), 2.7 million (2015), 3.4 million (2018)
**Number of RDTs distributed:** 1.6 million (2010), 2.5 million (2015), 3.5 million (2018)
**Number of ACT courses distributed:** 591 000 (2010), 1.3 million (2015), 1.7 million (2018)
**Number of any antimalarial treatment courses (incl. ACT) distributed:** 963 000 (2010), 1.4 million (2015), 1.7 million (2018)

## REPORTED CASES AND DEATHS IN PUBLIC SECTOR, 2010-2018
**Total (presumed and confirmed) cases:** 1.6 million (2010), 704 000 (2015), 1.1 million (2018)
**Confirmed cases:** 260 000 (2010), 411 000 (2015), 634 000 (2018)
**Percentage of total cases confirmed:** 15.8% (2010), 58.3% (2015), 58.9% (2018)
**Deaths:** 910 (2010), 234 (2015), 254 (2018)

## ESTIMATED CASES AND DEATHS, 2010-2018
**Cases:** 1.8 million (2010), 1.4 million (2015), 2.0 million (2018); increase 2010-2018: 8%
**Deaths:** 3780 (2010), 2840 (2015), 3450 (2018); decrease 2010-2018: 9%

## ACCELERATION TO ELIMINATION
**Countries with subnational/territorial elimination programme:** Philippines
**Countries with nationwide elimination programme:** Cambodia, China, Lao People's Democratic Republic, Malaysia, Republic of Korea and Viet Nam
**Zero indigenous cases in 2018:** China and Malaysia

## THERAPEUTIC EFFICACY TESTS (CLINICAL AND PARASITOLOGICAL FAILURE, %)

| Medicine | Study years | No. of studies | Min. | Median | Max. | Percentile 25 | Percentile 75 |
|---|---|---|---|---|---|---|---|
| AL | 2010-2018 | 30 | 0.0 | 0.0 | 17.2 | 0.0 | 5.2 |
| AS-MQ | 2010-2018 | 21 | 0.0 | 0.0 | 11.1 | 0.0 | 1.4 |
| AS-PY | 2014-2018 | 13 | 0.0 | 1.7 | 18.0 | 0.0 | 7.7 |
| DHA-PPQ | 2010-2017 | 75 | 0.0 | 0.8 | 62.5 | 0.0 | 12.3 |

AL: artemether-lumefantrine; AS-MQ: artesunate-mefloquine; AS-PY: artesunate-pyronaridine; DHA-PPQ: dihydroartemisinin-piperaquine.

## STATUS OF INSECTICIDE RESISTANCE[a] PER INSECTICIDE CLASS (2010-2018) AND USE OF EACH CLASS FOR MALARIA VECTOR CONTROL (2018)

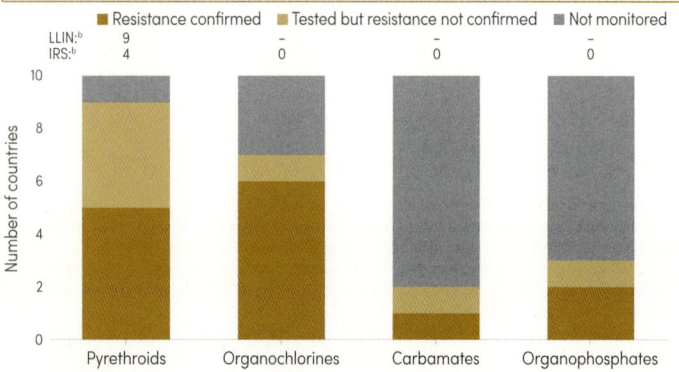

[a] Resistance is considered confirmed when it was detected to one insecticide in the class, in at least one malaria vector from one collection site.
[b] Number of countries that reported using the insecticide class for malaria vector control (2018).

### A. Confirmed malaria cases per 1000 population, 2018

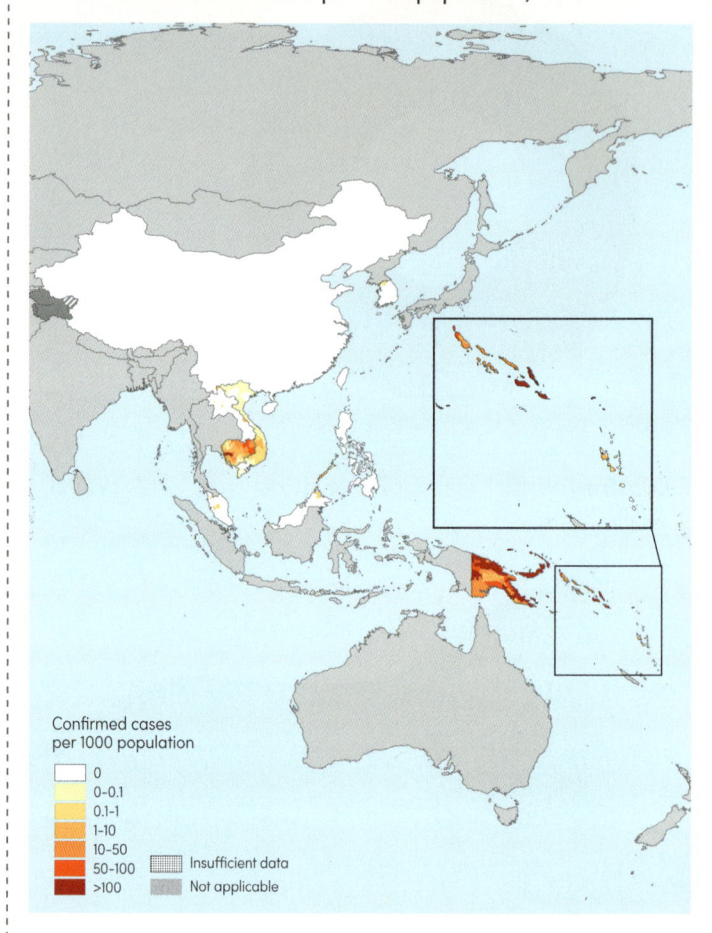

### B. Malaria funding* by source, 2010-2018

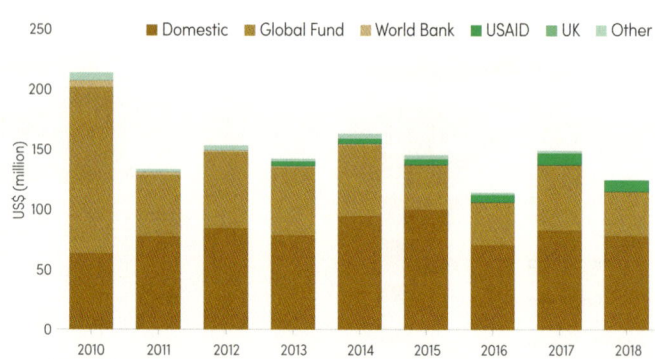

Global Fund: Global Fund to Fight AIDS, Tuberculosis and Malaria; UK: United Kingdom of Great Britain and Northern Ireland; USAID: United States Agency for International Development.
* Excludes patient service delivery costs and out-of-pocket expenditure.

### C. Malaria funding* per person at risk, 2016-2018

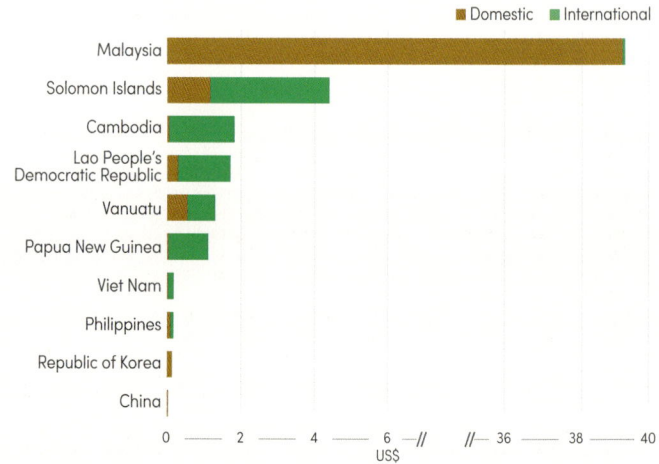

* Excludes costs related to health staff, costs at subnational level and out-of-pocket expenditure.
** Only domestic funding in China and the Republic of Korea.

## D. Share of estimated malaria cases, 2018

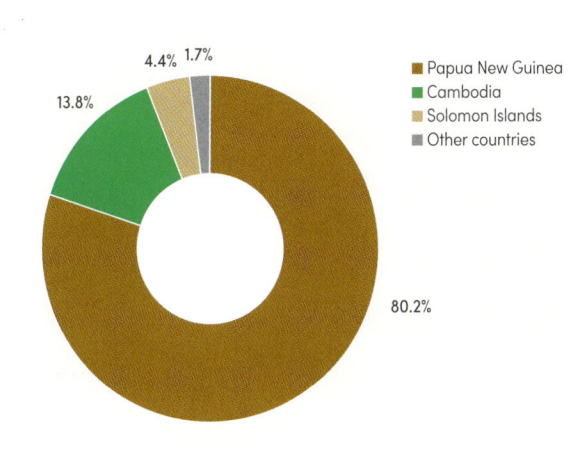

- Papua New Guinea: 80.2%
- Cambodia: 13.8%
- Solomon Islands: 4.4%
- Other countries: 1.7%

*Countries with zero cases: China and Malaysia.

## E. Percentage of Plasmodium species from indigenous cases, 2010 and 2018

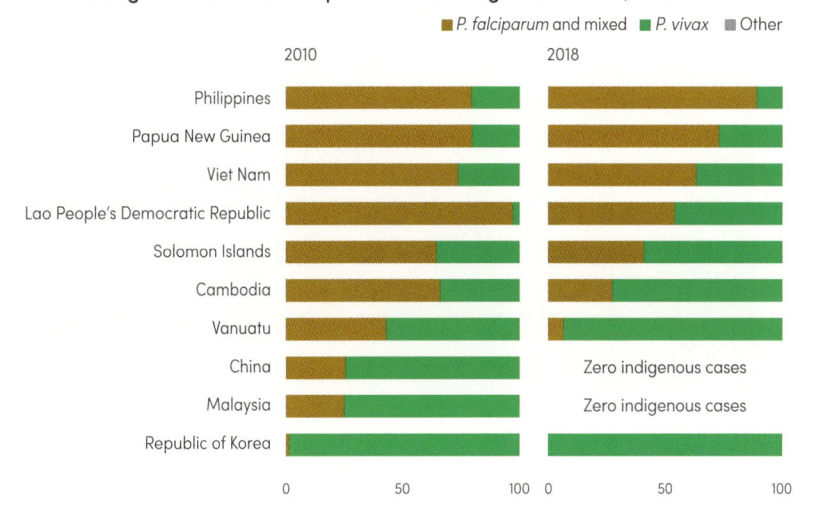

*P. falciparum* and mixed ■ *P. vivax* ■ Other

2010 and 2018 data shown for: Philippines, Papua New Guinea, Viet Nam, Lao People's Democratic Republic, Solomon Islands, Cambodia, Vanuatu, China (Zero indigenous cases in 2018), Malaysia (Zero indigenous cases in 2018), Republic of Korea.

## F. Countries on track to reduce case incidence by ≥40% by 2020

China, Malaysia, Vietnam, Lao People's Democratic Republic, Philippines — Baseline (2015)

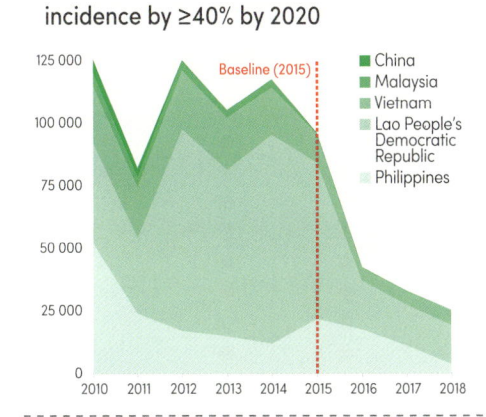

## G. Countries likely to reduce case incidence by <40% by 2020

Republic of Korea — Baseline (2015)

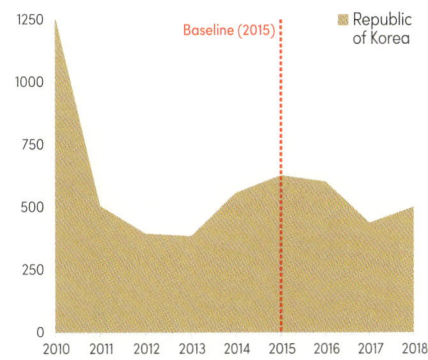

## H. Countries with an increase in case incidence, 2015–2018

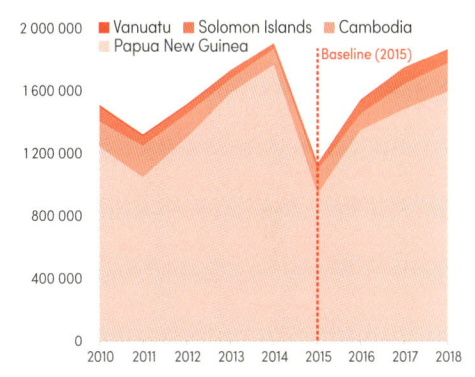

Vanuatu, Solomon Islands, Cambodia, Papua New Guinea — Baseline (2015)

## I. Change in estimated malaria incidence and mortality rates, 2015–2018

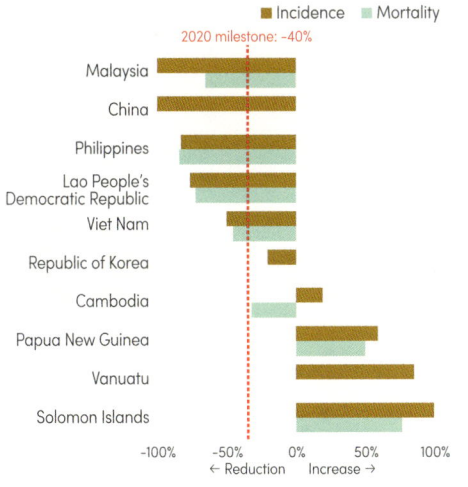

■ Incidence ■ Mortality; 2020 milestone: −40%

Countries: Malaysia, China, Philippines, Lao People's Democratic Republic, Viet Nam, Republic of Korea, Cambodia, Papua New Guinea, Vanuatu, Solomon Islands

*China, Republic of Korea and Vanuatu already achieved the 40% reduction in mortality rate in 2015; since then there has been no change.

## J. Percentage of total confirmed cases investigated, 2018

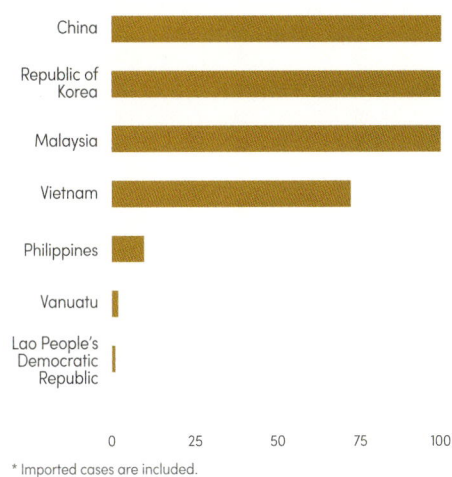

China, Republic of Korea, Malaysia, Vietnam, Philippines, Vanuatu, Lao People's Democratic Republic

*Imported cases are included.

## K. Reported indigenous cases in countries with national elimination activities, 2015 versus 2018

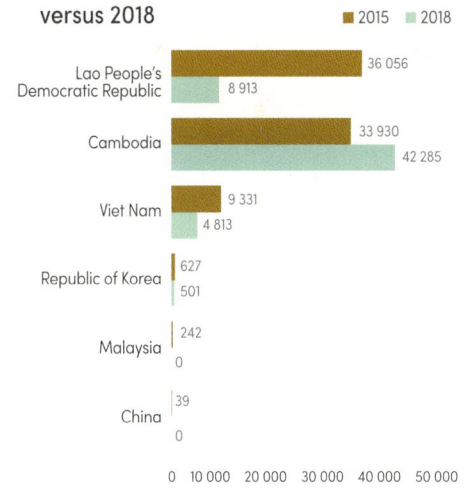

■ 2015 ■ 2018

| Country | 2015 | 2018 |
|---|---|---|
| Lao People's Democratic Republic | 36 056 | 8 913 |
| Cambodia | 33 930 | 42 285 |
| Viet Nam | 9 331 | 4 813 |
| Republic of Korea | 627 | 501 |
| Malaysia | 242 | 0 |
| China | 39 | 0 |

# KEY MESSAGES

- About 762 million people in 10 countries are at risk of malaria; infections are predominantly caused by *P. falciparum*, with about one third due to *P. vivax*. In 2018, the region had almost 2 million malaria cases and about 3500 estimated deaths – an 8% increase and a 9% decrease compared with 2010, respectively. Most of the cases were in Papua New Guinea (80%); when taken together with Cambodia and Solomon Islands, the three countries comprise 98% of the estimated cases. In the public health sector, just over 1 million cases were reported, of which 59% were confirmed. The proportion of total cases that were confirmed improved substantially between 2010 and 2015, from 15.8% to 58.3%, but since 2015 there has been little improvement. There were only about 250 reported deaths due to malaria.

- Five out of the 10 malaria endemic countries in the region are on target to achieve more than a 40% reduction in case incidence by 2020, and the Republic of Korea is on track for a 20–40% reduction. Cambodia, Papua New Guinea, Solomon Islands and Vanuatu have seen an increase in estimated cases since 2015: 18.8%, 40.2%, 99.6% and 37.3%, respectively. All countries are on track to reduce the malaria mortality rate by at least 40% by 2020, except Papua New Guinea and Solomon Islands.

- China and Malaysia are on course for elimination by 2020. China has reported zero indigenous cases for 2 consecutive years, and Malaysia reported zero indigenous human malaria cases for the first time in 2018. However, Malaysia is facing increasing cases of the zoonotic malaria *P. knowlesi*, which increased from 1600 to over 4000 between 2016 and 2018, and resulted in 12 deaths this year. The Republic of Korea is facing the challenge of malaria transmission in military personnel along the northern border. Philippines has initiated subnational elimination, reporting zero indigenous cases in 78 out of 81 provinces in 2018.

- Three countries of the GMS (Cambodia, Lao People's Democratic Republic and Viet Nam) aim to eliminate *P. falciparum* by 2020 and all species of malaria by 2030, through support from a Global Fund financed regional artemisinin-resistance initiative. The percentage of cases in Cambodia due to *P. falciparum* has fallen significantly, from 61% in 2015 to 27% in 2018, owing to intensified efforts in community outreach and active case detection to reduce *P. falciparum*. Although the goal of *P. falciparum* elimination will not be met by 2020, much progress has been made. Reducing *P. falciparum* cases in Lao People's Democratic Republic and Viet Nam has been more challenging, and from 2015 to 2018 they saw increases of 12% and 14%, respectively, due to sporadic outbreaks in 2017 and 2018.

- Vector resistance to pyrethroids was confirmed in half of the countries. Resistance to organochlorines was confirmed in more than half of the countries, although there are significant gaps in standard resistance monitoring for this class. Almost no standard resistance monitoring was reported for carbamates or organophosphates, other than in China, Philippines and Solomon Islands.

- Challenges include decreased funding, multiple ACT treatment failures, vector resistance to pyrethroids (in Cambodia, Lao People's Democratic Republic, Philippines and Viet Nam), resurgence of malaria in Cambodia and Solomon Islands, and sustained high levels of malaria in Papua New Guinea due to health system strengthening challenges. Recent efforts are underway to improve access to services and case-based surveillance to accelerate elimination in Cambodia, Lao People's Democratic Republic, Malaysia, Philippines, Republic of Korea, Vanuatu and Viet Nam.

# Annex 3 – A. Policy adoption, 2018

Legend: ● = black dot · ○ = grey dot · 🔴 = red/orange dot

| WHO region Country/area | Insecticide-treated mosquito nets | | | | Indoor residual spraying | | Chemoprevention | |
|---|---|---|---|---|---|---|---|---|
| | ITNs/LLINs are distributed free of charge | ITNs/LLINs are distributed through ANC | ITNs/LLINs distributed through EPI/well baby clinic | ITNs/LLINs distributed through mass campaigns | IRS is recommended by malaria control programme | DDT is used for IRS | IPTp is used to prevent malaria during pregnancy | Seasonal malaria chemoprevention (SMC or IPTc) is used |
| **AFRICAN** | | | | | | | | |
| Algeria | NA | NA | NA | NA | ○ | 🔴 | NA | NA |
| Angola | ● | ● | ● | ● | ○ | 🔴 | ● | NA |
| Benin | ● | ● | ● | ○ | ● | 🔴 | ● | 🔴 |
| Botswana | ○ | NA | NA | NA | ● | ● | 🔴 | NA |
| Burkina Faso | ● | ● | ● | ○ | ● | 🔴 | ● | ● |
| Burundi | ● | ● | ● | ○ | ● | 🔴 | ● | NA |
| Cabo Verde | NA | NA | NA | NA | ● | 🔴 | NA | NA |
| Cameroon | ● | ● | 🔴 | ○ | ● | 🔴 | ● | ● |
| Central African Republic | ● | ● | ● | ● | ○ | 🔴 | ● | NA |
| Chad | ● | ● | ● | ○ | ○ | 🔴 | ● | ● |
| Comoros | ● | ● | ● | ● | ○ | 🔴 | ● | NA |
| Congo | ● | ● | 🔴 | ● | ○ | 🔴 | ● | NA |
| Côte d'Ivoire | ● | ● | ● | ● | 🔴 | 🔴 | ● | NA |
| Democratic Republic of the Congo | ● | ● | ● | ● | ○ | 🔴 | ● | NA |
| Equatorial Guinea | ● | ● | 🔴 | ● | ● | 🔴 | ● | NA |
| Eritrea | ● | ● | ● | ● | ● | 🔴 | 🔴 | NA |
| Eswatini | ● | NA | NA | ● | ● | ● | NA | NA |
| Ethiopia | ● | 🔴 | 🔴 | ● | ● | 🔴 | 🔴 | NA |
| Gabon | ○ | ○ | ○ | ○ | ○ | 🔴 | ● | NA |
| Gambia | ● | ● | ● | ○ | ● | ○ | ● | ● |
| Ghana | ● | ● | ● | ● | ● | 🔴 | ● | ● |
| Guinea | ● | ● | ● | ○ | ○ | 🔴 | ● | ● |
| Guinea-Bissau | ● | ● | ● | ● | 🔴 | 🔴 | ● | ● |
| Kenya | ● | ● | ● | ● | ○ | 🔴 | ● | NA |
| Liberia | ○ | ● | 🔴 | ● | ○ | 🔴 | ● | NA |
| Madagascar | ● | ● | ● | ● | ○ | 🔴 | ● | NA |
| Malawi | ● | ● | ● | ● | ○ | 🔴 | ● | NA |
| Mali | ● | ● | ● | ● | ● | 🔴 | ● | ● |
| Mauritania | ● | ● | ● | ● | ○ | 🔴 | ● | 🔴 |
| Mayotte | ○ | – | – | – | – | 🔴 | NA | NA |
| Mozambique | ● | ● | 🔴 | ● | ● | ○ | ● | NA |
| Namibia | ● | NA | NA | ● | ● | ● | 🔴 | NA |
| Niger | ● | ● | ● | ● | ○ | 🔴 | ● | ● |
| Nigeria | ● | ● | ● | ● | ○ | 🔴 | ● | ● |
| Rwanda | ● | ● | ● | ○ | ● | 🔴 | 🔴 | NA |
| Sao Tome and Principe | ● | ● | ● | ● | ○ | 🔴 | ○ | NA |
| Senegal | ● | ● | 🔴 | ○ | ○ | 🔴 | ● | ○ |
| Sierra Leone | ● | ● | ● | ● | ○ | 🔴 | ● | NA |
| South Africa | NA | 🔴 | 🔴 | 🔴 | ● | ● | 🔴 | NA |
| South Sudan[2] | ● | ● | ● | ● | ○ | 🔴 | ● | NA |
| Togo | ● | ● | ● | ● | ● | 🔴 | ● | ● |
| Uganda | ● | ● | ● | ● | ● | 🔴 | ● | NA |
| United Republic of Tanzania[3] | | | | | | | | NA |
|   Mainland | ● | ● | ● | ● | ● | 🔴 | ● | NA |
|   Zanzibar | ● | ● | ● | 🔴 | ● | 🔴 | ○ | NA |
| Zambia | ● | ● | ● | ○ | ● | ○ | ● | NA |
| Zimbabwe | ● | ● | ● | ● | ● | ● | ● | NA |
| **AMERICAS** | | | | | | | | |
| Argentina | NA | 🔴 | 🔴 | 🔴 | ● | 🔴 | NA | NA |
| Belize | ● | ○ | 🔴 | ● | ● | 🔴 | NA | NA |
| Bolivia (Plurinational State of) | ● | ● | 🔴 | ○ | ● | 🔴 | NA | NA |
| Brazil | ● | 🔴 | 🔴 | ● | ● | 🔴 | NA | NA |
| Colombia | ● | 🔴 | ● | ○ | ● | 🔴 | NA | NA |

# Annex 3 – A. Policy adoption, 2018

Legend: ● = black dot, ◉ = orange/red dot, ○ = grey dot

| WHO region Country/area | ITNs/LLINs are distributed free of charge | ITNs/LLINs are distributed through ANC | ITNs/LLINs distributed through EPI/well baby clinic | ITNs/LLINs distributed through mass campaigns | IRS is recommended by malaria control programme | DDT is used for IRS | IPTp is used to prevent malaria during pregnancy | Seasonal malaria chemo-prevention (SMC or IPTc) is used |
|---|---|---|---|---|---|---|---|---|
| **AMERICAS** | | | | | | | | |
| Costa Rica | ● | ◉ | ◉ | ○ | ● | ◉ | NA | NA |
| Dominican Republic | ● | ◉ | ◉ | ● | ● | ◉ | NA | NA |
| Ecuador | ● | ◉ | ◉ | ● | ● | ◉ | NA | NA |
| El Salvador | ● | ◉ | ◉ | ● | ● | ◉ | NA | NA |
| French Guiana | ● | ○ | ○ | ● | ● | ◉ | NA | NA |
| Guatemala | ● | ◉ | ◉ | ● | ● | ◉ | NA | NA |
| Guyana | ● | ○ | ○ | ● | ● | ◉ | NA | NA |
| Haiti | ● | ◉ | ◉ | ● | ● | ◉ | NA | NA |
| Honduras | ● | ◉ | ◉ | ● | ● | ◉ | NA | NA |
| Mexico | ● | ◉ | ◉ | ● | ● | ◉ | NA | NA |
| Nicaragua | ● | ◉ | ◉ | ● | ● | ◉ | NA | NA |
| Panama | ◉ | ◉ | ◉ | ◉ | ● | ◉ | NA | NA |
| Peru | ● | ◉ | ◉ | ● | ● | ◉ | NA | NA |
| Suriname | ● | ◉ | ◉ | ● | ○ | ◉ | NA | NA |
| Venezuela (Bolivarian Republic of) | ● | ◉ | ◉ | ● | ○ | ◉ | NA | NA |
| **EASTERN MEDITERRANEAN** | | | | | | | | |
| Afghanistan | ● | ● | ◉ | ● | ○ | ◉ | NA | NA |
| Djibouti | ● | ○ | ○ | ○ | ● | ◉ | NA | NA |
| Iran (Islamic Republic of) | ○ | ◉ | ◉ | ● | ● | ◉ | NA | NA |
| Pakistan | ● | ◉ | ◉ | ● | ● | ◉ | NA | NA |
| Saudi Arabia | ● | ◉ | ◉ | ○ | ● | ◉ | NA | NA |
| Somalia | ● | ● | ○ | ● | ● | ◉ | ○ | NA |
| Sudan | ● | ● | ● | ● | ● | ◉ | ◉ | NA |
| Yemen | ● | ● | ○ | ● | ● | ◉ | NA | NA |
| **SOUTH-EAST ASIA** | | | | | | | | |
| Bangladesh | ● | ◉ | ◉ | ● | ● | ◉ | NA | NA |
| Bhutan | ○ | ◉ | ◉ | ● | ● | ◉ | NA | NA |
| Democratic People's Republic of Korea | ● | ◉ | ◉ | ● | ● | ◉ | NA | NA |
| India | ○ | ○ | ○ | ● | ● | ○ | NA | NA |
| Indonesia | ● | ● | ◉ | ● | ● | ◉ | NA | NA |
| Myanmar | ○ | ◉ | ◉ | ○ | ● | ◉ | NA | NA |
| Nepal | ● | ● | ● | ● | ● | ◉ | NA | NA |
| Thailand | ● | ◉ | ◉ | ● | ● | ◉ | NA | NA |
| Timor-Leste | ● | ● | ◉ | ● | ● | ◉ | NA | NA |
| **WESTERN PACIFIC** | | | | | | | | |
| Cambodia | ○ | ◉ | ◉ | ○ | ◉ | ◉ | NA | NA |
| China | ○ | ◉ | ◉ | ◉ | ● | ◉ | NA | NA |
| Lao People's Democratic Republic | ● | ● | ◉ | ○ | ● | ◉ | NA | NA |
| Malaysia | ○ | ◉ | ◉ | ● | ● | ◉ | NA | NA |
| Papua New Guinea | ● | ● | ● | ● | ○ | ◉ | ○ | NA |
| Philippines | ● | ● | ● | ● | ● | ◉ | NA | NA |
| Republic of Korea | ◉ | ◉ | ◉ | ○ | ● | ◉ | NA | NA |
| Solomon Islands | ● | ● | ● | ● | ○ | ◉ | NA | NA |
| Vanuatu | ● | ○ | ◉ | ● | ○ | ◉ | NA | NA |
| Viet Nam | ● | ● | ◉ | ● | ● | ◉ | NA | NA |

ACT: artemisinin-based combination therapy; ANC: antenatal care; DDT: dichloro-diphenyl-trichloroethane; EPI: Expanded Programme on Immunization; G6PD: glucose-6-phosphate dehydrogenase; IM: intramuscular; IPTc: intermittent preventive treatment in children; IPTp: intermittent preventive treatment in pregnancy; IRS: indoor residual spraying; ITN: insecticide-treated mosquito net; LLIN: long-lasting insecticidal net; RDT: rapid diagnostic test; SMC: seasonal malaria chemoprevention; WHO: World Health Organization.

[1] Single dose of primaquine (0.75 mg base/kg) for countries in the WHO Region of the Americas.

[2] In May 2013, South Sudan was reassigned to the WHO African Region (WHA resolution 66.21, https://apps.who.int/gb/ebwha/pdf_files/WHA66/A66_R21-en.pdf).

[3] Where national data for the United Republic of Tanzania are unavailable, refer to Mainland and Zanzibar.

| Testing | | | | Treatment | | | | |
|---|---|---|---|---|---|---|---|---|
| Patients of all ages should get diagnostic test | Malaria diagnosis is free of charge in the public sector | RDTs are used at community level | G6PD test is recommended before treatment with primaquine is used for treatment of P. vivax cases | ACT for treatment of P. falciparum | Pre-referral treatment with quinine or artemether IM or artesunate suppositories | Single dose of primaquine is used as gametocidal medicine for P. falciparum[1] | Primaquine is used for radical treatment of P. vivax cases | Directly observed treatment with primaquine is undertaken |

Data as of 26 November 2019

● = Policy adopted and implemented this year. Available data from the world malaria report data collection form provides evidence for implementation.

● = Policy adopted but not implemented this year (2018) or no supportive available data reported to WHO.

● = Policy not adopted.

NA = Question not applicable.

– = Question not answered and there is no information from previous years.

* Free for children and/or pregnant women only.

# Annex 3 – B. Antimalarial drug policy, 2018

| WHO region Country/area | P. falciparum | | | | P. vivax |
|---|---|---|---|---|---|
| | Uncomplicated unconfirmed | Uncomplicated confirmed | Severe | Prevention during pregnancy | Treatment |
| **AFRICAN** | | | | | |
| Algeria | - | - | - | - | PQ |
| Angola | AL | AL | AS; QN | SP(IPT) | - |
| Benin | AL | AL | AS; QN | SP(IPT) | - |
| Botswana | AL | AL | QN | - | - |
| Burkina Faso | AL; AS+AQ | AL; AS+AQ | AS; QN | SP(IPT) | - |
| Burundi | AS+AQ | AS+AQ | AS; QN | SP(IPT) | - |
| Cabo Verde | AL | AL | QN | - | - |
| Cameroon | AS+AQ | AS+AQ | AS; AM; QN | SP(IPT) | - |
| Central African Republic | AL | AL | AS; AM; QN | SP(IPT) | - |
| Chad | AL; AS+AQ | AL; AS+AQ | AS; QN | SP(IPT) | - |
| Comoros | AL | AL | AL | SP(IPT) | - |
| Congo | AS+AQ | AS+AQ | QN | SP(IPT) | - |
| Côte d'Ivoire | AS+AQ | AS+AQ | QN | SP(IPT) | - |
| Democratic Republic of the Congo | AS+AQ | AS+AQ | AS; QN | SP(IPT) | - |
| Equatorial Guinea | AS+AQ | AS+AQ | AS | SP(IPT) | - |
| Eritrea | AS+AQ | AS+AQ | QN | - | AS+AQ+PQ |
| Eswatini | - | AL | AS | - | - |
| Ethiopia | AL | AL | AS; AM; QN | - | CQ |
| Gabon | AS+AQ | AS+AQ | AS; AM; QN | SP(IPT) | - |
| Gambia | AL | AL | QN | SP(IPT) | - |
| Ghana | AS+AQ | AL; AS+AQ | AS; AM; QN | SP(IPT) | - |
| Guinea | AS+AQ | AS+AQ | AS | SP(IPT) | - |
| Guinea-Bissau | AL | AL | AS; QN | SP(IPT) | - |
| Kenya | AL | AL | AS; AM; QN | SP(IPT) | - |
| Liberia | AS+AQ | AS+AQ | AS; AM; QN | SP(IPT) | - |
| Madagascar | AS+AQ | AS+AQ | QN | SP(IPT) | - |
| Malawi | AL | AL | AS; QN | SP(IPT) | - |
| Mali | AS+AQ | AL; AS+AQ | QN | SP(IPT) | - |
| Mauritania | AS+AQ | AL; AS+AQ | QN | - | - |
| Mayotte | - | AL | QN; AS; QN+AS; AS+D; QN+D | - | CQ+PQ |
| Mozambique | AL | AL | AS; QN | SP(IPT) | - |
| Namibia | AL | AL | QN | - | AL |
| Niger | AL | AL | AS; QN | SP(IPT) | - |
| Nigeria | AL; AS+AQ | AL; AS+AQ | AS; AM; QN | SP(IPT) | - |
| Rwanda | AL | AL | AS; QN | - | - |
| Sao Tome and Principe | AS+AQ | AS+AQ | QN | - | - |
| Senegal | AL; AS+AQ; DHA-PPQ | AL; AS+AQ; DHA-PPQ | AS; QN | SP(IPT) | - |
| Sierra Leone | AS+AQ | AL; AS+AQ | AS; AM; QN | SP(IPT) | - |
| South Africa | - | AL; QN+CL; QN+D | QN | - | AL+PQ; CQ+PQ |
| South Sudan[1] | AS+AQ | AS+AQ | AM; AS; QN | - | AS+AQ+PQ |
| Togo | AL; AS+AQ | AL; AS+AQ | AS; AM; QN | SP(IPT) | - |
| Uganda | AL | AL | AS; QN | SP(IPT) | - |
| United Republic of Tanzania | AL; AS+AQ | AL; AS+AQ | AS; AM; QN | - | - |
|    Mainland | AL | AL | AS; AM; QN | SP(IPT) | - |
|    Zanzibar | AS+AQ | AS+AQ | AS; QN | SP(IPT) | - |
| Zambia | AL | AL | AS; AM; QN | SP(IPT) | - |
| Zimbabwe | AL | AL | QN | SP(IPT) | - |
| **AMERICAS** | | | | | |
| Argentina | - | AL | AS; AL | - | CQ + PQ |
| Belize | - | CQ+PQ | QN; AL | - | CQ+PQ |
| Bolivia (Plurinational State of) | - | AL | AS | - | CQ+PQ |
| Brazil | - | AL+PQ; AS+MQ+PQ | AS | - | CQ+PQ |
| Colombia | - | AL+PQ | AS | - | CQ+PQ |
| Costa Rica | - | CQ+PQ | AL | - | CQ+PQ |

| WHO region Country/area | P. falciparum | | | | P. vivax |
|---|---|---|---|---|---|
| | Uncomplicated unconfirmed | Uncomplicated confirmed | Severe | Prevention during pregnancy | Treatment |
| **AMERICAS** | | | | | |
| Dominican Republic | - | CQ+PQ | AS | - | CQ+PQ |
| Ecuador | - | AL+PQ | AS | - | CQ+PQ |
| El Salvador | - | CQ+PQ | AS | - | CQ+PQ |
| French Guiana | - | AL | AS | - | CQ+PQ |
| Guatemala | - | CQ+PQ | AS | - | CQ + PQ |
| Guyana | - | AL+PQ | AM | - | CQ+PQ |
| Haiti | - | CQ+PQ | QN | - | CQ+PQ |
| Honduras | - | CQ+PQ | QN; AS | - | CQ+PQ |
| Mexico | - | AL+PQ | AM; AL | - | CQ+PQ |
| Nicaragua | - | CQ+PQ | QN | - | CQ+PQ |
| Panama | - | AL+PQ | - | - | CQ+PQ |
| Paraguay | - | AL+PQ | AS | - | CQ+PQ |
| Peru | - | AS+MQ+PQ | AS+MQ | - | CQ+PQ |
| Suriname | - | AL+PQ | AS | - | CQ+PQ |
| Venezuela (Bolivarian Republic of) | - | AL+PQ | AS | - | CQ+PQ |
| **EASTERN MEDITERRANEAN** | | | | | |
| Afghanistan | CQ | AL+PQ | AS; AM; QN | - | CQ+PQ |
| Djibouti | AL | AL+PQ | AS | - | AL+PQ |
| Iran (Islamic Republic of) | - | AS+SP+PQ | AS; QN | - | CQ+PQ |
| Pakistan | CQ | AL+PQ | AS; QN | - | CQ+PQ |
| Saudi Arabia | - | AS+SP+PQ | AS; AM; QN | - | CQ+PQ |
| Somalia | AL | AL+PQ | AS; AM; QN | SP(IPT) | AL+PQ |
| Sudan | - | AL | AS; QN | - | AL+PQ |
| Yemen | AS+SP | AS+SP | AS, QN | - | CQ+PQ |
| **SOUTH-EAST ASIA** | | | | | |
| Bangladesh | - | AL | AS+AL; QN | - | CQ+PQ |
| Bhutan | - | AL | AM; QN | - | CQ+PQ |
| Democratic People's Republic of Korea | - | - | - | - | CQ+PQ |
| India | CQ | AS+SP+PQ; AL+PQ | AM; AS; QN | - | CQ+PQ |
| Indonesia | - | DHA-PPQ+PQ | AS; QN | - | DHA-PPQ+PQ |
| Myanmar | - | AL; AS+MQ; DHA-PPQ; PQ | AM; AS; QN | - | CQ+PQ |
| Nepal | - | AL+PQ | AS | - | CQ+PQ |
| Sri Lanka | - | AL+PQ | AS | - | CQ+PQ |
| Thailand | - | DHA-PPQ | AS | - | CQ+PQ |
| Timor-Leste | - | AL+PQ | AS; QN | - | AL+PQ |
| **WESTERN PACIFIC** | | | | | |
| Cambodia | - | AS+MQ | AM; AS; QN | - | AS+MQ+PQ |
| China | - | ART-PPQ; AS+AQ; DHA-PPQ; PYR | AM; AS; PYR | - | CQ+PQ; PQ+PPQ; ACTs+PQ; PYR |
| Lao People's Democratic Republic | AL+PQ | AL+PQ | AS+AL+PQ | - | AL+PQ; CQ+PQ |
| Malaysia | - | AS+MQ | AS+D; QN | - | ACT+PQ |
| Papua New Guinea | - | AL | AM; AS | SP(IPT) | AL+PQ |
| Philippines | AL | AL+PQ | QN+T; QN+D; QN+CL | SP(IPT) | CQ+PQ |
| Republic of Korea | CQ | - | QN | - | CQ+PQ |
| Solomon Islands | AL | AL | AS+AL; QN | CQ | AL+PQ |
| Vanuatu | - | AL | AS | CQ | AL+PQ |
| Viet Nam | DHA-PPQ | DHA-PPQ | AS; QN | - | CQ+PQ |

Data as of 26 November 2019

ACT: artemisinin-based combination therapy; AL: artemether-lumefantrine; AM: artemether; AQ: amodiaquine; ART: artemisinin; AS: artesunate; AT: atovaquone; CL: clindamycine; CQ: chloroquine; D: doxycycline; DHA: dihydroartemisinin; IPT: intermittent preventive treatment; MQ: mefloquine; NQ: naphroquine; PG: proguanil; PPQ: piperaquine; PQ: primaquine; PYR: pyronaridine; QN: quinine; SP: sulfadoxine-pyrimethamine; T: tetracycline; WHO: World Health Organization.

[1] In May 2013, South Sudan was reassigned to the WHO African Region (WHA resolution 66.21, http://apps.who.int/gb/ebwha/pdf_files/WHA66/A66_R21-en.pdf).

# Annex 3 - C. Funding for malaria control, 2016–2018

| WHO region Country/area | Year | Contributions reported by donors | | | |
|---|---|---|---|---|---|
| | | Global Fund[1] | PMI/USAID[2] | World Bank[3] | UK[4] |
| **AFRICAN** | | | | | |
| Algeria | 2016 | 0 | 0 | 0 | 0 |
| | 2017 | 0 | 0 | 0 | 0 |
| | 2018 | 0 | 0 | 0 | 0 |
| Angola | 2016 | 2 725 165 | 28 133 718 | 0 | 0 |
| | 2017 | 15 453 275 | 22 496 168 | 0 | 0 |
| | 2018 | 12 123 750 | 22 000 000 | 0 | 0 |
| Benin | 2016 | 2 476 172 | 17 192 827 | 0 | 0 |
| | 2017 | 25 699 563 | 16 360 849 | 0 | 0 |
| | 2018 | 4 743 095 | 16 000 000 | 0 | 0 |
| Botswana | 2016 | 0 | 0 | 0 | 0 |
| | 2017 | 1 654 745 | 0 | 0 | 0 |
| | 2018 | 1 475 705 | 0 | 0 | 0 |
| Burkina Faso | 2016 | 29 722 841 | 14 587 854 | 5 420 843 | 58 501 |
| | 2017 | 9 680 365 | 25 563 827 | 10 570 944 | 1 375 065 |
| | 2018 | 32 552 591 | 25 000 000 | 10 570 944 | 991 422 |
| Burundi | 2016 | 7 877 578 | 9 898 901 | 0 | 0 |
| | 2017 | 28 433 018 | 9 202 978 | 0 | 0 |
| | 2018 | 1 805 521 | 9 000 000 | 0 | 0 |
| Cabo Verde | 2016 | 32 723 | 0 | 0 | 0 |
| | 2017 | 237 164 | 0 | 0 | 0 |
| | 2018 | -19 013 | 0 | 0 | 0 |
| Cameroon | 2016 | 11 081 109 | 0 | 0 | 0 |
| | 2017 | 23 218 072 | 20 451 062 | 0 | 0 |
| | 2018 | 17 076 812 | 22 500 000 | 0 | 0 |
| Central African Republic | 2016 | 2 221 630 | 0 | 0 | 0 |
| | 2017 | 13 524 488 | 0 | 0 | 0 |
| | 2018 | 17 167 200 | 0 | 0 | 0 |
| Chad | 2016 | 34 361 246 | 0 | 0 | 0 |
| | 2017 | 14 272 836 | 0 | 0 | 0 |
| | 2018 | 18 323 111 | 0 | 0 | 0 |
| Comoros | 2016 | 3 017 257 | 0 | 0 | 0 |
| | 2017 | 860 330 | 0 | 0 | 0 |
| | 2018 | 2 298 799 | 0 | 0 | 0 |
| Congo | 2016 | 0 | 0 | 0 | 0 |
| | 2017 | 0 | 0 | 0 | 0 |
| | 2018 | 1 186 414 | 0 | 0 | 0 |
| Côte d'Ivoire | 2016 | 62 118 732 | 0 | 0 | 0 |
| | 2017 | 31 403 441 | 25 563 827 | 0 | 0 |
| | 2018 | 27 474 941 | 25 000 000 | 0 | 0 |
| Democratic Republic of the Congo | 2016 | 120 394 350 | 52 099 477 | 0 | 7 437 989 |
| | 2017 | 128 846 868 | 51 127 654 | 0 | 6 084 289 |
| | 2018 | 77 617 223 | 50 000 000 | 0 | 4 386 772 |
| Equatorial Guinea | 2016 | 0 | 0 | 0 | 0 |
| | 2017 | 0 | 0 | 0 | 0 |
| | 2018 | 0 | 0 | 0 | 0 |
| Eritrea | 2016 | 6 905 539 | 0 | 0 | 0 |
| | 2017 | 13 301 118 | 0 | 0 | 0 |
| | 2018 | 4 791 899 | 0 | 0 | 0 |
| Eswatini | 2016 | 897 122 | 0 | 0 | 0 |
| | 2017 | 1 686 517 | 0 | 0 | 0 |
| | 2018 | 579 780 | 0 | 0 | 0 |

|  | Contributions reported by countries | | | | | | |
|---|---|---|---|---|---|---|---|
| Government (NMP) | Global Fund | World Bank | PMI/USAID | Other bilaterals | WHO | UNICEF | Other contributions[7] |
| 1 743 483 | 0 | 0 | 0 | 0 |  | 0 | 0 |
| 1 748 498 | 0 | 0 | 0 | 0 | 43 809 | 0 | 0 |
| 1 812 462 | 0 | 0 | 0 | 0 | 9 214 | 0 | 0 |
| 50 874 556 [6] | 16 852 909 |  | 27 000 000 |  |  |  |  |
| 9 020 546 | 12 023 625 |  | 18 000 000 |  | 139 995 |  |  |
| 46 457 232 [5] | 9 578 147 |  | 22 000 000 |  | 88 217 |  |  |
| 17 540 458 [5] | 13 424 427 | 230 534 | 3 387 786 |  | 148 346 | 179 879 |  |
| 4 395 380 | 33 122 938 | 0 | 9 642 332 | 3 140 | 158 723 | 5 400 |  |
| 611 841 | 2 235 811 | 0 | 1 419 738 | 0 | 21 292 | 75 628 | 0 |
| 1 310 536 | 2 019 079 | 0 | 0 | 0 |  | 0 | 0 |
| 1 092 695 | 1 079 069 | 0 | 0 | 0 |  | 0 | 0 |
| 2 124 880 | 2 087 088 | 0 | 0 | 0 |  | 0 | 0 |
| 805 813 | 41 106 186 | 2 522 884 | 5 849 900 |  | 20 367 | 179 278 | 3 638 120 |
| 15 573 795 | 9 474 402 | 5 608 893 | 13 053 101 |  | 164 363 | 163 431 | 5 570 878 |
| 123 337 | 14 880 669 | 5 321 114 | 16 646 476 |  | 431 795 | 228 084 | 2 900 368 |
| 3 050 306 | 4 759 452 |  | 9 500 000 |  | 18 579 | 786 133 |  |
| 3 070 872 | 21 228 086 |  | 9 000 000 |  | 37 832 | 4 967 372 | 869 962 |
| 1 157 984 | 4 734 738 |  | 9 000 000 |  | 68 488 | 433 441 | 4 664 286 |
| 1 229 033 [5] | 315 038 |  |  |  | 59 219 |  |  |
| 4 627 843 | 466 244 |  |  |  | 29 000 |  |  |
| 621 612 | 221 609 |  |  |  | 25 641 |  |  |
| 1 989 500 | 14 478 500 |  |  |  | 747 500 |  | 2 024 000 |
| 2 288 193 [5] | 28 008 486 |  |  |  | 882 650 | 1 105 377 | 9 477 |
| 10 607 209 [5] | 47 200 683 |  | 29 913 228 |  |  |  |  |
| 530 000 | 4 724 918 |  |  |  | 150 000 |  |  |
| 530 000 | 443 466 |  |  |  | 70 419 |  |  |
| 675 455 | 8 399 445 |  |  |  | 50 000 | 306 968 |  |
| 1 000 000 [5] | 504 853 |  |  | 73 721 | 1 000 | 263 754 |  |
| 641 141 [6] | 34 927 891 |  |  |  | 416 | 540 870 | 867 119 |
| 534 407 [6] |  |  |  |  |  |  |  |
| 114 684 | 2 154 616 |  |  |  | 15 000 |  |  |
| 114 684 | 852 996 | 0 | 0 | 0 | 54 000 |  | 0 |
| 114 684 |  | 0 | 0 | 0 | 60 000 |  | 0 |
| 118 498 | 0 | 0 | 0 | 0 | 24 727 | 2 863 | 0 |
| 122 182 | 0 | 0 | 0 | 0 | 15 000 | 0 | 10 000 |
| 50 509 | 9 090 909 | 0 | 0 | 0 | 0 | 0 | 9 090 |
| 4 688 040 | 60 352 423 | 0 | 0 | 0 | 13 627 | 35 933 | 0 |
| 5 380 263 | 95 971 000 | 0 | 0 | 0 | 18 218 | 76 943 | 10 319 |
| 7 493 797 991 | 6 619 727 462 | 0 | 25 000 000 | 0 | 0 | 874 070 529 | 0 |
| 7 327 062 | 143 685 771 | 0 | 49 325 000 | 8 063 499 | 3 677 567 | 4 771 747 | 0 |
| 683 314 | 75 183 622 | 0 | 46 738 755 | 4 694 136 | 2 265 298 | 82 857 | 0 |
| 1 948 241 | 92 444 112 | 0 | 49 075 000 | 0 | 636 951 | 0 | 0 |
| 3 122 871 [6] |  |  |  |  |  |  |  |
| 3 153 487 [6] |  |  |  |  |  |  |  |
| 3 153 487 [6] |  |  |  |  |  |  |  |
| 397 657 [6] | 16 685 629 | 0 | 0 | 0 | 200 000 | 0 | 0 |
| 401 555 [6] | 9 150 700 | 0 | 0 | 0 | 80 450 | 0 |  |
| 401 555 [6] | 2 748 778 | 0 | 0 | 0 | 82 500 | 0 | 0 |
| 1 112 523 | 1 719 139 | 0 | 0 | 0 |  | 0 |  |
| 10 019 754 | 20 910 608 | 0 | 0 | 0 | 620 000 | 0 | 0 |
| 989 110 | 1 376 660 | 0 | 0 | 0 |  | 0 | 0 |

# Annex 3 - C. Funding for malaria control, 2016–2018

| WHO region Country/area | Year | Contributions reported by donors | | | |
|---|---|---|---|---|---|
| | | Global Fund[1] | PMI/USAID[2] | World Bank[3] | UK[4] |
| **AFRICAN** | | | | | |
| Ethiopia | 2016 | 26 310 036 | 41 679 582 | 0 | 0 |
| | 2017 | 73 672 826 | 37 834 464 | 0 | 0 |
| | 2018 | 36 485 376 | 36 000 000 | 0 | 0 |
| Gabon | 2016 | -574 | 0 | 0 | 0 |
| | 2017 | 0 | 0 | 0 | 0 |
| | 2018 | 0 | 0 | 0 | 0 |
| Gambia | 2016 | 3 171 117 | 0 | 0 | 336 595 |
| | 2017 | 10 403 537 | 0 | 0 | 0 |
| | 2018 | 7 988 886 | 0 | 0 | 0 |
| Ghana | 2016 | 39 257 572 | 29 175 707 | 0 | 5 224 120 |
| | 2017 | 40 834 747 | 28 631 486 | 0 | 1 136 043 |
| | 2018 | 44 164 622 | 28 000 000 | 0 | 819 087 |
| Guinea | 2016 | 29 160 172 | 15 629 843 | 255 449 | 0 |
| | 2017 | 14 405 410 | 15 338 296 | 535 378 | 0 |
| | 2018 | 12 534 176 | 15 000 000 | 535 378 | 0 |
| Guinea-Bissau | 2016 | 9 113 073 | 0 | 0 | 0 |
| | 2017 | 6 739 432 | 0 | 0 | 0 |
| | 2018 | 7 686 968 | 0 | 0 | 0 |
| Kenya | 2016 | 11 362 945 | 36 469 634 | 0 | 6 776 489 |
| | 2017 | 60 499 518 | 35 789 358 | 0 | 990 329 |
| | 2018 | 12 442 150 | 35 000 000 | 0 | 714 027 |
| Liberia | 2016 | 6 373 170 | 14 587 854 | 0 | 0 |
| | 2017 | 14 115 769 | 14 315 743 | 0 | 0 |
| | 2018 | 20 155 173 | 14 000 000 | 0 | 0 |
| Madagascar | 2016 | 12 460 235 | 27 091 728 | 0 | 0 |
| | 2017 | 14 309 923 | 26 586 380 | 0 | 0 |
| | 2018 | 40 366 061 | 26 000 000 | 0 | 0 |
| Malawi | 2016 | 16 538 845 | 22 923 770 | 0 | 3 783 827 |
| | 2017 | 11 926 740 | 22 496 168 | 0 | 0 |
| | 2018 | 30 542 662 | 24 000 000 | 0 | 0 |
| Mali | 2016 | 9 714 772 | 26 049 738 | 4 888 374 | 125 410 |
| | 2017 | 23 204 310 | 25 563 827 | 5 578 034 | 0 |
| | 2018 | 30 478 473 | 25 000 000 | 5 578 034 | 0 |
| Mauritania | 2016 | 1 861 629 | 0 | 0 | 0 |
| | 2017 | 4 592 194 | 0 | 0 | 0 |
| | 2018 | 4 020 544 | 0 | 0 | 0 |
| Mozambique | 2016 | 61 708 435 | 30 217 697 | 1 431 916 | 0 |
| | 2017 | 63 584 965 | 29 654 039 | 1 995 892 | 7 668 217 |
| | 2018 | 35 773 022 | 29 000 000 | 1 995 892 | 5 528 785 |
| Namibia | 2016 | 2 212 537 | 0 | 0 | 0 |
| | 2017 | 2 707 554 | 0 | 0 | 0 |
| | 2018 | 742 672 | 0 | 0 | 0 |
| Niger | 2016 | 9 226 298 | 0 | 3 837 140 | 0 |
| | 2017 | 24 712 609 | 18 405 955 | 6 472 782 | 0 |
| | 2018 | 28 316 962 | 18 000 000 | 6 472 782 | 0 |
| Nigeria | 2016 | 106 477 832 | 78 149 215 | 13 526 155 | 2 946 514 |
| | 2017 | 121 497 648 | 76 691 481 | 0 | 0 |
| | 2018 | 66 607 410 | 70 000 000 | 0 | 0 |
| Rwanda | 2016 | 22 669 934 | 18 755 812 | 0 | 0 |
| | 2017 | 17 066 738 | 18 405 955 | 0 | 0 |
| | 2018 | 9 931 433 | 18 000 000 | 0 | 0 |

| | Contributions reported by countries | | | | | | |
|---|---|---|---|---|---|---|---|
| Government (NMP) | Global Fund | World Bank | PMI/USAID | Other bilaterals | WHO | UNICEF | Other contributions[7] |
| 18 947 911 | 49 500 000 | | 10 600 000 | | 0 | 30 000 | 13 500 000 |
| 19 401 447 | 31 604 918 | | 7 150 000 | | 0 | 30 000 | 13 500 000 |
| 20 758 465 | 44 800 000 | | 26 358 971 | | | | 14 000 000 |
| 1 410 426 [6] | 0 | 0 | 0 | 0 | | 0 | |
| 142 296 | 0 | 0 | 0 | 0 | 12 616 | 0 | 0 |
| 0 | 0 | 0 | 0 | 0 | 128 016 | 0 | 49 674 |
| 604 456 [6] | 9 352 149 | | | | 0 | 0 | 1 031 868 |
| 610 382 [6] | 9 557 650 | | | | 14 400 | 33 839 | 117 749 |
| 1 327 049 | 8 376 620 | | | | 39 000 | 50 414 | 176 987 |
| 9 856 505 | 36 596 848 | 0 | 28 000 000 | 9 883 185 | 300 000 | 0 | 0 |
| 683 179 | 40 951 105 | 0 | 22 445 306 | | 140 000 | 0 | 0 |
| 140 392 544 | 47 579 039 | 0 | 30 634 694 | 7 560 000 | 300 000 | 0 | 0 |
| 4 229 893 | 36 810 868 | | 15 000 000 | 2 235 000 | 91 500 | 5 001 | 636 998 |
| 14 796 [5] | 9 251 505 | 125 000 | 12 500 000 | | 65 000 | | |
| 6 438 381 | 12 000 000 | 156 000 | 14 000 000 | | 45 000 | | |
| 241 163 | 8 972 945 | 0 | 0 | 0 | | 0 | 269 981 |
| 1 655 769 | 9 086 476 | 0 | 0 | 0 | | 0 | 256 659 |
| 651 820 | 3 199 732 | 0 | 0 | 0 | | 0 | 0 |
| 1 633 148 [6] | | | | | | | |
| 1 649 159 [6] | | | | | | | |
| 1 649 159 [6] | | | | | | | |
| 305 428 [6] | | | | | | | |
| 308 423 [6] | 18 526 566 | | 14 000 000 | | | | |
| 308 423 [6] | | | | | | | |
| 32 100 | 6 395 563 | 0 | 26 000 000 | 0 | 486 635 | | |
| 37 214 | 43 205 989 | 0 | 26 000 000 | 0 | 220 000 | 0 | 0 |
| 13 007 | 33 200 289 | 0 | 26 000 000 | | 46 000 | | |
| 347 710 [5] | | | 22 000 000 | | | | |
| 291 194 [5] | 16 282 087 | | 22 000 000 | | | | |
| 282 401 | 33 049 389 | | 20 000 000 | | | | |
| 3 263 366 | 16 374 449 | | 25 500 000 | | 4 983 | 2 203 890 | |
| 4 382 069 | 19 288 748 | 3 226 759 | 25 500 000 | 0 | 140 713 | 854 199 | |
| 14 329 420 | 54 053 651 | 6 406 499 | 25 000 000 | | | 337 884 | |
| 2 450 845 | | 3 500 400 | | | 220 | 384 900 | |
| 605 079 [5] | 6 957 945 | | | | 47 950 | | 13 944 |
| 2 191 549 | 164 778 | | | | | | |
| 1 237 214 | 190 374 239 | | 29 000 000 | | 325 000 | 1 250 640 | |
| 76 074 | 58 222 077 | | 29 000 000 | | 240 000 | 3 848 028 | 10 995 |
| 2 136 147 | 45 915 417 | | 29 000 000 | | | 1 590 000 | 4 361 414 |
| 5 218 841 | 4 227 559 | 0 | 0 | 0 | 100 000 | 0 | 878 882 |
| 5 166 667 | 1 096 657 | 0 | 0 | 0 | 100 000 | 0 | 789 566 |
| 11 216 160 | 908 515 | 0 | 0 | 0 | 100 000 | 100 000 | 1 148 515 |
| 2 672 787 | 14 911 144 | 641 402 | 106 000 | 0 | 75 586 | 39 712 | 39 712 |
| 4 454 320 | 22 404 758 | 2 177 698 | 220 000 | 0 | 328 594 | 805 598 | 476 444 |
| 7 363 777 | 20 159 800 | 4 490 567 | 18 000 000 | 0 | 220 356 | 674 811 | 0 |
| 476 077 607 | 372 939 170 | | 75 000 000 | 2 967 421 | | | |
| 107 005 355 | 198 176 039 | | 75 000 000 | | | | |
| 2 232 700 [6] | 43 206 463 | | 70 000 000 | | | | |
| 16 853 782 | 30 497 401 | | 18 000 000 | | 72 000 | | |
| 13 704 611 | 11 440 292 | | 18 000 000 | | 270 000 | | |
| 13 460 220 | 27 505 974 | | 18 000 000 | | | | |

# Annex 3 - C. Funding for malaria control, 2016–2018

| WHO region Country/area | Year | Contributions reported by donors | | | |
|---|---|---|---|---|---|
| | | Global Fund[1] | PMI/USAID[2] | World Bank[3] | UK[4] |
| **AFRICAN** | | | | | |
| Sao Tome and Principe | 2016 | 2 945 763 | 0 | 0 | 0 |
| | 2017 | 2 978 337 | 0 | 0 | 0 |
| | 2018 | 0 | 0 | 0 | 0 |
| Senegal | 2016 | 10 227 184 | 25 007 749 | 0 | 0 |
| | 2017 | 5 941 567 | 25 563 827 | 0 | 0 |
| | 2018 | 12 400 978 | 24 000 000 | 0 | 0 |
| Sierra Leone | 2016 | 5 776 307 | 0 | 0 | 7 657 486 |
| | 2017 | 1 521 619 | 15 338 296 | 0 | 1 264 107 |
| | 2018 | 1 442 219 | 15 000 000 | 0 | 911 421 |
| South Africa | 2016 | 0 | 0 | 0 | 48 271 |
| | 2017 | 0 | 0 | 0 | 0 |
| | 2018 | 0 | 0 | 0 | 0 |
| South Sudan[8] | 2016 | 6 625 486 | 6 251 937 | 0 | 21 105 454 |
| | 2017 | 23 225 030 | 0 | 0 | 13 351 190 |
| | 2018 | 11 119 479 | 0 | 0 | 9 626 208 |
| Togo | 2016 | 4 909 746 | 0 | 1 868 045 | 0 |
| | 2017 | 18 204 847 | 0 | 2 334 730 | 0 |
| | 2018 | 6 564 615 | 0 | 2 334 730 | 0 |
| Uganda | 2016 | 76 258 031 | 35 427 644 | 0 | 30 424 581 |
| | 2017 | 54 107 401 | 33 744 252 | 0 | 7 293 653 |
| | 2018 | 64 750 030 | 33 000 000 | 0 | 5 258 724 |
| United Republic of Tanzania[9] | 2016 | 62 681 243 | 0 | 0 | 0 |
| | 2017 | 72 183 435 | 0 | 0 | 0 |
| | 2018 | 0 | 0 | 0 | 0 |
| Mainland | 2016 | 61 652 875 | 0 | 0 | 0 |
| | 2017 | 69 674 305 | 0 | 0 | 0 |
| | 2018 | 0 | 0 | 0 | 0 |
| Zanzibar | 2016 | 1 028 368 | 0 | 0 | 0 |
| | 2017 | 2 509 129 | 0 | 0 | 0 |
| | 2018 | 0 | 0 | 0 | 0 |
| Zambia | 2016 | 27 622 155 | 26 049 738 | 286 668 | 28 080 |
| | 2017 | 40 378 684 | 30 676 592 | 606 731 | 0 |
| | 2018 | 22 106 638 | 30 000 000 | 606 731 | 0 |
| Zimbabwe | 2016 | 17 000 019 | 15 629 843 | 0 | 0 |
| | 2017 | 17 503 053 | 15 338 296 | 0 | 0 |
| | 2018 | 12 952 709 | 15 000 000 | 0 | 0 |
| **AMERICAS** | | | | | |
| Belize | 2016 | 0 | 0 | 0 | 0 |
| | 2017 | 0 | 0 | 0 | 0 |
| | 2018 | 0 | 0 | 0 | 0 |
| Bolivia (Plurinational State of) | 2016 | 4 324 861 | 0 | 0 | 0 |
| | 2017 | 2 805 373 | 0 | 0 | 0 |
| | 2018 | 3 347 788 | 0 | 0 | 0 |
| Brazil | 2016 | 0 | 0 | 0 | 0 |
| | 2017 | 0 | 0 | 0 | 0 |
| | 2018 | 0 | 0 | 0 | 0 |
| Colombia | 2016 | 0 | 0 | 0 | 0 |
| | 2017 | 0 | 0 | 0 | 0 |
| | 2018 | 0 | 0 | 0 | 0 |

| | | | Contributions reported by countries | | | | |
|---|---|---|---|---|---|---|---|
| Government (NMP) | Global Fund | World Bank | PMI/USAID | Other bilaterals | WHO | UNICEF | Other contributions[7] |
| 1 745 437 | 2 261 202 | 0 | 0 | 1 000 000 | 52 985 | 2 826 | 4 584 |
| 2 044 439 | 3 296 207 | 0 | 0 | 0 | 89 244 | 0 | 0 |
| 0 [6] | | | | | | | |
| 4 816 000 | 1 865 570 | 0 | 24 000 000 | 0 | 7 828 | 28 795 | 24 167 |
| 4 931 741 | 3 039 725 | 0 | 24 000 000 | 0 | 0 | 0 | 4 500 000 |
| 4 931 741 | 11 602 821 | 0 | 24 000 000 | 11 602 821 | 0 | 0 | 0 |
| 346 772 [5] | 5 389 748 | | | | 36 569 | 55 295 | |
| 807 592 [6] | 19 300 000 | | | | 72 812 | 3 464 362 | |
| 65 189 [5] | 8 728 599 | | 15 000 000 | | 70 000 | 148 214 | 2 742 |
| 15 428 406 | 0 | 0 | 0 | 0 | 0 | 0 | 75 061 |
| 10 656 029 | 27 226 495 | 0 | 0 | 0 | 20 000 | 0 | 0 |
| 16 954 533 | 4 197 290 | 0 | 0 | 0 | 50 000 | 0 | |
| 8 919 615 [5] | 20 288 506 | 7 000 000 | 6 000 000 | 6 000 808 | 4 779 900 | 12 812 860 | 6 758 505 |
| 2 603 242 [5] | 16 478 112 | 0 | 6 000 000 | 6 654 000 | 200 000 | | 5 249 000 |
| 2 658 638 [6] | | | | | | | |
| 68 213 | 2 973 548 | 943 022 | 0 | 0 | 7 158 | 169 496 | 10 650 |
| 1 847 898 | 24 435 381 | 1 014 708 | 0 | 0 | 7 765 | 556 712 | 5 238 461 |
| 64 103 | 23 830 061 | 440 567 | 0 | 0 | 4 715 | 553 567 | 0 |
| 7 585 730 | 31 501 450 | 0 | 33 000 000 | 29 246 018 | | 743 791 | 3 772 657 |
| 7 280 412 | 150 649 446 | 0 | 34 000 000 | 8 974 881 | | 743 791 | 4 335 860 |
| 7 243 128 | 47 530 743 | 0 | 33 000 000 | 14 073 138 | | 743 791 | 0 |
| 5 873 258 [6] | 104 603 541 | 37 578 250 | 2 888 539 | 5 466 569 | 0 | 0 | 0 |
| 70 283 449 [6] | 73 235 141 | 0 | 978 962 | | 52 000 | | |
| 145 338 516 [6] | 146 767 363 | 0 | 16 104 693 | 0 | 14 574 | 0 | 12 168 |
| 5 858 187 | 103 964 466 | 37 578 250 | 2 025 000 | 4 982 394 | 0 | 0 | 0 |
| 70 274 555 | 70 274 555 | | | | 42 000 | | |
| 145 258 808 | 145 258 808 | | 713 228 | | | | 12 168 |
| 15 071 | 639 075 | 0 | 863 539 | 484 175 | 0 | 0 | 0 |
| 8 894 | 2 960 586 | 0 | 978 962 | | 10 000 | | |
| 79 708 | 1 508 555 | 0 | 15 391 465 | 0 | 14 574 | 0 | 0 |
| 25 500 000 | 20 134 623 | | 24 000 000 | | 200 000 | | |
| 27 928 587 | 45 468 736 | | 25 000 000 | | 200 000 | | |
| 18 159 340 | 24 605 077 | | 3 000 000 | | 200 000 | | 3 692 991 |
| 675 000 | 21 823 373 | | 12 000 000 | | 46 698 | | |
| 782 250 | 17 407 287 | | 15 120 000 | | | | 224 970 |
| 2 786 540 | 16 973 379 | 0 | 11 000 000 | 0 | 118 000 | 0 | 0 |
| | | | | | | | |
| 248 000 | 0 | 0 | 1 419 | 0 | 0 | 0 | 0 |
| 250 000 | 0 | 0 | 9 778 | 0 | 0 | 0 | 0 |
| 252 000 | 11 122 | 0 | 3 234 | 0 | 5 609 | 0 | 0 |
| 425 405 | 2 846 786 | 0 | 0 | 0 | | 0 | |
| 451 993 | | 0 | 0 | 0 | | 0 | 0 |
| 416 666 | | | | | | | |
| 44 240 812 [5] | | 0 | 0 | | 0 | | 0 |
| 54 904 744 [5] | | 0 | | | 0 | | 0 |
| 61 816 864 [5] | | 0 | 82 861 | | 0 | | |
| 10 159 785 | 0 | 0 | 147 210 | 0 | 14 660 | 0 | 0 |
| 10 897 170 | 0 | 0 | 2 872 | 0 | 0 | 0 | 0 |
| 3 237 708 | 0 | 0 | 70 647 | | | | |

# Annex 3 - C. Funding for malaria control, 2016–2018

| WHO region Country/area | Year | Contributions reported by donors | | | |
|---|---|---|---|---|---|
| | | Global Fund[1] | PMI/USAID[2] | World Bank[3] | UK[4] |
| **AMERICAS** | | | | | |
| Costa Rica | 2016 | 0 | 0 | 0 | 0 |
| | 2017 | 0 | 0 | 0 | 0 |
| | 2018 | 0 | 0 | 0 | 0 |
| Dominican Republic | 2016 | 0 | 0 | 0 | 0 |
| | 2017 | 0 | 0 | 0 | 0 |
| | 2018 | 0 | 0 | 0 | 0 |
| Ecuador | 2016 | 0 | 0 | 0 | 0 |
| | 2017 | -598 176 | 0 | 0 | 0 |
| | 2018 | 0 | 0 | 0 | 0 |
| El Salvador | 2016 | 0 | 0 | 0 | 0 |
| | 2017 | 0 | 0 | 0 | 0 |
| | 2018 | 636 619 | 0 | 0 | 0 |
| French Guiana | 2016 | 0 | 0 | 0 | 0 |
| | 2017 | 0 | 0 | 0 | 0 |
| | 2018 | 0 | 0 | 0 | 0 |
| Guatemala | 2016 | 1 859 389 | 0 | 0 | 0 |
| | 2017 | 2 296 407 | 0 | 0 | 0 |
| | 2018 | 2 190 728 | 0 | 0 | 0 |
| Guyana | 2016 | -61 194 | 0 | 0 | 0 |
| | 2017 | 761 382 | 0 | 0 | 0 |
| | 2018 | 58 421 | 0 | 0 | 0 |
| Haiti | 2016 | 6 410 459 | 0 | 0 | 0 |
| | 2017 | 10 667 044 | 0 | 0 | 0 |
| | 2018 | 5 481 055 | 0 | 0 | 0 |
| Honduras | 2016 | 1 227 533 | 0 | 0 | 0 |
| | 2017 | 1 231 343 | 0 | 0 | 0 |
| | 2018 | 1 115 139 | 0 | 0 | 0 |
| Mexico | 2016 | 0 | 0 | 0 | 0 |
| | 2017 | 0 | 0 | 0 | 0 |
| | 2018 | 0 | 0 | 0 | 0 |
| Nicaragua | 2016 | 5 281 217 | 0 | 0 | 0 |
| | 2017 | 2 491 441 | 0 | 0 | 0 |
| | 2018 | 2 289 236 | 0 | 0 | 0 |
| Panama | 2016 | 0 | 0 | 0 | 0 |
| | 2017 | 0 | 0 | 0 | 0 |
| | 2018 | 0 | 0 | 0 | 0 |
| Paraguay | 2016 | 1 547 843 | 0 | 0 | 0 |
| | 2017 | 334 089 | 0 | 0 | 0 |
| | 2018 | 0 | 0 | 0 | 0 |
| Peru | 2016 | 0 | 0 | 0 | 0 |
| | 2017 | 0 | 0 | 0 | 0 |
| | 2018 | 0 | 0 | 0 | 0 |
| Suriname | 2016 | 170 752 | 0 | 0 | 0 |
| | 2017 | 1 168 802 | 0 | 0 | 0 |
| | 2018 | 819 904 | 0 | 0 | 0 |
| Venezuela (Bolivarian Republic of)[10] | 2016 | 0 | 0 | 0 | 0 |
| | 2017 | 0 | 0 | 0 | 0 |
| | 2018 | 0 | 0 | 0 | 0 |

| | Contributions reported by countries | | | | | | |
|---|---|---|---|---|---|---|---|
| Government (NMP) | Global Fund | World Bank | PMI/USAID | Other bilaterals | WHO | UNICEF | Other contributions[7] |
| 5 090 000 [5] | 14 000 | 0 | 1 624 | 0 | 3 000 | 0 | 0 |
| 4 980 000 [5] | 0 | 0 | 0 | 0 | 9 770 | 0 | 0 |
| 5 000 000 [5] | 0 | 0 | 0 | 0 | 12 155 | 0 | 0 |
| 3 525 868 | 0 | 0 | 0 | 0 | 0 | 0 | 334 363 |
| 1 149 368 | 125 543 | 0 | 0 | 0 | 824 | 0 | 27 987 |
| 367 647 | 9 949 957 | 0 | 0 | 0 | 143 176 | 0 | 48 938 |
| 20 000 000 [5] | 0 | 0 | | 0 | 69 279 | 0 | 0 |
| 5 835 716 [5] | 0 | 0 | | 0 | 69 039 | 0 | 0 |
| 6 898 763 [5] | 0 | 0 | 0 | 0 | 85 733 | 0 | |
| 2 662 869 | 166 311 | 0 | 1 089 | 0 | 4 733 | 0 | 65 789 |
| 2 662 869 | 538 732 | 0 | 0 | 0 | 73 758 | 0 | 0 |
| 3 950 441 | 707 436 | 0 | 0 | 0 | 15 156 | 0 | 0 |
| 0 [6] | 0 | 0 | 0 | 0 | 0 | 0 | 0 |
| 0 [6] | 0 | 0 | 0 | 0 | 0 | 0 | 0 |
| 0 [6] | | | | | | | |
| 2 639 249 | 10 669 242 | 0 | | | 0 | 0 | |
| 3 374 612 | 2 231 020 | | 75 981 | | | | |
| 3 492 749 | 1 724 076 | 0 | 138 643 | 0 | | 0 | 580 000 |
| 521 018 | 338 772 | 0 | 98 000 | 0 | 50 000 | 0 | 0 |
| 1 473 101 | 1 009 615 | 0 | 8 015 | 0 | 9 793 | 0 | 0 |
| 1 503 535 | 340 471 | 0 | 211 698 | 0 | 0 | 0 | 0 |
| 362 174 [5] | 4 926 108 | 0 | 0 | 500 000 | 227 455 | | 330 566 |
| 381 452 [6] | 12 540 295 | 0 | 17 956 | 500 000 | 227 455 | | 196 777 |
| 408 174 [5] | 7 384 832 | 0 | 0 | 0 | 275 872 | | 514 271 |
| 543 312 | 3 413 845 | | 7 840 | 0 | 0 | 0 | |
| 543 312 | 2 594 856 | 0 | 54 475 | 0 | 0 | 0 | 554 378 |
| 543 312 | 1 929 881 | 0 | 46 855 | 0 | 36 961 | 0 | 714 145 |
| 43 376 321 | 0 | 0 | 0 | 0 | | 0 | 0 |
| 40 661 276 | 0 | 0 | 0 | 0 | | 0 | 0 |
| 37 544 836 | 0 | 0 | 0 | 0 | | 0 | 0 |
| 3 544 313 | 3 727 737 | 0 | | 0 | 8 250 | 0 | |
| 3 984 944 | 1 826 934 | | 23 971 | | 98 131 | | |
| 3 263 970 | 1 986 357 | | 13 254 | | 83 000 | | 401 133 |
| 3 822 596 | | 0 | 23 247 | 0 | 9 665 | 0 | |
| 3 671 002 | | | 49 705 | | 7 087 | | |
| 8 000 000 [5] | 0 | 0 | 59 277 | 0 | 18 823 | 0 | |
| 2 264 399 | 1 517 493 | 0 | 0 | 0 | 0 | 0 | 0 |
| 2 883 082 | 593 059 | 0 | 0 | 0 | 0 | 0 | 0 |
| – | | | | | | | |
| 180 563 | 0 | 0 | 183 809 | 0 | | 0 | 0 |
| 2 074 113 [6] | | | 39 886 | | 168 737 | | |
| 1 774 350 | | | 90 000 | | | | |
| 106 372 [6] | 945 713 | 0 | 16 151 | 0 | 60 176 | 0 | 0 |
| 61 800 | 1 041 205 | 0 | 52 213 | 0 | 12 920 | 0 | 0 |
| 63 194 [6] | | 0 | 22 037 | 0 | | 0 | |
| 2 200 925 | 945 713 | 0 | 0 | 0 | 21 411 | 0 | 0 |
| 29 452 393 982 [5] | | | 0 | | 85 193 | | |
| 573 136 589 | | | 0 | | 435 366 | | |

# Annex 3 - C. Funding for malaria control, 2016–2018

| WHO region Country/area | Year | Contributions reported by donors | | | |
|---|---|---|---|---|---|
| | | Global Fund[1] | PMI/USAID[2] | World Bank[3] | UK[4] |
| **EASTERN MEDITERRANEAN** | | | | | |
| Afghanistan | 2016 | 5 945 750 | 0 | 0 | 0 |
| | 2017 | 7 043 533 | 0 | 0 | 0 |
| | 2018 | 9 556 500 | 0 | 0 | 0 |
| Djibouti | 2016 | 4 738 086 | 0 | 138 717 | 0 |
| | 2017 | 2 617 141 | 0 | 230 220 | 0 |
| | 2018 | 652 220 | 0 | 230 220 | 0 |
| Iran (Islamic Republic of) | 2016 | 1 798 772 | 0 | 0 | 0 |
| | 2017 | 1 113 357 | 0 | 0 | 0 |
| | 2018 | 0 | 0 | 0 | 0 |
| Pakistan | 2016 | 11 332 383 | 0 | 0 | 0 |
| | 2017 | 16 609 001 | 0 | 0 | 0 |
| | 2018 | 13 590 722 | 0 | 0 | 0 |
| Saudi Arabia | 2016 | 0 | 0 | 0 | 0 |
| | 2017 | 0 | 0 | 0 | 0 |
| | 2018 | 0 | 0 | 0 | 0 |
| Somalia | 2016 | 9 829 626 | 0 | 0 | 0 |
| | 2017 | 16 327 923 | 0 | 0 | 0 |
| | 2018 | 7 501 955 | 0 | 0 | 0 |
| Sudan | 2016 | 55 654 840 | 0 | 0 | 0 |
| | 2017 | 10 485 931 | 0 | 0 | 0 |
| | 2018 | 34 723 839 | 0 | 0 | 0 |
| Yemen | 2016 | 4 706 687 | 0 | 0 | 0 |
| | 2017 | 3 664 258 | 0 | 1 553 074 | 0 |
| | 2018 | -7 248 | 0 | 0 | 0 |
| **SOUTH-EAST ASIA** | | | | | |
| Bangladesh | 2016 | 6 658 153 | 0 | 0 | 0 |
| | 2017 | 12 956 676 | 0 | 0 | 0 |
| | 2018 | 6 940 221 | 0 | 0 | 0 |
| Bhutan | 2016 | 455 891 | 0 | 0 | 0 |
| | 2017 | 572 637 | 0 | 0 | 0 |
| | 2018 | 326 974 | 0 | 0 | 0 |
| Democratic People's Republic of Korea | 2016 | 3 781 468 | 0 | 0 | 0 |
| | 2017 | 1 523 252 | 0 | 0 | 0 |
| | 2018 | 2 314 541 | 0 | 0 | 0 |
| India | 2016 | 4 248 221 | 0 | 0 | 0 |
| | 2017 | 67 799 731 | 0 | 0 | 0 |
| | 2018 | 270 626 | 0 | 0 | 0 |
| Indonesia | 2016 | 11 275 924 | 0 | 0 | 49 453 |
| | 2017 | 23 553 669 | 0 | 0 | 0 |
| | 2018 | 9 987 790 | 0 | 0 | 0 |
| Myanmar | 2016 | 35 058 903 | 10 419 895 | 0 | 12 914 507 |
| | 2017 | 40 780 480 | 10 225 531 | 0 | 3 913 209 |
| | 2018 | 17 007 953 | 10 000 000 | 0 | 2 821 423 |
| Nepal | 2016 | 3 101 226 | 0 | 0 | 0 |
| | 2017 | 5 165 221 | 0 | 0 | 0 |
| | 2018 | 1 408 576 | 0 | 0 | 0 |
| Thailand | 2016 | 9 107 668 | 0 | 0 | 0 |
| | 2017 | 10 956 433 | 0 | 0 | 0 |
| | 2018 | 6 040 728 | 0 | 0 | 0 |
| Timor-Leste | 2016 | 3 233 190 | 0 | 0 | 0 |
| | 2017 | 2 688 860 | 0 | 0 | 0 |
| | 2018 | 2 427 241 | 0 | 0 | 0 |

| | Contributions reported by countries | | | | | | |
|---|---|---|---|---|---|---|---|
| Government (NMP) | Global Fund | World Bank | PMI/USAID | Other bilaterals | WHO | UNICEF | Other contributions[7] |
| 944 566 [6] | 9 762 977 | | | | 12 905 | | |
| 921 528 [6] | 1 053 356 | | | | 85 814 | | |
| 200 000 [6] | 10 556 626 | | | | 26 571 | | |
| 4 547 153 [5] | 4 547 153 | 0 | | 1 000 000 | 25 000 | 25 000 | |
| 3 222 506 [5] | | 0 | | 0 | 51 000 | 0 | |
| 3 295 183 [6] | 871 414 | | | 0 | 30 000 | 0 | |
| 2 500 000 | 1 364 857 | | | | | | |
| 2 700 000 | | | | | 48 000 | | |
| 3 300 000 | 0 | 0 | 0 | | 38 286 | | |
| 16 400 000 | 11 536 047 | | | | 300 000 | | |
| 18 344 729 [6] | 22 635 097 | | | | 130 000 | | |
| 3 774 306 | 9 615 605 | | | | 196 378 | | |
| 30 000 000 | 0 | 0 | 0 | 0 | 7 500 | 0 | 0 |
| 30 000 000 | 0 | 0 | 0 | 0 | 100 000 | 0 | 0 |
| 30 000 000 | 0 | 0 | 0 | 0 | 10 000 | 0 | 0 |
| 81 200 | 9 946 059 | 0 | 0 | 0 | 135 000 | | 0 |
| 85 350 | 20 986 170 | 0 | 0 | 0 | 147 000 | | 0 |
| 90 726 | 5 534 919 | 0 | 0 | 0 | 56 000 | | 0 |
| 24 209 740 | 61 304 230 | 0 | 0 | 0 | 93 302 | 1 200 574 | 0 |
| 19 087 941 | 31 496 505 | 0 | 0 | 0 | 3 084 | 0 | 0 |
| 16 726 945 | 21 485 294 | 0 | 0 | 0 | 60 000 | 203 000 | 9 619 |
| 0 | 1 140 758 | 0 | 0 | 0 | 105 000 | 0 | |
| 0 | 7 933 620 | | | | 2 080 000 | 473 627 | |
| 0 [5] | 1 890 037 | | | | 1 427 948 | | |
| 1 162 970 | 9 734 466 | 0 | 0 | 0 | 188 000 | 0 | 0 |
| 1 493 690 | 8 821 888 | 0 | 0 | 0 | 210 000 | 0 | 0 |
| 2 496 429 | 6 835 307 | 0 | 0 | 0 | 250 000 | 0 | 0 |
| 163 046 | 550 197 | 0 | 0 | 0 | 40 273 | 0 | 72 424 |
| 179 470 | 586 015 | 0 | 0 | 0 | 35 212 | 0 | 121 212 |
| 176 791 | 577 403 | 0 | 0 | 0 | 34 687 | 0 | 0 |
| 2 080 000 | 3 775 232 | 0 | 0 | 0 | 35 000 | 0 | |
| 2 151 000 | 3 426 508 | 0 | 0 | 0 | 35 000 | 0 | 0 |
| 2 181 000 | 3 219 957 | 0 | 0 | 0 | | 0 | |
| 48 364 518 | 15 892 221 | 0 | 0 | 0 | | 0 | |
| 145 564 257 | 94 474 099 | 0 | 0 | 0 | | 0 | |
| 46 783 323 | 34 958 663 | 0 | 0 | 0 | | 0 | |
| 20 307 710 [5] | 10 821 533 | 0 | 0 | 0 | 228 000 | 1 938 220 | 0 |
| 17 686 075 [5] | 30 336 061 | | | | 147 033 | 1 385 855 | |
| 21 683 909 [5] | 12 272 515 | | | | 260 738 | 115 242 | |
| 6 437 430 [5] | 55 302 769 | | 9 000 000 | 6 607 886 | 25 000 | | |
| 6 780 092 [6] | 53 056 520 | 0 | 10 000 000 | 6 532 464 | 25 000 | 0 | 3 462 068 |
| 6 780 092 [6] | 29 581 578 | | 9 000 000 | 6 607 886 | 25 000 | | |
| 966 200 [5] | 10 228 041 | 0 | 69 334 | 0 | 23 000 | | |
| 263 262 | 102 424 | | | | 24 509 | | |
| 613 873 | 1 107 196 | 0 | 120 482 | 0 | 31 214 | 0 | 0 |
| 8 502 036 | 13 984 633 | 0 | 0 | 0 | 103 514 | 0 | 61 463 |
| 7 664 899 | 15 622 625 | 0 | | | 188 686 | | 49 859 |
| 7 131 736 | 8 337 877 | 0 | 1 308 800 | 0 | 78 056 | 0 | 93 546 |
| 1 523 993 | 3 261 859 | 0 | 0 | 0 | 45 868 | 0 | 20 000 |
| 1 115 484 | 4 039 622 | 0 | 0 | 0 | 42 456 | 0 | 20 000 |
| 1 121 287 | 1 573 936 | 0 | 0 | 0 | 26 600 | 0 | 5 000 |

# Annex 3 - C. Funding for malaria control, 2016–2018

| WHO region Country/area | Year | Contributions reported by donors | | | |
|---|---|---|---|---|---|
| | | Global Fund[1] | PMI/USAID[2] | World Bank[3] | UK[4] |
| **WESTERN PACIFIC** | | | | | |
| Cambodia | 2016 | 8 383 140 | 6 251 937 | 0 | 0 |
| | 2017 | 14 368 640 | 10 225 531 | 0 | 0 |
| | 2018 | 10 380 499 | 10 000 000 | 0 | 0 |
| China | 2016 | -317 097 | 0 | 0 | 0 |
| | 2017 | 0 | 0 | 0 | 0 |
| | 2018 | 0 | 0 | 0 | 0 |
| Lao People's Democratic Republic | 2016 | 5 920 486 | 0 | 0 | 0 |
| | 2017 | 3 667 214 | 0 | 0 | 0 |
| | 2018 | 3 901 819 | 0 | 0 | 0 |
| Malaysia | 2016 | 0 | 0 | 0 | 779 447 |
| | 2017 | 0 | 0 | 0 | 0 |
| | 2018 | 0 | 0 | 0 | 0 |
| Papua New Guinea | 2016 | 7 880 106 | 0 | 0 | 135 199 |
| | 2017 | 10 563 330 | 0 | 0 | 0 |
| | 2018 | 7 276 337 | 0 | 0 | 0 |
| Philippines | 2016 | 3 531 540 | 0 | 0 | 0 |
| | 2017 | 7 342 397 | 0 | 0 | 0 |
| | 2018 | 3 195 184 | 0 | 0 | 0 |
| Republic of Korea | 2016 | 0 | 0 | 0 | 0 |
| | 2017 | 0 | 0 | 0 | 0 |
| | 2018 | 0 | 0 | 0 | 0 |
| Solomon Islands | 2016 | 2 540 226 | 0 | 0 | 0 |
| | 2017 | 1 025 914 | 0 | 0 | 0 |
| | 2018 | 1 729 636 | 0 | 0 | 0 |
| Vanuatu | 2016 | 0 | 0 | 0 | 0 |
| | 2017 | 0 | 0 | 0 | 0 |
| | 2018 | 0 | 0 | 0 | 0 |
| Viet Nam | 2016 | 6 091 536 | 0 | 0 | 0 |
| | 2017 | 15 802 793 | 0 | 0 | 0 |
| | 2018 | 9 296 596 | 0 | 0 | 0 |

NMP: National Malaria Programme; PMI: United States President's Malaria Initiative; UK: United Kingdom of Great Britain and Northern Ireland government; UNICEF: United Nations Children's Fund; USAID: United States Agency for International Development; WHO: World Health Organization.

"–" refers to data not available.

[1] Source: Global Fund to Fight AIDS, Tuberculosis and Malaria.
[2] Source: www.foreignassistance.gov.
[3] Source: Organisation for Economic Co-operation and Development (OECD) creditor reporting system (CRS) database.
[4] Source: OECD CRS database.
[5] Budget not expediture.

| | Contributions reported by countries | | | | | | |
|---|---|---|---|---|---|---|---|
| Government (NMP) | Global Fund | World Bank | PMI/USAID | Other bilaterals | WHO | UNICEF | Other contributions[7] |
| 22 297 | 2 002 435 | 0 | 6 000 000 | 0 | 304 651 | 0 | |
| 663 526 | 8 045 144 | 0 | 6 000 000 | 0 | 579 738 | 0 | |
| 83 636 | 3 181 783 | 0 | 10 000 000 | 0 | 628 297 | 0 | |
| 18 929 499 [6] | | | | | | | |
| 19 115 082 [6] | | | | | | | |
| 19 602 589 [6] | | | | | | | |
| 260 975 | 5 050 407 | 0 | 340 021 | 184 632 | 75 000 | 0 | 45 199 |
| 1 008 060 | 1 728 818 | 0 | 604 000 | 0 | 256 734 | 0 | 1 066 089 |
| 1 914 750 | 3 725 427 | 0 | 500 000 | 0 | 288 108 | 0 | 1 783 267 |
| 39 703 616 | 0 | 0 | 0 | 0 | 0 | 0 | 0 |
| 48 365 863 | 0 | 0 | 0 | 0 | 0 | 0 | 0 |
| 49 561 180 | 0 | 0 | 0 | 0 | 0 | 0 | 0 |
| 181 200 | 5 900 000 | 0 | 0 | 0 | 56 000 | 0 | 0 |
| 753 771 | 10 330 449 | 0 | 0 | 0 | 95 000 | 0 | 911 770 |
| 108 100 | 7 407 034 | 0 | 0 | 0 | 86 500 | 0 | 1 083 168 |
| 6 720 000 [5] | 3 944 923 | 0 | 0 | 0 | 0 | 0 | 0 |
| 7 012 009 | 6 471 549 | 0 | 0 | 0 | 0 | 0 | 0 |
| 3 548 266 | 4 190 984 | 0 | 0 | 0 | 0 | 0 | 0 |
| 526 499 | 0 | 0 | 0 | 0 | 0 | 0 | 0 |
| 475 173 | 0 | 0 | 0 | 0 | 0 | 0 | 0 |
| 433 726 | 0 | 0 | 0 | 0 | 0 | 0 | 0 |
| 327 032 | 1 309 126 | 0 | 0 | 448 718 | 358 000 | 0 | 0 |
| 858 256 | 977 025 | 0 | 0 | 0 | 736 892 | 0 | 0 |
| 979 891 | 1 494 080 | | | | 79 770 | | |
| 196 760 | 927 486 | 0 | 0 | 249 071 | 148 217 | 0 | 0 |
| 139 254 | 285 333 | 0 | 0 | 206 575 | 21 918 | 0 | 0 |
| 128 194 | 131 786 | 0 | 0 | 92 363 | 9 367 | 0 | 0 |
| 801 554 | 11 088 506 | | | | 200 764 | | 200 000 |
| 3 022 523 | 9 324 657 | 0 | 0 | 0 | 200 000 | 0 | 500 000 |
| 1 813 863 | 7 901 624 | 0 | 0 | 0 | 105 045 | 0 | 315 396 |

Data as of 26 November 2019

[6] WHO NMP funding estimates.

[7] Other contributions as reported by countries: NGOs, foundations, etc.

[8] South Sudan became an independent State on 9 July 2011 and a Member State of WHO on 27 September 2011. South Sudan and Sudan have distinct epidemiological profiles comprising high-transmission and low-transmission areas, respectively. For this reason data up to June 2011 from the high-transmission areas of Sudan (10 southern states which correspond to contemporary South Sudan) and low-transmission areas (15 northern states which correspond to contemporary Sudan) are reported separately.

[9] Where national totals for the United Republic of Tanzania are unavailable, refer to the sum of Mainland and Zanzibar.

[10] Government contributions for 2016, 2017 and 2018 are indicated in local currency during that period.

Note: Negative disbursements reflect recovery of funds on behalf of the financing organization.

# Annex 3 - D. Commodities distribution and coverage, 2016–2018

| WHO region Country/area | Year | No. of LLINs sold or delivered | Modelled percentage of population with access to an ITN | No. of people protected by IRS | No of RDTs distributed | Any first-line treatment courses delivered (including ACT) | ACT treatment courses delivered |
|---|---|---|---|---|---|---|---|
| **AFRICAN** | | | | | | | |
| Algeria | 2016 | 0 | – | – | 0 | 432 | – |
| | 2017 | 0 | – | – | 36 | 453 | – |
| | 2018 | 0 | – | – | 0 | 1 242 | – |
| Angola | 2016 | 3 507 740 | 21 | – | 3 000 000 | 4 000 000 | 4 000 000 |
| | 2017 | 2 924 769 | 32 | – | 397 882 | 3 090 761 | 3 090 761 |
| | 2018 | 3 863 521 | 38 | – | 2 000 350 | 1 950 000 | 1 950 000 |
| Benin | 2016 | 720 706 | 36 | 853 221 | 1 500 047 | 1 199 055 | 1 199 055 |
| | 2017 | 6 771 009 | 44 | 853 221 | 2 171 867 | 1 530 617 | 1 530 617 |
| | 2018 | 0 | 59 | 1 321 758 | 2 016 745 | 1 815 236 | 1 815 236 |
| Botswana | 2016 | 116 048 | – | 115 973 | 2 196 | 1 634 | 1 634 |
| | 2017 | 3 000 | – | 139 244 | 2 645 | 4 429 | 4 429 |
| | 2018 | – | – | 83 488 | 3 141 | 1 954 | 1 954 |
| Burkina Faso | 2016 | 10 924 031 | 62 | – | 11 974 810 | 9 519 568 | 9 519 568 |
| | 2017 | 986 164 | 68 | – | 12 853 861 | 10 457 752 | 10 457 752 |
| | 2018 | 1 946 047 | 48 | 766 374 | 13 026 870 | 11 968 368 | 11 968 368 |
| Burundi | 2016 | 755 182 | 49 | – | 8 077 703 | 8 277 026 | 8 031 773 |
| | 2017 | 6 717 994 | 58 | 848 441 | 10 046 047 | 7 978 264 | 7 613 646 |
| | 2018 | 986 025 | 81 | 1 754 679 | 7 012 203 | 5 149 436 | 5 032 209 |
| Cabo Verde | 2016 | 0 | – | 349 126 | 8 906 | 71 | 71 |
| | 2017 | 80 | – | 495 313 | 16 573 | 420 | 420 |
| | 2018 | 21 | – | – | 9 588 | 21 | 21 |
| Cameroon | 2016 | 9 588 733 | 56 | – | 1 380 725 | 1 093 036 | 1 093 036 |
| | 2017 | 362 629 | 67 | – | 1 589 218 | 879 039 | 785 765 |
| | 2018 | 573 843 | 55 | – | 1 739 286 | 1 064 668 | 918 505 |
| Central African Republic | 2016 | 57 110 | 59 | – | 1 651 645 | 1 714 647 | 1 714 647 |
| | 2017 | 857 198 | 59 | – | 806 218 | 947 205 | 947 205 |
| | 2018 | 753 889 | 63 | – | 1 189 881 | 1 773 072 | 1 773 072 |
| Chad | 2016 | 384 606 | 15 | – | 882 617 | – | – |
| | 2017 | 6 886 534 | 45 | – | 1 287 405 | 1 486 086 | 1 486 086 |
| | 2018 | – | 65 | – | – | – | – |
| Comoros | 2016 | 451 358 | 73 | – | 61 600 | 1 373 | 1 373 |
| | 2017 | 34 590 | 89 | – | 21 988 | 2 794 | 2 794 |
| | 2018 | 31 012 | 77 | – | – | – | – |
| Congo | 2016 | 1 291 | 39 | – | 45 000 | 0 | 0 |
| | 2017 | 2 223 | 27 | – | 0 | 0 | 0 |
| | 2018 | 4 641 | 29 | – | 0 | 0 | 0 |
| Côte d'Ivoire | 2016 | 1 177 906 | 69 | – | 5 351 325 | 4 964 065 | 4 964 065 |
| | 2017 | 13 216 468 | 70 | – | 6 986 825 | 5 373 545 | 5 373 545 |
| | 2018 | 15 875 381 | 80 | – | 6 069 250 | 6 799 565 | 6 799 565 |
| Democratic Republic of the Congo | 2016 | 31 439 920 | 70 | 916 524 | 18 630 636 | 17 258 290 | 17 258 290 |
| | 2017 | 8 412 959 | 75 | 232 181 | 18 994 861 | 17 250 728 | 17 250 728 |
| | 2018 | 16 919 441 | 71 | 111 735 | 18 549 327 | 16 917 207 | 16 917 207 |
| Equatorial Guinea | 2016 | 66 232 | 34 | 82 749 | 62 133 | 18 072 | 18 072 |
| | 2017 | 42 317 | 34 | 64 617 | 60 798 | 15 341 | 15 341 |
| | 2018 | 120 376 | 34 | 74 416 | 78 695 | 15 633 | 15 633 |
| Eritrea | 2016 | 156 553 | 46 | 364 007 | 0 | 177 525 | 177 525 |
| | 2017 | 1 724 972 | 50 | 375 696 | 481 600 | 296 399 | 296 399 |
| | 2018 | 60 083 | 58 | 376 143 | 400 900 | 301 525 | 301 525 |
| Eswatini | 2016 | 4 758 | – | 24 179 | 56 780 | 600 | 600 |
| | 2017 | 0 | – | 21 316 | 59 760 | 900 | 861 |
| | 2018 | 0 | – | 39 144 | 61 974 | 631 | 579 |
| Ethiopia | 2016 | 13 266 926 | 62 | 15 050 413 | 9 742 450 | 6 530 973 | 5 239 080 |
| | 2017 | 2 755 700 | 55 | 17 628 133 | 6 400 000 | 8 470 000 | 7 300 000 |
| | 2018 | 11 100 000 | 39 | 10 486 854 | 4 053 200 | 3 773 179 | 3 036 690 |

| WHO region Country/area | Year | No. of LLINs sold or delivered | Modelled percentage of population with access to an ITN | No. of people protected by IRS | No of RDTs distributed | Any first-line treatment courses delivered (including ACT) | ACT treatment courses delivered |
|---|---|---|---|---|---|---|---|
| **AFRICAN** | | | | | | | |
| Gabon | 2016 | 9 660 | 9 | 0 | 0 | 0 | 0 |
| | 2017 | – | 8 | – | 0 | 0 | 0 |
| | 2018 | 4 582 | 7 | – | 71 787 | – | 208 953 |
| Gambia | 2016 | 113 385 | 55 | 399 176 | 1 017 889 | 272 895 | 272 895 |
| | 2017 | 1 051 391 | 64 | 396 546 | 767 984 | 174 556 | 174 166 |
| | 2018 | 115 801 | 77 | 426 788 | 678 621 | 113 563 | 113 563 |
| Ghana | 2016 | 5 962 179 | 68 | 1 409 967 | 4 823 250 | 2 289 145 | 2 289 145 |
| | 2017 | 3 059 363 | 66 | 1 868 861 | 7 051 875 | 4 522 410 | 4 522 410 |
| | 2018 | 16 839 135 | 75 | 1 855 326 | 13 119 275 | 5 253 298 | 5 253 298 |
| Guinea | 2016 | 8 236 154 | 65 | – | 2 138 494 | 3 362 668 | 3 362 668 |
| | 2017 | 523 328 | 68 | – | 2 920 298 | 2 673 947 | 2 673 947 |
| | 2018 | 645 980 | 59 | – | 2 741 607 | 1 886 685 | 1 886 685 |
| Guinea-Bissau | 2016 | 71 500 | 77 | – | 238 412 | 133 647 | 115 361 |
| | 2017 | 1 222 428 | 73 | – | 303 651 | 136 507 | 110 508 |
| | 2018 | 93 859 | 72 | – | 320 217 | 162 773 | 147 927 |
| Kenya | 2016 | 2 005 477 | 68 | 0 | 8 352 950 | 11 327 340 | 11 327 340 |
| | 2017 | 15 621 773 | 70 | 906 388 | 11 337 850 | 10 696 827 | 10 696 827 |
| | 2018 | 2 673 730 | 74 | 1 833 860 | – | – | – |
| Liberia | 2016 | – | 59 | – | – | – | – |
| | 2017 | 157 954 | 30 | – | – | – | – |
| | 2018 | 2 500 796 | 34 | – | – | 994 008 | 994 008 |
| Madagascar | 2016 | 464 407 | 63 | 2 856 873 | 1 352 225 | 757 613 | 757 613 |
| | 2017 | 764 022 | 41 | 2 008 963 | 2 465 600 | 1 620 050 | 1 620 050 |
| | 2018 | 184 859 | 31 | – | 4 731 125 | 2 165 450 | 2 165 450 |
| Malawi | 2016 | 9 093 657 | 61 | – | 8 746 750 | 6 799 354 | 6 440 490 |
| | 2017 | 994 136 | 60 | – | 15 060 625 | 10 177 530 | 10 177 530 |
| | 2018 | 11 805 392 | 60 | – | 13 003 518 | 8 948 286 | 9 186 040 |
| Mali | 2016 | 2 189 027 | 69 | 788 711 | 3 250 000 | 3 511 970 | 3 511 970 |
| | 2017 | 4 148 911 | 66 | 823 201 | 4 164 041 | 3 746 616 | 3 746 616 |
| | 2018 | 4 993 868 | 68 | 665 581 | 6 105 500 | 3 558 964 | 3 558 964 |
| Mauritania | 2016 | 51 000 | 11 | – | 208 650 | 174 420 | 84 000 |
| | 2017 | 921 245 | 37 | – | 234 520 | 101 450 | – |
| | 2018 | 478 230 | 65 | – | 117 000 | 25 890 | 25 890 |
| Mayotte | 2016 | – | – | – | – | – | – |
| | 2017 | – | – | – | – | – | – |
| | 2018 | – | – | – | – | 44 | 44 |
| Mozambique | 2016 | 4 527 936 | 53 | 4 375 512 | 19 822 825 | 14 136 250 | 14 136 250 |
| | 2017 | 15 482 093 | 62 | 5 349 948 | 19 662 975 | 15 996 892 | 15 996 892 |
| | 2018 | 1 337 905 | 60 | 4 211 138 | 21 180 223 | 16 293 318 | 16 293 318 |
| Namibia | 2016 | 0 | – | 485 730 | 379 625 | 21 519 | 21 519 |
| | 2017 | 0 | – | 753 281 | 914 175 | 79 316 | 79 316 |
| | 2018 | 15 000 | – | 549 243 | 49 852 | 35 355 | 1 721 |
| Niger | 2016 | 746 469 | 64 | 0 | 4 622 433 | 3 257 506 | 3 257 506 |
| | 2017 | 981 423 | 56 | 0 | 3 909 600 | 2 697 115 | 2 161 440 |
| | 2018 | 4 015 529 | 58 | – | 5 149 981 | 3 536 000 | 3 536 000 |
| Nigeria | 2016 | 9 896 250 | 56 | 130 061 | 11 178 434 | 9 177 309 | 9 177 309 |
| | 2017 | 21 978 907 | 53 | – | 9 701 771 | 7 752 372 | 7 752 372 |
| | 2018 | 27 004 605 | 49 | – | 18 662 105 | 32 707 785 | 32 707 785 |
| Rwanda | 2016 | 2 882 445 | 66 | 2 484 672 | 6 013 020 | 7 639 177 | 7 603 560 |
| | 2017 | 2 816 586 | 73 | 1 753 230 | 4 960 020 | 6 300 445 | 6 265 890 |
| | 2018 | 974 847 | 70 | 1 621 955 | 5 364 990 | 5 233 680 | 5 214 330 |
| Sao Tome and Principe | 2016 | 11 922 | – | 149 930 | 117 676 | 2 121 | 2 121 |
| | 2017 | 15 151 | – | 138 000 | 96 826 | 2 410 | 2 410 |
| | 2018 | 142 894 | – | – | – | – | – |

# Annex 3 - D. Commodities distribution and coverage, 2016–2018

| WHO region Country/area | Year | No. of LLINs sold or delivered | Modelled percentage of population with access to an ITN | No. of people protected by IRS | No of RDTs distributed | Any first-line treatment courses delivered (including ACT) | ACT treatment courses delivered |
|---|---|---|---|---|---|---|---|
| **AFRICAN** | | | | | | | |
| Senegal | 2016 | 8 960 663 | 66 | 496 728 | 1 823 405 | 709 394 | 709 394 |
| | 2017 | 448 305 | 71 | 619 578 | 2 391 311 | 958 473 | 958 473 |
| | 2018 | 617 470 | 50 | 0 | 2 646 144 | 1 606 813 | 1 490 147 |
| Sierra Leone | 2016 | 452 608 | 42 | – | 3 093 725 | 4 714 900 | 4 714 900 |
| | 2017 | 4 611 638 | 53 | – | 2 611 550 | 2 504 960 | 2 504 960 |
| | 2018 | 502 834 | 73 | – | 4 316 420 | 3 415 480 | 3 415 480 |
| South Africa | 2016 | 0 | – | 1 165 955 | 227 325 | 12 677 | 12 677 |
| | 2017 | 0 | – | 1 550 235 | 865 050 | 72 439 | 72 439 |
| | 2018 | 0 | – | 1 600 747 | 887 300 | 51 142 | 51 142 |
| South Sudan[1] | 2016 | 2 759 527 | 65 | 281 998 | 5 147 954 | 13 617 422 | 13 617 422 |
| | 2017 | 1 902 020 | 75 | 153 285 | 1 945 875 | 12 188 601 | 12 188 601 |
| | 2018 | – | 73 | – | – | 2 680 776 | 2 680 776 |
| Togo | 2016 | 155 660 | 64 | – | 1 428 696 | 1 064 876 | 1 049 903 |
| | 2017 | 4 706 417 | 68 | – | 1 613 393 | 1 355 640 | 1 196 518 |
| | 2018 | 224 265 | 80 | – | 2 485 086 | 1 988 845 | 2 055 831 |
| Uganda | 2016 | 899 823 | 65 | 3 811 484 | 27 230 375 | 29 667 150 | 29 667 150 |
| | 2017 | 23 797 483 | 76 | 3 223 800 | 24 620 100 | 27 396 300 | 27 396 300 |
| | 2018 | 11 220 492 | 88 | 4 436 156 | 28 200 125 | 25 606 514 | 25 606 514 |
| United Republic of Tanzania[2] | 2016 | – | 59 | – | – | – | – |
| | 2017 | 5 335 910 | 60 | 2 568 522 | | | |
| | 2018 | – | 59 | – | | | |
| Mainland | 2016 | 11 731 272 | 59 | 2 377 403 | 23 223 400 | 13 786 620 | 13 786 620 |
| | 2017 | 5 335 910 | 60 | 2 377 403 | 34 649 050 | 20 895 180 | 20 895 180 |
| | 2018 | 6 200 375 | 59 | 2 507 920 | 29 906 950 | 16 420 560 | 16 420 560 |
| Zanzibar | 2016 | 756 445 | – | 27 664 | 24 026 | 11 100 | 10 020 |
| | 2017 | 0 | – | 191 119 | 459 957 | 8 506 | 8 506 |
| | 2018 | 177 794 | – | 334 715 | 356 775 | 5 050 | 4 650 |
| Zambia | 2016 | 1 292 400 | 58 | 6 737 918 | 15 286 570 | 19 084 818 | 19 084 818 |
| | 2017 | 10 759 947 | 64 | 7 717 767 | 18 884 600 | 17 460 232 | 17 460 232 |
| | 2018 | – | 79 | 6 436 719 | 17 868 550 | 27 071 994 | 27 071 994 |
| Zimbabwe | 2016 | 1 752 855 | 43 | 3 674 932 | 3 154 200 | 934 580 | 934 580 |
| | 2017 | 513 300 | 44 | 3 673 311 | 875 713 | 549 083 | 553 953 |
| | 2018 | 171 038 | 32 | 3 020 032 | 1 484 134 | 607 379 | 615 359 |
| **AMERICAS** | | | | | | | |
| Argentina | 2016 | 0 | – | 0 | 0 | 30 | 0 |
| | 2017 | 0 | – | 4 208 | 0 | 39 | 9 |
| | 2018 | 0 | – | 155 | 0 | 213 | 92 |
| Belize | 2016 | 4 000 | – | 35 264 | 0 | 5 | 0 |
| | 2017 | 0 | – | 37 466 | 0 | 9 | 1 |
| | 2018 | 2 619 | – | 36 688 | 0 | 7 | 0 |
| Bolivia (Plurinational State of) | 2016 | 84 000 | – | 12 689 | – | 5 553 | 5 553 |
| | 2017 | 23 500 | – | 20 000 | 3 500 | 0 | 0 |
| | 2018 | 23 500 | – | 2 000 | – | – | – |
| Brazil | 2016 | 0 | – | 98 593 | 68 650 | 567 842 | 103 428 |
| | 2017 | 0 | – | 83 990 | 72 200 | 651 274 | 69 960 |
| | 2018 | 300 000 | – | 99 321 | 114 775 | 634 935 | 79 200 |
| Colombia | 2016 | 306 498 | – | 1 180 400 | 21 575 | 202 175 | 94 494 |
| | 2017 | 295 250 | – | 153 690 | 265 250 | 95 570 | 56 030 |
| | 2018 | 0 | – | 60 000 | 13 252 | 46 217 | 26 507 |
| Costa Rica | 2016 | 206 | – | 430 | 0 | 13 | 3 |
| | 2017 | 104 | – | 8 479 | 0 | 25 | 7 |
| | 2018 | 3 100 | – | 4 095 | 700 | 108 | 5 |

| WHO region Country/area | Year | No. of LLINs sold or delivered | Modelled percentage of population with access to an ITN | No. of people protected by IRS | No of RDTs distributed | Any first-line treatment courses delivered (including ACT) | ACT treatment courses delivered |
|---|---|---|---|---|---|---|---|
| **AMERICAS** | | | | | | | |
| Dominican Republic | 2016 | 1 483 | – | 40 510 | 89 800 | 755 | 40 |
| | 2017 | 0 | – | 30 361 | 48 850 | 398 | – |
| | 2018 | 5 052 | – | 36 891 | 42 425 | 484 | 9 |
| Ecuador | 2016 | 51 795 | – | – | – | 1 191 | 403 |
| | 2017 | 72 015 | – | 667 111 | – | 1 380 | 371 |
| | 2018 | 50 000 | – | 775 884 | 51 200 | 1 806 | 191 |
| El Salvador | 2016 | 2 578 | – | 27 338 | 0 | 14 | 0 |
| | 2017 | 2 925 | – | 19 167 | 0 | 4 | 0 |
| | 2018 | 4 817 | – | 32 691 | 0 | 2 | 1 |
| French Guiana | 2016 | 4 455 | – | – | – | – | – |
| | 2017 | – | – | – | – | – | – |
| | 2018 | – | – | – | – | – | – |
| Guatemala | 2016 | 485 010 | – | – | 92 100 | 0 | 0 |
| | 2017 | 83 258 | – | 6 245 | 170 325 | 9 995 | 0 |
| | 2018 | 310 218 | – | 15 358 | 75 300 | 3 246 | – |
| Guyana | 2016 | 8 320 | – | 0 | 8 268 | 10 979 | 3 759 |
| | 2017 | 5 534 | – | – | – | 13 936 | 5 141 |
| | 2018 | 43 181 | – | – | – | 11 767 | 3 073 |
| Haiti | 2016 | 10 000 | – | – | 274 404 | 19 702 | – |
| | 2017 | 709 720 | – | – | 261 600 | 18 772 | – |
| | 2018 | 1 919 | – | 42 130 | 207 800 | 8 083 | – |
| Honduras | 2016 | 81 470 | – | 360 553 | 27 300 | 43 097 | 45 |
| | 2017 | 24 092 | – | 225 027 | 29 710 | – | – |
| | 2018 | 53 944 | – | 338 730 | 15 000 | – | 45 |
| Mexico | 2016 | 61 000 | – | 112 184 | 0 | 596 | 13 |
| | 2017 | 5 695 | – | – | 0 | 765 | 14 |
| | 2018 | 17 891 | – | 48 608 | 0 | 803 | 10 |
| Nicaragua | 2016 | 191 178 | – | 147 801 | 20 840 | 6 284 | – |
| | 2017 | 103 676 | – | 182 602 | 46 500 | 49 085 | 50 |
| | 2018 | 47 301 | – | 183 098 | 117 350 | 86 195 | – |
| Panama | 2016 | 0 | – | 9 675 | 0 | 811 | 0 |
| | 2017 | – | – | 3 921 | 16 000 | 689 | 144 |
| | 2018 | 0 | – | 19 500 | 20 000 | 715 | 3 |
| Paraguay | 2016 | 0 | – | 217 | 0 | 10 | 7 |
| | 2017 | 0 | – | 631 | 5 000 | 2 498 | 408 |
| | 2018 | – | – | – | – | – | – |
| Peru | 2016 | 430 | – | 30 499 | 150 000 | 74 554 | 6 500 |
| | 2017 | – | – | 62 804 | – | – | – |
| | 2018 | 83 220 | – | 23 420 | 180 000 | 65 000 | 14 500 |
| Suriname | 2016 | 37 000 | – | – | 13 825 | – | – |
| | 2017 | 6 022 | – | – | 14 325 | – | – |
| | 2018 | 15 000 | – | – | 13 575 | – | – |
| Venezuela (Bolivarian Republic of) | 2016 | 30 000 | – | 29 232 | 80 000 | 240 613 | 61 034 |
| | 2017 | 5 000 | – | 3 900 | – | – | – |
| | 2018 | 81 402 | – | – | 48 117 | 404 924 | 97 293 |
| **EASTERN MEDITERRANEAN** | | | | | | | |
| Afghanistan | 2016 | 992 319 | – | – | 758 675 | 93 335 | 89 500 |
| | 2017 | 2 372 354 | – | – | 514 875 | 27 850 | 27 850 |
| | 2018 | 649 383 | – | – | 28 915 | – | 47 665 |
| Djibouti | 2016 | 33 851 | 10 | – | – | – | – |
| | 2017 | 134 701 | 27 | – | 63 488 | 14 212 | – |
| | 2018 | 109 500 | 53 | – | 91 416 | 46 380 | 98 380 |

## Annex 3 – D. Commodities distribution and coverage, 2016–2018

| WHO region Country/area | Year | No. of LLINs sold or delivered | Modelled percentage of population with access to an ITN | No. of people protected by IRS | No of RDTs distributed | Any first-line treatment courses delivered (including ACT) | ACT treatment courses delivered |
|---|---|---|---|---|---|---|---|
| **EASTERN MEDITERRANEAN** | | | | | | | |
| Iran (Islamic Republic of) | 2016 | 6 393 | – | 172 666 | 120 000 | – | – |
| | 2017 | 4 218 | – | 126 111 | – | – | – |
| | 2018 | 4 500 | – | 117 174 | 128 650 | – | – |
| Pakistan | 2016 | 1 304 305 | – | 552 500 | 13 446 268 | 850 000 | 62 000 |
| | 2017 | 1 048 037 | – | 776 650 | 1 826 221 | 800 000 | 63 566 |
| | 2018 | 2 762 975 | – | 2 937 767 | 2 584 675 | 1 000 000 | 65 000 |
| Saudi Arabia | 2016 | 0 | – | 307 927 | – | 3 922 | 3 922 |
| | 2017 | 127 800 | – | 253 222 | – | 1 915 | 1 915 |
| | 2018 | 127 801 | – | 242 009 | – | 1 908 | 1 908 |
| Somalia | 2016 | 655 798 | 13 | 11 015 | 593 310 | 351 755 | 351 755 |
| | 2017 | 2 571 923 | 19 | 1 267 526 | 468 750 | 322 260 | 322 260 |
| | 2018 | 357 569 | 21 | 2 038 381 | 755 750 | 260 580 | 260 580 |
| Sudan | 2016 | 5 370 774 | 52 | 3 678 400 | 2 375 275 | 3 847 768 | 3 847 768 |
| | 2017 | 5 741 449 | 56 | 3 683 031 | 3 498 425 | 4 507 838 | 4 507 838 |
| | 2018 | 3 454 519 | 51 | 3 830 195 | 4 117 300 | 4 195 600 | 4 195 600 |
| Yemen | 2016 | 1 482 982 | – | 548 436 | 442 570 | 283 408 | 283 408 |
| | 2017 | 433 266 | – | 1 338 585 | 148 935 | 138 494 | 77 115 |
| | 2018 | 1 461 760 | – | 995 328 | 571 175 | 440 265 | 38 420 |
| **SOUTH-EAST ASIA** | | | | | | | |
| Bangladesh | 2016 | 41 255 | – | – | 420 049 | 28 407 | 24 431 |
| | 2017 | 2 242 527 | – | – | 373 138 | 29 916 | 24 790 |
| | 2018 | 1 559 423 | – | 72 000 | 500 440 | 10 762 | 8 609 |
| Bhutan | 2016 | 22 322 | – | 66 675 | 12 600 | 216 | 216 |
| | 2017 | 137 000 | – | 71 690 | 21 650 | 132 | 132 |
| | 2018 | 29 770 | – | 76 809 | 12 300 | 293 | 293 |
| Democratic People's Republic of Korea | 2016 | 0 | – | 1 152 402 | 182 980 | 23 231 | 0 |
| | 2017 | 0 | – | 1 147 548 | 176 612 | 17 038 | 0 |
| | 2018 | 500 815 | – | 169 841 | 657 050 | 3 698 | 0 |
| India | 2016 | 5 000 000 | – | 43 477 154 | 21 082 000 | 2 123 760 | 300 000 |
| | 2017 | 16 340 000 | – | 39 341 409 | 1 064 000 | 104 110 | 62 650 |
| | 2018 | 9 648 400 | – | 34 290 886 | 10 500 000 | 1 400 000 | 1 100 000 |
| Indonesia | 2016 | 2 977 539 | – | 6 240 | 1 382 208 | 438 178 | 438 178 |
| | 2017 | 4 376 636 | – | 3 320 | 1 783 498 | 607 965 | 607 965 |
| | 2018 | 340 074 | – | 305 493 | 255 300 | 670 603 | 670 603 |
| Myanmar | 2016 | 3 965 187 | – | 44 484 | 1 596 525 | 126 585 | 126 585 |
| | 2017 | 5 835 192 | – | – | 2 053 525 | 108 364 | 108 364 |
| | 2018 | 775 251 | – | 14 017 | 1 761 775 | 57 144 | 57 144 |
| Nepal | 2016 | 290 647 | – | 286 865 | 61 000 | 4 500 | 274 |
| | 2017 | 324 156 | – | 300 000 | 100 000 | 3 070 | 238 |
| | 2018 | 319 046 | – | 230 000 | 132 065 | 3 949 | 120 |
| Sri Lanka | 2016 | 16 465 | – | 57 111 | 31 950 | 41 | 19 |
| | 2017 | 18 019 | – | 10 317 | 27 500 | 57 | 27 |
| | 2018 | 21 759 | – | 15 707 | 11 150 | 48 | 15 |
| Thailand | 2016 | 465 600 | – | 237 398 | 68 500 | 40 801 | 14 321 |
| | 2017 | 358 400 | – | 207 250 | 173 425 | 21 540 | 7 540 |
| | 2018 | 131 425 | – | 165 580 | 30 550 | 25 292 | 9 892 |
| Timor-Leste | 2016 | 309 067 | – | 166 426 | 114 263 | 84 | 84 |
| | 2017 | 334 471 | – | 102 891 | 115 115 | 30 | 30 |
| | 2018 | 35 367 | – | 154 410 | 144 061 | 8 | 8 |

| WHO region Country/area | Year | No. of LLINs sold or delivered | Modelled percentage of population with access to an ITN | No. of people protected by IRS | No of RDTs distributed | Any first-line treatment courses delivered (including ACT) | ACT treatment courses delivered |
|---|---|---|---|---|---|---|---|
| **WESTERN PACIFIC** | | | | | | | |
| Cambodia | 2016 | 4 089 321 | – | – | 400 350 | 98 990 | 88 990 |
| | 2017 | 1 994 150 | – | – | 503 250 | 145 518 | 145 518 |
| | 2018 | 1 624 507 | – | – | – | – | – |
| China | 2016 | 26 562 | – | 272 108 | – | 6 290 | 4 130 |
| | 2017 | 11 349 | – | 352 731 | – | – | – |
| | 2018 | 5 987 | – | 161 224 | – | – | – |
| Lao People's Democratic Republic | 2016 | 1 213 755 | – | – | 270 950 | 63 889 | 62 994 |
| | 2017 | 242 405 | – | – | 333 675 | 42 972 | 39 272 |
| | 2018 | 50 403 | – | 2 052 | 34 387 | 8 931 | 34 765 |
| Malaysia | 2016 | 284 031 | – | 513 076 | 0 | 2 302 | 2 197 |
| | 2017 | 278 104 | – | 539 029 | 0 | 4 114 | 3 443 |
| | 2018 | 213 073 | – | – | 0 | 4 630 | 3 891 |
| Papua New Guinea | 2016 | 944 847 | – | – | 1 733 500 | 540 400 | 540 400 |
| | 2017 | 1 694 315 | – | – | 1 135 577 | 832 532 | 832 532 |
| | 2018 | 1 480 705 | – | – | 2 268 750 | 1 385 940 | 1 385 940 |
| Philippines | 2016 | 806 603 | – | 1 025 096 | 256 875 | 6 810 | 6 810 |
| | 2017 | 814 984 | – | 490 640 | 145 325 | 23 400 | 23 400 |
| | 2018 | 1 156 837 | – | 1 015 672 | 168 300 | 4 318 | 4 318 |
| Republic of Korea | 2016 | 0 | – | – | 4 625 | 673 | – |
| | 2017 | 0 | – | – | 0 | 515 | – |
| | 2018 | 0 | – | – | 0 | 576 | – |
| Solomon Islands | 2016 | 291 339 | – | 16 179 | 542 975 | 237 492 | 237 492 |
| | 2017 | 85 976 | – | 0 | 374 850 | 238 665 | 238 665 |
| | 2018 | 150 248 | – | – | 386 975 | 233 917 | 233 917 |
| Vanuatu | 2016 | 110 215 | – | – | 39 525 | 11 729 | 11 729 |
| | 2017 | 91 028 | – | – | 56 150 | 27 409 | 20 853 |
| | 2018 | 27 151 | – | – | 50 850 | 0 | 0 |
| Viet Nam | 2016 | 200 000 | – | 417 142 | 408 055 | 71 853 | 2 358 |
| | 2017 | 752 000 | – | 151 153 | 921 897 | 87 225 | 40 000 |
| | 2018 | 1 193 024 | – | 319 866 | 576 930 | 45 040 | 40 000 |

Data as of 19 December 2019

ACT: artemisinin-based combination therapy; IRS: indoor residual spraying; ITN: insecticide-treated mosquito net; LLIN: long-lasting insecticidal net; RDT: rapid diagnostic test; WHO: World Health Organization.

"–" refers to data not available.

[1] In May 2013, South Sudan was reassigned to the WHO African Region (WHA resolution 66.21, http://apps.who.int/gb/ebwha/pdf_files/WHA66/A66_R21-en.pdf).

[2] Where national data for the United Republic of Tanzania are unavailable, refer to Mainland and Zanzibar.

# Annex 3 - Ea. Household survey results, 2015–2018, compiled through STATcompiler

| WHO region Country/area | Source | % of households | | | | | % of population | |
|---|---|---|---|---|---|---|---|---|
| | | with at least one ITN | with at least one ITN for every two persons who stayed in the household the previous night | with IRS in last 12 months | with at least one ITN and/or IRS in the past 12 months | with at least one ITN for every two persons and/or IRS in the past 12 months | with access to an ITN | who slept under an ITN last night |
| **AFRICAN** | | | | | | | | |
| Angola | 2015–16 DHS | 30.9 | 11.3 | 1.6 | 31.8 | 12.5 | 19.7 | 17.6 |
| Benin | 2017–18 DHS | 91.5 | 60.5 | 8.7 | 92.0 | 63.8 | 77.2 | 71.1 |
| Burkina Faso | 2017–18 MIS | 75.3 | 32.8 | – | – | – | 54.5 | 44.1 |
| Burundi | 2016–17 DHS | 46.2 | 17.1 | 1.0 | 46.8 | 17.9 | 32.3 | 34.7 |
| Chad | 2014–15 DHS | 77.3 | 42.4 | 0.6 | 77.3 | 42.4 | 61.2 | 33.3 |
| Ethiopia | 2016 DHS | – | – | – | – | – | – | – |
| Ghana | 2016 MIS | 73.0 | 50.9 | 8.1 | 74.1 | 53.6 | 65.8 | 41.7 |
| Kenya | 2015 MIS | 62.5 | 40.0 | – | 62.5 | 39.7 | 52.5 | 47.6 |
| Liberia | 2016 MIS | 61.5 | 25.2 | 1.2 | 62.1 | 25.9 | 41.5 | 39.3 |
| Madagascar | 2016 MIS | 79.5 | 44.4 | 6.9 | 80.9 | 47.9 | 62.1 | 68.2 |
| Malawi | 2015–16 DHS | 56.9 | 23.5 | 4.9 | 58.6 | 27.0 | 38.8 | 33.9 |
| Malawi | 2017 MIS | 82.1 | 41.7 | – | – | – | 63.1 | 55.4 |
| Mali | 2015 MIS | 93.0 | 39.3 | 4.0 | 93.6 | 41.8 | 69.5 | 63.9 |
| Mali | 2018 DHS | 89.8 | 54.8 | – | – | – | 75.2 | 72.9 |
| Mozambique | 2015 AIS | 66.0 | 38.9 | 11.2 | 68.7 | 45.3 | 53.8 | 45.4 |
| Mozambique | 2018 MIS | 82.2 | 51.2 | – | – | – | 68.5 | 68.4 |
| Nigeria | 2015 MIS | 68.8 | 34.9 | 1.3 | 69.0 | 35.5 | 54.7 | 37.3 |
| Rwanda | 2014–15 DHS | 80.6 | 42.6 | – | 80.6 | 42.5 | 63.8 | 61.4 |
| Rwanda | 2017 MIS | 84.1 | 55.1 | 19.6 | 89.2 | 66.9 | 71.9 | 63.9 |
| Senegal | 2015 DHS | 76.8 | 40.5 | 4.8 | 77.1 | 43.0 | 66.0 | 51.0 |
| Senegal | 2016 DHS | 82.4 | 56.4 | 5.3 | 82.9 | 58.0 | 75.7 | 63.1 |
| Senegal | 2017 DHS | 84.2 | 50.4 | 4.2 | 84.5 | 52.3 | 72.8 | 56.9 |
| Sierra Leone | 2016 MIS | 60.3 | 16.2 | 1.7 | 61.1 | 17.7 | 37.1 | 38.6 |
| Togo | 2017 MIS | 85.2 | 71.4 | – | – | – | 82.3 | 62.5 |
| Uganda | 2014–15 MIS | 90.2 | 62.3 | 4.9 | 90.5 | 64.0 | 78.8 | 68.6 |
| Uganda | 2016 DHS | 78.4 | 51.1 | – | – | – | 64.6 | 55.0 |
| United Republic of Tanzania | 2015–16 DHS | 65.6 | 38.8 | 5.5 | 66.2 | 41.0 | 55.9 | 49.0 |
| United Republic of Tanzania | 2017 MIS | 77.9 | 45.4 | – | – | – | 62.5 | 52.2 |
| Zimbabwe | 2015 DHS | 47.9 | 26.4 | 21.3 | 54.9 | 39.4 | 37.2 | 8.5 |
| **AMERICAS** | | | | | | | | |
| Haiti | 2016–17 DHS | 30.7 | 12.3 | 2.2 | 32.0 | 14.1 | 19.9 | 13.0 |
| **EASTERN MEDITERRANEAN** | | | | | | | | |
| Afghanistan | 2015 DHS | 26.0 | 2.9 | | | | 13.2 | 3.9 |
| Pakistan | 2017–18 DHS | 3.6 | 0.6 | 5.1 | 8.4 | 5.7 | 2.0 | 0.2 |
| **SOUTH-EAST ASIA** | | | | | | | | |
| India | 2015–16 DHS | 0.9 | 0.4 | – | – | – | 0.6 | 4.1 |
| Myanmar | 2015–16 DHS | 26.8 | 14.1 | – | – | – | 21.2 | 15.6 |
| Timor-Leste | 2016 DHS | 63.6 | 32.7 | – | – | – | 48.1 | 47.3 |

ACT: artemisinin-based combination therapy; AIS: AIDS indicator survey; DHS: demographic and health survey; IPTp: intermittent preventive treatment in pregnancy; IRS: indoor residual spraying; ITN: insecticide-treated mosquito net; MIS: malaria indicator survey.

"–" refers to not applicable or data not available.

Sources: Nationally representative household survey data from DHS and MIS, compiled through STATcompiler – https://www.statcompiler.com/.

| % of ITNs | % of pregnant women | | % of children <5 years | | | | % of children <5 years with fever in last 2 weeks | | | |
|---|---|---|---|---|---|---|---|---|---|---|
| that were used last night | who slept under an ITN | who took 3+ doses of IPTp | who slept under an ITN | with moderate or severe anaemia | with a positive RDT | with a positive microscopy blood smear | for whom advice or treatment was sought | who had blood taken from a finger or heel for testing | who took antimalarial drugs | who took an ACT among those who received any antimalarial |
| 71.0 | 23.0 | 20.0 | 21.7 | 34.0 | 13.5 | – | 50.8 | 34.3 | 18.1 | 76.7 |
| 73.4 | 79.3 | 13.7 | 76.3 | 43.8 | 36.3 | 39.1 | 53.1 | 17.7 | 17.5 | 37.0 |
| 76.0 | 58.2 | 57.7 | 54.4 | 50.1 | 20.2 | 16.9 | 73.5 | 48.8 | 51.1 | 79.4 |
| 86.9 | 43.9 | 12.9 | 39.9 | 36.3 | 37.9 | 26.8 | 69.6 | 66.4 | 47.0 | 11.3 |
| 48.6 | 34.7 | 8.5 | 36.4 | – | – | – | 36.9 | 12.9 | 26.9 | 10.0 |
| – | – | – | – | 32.0 | – | – | 35.3 | | 7.7 | 11.5 |
| 47.7 | 50.0 | 59.6 | 52.2 | 35.2 | 27.9 | 20.6 | 71.8 | 30.3 | 50.1 | 58.8 |
| 75.2 | 57.8 | 22.9 | 56.1 | 16.2 | 9.1 | 5.0 | 71.9 | 39.2 | 27.1 | 91.6 |
| 71.2 | 39.5 | 23.1 | 43.7 | 49.2 | 44.9 | – | 78.2 | 49.8 | 65.5 | 81.1 |
| 78.7 | 68.5 | 10.6 | 73.4 | 20.5 | 5.1 | 6.9 | 55.5 | 15.5 | 10.1 | 17.0 |
| 73.3 | 43.9 | 30.4 | 42.7 | 36.1 | – | – | 67.0 | 52.0 | 37.6 | 91.8 |
| 76.8 | 62.5 | 41.1 | 67.5 | 37.1 | 36.0 | 24.3 | 54.4 | 37.6 | 29.4 | 96.4 |
| 90.7 | 77.9 | 21.0 | 71.2 | 63.0 | 32.4 | 35.7 | 49.2 | 14.2 | 28.7 | 28.9 |
| 88.7 | 83.7 | 28.3 | 79.1 | 56.7 | 18.9 | – | 52.8 | 16.4 | 18.7 | 31.0 |
| 70.9 | 52.1 | 23.3 | 47.9 | 36.7 | 40.2 | – | 62.7 | 39.6 | 38.4 | 92.6 |
| 85.4 | 76.4 | 40.6 | 72.7 | 55.2 | 38.9 | – | 68.6 | 47.9 | 32.7 | 98.6 |
| 60.8 | 49.0 | 21.4 | 43.6 | 43.1 | 45.1 | 27.4 | 66.1 | 12.6 | 41.2 | 37.6 |
| 77.4 | 72.9 | – | 67.7 | 15.7 | 7.8 | 2.2 | 56.7 | 36.1 | 11.4 | 98.7 |
| 71.0 | 68.5 | – | 68.0 | – | 11.8 | 7.2 | 55.6 | 38.1 | 19.6 | 98.7 |
| 70.0 | 51.8 | 11.2 | 55.4 | 38.0 | 0.6 | 0.3 | 49.3 | 9.5 | 3.4 | 12.5 |
| 68.2 | 69.0 | 22.1 | 66.6 | 36.7 | 0.9 | 0.9 | 49.5 | 13.0 | 1.7 | 85.0 |
| 68.6 | 61.8 | 22 | 60.7 | 41.8 | 0.9 | 0.4 | 51.4 | 16.1 | 4.7 | 65.5 |
| 89.0 | 44.0 | 31.1 | 44.1 | 49.2 | 52.7 | 40.1 | 71.4 | 51.1 | 57.0 | 96.0 |
| 52.3 | 69.0 | 41.7 | 69.7 | 47.8 | 43.9 | 28.3 | 55.9 | 29.3 | 31.1 | 76.3 |
| 74.4 | 75.4 | 27.5 | 74.3 | 28.8 | 31.7 | 20.0 | 82.0 | 35.8 | 76.9 | 86.7 |
| 74.0 | 64.1 | 17.2 | 62.0 | 29.2 | 30.4 | – | 81.2 | 49.0 | 71.5 | 87.8 |
| 69.4 | 53.9 | 8.0 | 54.4 | 31.2 | 14.4 | 5.6 | 80.1 | 35.9 | 51.1 | 84.9 |
| 66.7 | 51.4 | 25.8 | 54.6 | 30.5 | 7.3 | – | 75.4 | 43.1 | 36.2 | 89.4 |
| 18.8 | 6.1 | – | 9.0 | 14.9 | – | – | 50.5 | 12.7 | 1.0 | – |
| 62.3 | 16.0 | – | 18.2 | 37.5 | – | – | 40.3 | 15.8 | 1.1 | – |
| 21.4 | 4.1 | – | 4.6 | – | – | – | 63.7 | 7.9 | 11.8 | 4.4 |
| 11.6 | 0.4 | – | 0.4 | – | – | – | 81.4 | – | 9.2 | 3.3 |
| 68.9 | 4.3 | – | 4.6 | 30.8 | – | – | 73.2 | 10.8 | 20.1 | 8.5 |
| 58.3 | 18.4 | – | 18.6 | 26.7 | – | – | 65.0 | 3.0 | 0.8 | – |
| 79.8 | 60.1 | – | 55.4 | 12.6 | – | – | 57.6 | 24.5 | 10.0 | 11.1 |

Data as of 23 October 2019

# Annex 3 - Eb. Household survey results, 2015–2018, compiled through WHO calculations

| WHO region Country/area | Survey | Fever prevalence | Health sector where treatment was sought | | | | | | | Diagnostic testing coverage in each health sector | |
|---|---|---|---|---|---|---|---|---|---|---|---|
| | | Overall | Public excluding community health workers | Community health workers | Formal medical private excluding pharmacies | Pharmacies or accredited drug stores | Informal private | No treatment seeking | Trained provider | Public excluding community health workers | Community health workers |
| **AFRICAN** | | | | | | | | | | | |
| Angola | 2015–16 DHS | 15% | 47% | – | 5% | 1% | 2% | 45% | 53% | 59% | – |
| Benin | 2017–18 DHS | 20% | 22% | – | 9% | 9% | 14% | 46% | 40% | 52% | – |
| Burkina Faso | 2017–18 MIS | 20% | 71% | 1% | 1% | 0% | 2% | 26% | 73% | 66% | – |
| Burundi | 2016–17 DHS | 40% | 54% | 3% | 10% | 5% | 1% | 30% | 69% | 87% | 95% |
| Ethiopia | 2016 DHS | 14% | 26% | – | 8% | 0% | 2% | 63% | 34% | – | – |
| Ghana | 2016 MIS | 31% | 34% | – | 15% | 10% | 12% | 28% | 60% | 59% | – |
| Kenya | 2015 MIS | 36% | 51% | – | 15% | 5% | 3% | 27% | 70% | 52% | – |
| Liberia | 2016 MIS | 39% | 46% | – | 13% | 14% | 8% | 22% | 71% | 77% | – |
| Madagascar | 2016 MIS | 16% | 36% | 7% | 10% | 1% | 7% | 40% | 53% | 31% | 37% |
| Malawi | 2017 MIS | 40% | 38% | 3% | 6% | 2% | 7% | 46% | 48% | 76% | – |
| Mali | 2018 DHS | 16% | 24% | 3% | 2% | 7% | 23% | 42% | 36% | 46% | 37% |
| Mozambique | 2018 MIS | 31% | 64% | 4% | 0% | 0% | 1% | 31% | 68% | 72% | 41% |
| Nigeria | 2015 MIS | 41% | 20% | 1% | 6% | 39% | 3% | 32% | 65% | 32% | – |
| Rwanda | 2017 MIS | 31% | 33% | 18% | 3% | 5% | 1% | 44% | 55% | 73% | 74% |
| Senegal | 2017 DHS | 21% | 39% | 1% | 4% | 6% | 3% | 48% | 49% | 32% | – |
| Sierra Leone | 2016 MIS | 27% | 63% | – | 4% | 4% | 2% | 28% | 70% | 74% | – |
| Togo | 2017 MIS | 24% | 26% | 5% | 7% | 3% | 16% | 43% | 42% | 78% | 76% |
| Uganda | 2016 DHS | 34% | 34% | 3% | 34% | 12% | 1% | 18% | 80% | 77% | 58% |
| United Republic of Tanzania | 2017 MIS | 21% | 46% | – | 13% | 17% | 1% | 25% | 75% | 66% | – |
| Zimbabwe | 2015 DHS | 14% | 35% | 1% | 9% | 0% | 6% | 49% | 45% | 26% | – |

ACT: artemisinin-based combination therapy; DHS: demographic and health survey; MIS: malaria indicator survey; WHO: World Health Organization. "–" refers to not applicable or data not available.

Note: Figures with fewer than 30 children in the denominator were removed.

Sources: Nationally representative household survey data from DHS and MIS, compiled through WHO calculations.

| Diagnostic testing coverage in each health sector | | | | Antimalarial treatment coverage in each health sector | | | | | | | ACT use among antimalarial treatment in each health sector | | |
|---|---|---|---|---|---|---|---|---|---|---|---|---|---|
| Formal medical private excluding pharmacies | Pharmacies or accredited drug stores | Informal private | Trained provider | Public excluding community health workers | Community health workers | Formal medical private excluding pharmacies | Pharmacies or accredited drug stores | Self-treatment | No treatment seeking | Trained provider | Public | Private | Informal private |
| 82% | 27% | 23% | 60% | 27% | – | 40% | 23% | 10% | 7% | 28% | 74% | 88% | – |
| 30% | 9% | 8% | 37% | 38% | – | 34% | 23% | 12% | 7% | 34% | 44% | 28% | 40% |
| – | – | – | 66% | 69% | – | – | – | – | 10% | 68% | 80% | – | – |
| 86% | 36% | 54% | 84% | 69% | 93% | 55% | 32% | – | 9% | 66% | 12% | 10% | – |
| – | – | – | – | 16% | – | 19% | – | – | 4% | 17% | 14% | – | – |
| 60% | 11% | 0% | 50% | 64% | – | 49% | 56% | 61% | 29% | 59% | 57% | 63% | 40% |
| 57% | 9% | 25% | 49% | 31% | – | 30% | 44% | 29% | 19% | 31% | 93% | 91% | – |
| 82% | 35% | 14% | 70% | 84% | – | 75% | 76% | 62% | 21% | 81% | 87% | 71% | 80% |
| 7% | – | 3% | 27% | 13% | 19% | 13% | – | 18% | 5% | 14% | 9% | – | – |
| 76% | – | 4% | 73% | 55% | – | 55% | – | 21% | 7% | 54% | 98% | – | – |
| – | 8% | 5% | 36% | 61% | 56% | – | 17% | 5% | 4% | 50% | 35% | – | – |
| – | – | – | 70% | 47% | 57% | – | – | – | 10% | 47% | 98% | – | – |
| 29% | 6% | 7% | 16% | 48% | 47% | 56% | 48% | 20% | 28% | 48% | 46% | 37% | – |
| 70% | 14% | – | 67% | 30% | 60% | 13% | 31% | – | 2% | 37% | 99% | – | – |
| 23% | 6% | 20% | 28% | 9% | – | 11% | 3% | 8% | 1% | 8% | 68% | – | – |
| 72% | 13% | – | 71% | 77% | – | 77% | 41% | – | 19% | 75% | 98% | 92% | – |
| 45% | – | 4% | 66% | 70% | 83% | 54% | – | 10% | 7% | 66% | 82% | – | – |
| 49% | 22% | 36% | 57% | 82% | 87% | 79% | 78% | 67% | 43% | 80% | 91% | 84% | 96% |
| 76% | 13% | – | 55% | 34% | – | 49% | 57% | – | 24% | 42% | 96% | 83% | – |
| 13% | – | 9% | 23% | 2% | – | 1% | – | 0% | 1% | 1% | – | – | – |

Data as of 23 October 2019

# Annex 3 - F. Population at risk and estimated malaria cases and deaths, 2010–2018

| WHO region Country/area | Year | Population at risk | Cases | | | Deaths | | |
|---|---|---|---|---|---|---|---|---|
| | | | Lower | Point | Upper | Lower | Point | Upper |
| **AFRICAN** | | | | | | | | |
| Algeria[1,2,3] | 2010 | 2 113 135 | – | 1 | – | – | 1 | – |
| | 2011 | 2 153 309 | – | 1 | – | – | 0 | – |
| | 2012 | 2 195 743 | – | 55 | – | – | 0 | – |
| | 2013 | 2 240 160 | – | 8 | – | – | 0 | – |
| | 2014 | 2 286 182 | – | 0 | – | – | 0 | – |
| | 2015 | 2 333 425 | – | 0 | – | – | 0 | – |
| | 2016 | 2 381 786 | – | 0 | – | – | 0 | – |
| | 2017 | 2 431 200 | – | 0 | – | – | 0 | – |
| | 2018 | 2 480 497 | – | 0 | – | – | 0 | – |
| Angola | 2010 | 23 356 247 | 3 209 000 | 4 332 945 | 5 712 000 | 11 000 | 13 387 | 16 500 |
| | 2011 | 24 220 660 | 3 171 000 | 4 262 568 | 5 614 000 | 10 400 | 12 803 | 16 100 |
| | 2012 | 25 107 925 | 3 241 000 | 4 379 690 | 5 807 000 | 9 930 | 12 408 | 15 900 |
| | 2013 | 26 015 786 | 3 464 000 | 4 706 326 | 6 229 000 | 9 700 | 12 229 | 15 900 |
| | 2014 | 26 941 773 | 3 762 000 | 5 063 524 | 6 625 000 | 9 780 | 12 484 | 16 600 |
| | 2015 | 27 884 380 | 4 238 000 | 5 576 653 | 7 193 000 | 10 100 | 13 118 | 17 800 |
| | 2016 | 28 842 482 | 4 852 000 | 6 345 114 | 8 177 000 | 10 100 | 13 252 | 18 200 |
| | 2017 | 29 816 769 | 5 109 000 | 6 825 325 | 8 998 000 | 10 100 | 13 345 | 18 500 |
| | 2018 | 30 809 787 | 5 261 000 | 7 052 636 | 9 225 000 | 10 200 | 13 425 | 18 800 |
| Benin | 2010 | 9 199 254 | 2 734 000 | 3 567 057 | 4 589 000 | 7 530 | 8 048 | 8 610 |
| | 2011 | 9 460 829 | 2 707 000 | 3 501 513 | 4 472 000 | 6 830 | 7 303 | 7 830 |
| | 2012 | 9 729 254 | 2 894 000 | 3 677 978 | 4 636 000 | 6 270 | 6 720 | 7 210 |
| | 2013 | 10 004 594 | 3 123 000 | 3 951 788 | 4 930 000 | 5 930 | 6 362 | 6 840 |
| | 2014 | 10 286 839 | 3 233 000 | 4 106 892 | 5 127 000 | 5 950 | 6 404 | 6 910 |
| | 2015 | 10 575 962 | 3 467 000 | 4 355 431 | 5 386 000 | 6 140 | 6 655 | 7 220 |
| | 2016 | 10 872 072 | 3 692 000 | 4 583 409 | 5 611 000 | 6 340 | 6 915 | 7 530 |
| | 2017 | 11 175 192 | 3 571 000 | 4 465 137 | 5 509 000 | 6 480 | 7 115 | 7 810 |
| | 2018 | 11 485 035 | 3 489 000 | 4 435 318 | 5 556 000 | 6 370 | 7 081 | 7 870 |
| Botswana | 2010 | 1 317 417 | 1 300 | 2 229 | 3 900 | 0 | 5 | 13 |
| | 2011 | 1 336 179 | 520 | 682 | 1 000 | 0 | 1 | 3 |
| | 2012 | 1 352 187 | 230 | 304 | 410 | 0 | 0 | 1 |
| | 2013 | 1 367 436 | 570 | 729 | 980 | 0 | 1 | 3 |
| | 2014 | 1 384 718 | 1 600 | 2 075 | 2 800 | 0 | 5 | 10 |
| | 2015 | 1 405 998 | 400 | 521 | 700 | 0 | 1 | 2 |
| | 2016 | 1 431 993 | 890 | 1 154 | 1 500 | 0 | 2 | 5 |
| | 2017 | 1 461 921 | 2 300 | 2 999 | 4 000 | 0 | 7 | 14 |
| | 2018 | 1 494 401 | 680 | 879 | 1 200 | 0 | 2 | 4 |
| Burkina Faso | 2010 | 15 605 211 | 6 884 000 | 8 602 187 | 10 590 000 | 28 000 | 30 750 | 33 800 |
| | 2011 | 16 081 915 | 6 968 000 | 8 677 204 | 10 710 000 | 25 200 | 27 994 | 31 200 |
| | 2012 | 16 571 252 | 7 043 000 | 8 742 005 | 10 760 000 | 18 500 | 20 916 | 23 700 |
| | 2013 | 17 072 791 | 6 694 000 | 8 323 401 | 10 230 000 | 17 200 | 19 930 | 23 100 |
| | 2014 | 17 586 029 | 6 151 000 | 7 668 618 | 9 439 000 | 15 300 | 18 144 | 21 500 |
| | 2015 | 18 110 616 | 5 741 000 | 7 245 827 | 9 025 000 | 13 100 | 15 940 | 19 300 |
| | 2016 | 18 646 350 | 5 249 000 | 7 490 818 | 10 340 000 | 11 400 | 14 072 | 17 500 |
| | 2017 | 19 193 236 | 5 406 000 | 7 676 215 | 10 590 000 | 10 300 | 12 955 | 16 600 |
| | 2018 | 19 751 466 | 5 551 000 | 7 875 575 | 10 960 000 | 9 860 | 12 725 | 16 700 |
| Burundi | 2010 | 8 675 606 | 1 321 000 | 1 823 594 | 2 488 000 | 4 390 | 4 720 | 5 090 |
| | 2011 | 8 958 406 | 1 193 000 | 1 649 646 | 2 226 000 | 4 300 | 4 636 | 5 020 |
| | 2012 | 9 245 992 | 1 037 000 | 1 423 214 | 1 903 000 | 4 390 | 4 776 | 5 230 |
| | 2013 | 9 540 302 | 936 000 | 1 341 256 | 1 858 000 | 4 330 | 4 754 | 5 260 |
| | 2014 | 9 844 301 | 967 000 | 1 393 043 | 1 969 000 | 4 370 | 4 850 | 5 480 |
| | 2015 | 10 160 034 | 1 167 000 | 1 681 495 | 2 322 000 | 4 380 | 4 917 | 5 640 |
| | 2016 | 10 488 002 | 1 739 000 | 2 367 597 | 3 150 000 | 4 410 | 5 020 | 5 870 |
| | 2017 | 10 827 010 | 2 009 000 | 2 709 703 | 3 557 000 | 4 420 | 5 097 | 6 060 |
| | 2018 | 11 175 379 | 2 079 000 | 2 796 890 | 3 682 000 | 4 410 | 5 118 | 6 170 |
| Cabo Verde[1,2] | 2010 | 128 087 | – | 47 | – | – | 1 | – |
| | 2011 | 129 703 | – | 7 | – | – | 1 | – |
| | 2012 | 131 362 | – | 1 | – | – | 0 | – |
| | 2013 | 133 052 | – | 22 | – | – | 0 | – |
| | 2014 | 134 751 | – | 26 | – | – | 1 | – |
| | 2015 | 136 432 | – | 7 | – | – | 0 | – |
| | 2016 | 138 096 | – | 48 | – | – | 1 | – |
| | 2017 | 139 749 | – | 423 | – | – | 1 | – |
| | 2018 | 141 378 | – | 2 | – | – | 0 | – |
| Cameroon | 2010 | 20 341 236 | 4 436 000 | 6 011 372 | 7 914 000 | 11 400 | 12 409 | 13 600 |
| | 2011 | 20 906 392 | 4 204 000 | 5 542 323 | 7 153 000 | 10 900 | 11 903 | 13 100 |
| | 2012 | 21 485 267 | 3 993 000 | 5 266 733 | 6 827 000 | 11 200 | 12 317 | 13 600 |
| | 2013 | 22 077 300 | 3 839 000 | 5 365 639 | 7 162 000 | 11 300 | 12 481 | 13 800 |
| | 2014 | 22 681 853 | 3 808 000 | 5 536 236 | 7 750 000 | 11 300 | 12 547 | 14 000 |
| | 2015 | 23 298 376 | 4 059 000 | 5 929 407 | 8 411 000 | 10 900 | 12 276 | 13 900 |
| | 2016 | 23 926 549 | 4 011 000 | 6 324 089 | 9 433 000 | 10 300 | 11 886 | 13 700 |
| | 2017 | 24 566 070 | 3 807 000 | 6 441 846 | 10 160 000 | 9 700 | 11 371 | 13 400 |
| | 2018 | 25 216 261 | 3 644 000 | 6 228 154 | 9 831 000 | 9 360 | 11 192 | 13 500 |

| WHO region Country/area | Year | Population at risk | Cases | | | Deaths | | |
|---|---|---|---|---|---|---|---|---|
| | | | Lower | Point | Upper | Lower | Point | Upper |
| **AFRICAN** | | | | | | | | |
| Central African Republic | 2010 | 4 386 765 | 1 393 000 | 1 906 095 | 2 567 000 | 5 890 | 7 378 | 9 320 |
| | 2011 | 4 418 639 | 1 304 000 | 1 852 888 | 2 559 000 | 5 020 | 6 389 | 8 270 |
| | 2012 | 4 436 411 | 1 289 000 | 1 832 621 | 2 527 000 | 4 490 | 5 845 | 7 750 |
| | 2013 | 4 447 945 | 1 265 000 | 1 809 535 | 2 499 000 | 3 770 | 5 053 | 6 880 |
| | 2014 | 4 464 171 | 1 218 000 | 1 754 603 | 2 434 000 | 3 420 | 4 721 | 6 620 |
| | 2015 | 4 493 171 | 1 183 000 | 1 707 013 | 2 394 000 | 3 060 | 4 302 | 6 200 |
| | 2016 | 4 537 683 | 1 094 000 | 1 642 736 | 2 373 000 | 2 730 | 3 949 | 5 860 |
| | 2017 | 4 596 023 | 1 050 000 | 1 596 323 | 2 318 000 | 2 530 | 3 739 | 5 700 |
| | 2018 | 4 666 375 | 1 078 000 | 1 620 758 | 2 361 000 | 2 410 | 3 654 | 5 730 |
| Chad | 2010 | 11 821 305 | 1 610 000 | 2 670 920 | 4 135 000 | 12 600 | 13 692 | 14 900 |
| | 2011 | 12 225 682 | 1 584 000 | 2 573 306 | 3 958 000 | 11 600 | 12 672 | 13 800 |
| | 2012 | 12 644 806 | 1 514 000 | 2 469 991 | 3 805 000 | 10 400 | 11 499 | 12 600 |
| | 2013 | 13 075 722 | 1 297 000 | 2 345 147 | 3 920 000 | 9 580 | 10 607 | 11 700 |
| | 2014 | 13 514 000 | 1 242 000 | 2 301 093 | 3 969 000 | 8 680 | 9 685 | 10 800 |
| | 2015 | 13 956 512 | 1 268 000 | 2 334 698 | 3 924 000 | 8 160 | 9 190 | 10 300 |
| | 2016 | 14 402 266 | 1 288 000 | 2 447 429 | 4 300 000 | 7 780 | 8 862 | 10 100 |
| | 2017 | 14 852 327 | 1 248 000 | 2 559 078 | 4 687 000 | 7 510 | 8 693 | 10 000 |
| | 2018 | 15 308 245 | 1 253 000 | 2 523 288 | 4 594 000 | 7 370 | 8 693 | 10 300 |
| Comoros[1] | 2010 | 689 696 | – | 36 538 | – | 3 | 89 | 140 |
| | 2011 | 706 578 | – | 24 856 | – | 2 | 61 | 95 |
| | 2012 | 723 865 | – | 49 840 | – | 4 | 125 | 200 |
| | 2013 | 741 511 | – | 53 156 | – | 5 | 134 | 210 |
| | 2014 | 759 390 | – | 2 203 | – | 0 | 5 | 8 |
| | 2015 | 777 435 | – | 1 300 | – | 0 | 3 | 5 |
| | 2016 | 795 597 | – | 1 143 | – | 0 | 2 | 4 |
| | 2017 | 813 890 | – | 3 230 | – | 0 | 8 | 12 |
| | 2018 | 832 322 | – | 15 613 | – | 1 | 39 | 62 |
| Congo | 2010 | 4 273 738 | 593 000 | 944 174 | 1 442 000 | 1 800 | 1 894 | 2 000 |
| | 2011 | 4 394 842 | 628 000 | 986 118 | 1 500 000 | 1 770 | 1 883 | 2 000 |
| | 2012 | 4 510 197 | 650 000 | 1 013 105 | 1 499 000 | 1 770 | 1 899 | 2 040 |
| | 2013 | 4 622 757 | 694 000 | 1 068 018 | 1 580 000 | 1 790 | 1 955 | 2 150 |
| | 2014 | 4 736 965 | 724 000 | 1 098 243 | 1 597 000 | 1 790 | 1 972 | 2 220 |
| | 2015 | 4 856 093 | 703 000 | 1 100 944 | 1 635 000 | 1 730 | 1 907 | 2 160 |
| | 2016 | 4 980 996 | 679 000 | 1 162 467 | 1 855 000 | 1 760 | 1 948 | 2 250 |
| | 2017 | 5 110 701 | 697 000 | 1 229 822 | 2 053 000 | 1 750 | 1 938 | 2 260 |
| | 2018 | 5 244 363 | 703 000 | 1 232 815 | 2 017 000 | 1 760 | 1 961 | 2 310 |
| Côte d'Ivoire | 2010 | 20 532 944 | 7 829 000 | 9 635 484 | 11 700 000 | 15 400 | 16 488 | 17 700 |
| | 2011 | 21 028 652 | 7 612 000 | 9 296 942 | 11 240 000 | 13 500 | 14 492 | 15 600 |
| | 2012 | 21 547 188 | 6 845 000 | 8 538 623 | 10 460 000 | 11 300 | 12 157 | 13 100 |
| | 2013 | 22 087 506 | 5 714 000 | 7 484 764 | 9 688 000 | 9 830 | 10 548 | 11 400 |
| | 2014 | 22 647 672 | 5 354 000 | 7 135 696 | 9 284 000 | 8 840 | 9 486 | 10 200 |
| | 2015 | 23 226 148 | 5 561 000 | 7 433 189 | 9 805 000 | 8 800 | 9 501 | 10 300 |
| | 2016 | 23 822 726 | 6 048 000 | 8 448 875 | 11 500 000 | 8 530 | 9 275 | 10 100 |
| | 2017 | 24 437 475 | 6 128 000 | 8 855 281 | 12 340 000 | 8 460 | 9 263 | 10 200 |
| | 2018 | 25 069 226 | 5 381 000 | 8 287 840 | 12 270 000 | 8 410 | 9 297 | 10 300 |
| Democratic Republic of the Congo | 2010 | 64 563 853 | 22 370 000 | 27 653 200 | 33 780 000 | 54 100 | 63 385 | 74 000 |
| | 2011 | 66 755 151 | 21 440 000 | 26 674 386 | 32 590 000 | 40 900 | 48 721 | 57 500 |
| | 2012 | 69 020 749 | 19 980 000 | 25 054 526 | 30 890 000 | 38 500 | 46 851 | 56 100 |
| | 2013 | 71 358 804 | 18 320 000 | 23 378 784 | 29 300 000 | 35 500 | 43 955 | 53 500 |
| | 2014 | 73 767 445 | 17 600 000 | 22 748 873 | 28 730 000 | 36 600 | 46 394 | 57 900 |
| | 2015 | 76 244 532 | 17 940 000 | 23 546 242 | 30 470 000 | 34 700 | 44 994 | 57 300 |
| | 2016 | 78 789 130 | 18 860 000 | 25 430 848 | 33 900 000 | 30 800 | 40 491 | 53 100 |
| | 2017 | 81 398 765 | 19 410 000 | 26 790 666 | 35 990 000 | 33 100 | 44 991 | 60 700 |
| | 2018 | 84 068 092 | 19 600 000 | 26 888 424 | 35 910 000 | 32 200 | 44 615 | 62 000 |
| Equatorial Guinea | 2010 | 943 640 | 207 000 | 320 824 | 481 000 | 860 | 1 058 | 1 290 |
| | 2011 | 986 861 | 224 000 | 337 903 | 489 000 | 860 | 1 078 | 1 340 |
| | 2012 | 1 031 191 | 276 000 | 368 909 | 488 000 | 810 | 1 054 | 1 340 |
| | 2013 | 1 076 412 | 306 000 | 393 693 | 495 000 | 760 | 1 012 | 1 320 |
| | 2014 | 1 122 273 | 313 000 | 405 084 | 514 000 | 660 | 906 | 1 210 |
| | 2015 | 1 168 575 | 288 000 | 396 704 | 537 000 | 540 | 760 | 1 040 |
| | 2016 | 1 215 181 | 216 000 | 373 026 | 604 000 | 470 | 662 | 930 |
| | 2017 | 1 262 008 | 180 000 | 360 585 | 652 000 | 460 | 662 | 950 |
| | 2018 | 1 308 966 | 183 000 | 352 124 | 623 000 | 440 | 659 | 970 |
| Eritrea | 2010 | 3 170 437 | 53 000 | 83 471 | 118 000 | 8 | 161 | 320 |
| | 2011 | 3 213 969 | 49 000 | 76 678 | 107 000 | 8 | 141 | 280 |
| | 2012 | 3 250 104 | 33 000 | 52 483 | 76 000 | 6 | 85 | 170 |
| | 2013 | 3 281 453 | 31 000 | 49 309 | 70 000 | 5 | 88 | 180 |
| | 2014 | 3 311 444 | 70 000 | 109 689 | 153 000 | 11 | 227 | 460 |
| | 2015 | 3 342 818 | 41 000 | 64 176 | 90 000 | 6 | 128 | 260 |
| | 2016 | 3 376 558 | 47 000 | 86 561 | 137 000 | 6 | 198 | 440 |
| | 2017 | 3 412 894 | 74 000 | 115 928 | 161 000 | 12 | 221 | 450 |
| | 2018 | 3 452 797 | 64 000 | 99 716 | 139 000 | 10 | 196 | 390 |

# Annex 3 - F. Population at risk and estimated malaria cases and deaths, 2010–2018

| WHO region Country/area | Year | Population at risk | Cases | | | Deaths | | |
|---|---|---|---|---|---|---|---|---|
| | | | Lower | Point | Upper | Lower | Point | Upper |
| **AFRICAN** | | | | | | | | |
| Eswatini[1] | 2010 | 298 155 | – | 268 | – | 0 | 0 | 1 |
| | 2011 | 300 168 | – | 549 | – | 0 | 1 | 2 |
| | 2012 | 302 199 | – | 562 | – | 0 | 1 | 2 |
| | 2013 | 304 316 | – | 962 | – | 0 | 2 | 3 |
| | 2014 | 306 606 | – | 711 | – | 0 | 1 | 2 |
| | 2015 | 309 130 | – | 157 | – | – | 0 | – |
| | 2016 | 311 918 | – | 350 | – | 0 | 0 | 1 |
| | 2017 | 314 946 | – | 724 | – | 0 | 1 | 2 |
| | 2018 | 318 156 | – | 268 | – | 0 | 0 | 1 |
| Ethiopia | 2010 | 59 595 174 | 470 000 | 7 652 137 | 26 680 000 | 63 | 14 424 | 62 900 |
| | 2011 | 61 295 151 | 415 000 | 7 118 302 | 24 110 000 | 55 | 11 571 | 47 600 |
| | 2012 | 63 054 347 | 431 000 | 7 326 062 | 24 490 000 | 58 | 12 042 | 49 800 |
| | 2013 | 64 862 339 | 431 000 | 7 238 627 | 22 650 000 | 56 | 13 081 | 52 700 |
| | 2014 | 66 704 099 | 432 000 | 3 809 119 | 10 240 000 | 57 | 6 665 | 23 600 |
| | 2015 | 68 568 108 | 513 000 | 3 618 580 | 9 267 000 | 80 | 6 769 | 22 600 |
| | 2016 | 70 450 353 | 515 000 | 2 917 544 | 7 035 000 | 80 | 5 687 | 17 900 |
| | 2017 | 72 351 949 | 537 000 | 2 658 314 | 6 225 000 | 78 | 5 352 | 16 400 |
| | 2018 | 74 272 598 | 474 000 | 2 362 979 | 5 553 000 | 74 | 4 757 | 14 700 |
| Gabon | 2010 | 1 624 146 | 122 000 | 288 810 | 597 000 | 400 | 424 | 450 |
| | 2011 | 1 684 629 | 167 000 | 358 358 | 686 000 | 420 | 448 | 490 |
| | 2012 | 1 749 677 | 231 000 | 429 606 | 730 000 | 430 | 469 | 520 |
| | 2013 | 1 817 070 | 285 000 | 495 758 | 799 000 | 450 | 497 | 550 |
| | 2014 | 1 883 801 | 317 000 | 538 273 | 864 000 | 460 | 514 | 580 |
| | 2015 | 1 947 690 | 316 000 | 553 999 | 902 000 | 470 | 523 | 600 |
| | 2016 | 2 007 882 | 284 000 | 543 480 | 933 000 | 460 | 510 | 590 |
| | 2017 | 2 064 812 | 264 000 | 524 958 | 937 000 | 460 | 521 | 610 |
| | 2018 | 2 119 275 | 276 000 | 526 060 | 922 000 | 470 | 528 | 620 |
| Gambia | 2010 | 1 793 199 | 402 000 | 518 727 | 651 000 | 560 | 618 | 690 |
| | 2011 | 1 848 142 | 384 000 | 475 455 | 575 000 | 570 | 629 | 710 |
| | 2012 | 1 905 020 | 420 000 | 523 533 | 637 000 | 580 | 637 | 720 |
| | 2013 | 1 963 708 | 366 000 | 465 386 | 575 000 | 580 | 645 | 740 |
| | 2014 | 2 024 037 | 228 000 | 287 463 | 354 000 | 590 | 654 | 760 |
| | 2015 | 2 085 860 | 321 000 | 406 835 | 499 000 | 590 | 661 | 770 |
| | 2016 | 2 149 134 | 199 000 | 250 439 | 308 000 | 600 | 668 | 780 |
| | 2017 | 2 213 900 | 93 000 | 117 383 | 144 000 | 600 | 677 | 800 |
| | 2018 | 2 280 092 | 119 000 | 150 480 | 184 000 | 610 | 688 | 820 |
| Ghana | 2010 | 24 779 614 | 7 354 000 | 9 023 507 | 10 910 000 | 14 300 | 14 866 | 15 500 |
| | 2011 | 25 387 713 | 7 904 000 | 9 635 269 | 11 650 000 | 14 100 | 14 626 | 15 200 |
| | 2012 | 25 996 454 | 8 005 000 | 9 730 304 | 11 800 000 | 13 500 | 14 092 | 14 700 |
| | 2013 | 26 607 641 | 7 532 000 | 9 293 452 | 11 290 000 | 12 900 | 13 469 | 14 000 |
| | 2014 | 27 224 480 | 6 872 000 | 8 596 537 | 10 630 000 | 12 100 | 12 558 | 13 100 |
| | 2015 | 27 849 203 | 6 040 000 | 7 719 431 | 9 709 000 | 11 300 | 11 757 | 12 300 |
| | 2016 | 28 481 947 | 5 190 000 | 6 721 686 | 8 620 000 | 10 800 | 11 277 | 11 800 |
| | 2017 | 29 121 464 | 4 570 000 | 6 190 041 | 8 182 000 | 10 600 | 11 003 | 11 500 |
| | 2018 | 29 767 108 | 4 187 000 | 6 678 000 | 10 100 000 | 10 600 | 11 070 | 11 700 |
| Guinea | 2010 | 10 192 168 | 3 284 000 | 4 226 309 | 5 365 000 | 12 300 | 13 400 | 14 700 |
| | 2011 | 10 420 459 | 3 599 000 | 4 448 442 | 5 435 000 | 11 800 | 13 003 | 14 300 |
| | 2012 | 10 652 032 | 3 751 000 | 4 556 901 | 5 474 000 | 10 900 | 12 084 | 13 500 |
| | 2013 | 10 892 821 | 3 534 000 | 4 445 128 | 5 537 000 | 9 800 | 11 017 | 12 400 |
| | 2014 | 11 150 970 | 3 216 000 | 4 249 538 | 5 529 000 | 8 840 | 10 017 | 11 500 |
| | 2015 | 11 432 096 | 2 945 000 | 4 077 155 | 5 512 000 | 8 050 | 9 223 | 10 700 |
| | 2016 | 11 738 434 | 2 614 000 | 3 890 993 | 5 570 000 | 7 400 | 8 573 | 10 200 |
| | 2017 | 12 067 516 | 2 312 000 | 3 759 396 | 5 708 000 | 7 020 | 8 234 | 9 900 |
| | 2018 | 12 414 292 | 2 055 000 | 3 524 261 | 5 625 000 | 6 880 | 8 203 | 10 100 |
| Guinea-Bissau | 2010 | 1 522 603 | 133 000 | 204 588 | 303 000 | 610 | 651 | 710 |
| | 2011 | 1 562 996 | 135 000 | 219 683 | 337 000 | 600 | 651 | 710 |
| | 2012 | 1 604 981 | 114 000 | 206 635 | 343 000 | 600 | 646 | 710 |
| | 2013 | 1 648 259 | 86 000 | 186 899 | 355 000 | 590 | 646 | 710 |
| | 2014 | 1 692 433 | 64 000 | 158 919 | 331 000 | 590 | 647 | 720 |
| | 2015 | 1 737 207 | 57 000 | 138 573 | 290 000 | 580 | 637 | 710 |
| | 2016 | 1 782 434 | 44 000 | 127 177 | 292 000 | 600 | 671 | 760 |
| | 2017 | 1 828 146 | 41 000 | 143 200 | 377 000 | 610 | 674 | 770 |
| | 2018 | 1 874 304 | 66 000 | 231 124 | 593 000 | 610 | 680 | 780 |
| Kenya | 2010 | 42 030 684 | 1 658 000 | 2 845 913 | 4 638 000 | 11 100 | 11 456 | 11 800 |
| | 2011 | 43 178 270 | 1 696 000 | 2 930 265 | 4 795 000 | 11 500 | 11 874 | 12 300 |
| | 2012 | 44 343 469 | 1 866 000 | 3 252 855 | 5 394 000 | 11 600 | 12 007 | 12 400 |
| | 2013 | 45 519 986 | 2 112 000 | 3 754 660 | 6 340 000 | 11 700 | 12 106 | 12 600 |
| | 2014 | 46 700 063 | 2 201 000 | 3 916 556 | 6 580 000 | 11 700 | 12 195 | 12 700 |
| | 2015 | 47 878 339 | 1 922 000 | 3 455 175 | 5 783 000 | 11 800 | 12 241 | 12 900 |
| | 2016 | 49 051 531 | 1 921 000 | 3 452 117 | 5 758 000 | 11 800 | 12 280 | 13 000 |
| | 2017 | 50 221 146 | 1 964 000 | 3 520 384 | 5 866 000 | 11 800 | 12 307 | 13 100 |
| | 2018 | 51 392 570 | 2 017 000 | 3 602 498 | 5 997 000 | 11 800 | 12 416 | 13 200 |

| WHO region Country/area | Year | Population at risk | Cases | | | Deaths | | |
|---|---|---|---|---|---|---|---|---|
| | | | Lower | Point | Upper | Lower | Point | Upper |
| **AFRICAN** | | | | | | | | |
| Liberia | 2010 | 3 891 357 | 1 025 000 | 1 345 523 | 1 736 000 | 2 410 | 2 583 | 2 780 |
| | 2011 | 4 017 446 | 1 009 000 | 1 327 415 | 1 718 000 | 2 260 | 2 437 | 2 640 |
| | 2012 | 4 135 662 | 918 000 | 1 273 383 | 1 726 000 | 2 120 | 2 310 | 2 530 |
| | 2013 | 4 248 337 | 916 000 | 1 347 912 | 1 924 000 | 1 970 | 2 157 | 2 390 |
| | 2014 | 4 359 508 | 1 011 000 | 1 471 653 | 2 094 000 | 1 900 | 2 110 | 2 380 |
| | 2015 | 4 472 229 | 1 140 000 | 1 551 740 | 2 039 000 | 1 730 | 1 928 | 2 190 |
| | 2016 | 4 586 788 | 1 422 000 | 1 771 898 | 2 180 000 | 1 770 | 2 001 | 2 330 |
| | 2017 | 4 702 224 | 1 465 000 | 1 886 107 | 2 378 000 | 1 750 | 2 004 | 2 380 |
| | 2018 | 4 818 976 | 1 182 000 | 1 742 079 | 2 447 000 | 1 730 | 2 006 | 2 420 |
| Madagascar | 2010 | 21 151 640 | 523 000 | 893 540 | 1 425 000 | 68 | 2 208 | 5 000 |
| | 2011 | 21 743 970 | 486 000 | 794 810 | 1 161 000 | 61 | 1 964 | 4 140 |
| | 2012 | 22 346 641 | 967 000 | 1 594 592 | 2 516 000 | 130 | 3 941 | 8 730 |
| | 2013 | 22 961 259 | 966 000 | 1 497 292 | 2 298 000 | 120 | 3 701 | 8 010 |
| | 2014 | 23 589 897 | 768 000 | 1 079 845 | 1 448 000 | 93 | 2 669 | 5 200 |
| | 2015 | 24 234 080 | 1 705 000 | 2 358 382 | 3 106 000 | 200 | 5 830 | 11 200 |
| | 2016 | 24 894 370 | 1 034 000 | 1 408 502 | 1 857 000 | 120 | 3 482 | 6 650 |
| | 2017 | 25 570 511 | 1 442 000 | 1 934 794 | 2 488 000 | 170 | 4 783 | 9 020 |
| | 2018 | 26 262 313 | 1 618 000 | 2 163 930 | 2 775 000 | 190 | 5 350 | 10 100 |
| Malawi | 2010 | 14 539 609 | 4 482 000 | 5 612 558 | 6 919 000 | 8 650 | 9 139 | 9 680 |
| | 2011 | 14 962 118 | 4 282 000 | 5 427 890 | 6 785 000 | 8 220 | 8 674 | 9 170 |
| | 2012 | 15 396 010 | 3 741 000 | 4 834 579 | 6 111 000 | 7 960 | 8 420 | 8 940 |
| | 2013 | 15 839 287 | 3 273 000 | 4 242 633 | 5 435 000 | 7 240 | 7 682 | 8 210 |
| | 2014 | 16 289 550 | 2 937 000 | 3 860 686 | 4 953 000 | 6 700 | 7 192 | 7 770 |
| | 2015 | 16 745 305 | 2 752 000 | 3 634 338 | 4 682 000 | 6 310 | 6 846 | 7 520 |
| | 2016 | 17 205 253 | 2 694 000 | 3 624 533 | 4 730 000 | 6 020 | 6 614 | 7 370 |
| | 2017 | 17 670 193 | 2 880 000 | 3 821 420 | 4 982 000 | 5 850 | 6 495 | 7 340 |
| | 2018 | 18 143 215 | 2 678 000 | 3 876 121 | 5 471 000 | 5 780 | 6 478 | 7 460 |
| Mali | 2010 | 15 049 352 | 4 132 000 | 5 772 983 | 7 951 000 | 15 700 | 16 884 | 18 200 |
| | 2011 | 15 514 593 | 4 471 000 | 6 279 267 | 8 582 000 | 17 300 | 18 737 | 20 300 |
| | 2012 | 15 979 492 | 4 942 000 | 6 961 475 | 9 455 000 | 17 700 | 19 306 | 21 000 |
| | 2013 | 16 449 854 | 5 334 000 | 7 448 756 | 10 240 000 | 17 400 | 19 142 | 21 000 |
| | 2014 | 16 934 213 | 5 365 000 | 7 468 113 | 10 370 000 | 15 800 | 17 513 | 19 400 |
| | 2015 | 17 438 772 | 4 827 000 | 6 833 022 | 9 671 000 | 13 800 | 15 478 | 17 400 |
| | 2016 | 17 965 448 | 4 860 000 | 6 902 717 | 9 818 000 | 12 000 | 13 602 | 15 500 |
| | 2017 | 18 512 429 | 5 057 000 | 7 160 192 | 10 190 000 | 10 400 | 12 017 | 13 800 |
| | 2018 | 19 077 755 | 5 200 000 | 7 378 847 | 10 480 000 | 10 100 | 11 848 | 13 800 |
| Mauritania | 2010 | 3 494 200 | 21 000 | 135 686 | 297 000 | 1 030 | 1 155 | 1 350 |
| | 2011 | 3 598 646 | 40 000 | 171 207 | 359 000 | 1 060 | 1 199 | 1 420 |
| | 2012 | 3 706 555 | 24 000 | 105 342 | 233 000 | 1 080 | 1 241 | 1 490 |
| | 2013 | 3 817 497 | 39 000 | 126 803 | 264 000 | 1 100 | 1 260 | 1 530 |
| | 2014 | 3 930 894 | 67 000 | 193 411 | 380 000 | 1 130 | 1 315 | 1 630 |
| | 2015 | 4 046 304 | 98 000 | 249 288 | 468 000 | 1 160 | 1 350 | 1 700 |
| | 2016 | 4 163 532 | 132 000 | 297 695 | 546 000 | 1 170 | 1 365 | 1 740 |
| | 2017 | 4 282 582 | 94 000 | 237 631 | 453 000 | 1 180 | 1 380 | 1 770 |
| | 2018 | 4 403 312 | 81 000 | 173 555 | 298 000 | 1 190 | 1 397 | 1 800 |
| Mozambique | 2010 | 23 531 567 | 7 707 000 | 9 375 217 | 11 280 000 | 15 500 | 16 896 | 18 500 |
| | 2011 | 24 187 500 | 7 749 000 | 9 431 228 | 11 370 000 | 15 400 | 16 935 | 18 800 |
| | 2012 | 24 862 673 | 7 716 000 | 9 492 059 | 11 490 000 | 15 200 | 16 940 | 19 100 |
| | 2013 | 25 560 752 | 7 710 000 | 9 635 885 | 11 850 000 | 14 900 | 16 919 | 19 600 |
| | 2014 | 26 286 192 | 7 778 000 | 9 590 106 | 11 670 000 | 14 300 | 16 451 | 19 400 |
| | 2015 | 27 042 001 | 7 905 000 | 9 623 584 | 11 580 000 | 13 400 | 15 644 | 18 800 |
| | 2016 | 27 829 930 | 7 844 000 | 9 596 334 | 11 620 000 | 12 700 | 14 951 | 18 300 |
| | 2017 | 28 649 007 | 7 505 000 | 9 350 958 | 11 590 000 | 12 100 | 14 412 | 18 000 |
| | 2018 | 29 496 009 | 7 159 000 | 9 006 864 | 11 160 000 | 11 900 | 14 426 | 18 400 |
| Namibia | 2010 | 1 681 850 | 800 | 2 590 | 6 200 | 0 | 6 | 20 |
| | 2011 | 1 711 870 | 2 600 | 3 654 | 5 400 | 0 | 9 | 19 |
| | 2012 | 1 742 095 | 2 700 | 5 861 | 9 700 | 0 | 15 | 36 |
| | 2013 | 1 772 836 | 6 400 | 8 068 | 9 800 | 0 | 20 | 37 |
| | 2014 | 1 804 522 | 21 000 | 26 144 | 32 000 | 2 | 66 | 120 |
| | 2015 | 1 837 443 | 16 000 | 19 990 | 24 000 | 1 | 51 | 93 |
| | 2016 | 1 871 687 | 33 000 | 41 397 | 51 000 | 3 | 105 | 190 |
| | 2017 | 1 907 082 | 71 000 | 89 155 | 109 000 | 7 | 228 | 420 |
| | 2018 | 1 943 338 | 41 000 | 51 898 | 64 000 | 4 | 132 | 240 |
| Niger | 2010 | 16 464 025 | 3 841 000 | 7 007 707 | 10 720 000 | 18 900 | 21 543 | 24 600 |
| | 2011 | 17 114 770 | 4 112 000 | 7 323 097 | 11 180 000 | 18 800 | 21 975 | 25 600 |
| | 2012 | 17 795 209 | 4 442 000 | 7 660 985 | 11 850 000 | 18 100 | 21 678 | 25 900 |
| | 2013 | 18 504 287 | 4 425 000 | 7 780 901 | 12 250 000 | 17 000 | 20 907 | 25 700 |
| | 2014 | 19 240 182 | 4 185 000 | 7 700 900 | 12 430 000 | 15 700 | 19 775 | 25 000 |
| | 2015 | 20 001 663 | 3 920 000 | 7 397 212 | 12 220 000 | 14 200 | 18 392 | 24 000 |
| | 2016 | 20 788 789 | 3 908 000 | 7 457 829 | 12 450 000 | 13 700 | 18 164 | 24 400 |
| | 2017 | 21 602 388 | 4 050 000 | 7 702 777 | 12 850 000 | 12 700 | 17 120 | 23 700 |
| | 2018 | 22 442 831 | 4 215 000 | 8 002 454 | 13 360 000 | 12 300 | 17 084 | 24 200 |

# Annex 3 - F. Population at risk and estimated malaria cases and deaths, 2010–2018

| WHO region Country/area | Year | Population at risk | Cases Lower | Cases Point | Cases Upper | Deaths Lower | Deaths Point | Deaths Upper |
|---|---|---|---|---|---|---|---|---|
| **AFRICAN** | | | | | | | | |
| Nigeria | 2010 | 158 503 203 | 51 570 000 | 63 227 343 | 77 010 000 | 142 000 | 153 437 | 166 000 |
| | 2011 | 162 805 080 | 49 400 000 | 60 654 202 | 73 960 000 | 132 000 | 143 660 | 157 000 |
| | 2012 | 167 228 803 | 46 370 000 | 58 151 864 | 72 090 000 | 124 000 | 136 386 | 150 000 |
| | 2013 | 171 765 819 | 44 150 000 | 56 451 623 | 70 980 000 | 112 000 | 123 585 | 137 000 |
| | 2014 | 176 404 931 | 43 450 000 | 55 462 568 | 69 290 000 | 108 000 | 121 382 | 137 000 |
| | 2015 | 181 137 454 | 42 460 000 | 53 631 431 | 66 830 000 | 98 300 | 111 554 | 128 000 |
| | 2016 | 185 960 244 | 38 610 000 | 52 324 868 | 68 990 000 | 90 600 | 104 403 | 122 000 |
| | 2017 | 190 873 247 | 37 020 000 | 54 029 359 | 76 150 000 | 82 100 | 95 916 | 115 000 |
| | 2018 | 195 874 685 | 38 940 000 | 57 184 148 | 81 230 000 | 80 800 | 95 844 | 117 000 |
| Rwanda | 2010 | 10 039 338 | 852 000 | 1 268 118 | 1 751 000 | 3 020 | 3 132 | 3 260 |
| | 2011 | 10 293 333 | 301 000 | 404 386 | 514 000 | 2 970 | 3 098 | 3 260 |
| | 2012 | 10 549 668 | 595 000 | 753 855 | 916 000 | 2 940 | 3 092 | 3 290 |
| | 2013 | 10 811 538 | 1 095 000 | 1 313 059 | 1 550 000 | 2 920 | 3 088 | 3 320 |
| | 2014 | 11 083 629 | 1 827 000 | 2 436 249 | 3 069 000 | 2 920 | 3 100 | 3 370 |
| | 2015 | 11 369 066 | 2 892 000 | 3 887 798 | 4 907 000 | 2 920 | 3 123 | 3 420 |
| | 2016 | 11 668 829 | 5 035 000 | 6 832 535 | 8 707 000 | 2 950 | 3 153 | 3 480 |
| | 2017 | 11 980 960 | 4 706 000 | 6 449 821 | 8 267 000 | 2 980 | 3 194 | 3 550 |
| | 2018 | 12 301 969 | 4 369 000 | 5 984 752 | 7 678 000 | 3 020 | 3 244 | 3 630 |
| Sao Tome and Principe[1,2] | 2010 | 180 372 | – | 2 740 | – | – | 14 | – |
| | 2011 | 184 521 | – | 8 442 | – | – | 19 | – |
| | 2012 | 188 394 | – | 10 701 | – | – | 7 | – |
| | 2013 | 192 076 | – | 9 243 | – | – | 11 | – |
| | 2014 | 195 727 | – | 1 754 | – | – | 0 | – |
| | 2015 | 199 439 | – | 2 058 | – | – | 0 | – |
| | 2016 | 203 221 | – | 2 238 | – | – | 1 | – |
| | 2017 | 207 086 | – | 2 239 | – | – | 1 | – |
| | 2018 | 211 032 | – | 2 937 | – | – | 0 | – |
| Senegal | 2010 | 12 678 143 | 526 000 | 751 511 | 1 001 000 | 4 090 | 4 194 | 4 310 |
| | 2011 | 13 033 814 | 455 000 | 650 480 | 867 000 | 4 080 | 4 187 | 4 310 |
| | 2012 | 13 401 990 | 522 000 | 762 806 | 1 032 000 | 4 060 | 4 166 | 4 290 |
| | 2013 | 13 782 429 | 659 000 | 935 859 | 1 238 000 | 4 050 | 4 159 | 4 290 |
| | 2014 | 14 174 740 | 410 000 | 560 097 | 732 000 | 4 140 | 4 279 | 4 450 |
| | 2015 | 14 578 450 | 692 000 | 1 017 535 | 1 381 000 | 4 170 | 4 331 | 4 530 |
| | 2016 | 14 993 514 | 468 000 | 684 544 | 920 000 | 4 190 | 4 373 | 4 600 |
| | 2017 | 15 419 354 | 561 000 | 807 277 | 1 072 000 | 4 220 | 4 418 | 4 680 |
| | 2018 | 15 854 324 | 618 000 | 883 919 | 1 163 000 | 4 260 | 4 480 | 4 780 |
| Sierra Leone | 2010 | 6 415 636 | 2 295 000 | 2 943 081 | 3 698 000 | 13 100 | 14 100 | 15 100 |
| | 2011 | 6 563 238 | 2 319 000 | 2 977 428 | 3 753 000 | 11 800 | 12 757 | 13 700 |
| | 2012 | 6 712 586 | 2 390 000 | 3 003 669 | 3 738 000 | 10 000 | 10 831 | 11 700 |
| | 2013 | 6 863 975 | 2 304 000 | 2 970 027 | 3 765 000 | 8 390 | 9 151 | 9 990 |
| | 2014 | 7 017 153 | 2 187 000 | 2 872 180 | 3 698 000 | 7 220 | 7 975 | 8 820 |
| | 2015 | 7 171 909 | 2 255 000 | 2 895 435 | 3 672 000 | 6 530 | 7 329 | 8 210 |
| | 2016 | 7 328 846 | 2 311 000 | 2 868 006 | 3 530 000 | 6 110 | 6 983 | 7 940 |
| | 2017 | 7 488 427 | 2 000 000 | 2 726 766 | 3 625 000 | 5 830 | 6 786 | 7 860 |
| | 2018 | 7 650 149 | 1 433 000 | 2 451 110 | 3 979 000 | 5 520 | 6 564 | 7 770 |
| South Africa[1,2] | 2010 | 5 121 696 | – | 8 060 | – | – | 83 | – |
| | 2011 | 5 200 375 | – | 9 866 | – | – | 54 | – |
| | 2012 | 5 283 265 | – | 6 621 | – | – | 72 | – |
| | 2013 | 5 368 712 | – | 8 645 | – | – | 105 | – |
| | 2014 | 5 454 418 | – | 11 705 | – | – | 174 | – |
| | 2015 | 5 538 636 | – | 1 157 | – | – | 110 | – |
| | 2016 | 5 620 764 | – | 4 323 | – | – | 34 | – |
| | 2017 | 5 700 975 | – | 22 517 | – | – | 301 | – |
| | 2018 | 5 779 252 | – | 9 540 | – | – | 69 | – |
| South Sudan[4] | 2010 | 9 508 372 | 1 464 000 | 2 319 793 | 3 495 000 | 4 360 | 5 010 | 5 810 |
| | 2011 | 9 830 695 | 1 428 000 | 2 318 780 | 3 552 000 | 4 180 | 4 841 | 5 660 |
| | 2012 | 10 113 648 | 1 449 000 | 2 353 290 | 3 599 000 | 4 020 | 4 678 | 5 520 |
| | 2013 | 10 355 030 | 1 485 000 | 2 427 031 | 3 747 000 | 3 980 | 4 695 | 5 620 |
| | 2014 | 10 554 882 | 1 531 000 | 2 492 468 | 3 867 000 | 4 080 | 4 910 | 6 080 |
| | 2015 | 10 715 657 | 1 576 000 | 2 575 568 | 3 926 000 | 4 100 | 5 056 | 6 440 |
| | 2016 | 10 832 520 | 1 598 000 | 2 649 109 | 4 068 000 | 4 120 | 5 188 | 6 800 |
| | 2017 | 10 910 774 | 1 627 000 | 2 681 845 | 4 161 000 | 4 130 | 5 328 | 7 230 |
| | 2018 | 10 975 924 | 1 578 000 | 2 589 443 | 4 048 000 | 4 080 | 5 356 | 7 490 |
| Togo | 2010 | 6 421 674 | 1 489 000 | 1 983 506 | 2 596 000 | 4 520 | 4 947 | 5 420 |
| | 2011 | 6 595 939 | 1 570 000 | 2 067 173 | 2 686 000 | 4 280 | 4 715 | 5 200 |
| | 2012 | 6 773 807 | 1 855 000 | 2 368 811 | 2 987 000 | 4 100 | 4 554 | 5 050 |
| | 2013 | 6 954 721 | 2 182 000 | 2 680 257 | 3 253 000 | 4 040 | 4 532 | 5 080 |
| | 2014 | 7 137 997 | 2 247 000 | 2 745 866 | 3 324 000 | 4 240 | 4 812 | 5 470 |
| | 2015 | 7 323 162 | 2 170 000 | 2 667 930 | 3 237 000 | 4 430 | 5 129 | 5 950 |
| | 2016 | 7 509 952 | 1 953 000 | 2 439 684 | 3 008 000 | 4 440 | 5 244 | 6 220 |
| | 2017 | 7 698 476 | 1 678 000 | 2 141 714 | 2 694 000 | 4 310 | 5 199 | 6 320 |
| | 2018 | 7 889 095 | 1 508 000 | 2 108 823 | 2 901 000 | 4 170 | 5 132 | 6 410 |

| WHO region Country/area | Year | Population at risk | Cases | | | Deaths | | |
|---|---|---|---|---|---|---|---|---|
| | | | Lower | Point | Upper | Lower | Point | Upper |
| **AFRICAN** | | | | | | | | |
| Uganda | 2010 | 32 428 164 | 10 870 000 | 13 533 746 | 16 620 000 | 19 300 | 20 412 | 21 700 |
| | 2011 | 33 476 772 | 10 210 000 | 12 912 102 | 16 120 000 | 16 400 | 17 358 | 18 500 |
| | 2012 | 34 558 700 | 8 748 000 | 11 465 552 | 14 640 000 | 14 000 | 14 920 | 15 900 |
| | 2013 | 35 694 519 | 6 542 000 | 9 074 826 | 12 200 000 | 12 600 | 13 402 | 14 300 |
| | 2014 | 36 911 530 | 5 749 000 | 8 143 369 | 11 020 000 | 12 100 | 13 029 | 14 000 |
| | 2015 | 38 225 447 | 6 554 000 | 9 025 492 | 12 200 000 | 11 800 | 12 800 | 14 000 |
| | 2016 | 39 649 173 | 9 342 000 | 12 069 689 | 15 300 000 | 11 800 | 13 036 | 14 500 |
| | 2017 | 41 166 588 | 10 840 000 | 13 863 230 | 17 470 000 | 11 800 | 13 272 | 15 000 |
| | 2018 | 42 729 032 | 7 623 000 | 12 356 577 | 18 970 000 | 11 700 | 13 203 | 15 200 |
| United Republic of Tanzania | 2010 | 44 346 532 | 4 688 000 | 6 450 494 | 8 725 000 | 18 600 | 19 241 | 20 000 |
| | 2011 | 45 673 520 | 4 389 000 | 6 050 835 | 8 096 000 | 18 500 | 19 107 | 19 800 |
| | 2012 | 47 053 033 | 3 992 000 | 5 469 691 | 7 351 000 | 18 400 | 19 127 | 19 900 |
| | 2013 | 48 483 132 | 3 944 000 | 5 419 407 | 7 268 000 | 19 100 | 19 946 | 20 900 |
| | 2014 | 49 960 563 | 4 368 000 | 5 942 515 | 7 966 000 | 19 300 | 20 253 | 21 300 |
| | 2015 | 51 482 638 | 4 569 000 | 6 267 687 | 8 287 000 | 19 600 | 20 624 | 21 900 |
| | 2016 | 53 049 231 | 4 818 000 | 6 555 045 | 8 675 000 | 19 800 | 20 922 | 22 400 |
| | 2017 | 54 660 345 | 5 025 000 | 6 775 567 | 8 955 000 | 19 900 | 21 163 | 22 900 |
| | 2018 | 56 313 444 | 4 677 000 | 6 997 809 | 10 090 000 | 20 100 | 21 550 | 23 500 |
| Zambia | 2010 | 13 605 986 | 1 885 000 | 2 408 568 | 3 042 000 | 6 080 | 6 286 | 6 520 |
| | 2011 | 14 023 199 | 2 067 000 | 2 618 128 | 3 274 000 | 6 250 | 6 479 | 6 740 |
| | 2012 | 14 465 148 | 2 270 000 | 2 937 598 | 3 724 000 | 6 480 | 6 739 | 7 030 |
| | 2013 | 14 926 551 | 2 599 000 | 3 369 958 | 4 296 000 | 6 640 | 6 935 | 7 270 |
| | 2014 | 15 399 793 | 2 632 000 | 3 433 829 | 4 420 000 | 6 930 | 7 303 | 7 720 |
| | 2015 | 15 879 370 | 2 410 000 | 3 216 354 | 4 211 000 | 6 960 | 7 389 | 7 890 |
| | 2016 | 16 363 449 | 2 042 000 | 2 968 175 | 4 180 000 | 6 930 | 7 417 | 8 030 |
| | 2017 | 16 853 608 | 1 730 000 | 2 697 352 | 3 997 000 | 6 860 | 7 419 | 8 140 |
| | 2018 | 17 351 714 | 1 709 000 | 2 719 036 | 4 096 000 | 6 890 | 7 519 | 8 390 |
| Zimbabwe | 2010 | 9 998 533 | 606 000 | 1 094 108 | 1 709 000 | 73 | 2 800 | 6 220 |
| | 2011 | 10 153 338 | 468 000 | 717 620 | 989 000 | 52 | 1 837 | 3 690 |
| | 2012 | 10 327 222 | 402 000 | 590 910 | 793 000 | 44 | 1 512 | 3 010 |
| | 2013 | 10 512 448 | 613 000 | 861 512 | 1 122 000 | 66 | 2 205 | 4 280 |
| | 2014 | 10 698 542 | 805 000 | 1 090 113 | 1 397 000 | 86 | 2 790 | 5 320 |
| | 2015 | 10 878 022 | 717 000 | 1 062 200 | 1 448 000 | 80 | 2 719 | 5 430 |
| | 2016 | 11 047 866 | 489 000 | 726 722 | 995 000 | 54 | 1 860 | 3 740 |
| | 2017 | 11 210 282 | 805 000 | 1 216 876 | 1 710 000 | 90 | 3 115 | 6 410 |
| | 2018 | 11 369 510 | 393 000 | 579 888 | 789 000 | 43 | 1 484 | 2 960 |
| **AMERICAS** | | | | | | | | |
| Argentina[1,2,3] | 2010 | 204 478 | – | 14 | – | – | 0 | – |
| | 2011 | 206 602 | – | 0 | – | – | 0 | – |
| | 2012 | 208 775 | – | 0 | – | – | 0 | – |
| | 2013 | 210 980 | – | 0 | – | – | 0 | – |
| | 2014 | 213 187 | – | 0 | – | – | 0 | – |
| | 2015 | 215 377 | – | 0 | – | – | 0 | – |
| | 2016 | 217 542 | – | 0 | – | – | 0 | – |
| | 2017 | 219 685 | – | 0 | – | – | 0 | – |
| | 2018 | 221 805 | – | 0 | – | – | 0 | – |
| Belize[1,2] | 2010 | 222 500 | – | 150 | – | – | 0 | – |
| | 2011 | 227 862 | – | 72 | – | – | 0 | – |
| | 2012 | 233 220 | – | 33 | – | – | 0 | – |
| | 2013 | 238 537 | – | 20 | – | – | 0 | – |
| | 2014 | 243 822 | – | 19 | – | – | 0 | – |
| | 2015 | 249 038 | – | 9 | – | – | 0 | – |
| | 2016 | 254 195 | – | 4 | – | – | 0 | – |
| | 2017 | 259 284 | – | 7 | – | – | 0 | – |
| | 2018 | 264 318 | – | 3 | – | – | 0 | – |
| Bolivia (Plurinational State of) | 2010 | 4 558 757 | 15 000 | 18 659 | 23 000 | 2 | 10 | 18 |
| | 2011 | 4 633 319 | 7 600 | 9 680 | 12 000 | 1 | 4 | 8 |
| | 2012 | 4 708 051 | 8 600 | 10 972 | 13 000 | 1 | 4 | 8 |
| | 2013 | 4 782 769 | 8 500 | 10 804 | 13 000 | 1 | 6 | 11 |
| | 2014 | 4 857 236 | 8 500 | 10 952 | 13 000 | 1 | 4 | 8 |
| | 2015 | 4 931 282 | 7 300 | 9 315 | 11 000 | 1 | 3 | 6 |
| | 2016 | 5 004 817 | 5 900 | 7 510 | 9 200 | 0 | 2 | 5 |
| | 2017 | 5 077 861 | 4 800 | 6 195 | 7 600 | 0 | 2 | 4 |
| | 2018 | 5 150 579 | 5 700 | 7 239 | 8 900 | 0 | 2 | 4 |
| Brazil[2] | 2010 | 39 729 868 | 349 000 | 389 809 | 422 000 | – | 76 | – |
| | 2011 | 40 095 451 | 273 000 | 284 024 | 303 000 | – | 70 | – |
| | 2012 | 40 455 320 | 248 000 | 258 095 | 275 000 | – | 60 | – |
| | 2013 | 40 810 288 | 176 000 | 196 793 | 213 000 | – | 40 | – |
| | 2014 | 41 161 040 | 142 000 | 148 071 | 158 000 | – | 36 | – |
| | 2015 | 41 507 767 | 144 000 | 161 093 | 174 000 | – | 35 | – |
| | 2016 | 41 851 100 | 129 000 | 134 862 | 144 000 | – | 35 | – |
| | 2017 | 42 190 266 | 197 000 | 220 848 | 239 000 | – | 34 | – |
| | 2018 | 42 522 271 | 207 000 | 217 900 | 232 000 | – | 44 | – |

# Annex 3 – F. Population at risk and estimated malaria cases and deaths, 2010–2018

| WHO region Country/area | Year | Population at risk | Cases | | | Deaths | | |
|---|---|---|---|---|---|---|---|---|
| | | | Lower | Point | Upper | Lower | Point | Upper |
| **AMERICAS** | | | | | | | | |
| Colombia[2] | 2010 | 10 011 898 | 125 000 | 164 479 | 206 000 | – | 42 | – |
| | 2011 | 10 109 321 | 64 000 | 84 072 | 105 000 | – | 23 | – |
| | 2012 | 10 200 749 | 64 000 | 84 176 | 105 000 | – | 24 | – |
| | 2013 | 10 293 683 | 55 000 | 72 310 | 91 000 | – | 10 | – |
| | 2014 | 10 398 227 | 43 000 | 57 024 | 71 000 | – | 17 | – |
| | 2015 | 10 520 647 | 54 000 | 73 007 | 94 000 | – | 18 | – |
| | 2016 | 10 665 522 | 88 000 | 115 550 | 145 000 | – | 36 | – |
| | 2017 | 10 828 150 | 60 000 | 80 963 | 104 000 | – | 19 | – |
| | 2018 | 10 994 461 | 71 000 | 93 468 | 117 000 | – | 9 | – |
| Costa Rica[1,2] | 2010 | 1 602 079 | – | 110 | – | – | 0 | – |
| | 2011 | 1 621 580 | – | 10 | – | – | 0 | – |
| | 2012 | 1 640 801 | – | 6 | – | – | 0 | – |
| | 2013 | 1 659 738 | – | 0 | – | – | 0 | – |
| | 2014 | 1 678 386 | – | 0 | – | – | 0 | – |
| | 2015 | 1 696 731 | – | 0 | – | – | 0 | – |
| | 2016 | 1 714 767 | – | 4 | – | – | 0 | – |
| | 2017 | 1 732 484 | – | 12 | – | – | 0 | – |
| | 2018 | 1 749 805 | – | 70 | – | – | 0 | – |
| Dominican Republic | 2010 | 5 340 225 | 2 600 | 3 202 | 3 800 | 0 | 8 | 14 |
| | 2011 | 5 405 278 | 1 700 | 2 088 | 2 500 | 0 | 5 | 9 |
| | 2012 | 5 470 107 | 1 000 | 1 232 | 1 500 | 0 | 3 | 5 |
| | 2013 | 5 534 723 | 610 | 751 | 900 | 0 | 1 | 3 |
| | 2014 | 5 599 144 | 480 | 566 | 660 | 0 | 1 | 2 |
| | 2015 | 5 663 311 | 660 | 779 | 910 | 0 | 1 | 3 |
| | 2016 | 5 727 240 | 760 | 933 | 1 100 | 0 | 2 | 4 |
| | 2017 | 5 790 831 | 300 | 349 | 400 | 0 | 0 | 1 |
| | 2018 | 5 853 645 | 600 | 704 | 820 | 0 | 1 | 3 |
| Ecuador[1,2] | 2010 | 437 453 | – | 1 871 | – | – | 0 | – |
| | 2011 | 444 237 | – | 1 219 | – | – | 0 | – |
| | 2012 | 450 946 | – | 544 | – | – | 0 | – |
| | 2013 | 457 747 | – | 368 | – | – | 0 | – |
| | 2014 | 464 868 | – | 242 | – | – | 0 | – |
| | 2015 | 472 450 | – | 618 | – | – | 0 | – |
| | 2016 | 480 584 | – | 1 191 | – | – | 0 | – |
| | 2017 | 489 125 | – | 1 275 | – | – | 0 | – |
| | 2018 | 497 838 | – | 1 653 | – | – | 0 | – |
| El Salvador[1,2] | 2010 | 1 255 327 | – | 19 | – | – | 0 | – |
| | 2011 | 1 260 745 | – | 10 | – | – | 0 | – |
| | 2012 | 1 266 298 | – | 13 | – | – | 0 | – |
| | 2013 | 1 272 013 | – | 6 | – | – | 0 | – |
| | 2014 | 1 277 910 | – | 6 | – | – | 0 | – |
| | 2015 | 1 283 999 | – | 2 | – | – | 0 | – |
| | 2016 | 1 290 295 | – | 12 | – | – | 0 | – |
| | 2017 | 1 296 789 | – | 0 | – | – | 0 | – |
| | 2018 | 1 303 410 | – | 0 | – | – | 0 | – |
| French Guiana | 2010 | 128 915 | 1 800 | 2 260 | 2 900 | 0 | 4 | 8 |
| | 2011 | 131 893 | 1 300 | 1 412 | 1 600 | 0 | 2 | 4 |
| | 2012 | 134 816 | 940 | 1 052 | 1 200 | 0 | 2 | 3 |
| | 2013 | 137 797 | 960 | 1 123 | 1 300 | 0 | 2 | 3 |
| | 2014 | 140 961 | 480 | 541 | 620 | 0 | 0 | 1 |
| | 2015 | 144 406 | 410 | 460 | 530 | – | 0 | – |
| | 2016 | 148 180 | 240 | 267 | 310 | – | 0 | – |
| | 2017 | 152 257 | 610 | 681 | 780 | – | 0 | – |
| | 2018 | 156 543 | 230 | 444 | 710 | – | 0 | – |
| Guatemala | 2010 | 11 044 796 | 7 900 | 9 657 | 12 000 | 1 | 3 | 6 |
| | 2011 | 11 285 142 | 7 100 | 7 961 | 9 200 | 1 | 2 | 5 |
| | 2012 | 11 528 212 | 5 600 | 6 251 | 7 200 | 0 | 2 | 3 |
| | 2013 | 11 773 597 | 6 500 | 7 263 | 8 400 | 0 | 2 | 4 |
| | 2014 | 12 020 770 | 5 900 | 6 625 | 7 600 | 0 | 2 | 4 |
| | 2015 | 12 269 280 | 7 100 | 7 967 | 9 200 | 1 | 2 | 5 |
| | 2016 | 12 518 897 | 5 100 | 5 656 | 6 500 | 0 | 2 | 3 |
| | 2017 | 12 769 455 | 3 900 | 4 380 | 5 000 | 0 | 1 | 2 |
| | 2018 | 13 020 750 | 3 100 | 3 521 | 4 000 | 0 | 1 | 2 |
| Guyana | 2010 | 749 430 | 26 000 | 32 823 | 41 000 | 3 | 56 | 100 |
| | 2011 | 752 029 | 34 000 | 41 096 | 49 000 | 4 | 76 | 130 |
| | 2012 | 755 388 | 36 000 | 43 584 | 52 000 | 5 | 76 | 130 |
| | 2013 | 759 281 | 43 000 | 57 459 | 79 000 | 7 | 90 | 170 |
| | 2014 | 763 371 | 17 000 | 22 310 | 31 000 | 2 | 27 | 53 |
| | 2015 | 767 433 | 14 000 | 18 030 | 25 000 | 1 | 22 | 41 |
| | 2016 | 771 363 | 14 000 | 19 269 | 26 000 | 2 | 24 | 46 |
| | 2017 | 775 218 | 19 000 | 25 235 | 35 000 | 3 | 33 | 63 |
| | 2018 | 779 007 | 26 000 | 34 565 | 47 000 | 4 | 43 | 83 |

| WHO region Country/area | Year | Population at risk | Cases | | | Deaths | | |
|---|---|---|---|---|---|---|---|---|
| | | | Lower | Point | Upper | Lower | Point | Upper |
| **AMERICAS** | | | | | | | | |
| Haiti | 2010 | 8 888 919 | 44 000 | 77 638 | 125 000 | 5 | 198 | 450 |
| | 2011 | 9 023 827 | 50 000 | 81 483 | 127 000 | 5 | 208 | 460 |
| | 2012 | 9 158 378 | 36 000 | 59 798 | 92 000 | 4 | 153 | 340 |
| | 2013 | 9 292 168 | 30 000 | 49 387 | 77 000 | 3 | 126 | 280 |
| | 2014 | 9 424 693 | 22 000 | 32 932 | 45 000 | 2 | 84 | 170 |
| | 2015 | 9 555 609 | 22 000 | 32 829 | 44 000 | 2 | 84 | 170 |
| | 2016 | 9 684 651 | 24 000 | 36 765 | 50 000 | 2 | 94 | 190 |
| | 2017 | 9 811 866 | 23 000 | 34 878 | 47 000 | 2 | 89 | 180 |
| | 2018 | 9 937 674 | 11 000 | 16 000 | 22 000 | 1 | 40 | 81 |
| Honduras | 2010 | 7 533 978 | 10 000 | 13 306 | 16 000 | 2 | 7 | 13 |
| | 2011 | 7 681 807 | 8 000 | 10 124 | 12 000 | 1 | 5 | 8 |
| | 2012 | 7 826 756 | 6 800 | 8 677 | 11 000 | 1 | 4 | 7 |
| | 2013 | 7 969 720 | 5 700 | 7 317 | 8 900 | 1 | 5 | 10 |
| | 2014 | 8 111 981 | 3 600 | 4 553 | 5 600 | 0 | 3 | 5 |
| | 2015 | 8 254 486 | 3 800 | 4 849 | 5 900 | 0 | 4 | 7 |
| | 2016 | 8 397 503 | 4 800 | 6 230 | 7 800 | 0 | 6 | 11 |
| | 2017 | 8 540 802 | 1 500 | 1 876 | 2 300 | 0 | 0 | 1 |
| | 2018 | 8 684 378 | 900 | 1 154 | 1 400 | – | 0 | – |
| Mexico[1,2] | 2010 | 2 419 227 | – | 1 226 | – | – | 0 | – |
| | 2011 | 2 453 206 | – | 1 124 | – | – | 0 | – |
| | 2012 | 2 486 681 | – | 833 | – | – | 0 | – |
| | 2013 | 2 519 611 | – | 495 | – | – | 0 | – |
| | 2014 | 2 552 010 | – | 656 | – | – | 0 | – |
| | 2015 | 2 583 882 | – | 517 | – | – | 0 | – |
| | 2016 | 2 615 160 | – | 551 | – | – | 0 | – |
| | 2017 | 2 645 279 | – | 736 | – | – | 0 | – |
| | 2018 | 2 675 244 | – | 803 | – | – | 0 | – |
| Nicaragua | 2010 | 2 542 195 | 730 | 876 | 1 000 | – | 0 | – |
| | 2011 | 2 576 668 | 970 | 1 171 | 1 400 | – | 0 | – |
| | 2012 | 2 611 368 | 1 300 | 1 564 | 1 800 | 0 | 0 | 1 |
| | 2013 | 2 646 258 | 1 200 | 1 471 | 1 700 | 0 | 0 | 1 |
| | 2014 | 2 681 297 | 1 200 | 1 446 | 1 700 | – | 0 | – |
| | 2015 | 2 716 435 | 2 400 | 2 886 | 3 400 | 0 | 1 | 2 |
| | 2016 | 2 751 676 | 6 600 | 7 943 | 9 400 | 1 | 6 | 10 |
| | 2017 | 2 786 983 | 12 000 | 13 866 | 16 000 | 2 | 10 | 16 |
| | 2018 | 2 822 191 | 17 000 | 20 158 | 24 000 | 3 | 10 | 18 |
| Panama[2] | 2010 | 3 524 055 | 420 | 440 | 470 | – | 1 | – |
| | 2011 | 3 585 766 | 360 | 372 | 400 | – | 0 | – |
| | 2012 | 3 647 832 | 860 | 888 | 950 | – | 1 | – |
| | 2013 | 3 710 534 | 720 | 751 | 800 | – | 0 | – |
| | 2014 | 3 774 253 | 960 | 1 007 | 1 100 | – | 0 | – |
| | 2015 | 3 839 244 | 550 | 575 | 610 | – | 0 | – |
| | 2016 | 3 905 593 | 780 | 809 | 860 | – | 0 | – |
| | 2017 | 3 973 006 | 760 | 801 | 860 | – | 0 | – |
| | 2018 | 4 040 827 | 750 | 786 | 840 | – | 0 | – |
| Paraguay[1,2,3] | 2010 | 224 928 | – | 18 | – | – | 0 | – |
| | 2011 | 228 023 | – | 1 | – | – | 0 | – |
| | 2012 | 231 174 | – | 0 | – | – | 0 | – |
| | 2013 | 234 369 | – | 0 | – | – | 0 | – |
| | 2014 | 237 582 | – | 0 | – | – | 0 | – |
| | 2015 | 240 794 | – | 0 | – | – | 0 | – |
| | 2016 | 244 003 | – | 0 | – | – | 0 | – |
| | 2017 | 247 214 | – | 0 | – | – | 0 | – |
| | 2018 | 250 418 | – | 0 | – | – | 0 | – |
| Peru[2] | 2010 | 11 400 969 | 33 000 | 37 849 | 43 000 | – | 0 | – |
| | 2011 | 11 493 910 | 26 000 | 30 924 | 36 000 | – | 1 | – |
| | 2012 | 11 589 145 | 33 000 | 40 437 | 48 000 | – | 7 | – |
| | 2013 | 11 694 090 | 51 000 | 62 669 | 75 000 | – | 4 | – |
| | 2014 | 11 818 354 | 69 000 | 83 936 | 100 000 | – | 4 | – |
| | 2015 | 11 967 748 | 76 000 | 93 936 | 113 000 | – | 5 | – |
| | 2016 | 12 146 571 | 60 000 | 72 836 | 87 000 | – | 7 | – |
| | 2017 | 12 350 062 | 59 000 | 72 518 | 86 000 | – | 10 | – |
| | 2018 | 12 564 103 | 48 000 | 58 455 | 70 000 | – | 4 | – |
| Suriname[1,2] | 2010 | 78 151 | – | 1 823 | – | – | 1 | – |
| | 2011 | 79 045 | – | 771 | – | – | 1 | – |
| | 2012 | 79 942 | – | 554 | – | – | 0 | – |
| | 2013 | 80 835 | – | 729 | – | – | 1 | – |
| | 2014 | 81 719 | – | 401 | – | – | 1 | – |
| | 2015 | 82 584 | – | 81 | – | – | 0 | – |
| | 2016 | 83 433 | – | 76 | – | – | 0 | – |
| | 2017 | 84 262 | – | 40 | – | – | 1 | – |
| | 2018 | 85 073 | – | 29 | – | – | 0 | – |

# Annex 3 - F. Population at risk and estimated malaria cases and deaths, 2010–2018

| WHO region Country/area | Year | Population at risk | Cases | | | Deaths | | |
|---|---|---|---|---|---|---|---|---|
| | | | Lower | Point | Upper | Lower | Point | Upper |
| **AMERICAS** | | | | | | | | |
| Venezuela (Bolivarian Republic of) | 2010 | 14 219 971 | 48 000 | 57 926 | 74 000 | 8 | 53 | 91 |
| | 2011 | 14 443 936 | 48 000 | 53 539 | 62 000 | 8 | 47 | 77 |
| | 2012 | 14 680 413 | 55 000 | 61 768 | 71 000 | 9 | 56 | 92 |
| | 2013 | 14 890 523 | 82 000 | 91 924 | 106 000 | 13 | 104 | 170 |
| | 2014 | 15 021 486 | 94 000 | 105 721 | 122 000 | 15 | 110 | 180 |
| | 2015 | 15 040 913 | 142 000 | 158 987 | 182 000 | 25 | 149 | 240 |
| | 2016 | 14 925 624 | 251 000 | 280 468 | 321 000 | 44 | 260 | 420 |
| | 2017 | 14 701 240 | 428 000 | 479 761 | 549 000 | 78 | 421 | 680 |
| | 2018 | 14 443 558 | 422 000 | 471 995 | 541 000 | 75 | 423 | 680 |
| **EASTERN MEDITERRANEAN** | | | | | | | | |
| Afghanistan | 2010 | 22 496 454 | 171 000 | 339 820 | 571 000 | 54 | 192 | 400 |
| | 2011 | 23 214 771 | 204 000 | 438 076 | 736 000 | 65 | 232 | 480 |
| | 2012 | 24 019 470 | 126 000 | 267 829 | 467 000 | 33 | 113 | 240 |
| | 2013 | 24 873 691 | 126 000 | 224 236 | 370 000 | 34 | 103 | 210 |
| | 2014 | 25 722 516 | 220 000 | 325 811 | 461 000 | 54 | 156 | 290 |
| | 2015 | 26 526 314 | 263 000 | 395 552 | 561 000 | 66 | 187 | 340 |
| | 2016 | 27 273 556 | 506 000 | 712 132 | 975 000 | 120 | 341 | 610 |
| | 2017 | 27 977 405 | 573 000 | 757 412 | 982 000 | 140 | 353 | 620 |
| | 2018 | 28 652 489 | 633 000 | 831 091 | 1 068 000 | 140 | 383 | 670 |
| Djibouti[1,2] | 2010 | 630 077 | – | 1 010 | – | – | 0 | – |
| | 2011 | 640 184 | 1 700 | 2 189 | 2 700 | – | 0 | – |
| | 2012 | 651 032 | 1 700 | 2 153 | 2 600 | – | 0 | – |
| | 2013 | 662 401 | – | 1 684 | – | – | 17 | – |
| | 2014 | 673 958 | – | 9 439 | – | – | 28 | – |
| | 2015 | 685 425 | – | 9 473 | – | – | 23 | – |
| | 2016 | 696 763 | – | 13 804 | – | – | 5 | – |
| | 2017 | 707 999 | – | 14 671 | – | – | 0 | – |
| | 2018 | 719 115 | – | 25 319 | – | – | 0 | – |
| Egypt[1,2] | 2010 | 82 761 244 | – | 0 | – | – | 0 | – |
| | 2011 | 84 529 251 | – | 0 | – | – | 0 | – |
| | 2012 | 86 422 240 | – | 0 | – | – | 0 | – |
| | 2013 | 88 404 652 | – | 0 | – | – | 0 | – |
| | 2014 | 90 424 668 | – | 0 | – | – | 0 | – |
| | 2015 | 92 442 549 | – | 0 | – | – | 0 | – |
| | 2016 | 94 447 071 | – | 0 | – | – | 0 | – |
| | 2017 | 96 442 590 | – | 0 | – | – | 0 | – |
| | 2018 | 98 423 602 | – | 0 | – | – | 0 | – |
| Iran (Islamic Republic of)[1,2] | 2010 | 753 410 | – | 1 847 | – | – | 0 | – |
| | 2011 | 762 321 | – | 1 632 | – | – | 0 | – |
| | 2012 | 771 564 | – | 756 | – | – | 0 | – |
| | 2013 | 781 186 | – | 479 | – | – | 0 | – |
| | 2014 | 791 235 | – | 358 | – | – | 0 | – |
| | 2015 | 801 719 | – | 167 | – | – | 0 | – |
| | 2016 | 812 666 | – | 81 | – | – | 0 | – |
| | 2017 | 823 680 | – | 60 | – | – | 0 | – |
| | 2018 | 835 180 | – | 0 | – | – | 0 | – |
| Morocco[1,2,3] | 2010 | 32 343 384 | – | 0 | – | – | 0 | – |
| | 2011 | 32 781 860 | – | 0 | – | – | 0 | – |
| | 2012 | 33 241 898 | – | 0 | – | – | 0 | – |
| | 2013 | 33 715 705 | – | 0 | – | – | 0 | – |
| | 2014 | 34 192 358 | – | 0 | – | – | 0 | – |
| | 2015 | 34 663 608 | – | 0 | – | – | 0 | – |
| | 2016 | 35 126 274 | – | 0 | – | – | 0 | – |
| | 2017 | 35 581 257 | – | 0 | – | – | 0 | – |
| | 2018 | 36 029 089 | – | 0 | – | – | 0 | – |
| Oman[1,2] | 2010 | 3 041 435 | – | 7 | – | – | 0 | – |
| | 2011 | 3 251 102 | – | 0 | – | – | 0 | – |
| | 2012 | 3 498 031 | – | 0 | – | – | 0 | – |
| | 2013 | 3 764 805 | – | 0 | – | – | 0 | – |
| | 2014 | 4 027 255 | – | 0 | – | – | 0 | – |
| | 2015 | 4 267 341 | – | 0 | – | – | 0 | – |
| | 2016 | 4 479 217 | – | 0 | – | – | 0 | – |
| | 2017 | 4 665 926 | – | 0 | – | – | 0 | – |
| | 2018 | 4 829 476 | – | 0 | – | – | 0 | – |
| Pakistan | 2010 | 176 393 981 | 640 000 | 1 445 704 | 3 037 000 | 190 | 1 616 | 4 280 |
| | 2011 | 180 243 369 | 918 000 | 1 905 938 | 3 739 000 | 280 | 1 814 | 4 360 |
| | 2012 | 184 116 776 | 774 000 | 1 652 576 | 3 284 000 | 220 | 1 703 | 4 270 |
| | 2013 | 188 030 212 | 750 000 | 1 419 225 | 2 716 000 | 220 | 1 047 | 2 420 |
| | 2014 | 192 006 115 | 724 000 | 1 373 305 | 2 723 000 | 220 | 897 | 2 100 |
| | 2015 | 196 058 432 | 526 000 | 992 598 | 2 028 000 | 160 | 716 | 1 780 |
| | 2016 | 200 191 818 | 800 000 | 1 202 476 | 1 996 000 | 200 | 1 012 | 2 110 |
| | 2017 | 204 394 674 | 707 000 | 970 992 | 1 468 000 | 160 | 756 | 1 430 |
| | 2018 | 208 643 752 | 545 000 | 705 532 | 987 000 | 120 | 495 | 880 |

| WHO region Country/area | Year | Population at risk | Cases | | | Deaths | | |
|---|---|---|---|---|---|---|---|---|
| | | | Lower | Point | Upper | Lower | Point | Upper |
| **EASTERN MEDITERRANEAN** | | | | | | | | |
| Saudi Arabia[1,2] | 2010 | 2 196 624 | – | 29 | – | – | 0 | – |
| | 2011 | 2 264 403 | – | 69 | – | – | 0 | – |
| | 2012 | 2 335 482 | – | 82 | – | – | 0 | – |
| | 2013 | 2 407 350 | – | 34 | – | – | 0 | – |
| | 2014 | 2 476 605 | – | 30 | – | – | 0 | – |
| | 2015 | 2 540 776 | – | 83 | – | – | 0 | – |
| | 2016 | 2 598 914 | – | 272 | – | – | 0 | – |
| | 2017 | 2 651 735 | – | 177 | – | – | 0 | – |
| | 2018 | 2 699 927 | – | 61 | – | – | 0 | – |
| Somalia | 2010 | 12 043 886 | 214 000 | 356 323 | 526 000 | 24 | 912 | 2 000 |
| | 2011 | 12 376 305 | 181 000 | 301 405 | 441 000 | 20 | 771 | 1 680 |
| | 2012 | 12 715 487 | 188 000 | 310 864 | 454 000 | 21 | 795 | 1 730 |
| | 2013 | 13 063 711 | 223 000 | 366 378 | 546 000 | 26 | 937 | 2 070 |
| | 2014 | 13 423 571 | 265 000 | 430 886 | 640 000 | 30 | 1 103 | 2 440 |
| | 2015 | 13 797 204 | 304 000 | 514 253 | 769 000 | 35 | 1 316 | 2 920 |
| | 2016 | 14 185 635 | 311 000 | 528 591 | 795 000 | 35 | 1 353 | 3 020 |
| | 2017 | 14 589 165 | 320 000 | 541 768 | 813 000 | 37 | 1 386 | 3 100 |
| | 2018 | 15 008 225 | 305 000 | 514 396 | 772 000 | 35 | 1 316 | 2 960 |
| Sudan | 2010 | 34 545 014 | 779 000 | 1 059 304 | 1 405 000 | 87 | 2 711 | 5 160 |
| | 2011 | 35 349 676 | 781 000 | 1 059 374 | 1 400 000 | 88 | 2 711 | 5 090 |
| | 2012 | 36 193 781 | 797 000 | 1 091 647 | 1 457 000 | 90 | 2 794 | 5 400 |
| | 2013 | 37 072 555 | 812 000 | 1 166 089 | 1 645 000 | 92 | 2 985 | 5 900 |
| | 2014 | 37 977 657 | 827 000 | 1 267 868 | 1 843 000 | 97 | 3 245 | 6 680 |
| | 2015 | 38 902 948 | 847 000 | 1 395 818 | 2 202 000 | 100 | 3 573 | 7 710 |
| | 2016 | 39 847 433 | 842 000 | 1 662 933 | 2 933 000 | 110 | 4 257 | 10 100 |
| | 2017 | 40 813 398 | 871 000 | 1 908 105 | 3 652 000 | 120 | 4 884 | 12 100 |
| | 2018 | 41 801 532 | 904 000 | 1 954 302 | 3 686 000 | 120 | 5 003 | 12 300 |
| Syrian Arab Republic[1,2] | 2010 | 21 362 541 | – | 0 | – | – | 0 | – |
| | 2011 | 21 081 814 | – | 0 | – | – | 0 | – |
| | 2012 | 20 438 861 | – | 0 | – | – | 0 | – |
| | 2013 | 19 578 466 | – | 0 | – | – | 0 | – |
| | 2014 | 18 710 711 | – | 0 | – | – | 0 | – |
| | 2015 | 17 997 411 | – | 0 | – | – | 0 | – |
| | 2016 | 17 465 567 | – | 0 | – | – | 0 | – |
| | 2017 | 17 095 669 | – | 0 | – | – | 0 | – |
| | 2018 | 16 945 062 | – | 0 | – | – | 0 | – |
| United Arab Emirates[1,2,3] | 2010 | 8 549 998 | – | 0 | – | – | 0 | – |
| | 2011 | 8 946 778 | – | 0 | – | – | 0 | – |
| | 2012 | 9 141 598 | – | 0 | – | – | 0 | – |
| | 2013 | 9 197 908 | – | 0 | – | – | 0 | – |
| | 2014 | 9 214 182 | – | 0 | – | – | 0 | – |
| | 2015 | 9 262 896 | – | 0 | – | – | 0 | – |
| | 2016 | 9 360 975 | – | 0 | – | – | 0 | – |
| | 2017 | 9 487 206 | – | 0 | – | – | 0 | – |
| | 2018 | 9 630 966 | – | 0 | – | – | 0 | – |
| Yemen | 2010 | 18 035 338 | 649 000 | 1 131 912 | 2 191 000 | 82 | 2 866 | 7 350 |
| | 2011 | 18 543 752 | 492 000 | 792 413 | 1 326 000 | 60 | 2 013 | 4 620 |
| | 2012 | 19 062 181 | 577 000 | 859 569 | 1 302 000 | 67 | 2 193 | 4 690 |
| | 2013 | 19 587 110 | 494 000 | 700 432 | 1 006 000 | 56 | 1 786 | 3 670 |
| | 2014 | 20 113 940 | 412 000 | 585 987 | 850 000 | 46 | 1 495 | 3 080 |
| | 2015 | 20 639 226 | 362 000 | 513 816 | 737 000 | 40 | 1 309 | 2 700 |
| | 2016 | 17 515 888 | 464 000 | 661 252 | 949 000 | 54 | 1 668 | 3 420 |
| | 2017 | 17 945 659 | 525 000 | 747 173 | 1 073 000 | 64 | 1 853 | 3 800 |
| | 2018 | 18 373 670 | 587 000 | 842 226 | 1 233 000 | 68 | 2 138 | 4 400 |
| **EUROPEAN** | | | | | | | | |
| Armenia[1,2,3] | 2010 | 2 877 314 | – | 0 | – | – | 0 | – |
| | 2011 | 2 876 536 | – | 0 | – | – | 0 | – |
| | 2012 | 2 884 239 | – | 0 | – | – | 0 | – |
| | 2013 | 2 897 593 | – | 0 | – | – | 0 | – |
| | 2014 | 2 912 403 | – | 0 | – | – | 0 | – |
| | 2015 | 2 925 559 | – | 0 | – | – | 0 | – |
| | 2016 | 2 936 147 | – | 0 | – | – | 0 | – |
| | 2017 | 2 944 789 | – | 0 | – | – | 0 | – |
| | 2018 | 2 951 741 | – | 0 | – | – | 0 | – |
| Azerbaijan[1,2] | 2010 | 207 746 | – | 50 | – | – | 0 | – |
| | 2011 | 210 364 | – | 4 | – | – | 0 | – |
| | 2012 | 213 087 | – | 3 | – | – | 0 | – |
| | 2013 | 215 865 | – | 0 | – | – | 0 | – |
| | 2014 | 218 629 | – | 0 | – | – | 0 | – |
| | 2015 | 221 323 | – | 0 | – | – | 0 | – |
| | 2016 | 223 928 | – | 0 | – | – | 0 | – |
| | 2017 | 226 442 | – | 0 | – | – | 0 | – |
| | 2018 | 228 839 | – | 0 | – | – | 0 | – |

# Annex 3 – F. Population at risk and estimated malaria cases and deaths, 2010–2018

| WHO region Country/area | Year | Population at risk | Cases | | | Deaths | | |
|---|---|---|---|---|---|---|---|---|
| | | | Lower | Point | Upper | Lower | Point | Upper |
| **EUROPEAN** | | | | | | | | |
| Georgia[1,2] | 2010 | 40 990 | – | 0 | – | – | 0 | – |
| | 2011 | 40 810 | – | 0 | – | – | 0 | – |
| | 2012 | 40 640 | – | 0 | – | – | 0 | – |
| | 2013 | 40 487 | – | 0 | – | – | 0 | – |
| | 2014 | 40 353 | – | 0 | – | – | 0 | – |
| | 2015 | 40 241 | – | 0 | – | – | 0 | – |
| | 2016 | 40 154 | – | 0 | – | – | 0 | – |
| | 2017 | 40 087 | – | 0 | – | – | 0 | – |
| | 2018 | 40 029 | – | 0 | – | – | 0 | – |
| Kazakhstan[1,2] | 2010 | 16 252 273 | – | 0 | – | – | 0 | – |
| | 2011 | 16 490 669 | – | 0 | – | – | 0 | – |
| | 2012 | 16 751 523 | – | 0 | – | – | 0 | – |
| | 2013 | 17 026 118 | – | 0 | – | – | 0 | – |
| | 2014 | 17 302 619 | – | 0 | – | – | 0 | – |
| | 2015 | 17 572 010 | – | 0 | – | – | 0 | – |
| | 2016 | 17 830 902 | – | 0 | – | – | 0 | – |
| | 2017 | 18 080 023 | – | 0 | – | – | 0 | – |
| | 2018 | 18 319 616 | – | 0 | – | – | 0 | – |
| Kyrgyzstan[1,2,3] | 2010 | 4 229 392 | – | 3 | – | – | 0 | – |
| | 2011 | 4 303 983 | – | 0 | – | – | 0 | – |
| | 2012 | 4 384 834 | – | 0 | – | – | 0 | – |
| | 2013 | 4 470 423 | – | 0 | – | – | 0 | – |
| | 2014 | 4 558 726 | – | 0 | – | – | 0 | – |
| | 2015 | 4 648 118 | – | 0 | – | – | 0 | – |
| | 2016 | 4 737 975 | – | 0 | – | – | 0 | – |
| | 2017 | 4 827 987 | – | 0 | – | – | 0 | – |
| | 2018 | 4 917 139 | – | 0 | – | – | 0 | – |
| Tajikistan[1,2] | 2010 | 2 514 150 | – | 111 | – | – | 0 | – |
| | 2011 | 2 570 967 | – | 65 | – | – | 0 | – |
| | 2012 | 2 630 195 | – | 18 | – | – | 0 | – |
| | 2013 | 2 691 967 | – | 3 | – | – | 0 | – |
| | 2014 | 2 756 444 | – | 2 | – | – | 0 | – |
| | 2015 | 2 823 642 | – | 0 | – | – | 0 | – |
| | 2016 | 2 893 634 | – | 0 | – | – | 0 | – |
| | 2017 | 2 966 010 | – | 0 | – | – | 0 | – |
| | 2018 | 3 039 682 | – | 0 | – | – | 0 | – |
| Turkey[1,2] | 2010 | 4 701 254 | – | 0 | – | – | 0 | – |
| | 2011 | 4 773 811 | – | 0 | – | – | 0 | – |
| | 2012 | 4 852 317 | – | 0 | – | – | 0 | – |
| | 2013 | 4 935 154 | – | 0 | – | – | 0 | – |
| | 2014 | 5 019 902 | – | 0 | – | – | 0 | – |
| | 2015 | 5 104 411 | – | 0 | – | – | 0 | – |
| | 2016 | 5 188 811 | – | 0 | – | – | 0 | – |
| | 2017 | 5 272 569 | – | 0 | – | – | 0 | – |
| | 2018 | 5 352 105 | – | 0 | – | – | 0 | – |
| Turkmenistan[1,2,3] | 2010 | 5 087 211 | – | 0 | – | – | 0 | – |
| | 2011 | 5 174 076 | – | 0 | – | – | 0 | – |
| | 2012 | 5 267 906 | – | 0 | – | – | 0 | – |
| | 2013 | 5 366 376 | – | 0 | – | – | 0 | – |
| | 2014 | 5 466 324 | – | 0 | – | – | 0 | – |
| | 2015 | 5 565 283 | – | 0 | – | – | 0 | – |
| | 2016 | 5 662 371 | – | 0 | – | – | 0 | – |
| | 2017 | 5 757 667 | – | 0 | – | – | 0 | – |
| | 2018 | 5 850 902 | – | 0 | – | – | 0 | – |
| Uzbekistan[1,2,3] | 2010 | 2 028 390 | – | 0 | – | – | 0 | – |
| | 2011 | 2 061 459 | – | 0 | – | – | 0 | – |
| | 2012 | 2 095 284 | – | 0 | – | – | 0 | – |
| | 2013 | 2 129 847 | – | 0 | – | – | 0 | – |
| | 2014 | 2 165 068 | – | 0 | – | – | 0 | – |
| | 2015 | 2 200 922 | – | 0 | – | – | 0 | – |
| | 2016 | 2 237 184 | – | 0 | – | – | 0 | – |
| | 2017 | 2 273 336 | – | 0 | – | – | 0 | – |
| | 2018 | 2273336 | – | 0 | – | – | 0 | – |
| **SOUTH-EAST ASIA** | | | | | | | | |
| Bangladesh | 2010 | 15 868 196 | 59 000 | 68 774 | 80 000 | 6 | 165 | 290 |
| | 2011 | 16 050 743 | 54 000 | 63 356 | 73 000 | 5 | 155 | 270 |
| | 2012 | 16 237 042 | 31 000 | 35 747 | 41 000 | 3 | 87 | 150 |
| | 2013 | 16 425 823 | 23 000 | 25 366 | 29 000 | 2 | 60 | 100 |
| | 2014 | 16 614 636 | 49 000 | 54 801 | 61 000 | 4 | 133 | 220 |
| | 2015 | 16 801 613 | 41 000 | 45 658 | 51 000 | 4 | 109 | 180 |
| | 2016 | 16 986 651 | 29 000 | 31 662 | 35 000 | 2 | 74 | 120 |
| | 2017 | 17 170 973 | 30 000 | 33 444 | 37 000 | 2 | 77 | 130 |
| | 2018 | 17 352 837 | 11 000 | 12 021 | 13 000 | 0 | 26 | 44 |

| WHO region Country/area | Year | Population at risk | Cases | | | Deaths | | |
|---|---|---|---|---|---|---|---|---|
| | | | Lower | Point | Upper | Lower | Point | Upper |
| **SOUTH-EAST ASIA** | | | | | | | | |
| Bhutan[1,2] | 2010 | 507 271 | – | 526 | – | – | 2 | – |
| | 2011 | 513 039 | – | 228 | – | – | 1 | – |
| | 2012 | 519 170 | – | 82 | – | – | 1 | – |
| | 2013 | 525 573 | – | 15 | – | – | 0 | – |
| | 2014 | 532 099 | – | 19 | – | – | 0 | – |
| | 2015 | 538 634 | – | 34 | – | – | 0 | – |
| | 2016 | 545 162 | – | 15 | – | – | 0 | – |
| | 2017 | 551 716 | – | 11 | – | – | 0 | – |
| | 2018 | 558 253 | – | 6 | – | – | 0 | – |
| Democratic People's Republic of Korea[1,2] | 2010 | 9 585 831 | – | 13 520 | – | – | 0 | – |
| | 2011 | 9 634 466 | – | 16 760 | – | – | 0 | – |
| | 2012 | 9 684 153 | – | 21 850 | – | – | 0 | – |
| | 2013 | 9 734 471 | – | 14 407 | – | – | 0 | – |
| | 2014 | 9 784 567 | – | 10 535 | – | – | 0 | – |
| | 2015 | 9 833 782 | – | 7 409 | – | – | 0 | – |
| | 2016 | 9 882 137 | – | 2 719 | – | – | 0 | – |
| | 2017 | 9 929 834 | – | 4 575 | – | – | 0 | – |
| | 2018 | 9 976 610 | – | 3 598 | – | – | 0 | – |
| India | 2010 | 1 153 311 084 | 14 840 000 | 20 200 000 | 28 480 000 | 2 730 | 30 495 | 57 800 |
| | 2011 | 1 168 267 799 | 12 770 000 | 17 240 000 | 24 290 000 | 2 370 | 25 574 | 48 300 |
| | 2012 | 1 182 743 793 | 10 290 000 | 14 020 000 | 19 840 000 | 1 920 | 20 433 | 38 800 |
| | 2013 | 1 196 817 595 | 8 172 000 | 10 960 000 | 15 210 000 | 1 490 | 16 706 | 31 200 |
| | 2014 | 1 210 608 062 | 8 383 000 | 11 140 000 | 15 520 000 | 1 350 | 20 128 | 37 700 |
| | 2015 | 1 224 205 084 | 8 941 000 | 11 840 000 | 16 220 000 | 1 470 | 21 667 | 40 900 |
| | 2016 | 1 237 627 593 | 8 826 000 | 12 370 000 | 17 930 000 | 1 550 | 22 316 | 44 500 |
| | 2017 | 1 250 859 582 | 6 832 000 | 9 348 000 | 13 250 000 | 1 210 | 16 310 | 31 700 |
| | 2018 | 1 263 908 949 | 4 659 000 | 6 737 000 | 9 541 000 | 930 | 9 620 | 18 300 |
| Indonesia | 2010 | 241 834 226 | 2 120 000 | 2 665 491 | 3 501 000 | 370 | 4 260 | 8 000 |
| | 2011 | 245 115 988 | 1 930 000 | 2 424 712 | 3 190 000 | 330 | 3 820 | 7 160 |
| | 2012 | 248 451 714 | 1 913 000 | 2 405 245 | 3 147 000 | 320 | 3 785 | 7 120 |
| | 2013 | 251 805 314 | 1 632 000 | 2 047 233 | 2 686 000 | 270 | 3 256 | 6 100 |
| | 2014 | 255 128 076 | 1 241 000 | 1 556 734 | 2 041 000 | 210 | 2 510 | 4 700 |
| | 2015 | 258 383 257 | 1 108 000 | 1 391 240 | 1 830 000 | 190 | 2 190 | 4 080 |
| | 2016 | 261 556 386 | 1 154 000 | 1 448 007 | 1 896 000 | 190 | 2 516 | 4 740 |
| | 2017 | 264 650 969 | 1 428 000 | 1 792 690 | 2 338 000 | 230 | 3 138 | 5 890 |
| | 2018 | 267 670 549 | 933 000 | 1 034 866 | 1 154 000 | 140 | 1 785 | 2 930 |
| Myanmar | 2010 | 30 116 448 | 1 384 000 | 2 017 346 | 3 108 000 | 230 | 3 882 | 8 320 |
| | 2011 | 30 348 439 | 1 014 000 | 1 319 917 | 1 761 000 | 160 | 2 466 | 4 620 |
| | 2012 | 30 600 253 | 1 355 000 | 1 892 905 | 2 749 000 | 220 | 3 680 | 7 500 |
| | 2013 | 30 861 393 | 455 000 | 611 838 | 840 000 | 74 | 1 169 | 2 290 |
| | 2014 | 31 116 339 | 281 000 | 383 705 | 535 000 | 46 | 729 | 1 440 |
| | 2015 | 31 354 355 | 220 000 | 272 329 | 328 000 | 34 | 482 | 850 |
| | 2016 | 31 571 282 | 131 000 | 161 570 | 195 000 | 20 | 273 | 480 |
| | 2017 | 31 772 208 | 98 000 | 120 755 | 145 000 | 15 | 209 | 370 |
| | 2018 | 31 966 116 | 88 000 | 108 815 | 131 000 | 14 | 172 | 300 |
| Nepal | 2010 | 7 841 339 | 15 000 | 30 320 | 63 000 | 3 | 27 | 70 |
| | 2011 | 7 849 471 | 14 000 | 23 802 | 45 000 | 3 | 9 | 23 |
| | 2012 | 7 834 359 | 12 000 | 18 349 | 33 000 | 2 | 9 | 20 |
| | 2013 | 7 813 353 | 7 000 | 10 222 | 18 000 | 1 | 6 | 14 |
| | 2014 | 7 810 214 | 3 000 | 4 885 | 9 800 | 0 | 3 | 8 |
| | 2015 | 7 841 869 | 2 500 | 4 483 | 9 600 | 0 | 2 | 7 |
| | 2016 | 7 913 973 | 2 300 | 3 372 | 5 900 | 0 | 2 | 4 |
| | 2017 | 8 021 214 | 2 500 | 3 104 | 4 100 | 0 | 1 | 2 |
| | 2018 | 8 155 623 | 2 600 | 3 588 | 5 300 | 0 | 1 | 2 |
| Sri Lanka[1,2,3] | 2010 | 4 660 199 | – | 684 | – | – | 0 | – |
| | 2011 | 4 691 654 | – | 124 | – | – | 0 | – |
| | 2012 | 4 722 497 | – | 23 | – | – | 0 | – |
| | 2013 | 4 752 502 | – | 0 | – | – | 0 | – |
| | 2014 | 4 781 357 | – | 0 | – | – | 0 | – |
| | 2015 | 4 808 845 | – | 0 | – | – | 0 | – |
| | 2016 | 4 834 870 | – | 0 | – | – | 0 | – |
| | 2017 | 4 859 446 | – | 0 | – | – | 0 | – |
| | 2018 | 4 882 614 | – | 0 | – | – | 0 | – |
| Thailand[1,2] | 2010 | 12 751 063 | – | 32 480 | – | – | 80 | – |
| | 2011 | 12 812 422 | – | 24 897 | – | – | 43 | – |
| | 2012 | 12 872 689 | – | 32 569 | – | – | 37 | – |
| | 2013 | 12 931 240 | – | 33 302 | – | – | 47 | – |
| | 2014 | 12 987 073 | – | 37 921 | – | – | 38 | – |
| | 2015 | 13 039 404 | – | 17 427 | – | – | 33 | – |
| | 2016 | 13 088 134 | – | 13 451 | – | – | 27 | – |
| | 2017 | 13 133 254 | – | 12 515 | – | – | 15 | – |
| | 2018 | 13 174 743 | – | 4 782 | – | – | 8 | – |

# Annex 3 - F. Population at risk and estimated malaria cases and deaths, 2010–2018

| WHO region Country/area | Year | Population at risk | Cases | | | Deaths | | |
|---|---|---|---|---|---|---|---|---|
| | | | Lower | Point | Upper | Lower | Point | Upper |
| **SOUTH-EAST ASIA** | | | | | | | | |
| Timor-Leste | 2010 | 1 028 463 | 72 000 | 102 579 | 136 000 | 11 | 198 | 380 |
| | 2011 | 1 046 931 | 26 000 | 32 736 | 41 000 | 3 | 69 | 130 |
| | 2012 | 1 065 599 | 6 500 | 7 740 | 9 100 | 0 | 10 | 17 |
| | 2013 | 1 084 678 | 1 400 | 1 692 | 2 000 | 0 | 2 | 3 |
| | 2014 | 1 104 471 | 480 | 568 | 660 | 0 | 0 | 1 |
| | 2015 | 1 125 125 | 120 | 139 | 160 | – | 0 | – |
| | 2016 | 1 146 752 | 110 | 130 | 150 | – | 0 | – |
| | 2017 | 1 169 297 | 31 | 37 | 43 | – | 0 | – |
| | 2018 | 1 192 542 | – | 0 | – | – | 0 | – |
| **WESTERN PACIFIC** | | | | | | | | |
| Cambodia | 2010 | 10 121 505 | 292 000 | 353 293 | 428 000 | 45 | 644 | 1 120 |
| | 2011 | 10 283 605 | 321 000 | 368 041 | 426 000 | 47 | 641 | 1 080 |
| | 2012 | 10 452 648 | 226 000 | 260 016 | 301 000 | 35 | 383 | 640 |
| | 2013 | 10 626 530 | 147 000 | 168 806 | 196 000 | 23 | 231 | 380 |
| | 2014 | 10 802 038 | 208 000 | 240 449 | 282 000 | 31 | 399 | 670 |
| | 2015 | 10 976 665 | 189 000 | 218 837 | 255 000 | 28 | 374 | 630 |
| | 2016 | 11 149 825 | 107 000 | 124 137 | 145 000 | 16 | 204 | 340 |
| | 2017 | 11 321 696 | 175 000 | 202 696 | 237 000 | 27 | 336 | 560 |
| | 2018 | 11 491 692 | 235 000 | 272 272 | 320 000 | 42 | 265 | 430 |
| China[1,2] | 2010 | 575 598 390 | – | 4 990 | – | – | 19 | – |
| | 2011 | 578 835 356 | – | 3 367 | – | – | 33 | – |
| | 2012 | 582 081 652 | – | 244 | – | – | 0 | – |
| | 2013 | 585 315 386 | – | 86 | – | – | 0 | – |
| | 2014 | 588 506 114 | – | 56 | – | – | 0 | – |
| | 2015 | 591 624 804 | – | 39 | – | – | 0 | – |
| | 2016 | 594 665 143 | – | 3 | – | – | 0 | – |
| | 2017 | 597 615 756 | – | 0 | – | – | 0 | – |
| | 2018 | 600 418 023 | – | 0 | – | – | 0 | – |
| Lao People's Democratic Republic | 2010 | 3 251 667 | 36 000 | 51 184 | 69 000 | 3 | 127 | 250 |
| | 2011 | 3 302 866 | 26 000 | 35 886 | 48 000 | 2 | 85 | 160 |
| | 2012 | 3 353 319 | 70 000 | 96 451 | 127 000 | 9 | 211 | 400 |
| | 2013 | 3 403 674 | 58 000 | 79 309 | 105 000 | 9 | 145 | 280 |
| | 2014 | 3 454 907 | 75 000 | 103 303 | 137 000 | 13 | 157 | 300 |
| | 2015 | 3 507 668 | 57 000 | 78 225 | 103 000 | 10 | 100 | 190 |
| | 2016 | 3 562 141 | 20 000 | 27 668 | 37 000 | 3 | 33 | 62 |
| | 2017 | 3 617 940 | 15 000 | 20 357 | 27 000 | 2 | 29 | 56 |
| | 2018 | 3 674 379 | 11 000 | 15 437 | 20 000 | 1 | 23 | 44 |
| Malaysia[1,2] | 2010 | 1 128 321 | – | 5 194 | – | – | 13 | – |
| | 2011 | 1 146 038 | – | 3 954 | – | – | 12 | – |
| | 2012 | 1 162 727 | – | 3 662 | – | – | 12 | – |
| | 2013 | 1 178 756 | – | 2 921 | – | – | 10 | – |
| | 2014 | 1 194 664 | – | 3 147 | – | – | 4 | – |
| | 2015 | 1 210 838 | – | 242 | – | – | 4 | – |
| | 2016 | 1 227 386 | – | 266 | – | – | 2 | – |
| | 2017 | 1 244 186 | – | 85 | – | – | 10 | – |
| | 2018 | 1 261 121 | – | 0 | – | – | 12 | – |
| Papua New Guinea | 2010 | 7 310 512 | 463 000 | 1 240 109 | 2 159 000 | 110 | 2 633 | 6 270 |
| | 2011 | 7 472 196 | 389 000 | 1 045 967 | 1 826 000 | 87 | 2 344 | 5 580 |
| | 2012 | 7 631 003 | 420 000 | 1 296 356 | 2 600 000 | 100 | 2 793 | 7 230 |
| | 2013 | 7 788 388 | 952 000 | 1 677 722 | 2 572 000 | 140 | 4 043 | 8 660 |
| | 2014 | 7 946 733 | 1 177 000 | 1 931 287 | 2 943 000 | 220 | 3 728 | 7 750 |
| | 2015 | 8 107 772 | 739 000 | 1 066 533 | 1 461 000 | 120 | 2 227 | 4 310 |
| | 2016 | 8 271 766 | 1 056 000 | 1 469 150 | 1 965 000 | 160 | 3 108 | 5 970 |
| | 2017 | 8 438 038 | 1 036 000 | 1 500 657 | 2 077 000 | 170 | 3 053 | 5 970 |
| | 2018 | 8 606 324 | 1 096 000 | 1 587 573 | 2 180 000 | 180 | 3 124 | 6 060 |
| Philippines | 2010 | 54 570 270 | 37 000 | 53 401 | 71 000 | 5 | 112 | 220 |
| | 2011 | 55 501 350 | 17 000 | 23 891 | 31 000 | 2 | 47 | 90 |
| | 2012 | 56 455 267 | 14 000 | 19 138 | 25 000 | 1 | 35 | 67 |
| | 2013 | 57 418 668 | 13 000 | 17 518 | 23 000 | 1 | 35 | 68 |
| | 2014 | 58 371 999 | 11 000 | 14 543 | 19 000 | 0 | 31 | 59 |
| | 2015 | 59 301 223 | 20 000 | 28 020 | 37 000 | 2 | 62 | 120 |
| | 2016 | 60 201 722 | 12 000 | 17 491 | 23 000 | 1 | 38 | 74 |
| | 2017 | 61 078 122 | 13 000 | 18 685 | 25 000 | 1 | 41 | 81 |
| | 2018 | 61 936 730 | 7 700 | 10 947 | 15 000 | 0 | 24 | 48 |
| Republic of Korea[1,2] | 2010 | 3 468 194 | – | 1 267 | – | – | 1 | – |
| | 2011 | 3 485 030 | – | 505 | – | – | 2 | – |
| | 2012 | 3 504 244 | – | 394 | – | – | 0 | – |
| | 2013 | 3 524 200 | – | 383 | – | – | 0 | – |
| | 2014 | 3 542 553 | – | 557 | – | – | 0 | – |
| | 2015 | 3 557 616 | – | 627 | – | – | 0 | – |
| | 2016 | 3 568 841 | – | 602 | – | – | 0 | – |
| | 2017 | 3 576 748 | – | 436 | – | – | 0 | – |
| | 2018 | 3 582 019 | – | 501 | – | – | 0 | – |

| WHO region Country/area | Year | Population at risk | Cases | | | Deaths | | |
|---|---|---|---|---|---|---|---|---|
| | | | Lower | Point | Upper | Lower | Point | Upper |
| **WESTERN PACIFIC** | | | | | | | | |
| Solomon Islands | 2010 | 522 582 | 65 000 | 91 425 | 130 000 | 10 | 163 | 320 |
| | 2011 | 536 106 | 44 000 | 62 676 | 92 000 | 7 | 108 | 220 |
| | 2012 | 550 505 | 39 000 | 52 221 | 73 000 | 6 | 89 | 170 |
| | 2013 | 565 615 | 40 000 | 53 689 | 74 000 | 6 | 83 | 160 |
| | 2014 | 581 208 | 25 000 | 30 591 | 38 000 | 3 | 48 | 87 |
| | 2015 | 597 101 | 33 000 | 39 916 | 49 000 | 5 | 57 | 99 |
| | 2016 | 613 243 | 72 000 | 84 451 | 101 000 | 12 | 103 | 170 |
| | 2017 | 629 669 | 80 000 | 103 482 | 139 000 | 15 | 134 | 250 |
| | 2018 | 646 327 | 75 000 | 86 343 | 101 000 | 12 | 109 | 180 |
| Vanuatu | 2010 | 236 216 | 13 000 | 15 669 | 19 000 | 1 | 20 | 35 |
| | 2011 | 242 658 | 8 900 | 11 631 | 16 000 | 1 | 14 | 27 |
| | 2012 | 249 505 | 6 500 | 8 394 | 11 000 | – | 0 | – |
| | 2013 | 256 637 | 4 100 | 5 326 | 7 200 | – | 0 | – |
| | 2014 | 263 888 | 1 900 | 2 427 | 3 300 | – | 0 | – |
| | 2015 | 271 128 | 680 | 787 | 920 | – | 0 | – |
| | 2016 | 278 326 | 3 200 | 4 177 | 5 600 | – | 0 | – |
| | 2017 | 285 499 | 1 700 | 2 266 | 3 000 | – | 0 | – |
| | 2018 | 292 675 | 900 | 1 167 | 1 600 | – | 0 | – |
| Viet Nam | 2010 | 64 831 194 | 21 000 | 22 959 | 26 000 | 2 | 45 | 76 |
| | 2011 | 65 497 232 | 19 000 | 20 206 | 23 000 | 2 | 35 | 58 |
| | 2012 | 66 183 031 | 22 000 | 23 838 | 27 000 | 2 | 40 | 66 |
| | 2013 | 66 883 662 | 19 000 | 20 760 | 23 000 | 2 | 33 | 55 |
| | 2014 | 67 592 098 | 18 000 | 19 060 | 21 000 | 2 | 29 | 47 |
| | 2015 | 68 301 989 | 10 000 | 11 283 | 13 000 | 1 | 16 | 25 |
| | 2016 | 69 011 970 | 4 600 | 5 024 | 5 600 | 0 | 7 | 13 |
| | 2017 | 69 719 633 | 5 100 | 5 481 | 6 100 | 0 | 9 | 15 |
| | 2018 | 70 416 320 | 5 300 | 5 794 | 6 500 | 0 | 9 | 16 |

Data as of 19 November 2019

"–" refers to not applicable.

[1] The number of indigenous malaria cases registered by the NMPs is reported here without further adjustments.

[2] The number of indigenous malaria deaths registered by the NMPs is reported here without further adjustments.

[3] Certified malaria free countries are included in this listing for historical purposes.

[4] South Sudan became an independent state on 9 July 2011 and a Member State of WHO on 27 September 2011. South Sudan and Sudan have distinct epidemiological profiles comprising high-transmission and low-transmission areas respectively. For this reason, data up to June 2011 from the Sudanese high-transmission areas (10 southern states, which correspond to South Sudan) and low-transmission areas (15 northern states which correspond to contemporary Sudan) are reported separately.

# Annex 3 - F. Population at risk and estimated malaria cases and deaths, 2010–2018

| WHO region | Year | Population at risk | Cases | | | Deaths | | |
|---|---|---|---|---|---|---|---|---|
| | | | Lower | Point | Upper | Lower | Point | Upper |
| **REGIONAL SUMMARY** | | | | | | | | |
| African | 2010 | 742 051 480 | 199 000 000 | 219 000 000 | 245 000 000 | 507 000 | 533 000 | 588 000 |
| | 2011 | 763 387 315 | 194 000 000 | 213 000 000 | 237 000 000 | 469 000 | 493 000 | 537 000 |
| | 2012 | 785 260 919 | 190 000 000 | 209 000 000 | 233 000 000 | 444 000 | 469 000 | 514 000 |
| | 2013 | 807 674 747 | 185 000 000 | 204 000 000 | 229 000 000 | 419 000 | 444 000 | 493 000 |
| | 2014 | 830 636 558 | 181 000 000 | 198 000 000 | 218 000 000 | 408 000 | 428 000 | 462 000 |
| | 2015 | 854 147 991 | 184 000 000 | 199 000 000 | 219 000 000 | 391 000 | 411 000 | 448 000 |
| | 2016 | 878 208 734 | 189 000 000 | 206 000 000 | 229 000 000 | 371 000 | 389 000 | 425 000 |
| | 2017 | 902 801 325 | 192 000 000 | 212 000 000 | 240 000 000 | 364 000 | 383 000 | 423 000 |
| | 2018 | 927 888 238 | 191 000 000 | 213 000 000 | 244 000 000 | 361 000 | 380 000 | 425 000 |
| Americas | 2010 | 126 118 119 | 744 000 | 814 000 | 894 000 | 220 | 459 | 730 |
| | 2011 | 127 739 647 | 566 000 | 611 000 | 666 000 | 180 | 444 | 710 |
| | 2012 | 129 364 372 | 541 000 | 580 000 | 627 000 | 180 | 392 | 600 |
| | 2013 | 130 969 261 | 520 000 | 562 000 | 613 000 | 180 | 391 | 590 |
| | 2014 | 132 522 297 | 445 000 | 477 000 | 512 000 | 140 | 289 | 420 |
| | 2015 | 134 003 416 | 525 000 | 566 000 | 611 000 | 150 | 324 | 460 |
| | 2016 | 135 398 716 | 640 000 | 691 000 | 749 000 | 210 | 474 | 680 |
| | 2017 | 136 722 119 | 880 000 | 944 000 | 1 026 000 | 250 | 620 | 910 |
| | 2018 | 138 017 898 | 867 000 | 929 000 | 1 007 000 | 220 | 577 | 850 |
| Eastern Mediterranean | 2010 | 419 019 843 | 3 300 000 | 4 300 000 | 6 300 000 | 3 000 | 8 300 | 14 400 |
| | 2011 | 427 979 875 | 3 400 000 | 4 500 000 | 6 500 000 | 3 000 | 7 500 | 12 300 |
| | 2012 | 436 754 102 | 3 200 000 | 4 200 000 | 6 000 000 | 2 900 | 7 600 | 12 400 |
| | 2013 | 445 450 169 | 3 000 000 | 3 900 000 | 5 300 000 | 2 500 | 6 900 | 11 100 |
| | 2014 | 454 228 324 | 3 100 000 | 4 000 000 | 5 500 000 | 2 400 | 6 900 | 11 300 |
| | 2015 | 463 210 243 | 3 000 000 | 3 800 000 | 5 200 000 | 2 300 | 7 100 | 12 200 |
| | 2016 | 468 761 159 | 3 800 000 | 4 800 000 | 6 400 000 | 2 900 | 8 600 | 15 300 |
| | 2017 | 478 058 225 | 3 800 000 | 4 900 000 | 6 800 000 | 3 000 | 9 200 | 17 300 |
| | 2018 | 487 588 453 | 3 700 000 | 4 900 000 | 6 800 000 | 2 600 | 9 300 | 17 700 |
| European | 2010 | 37 906 443 | – | 170 | – | – | 0 | – |
| | 2011 | 38 469 606 | – | 69 | – | – | 0 | – |
| | 2012 | 39 086 200 | – | 21 | – | – | 0 | – |
| | 2013 | 39 739 267 | – | 3 | – | – | 0 | – |
| | 2014 | 40 405 247 | – | 2 | – | – | 0 | – |
| | 2015 | 41 065 655 | – | 0 | – | – | 0 | – |
| | 2016 | 41 714 844 | – | 0 | – | – | 0 | – |
| | 2017 | 42 352 758 | – | 0 | – | – | 0 | – |
| | 2018 | 42 973 389 | – | 0 | – | – | 0 | – |
| South-East Asia | 2010 | 1 477 504 120 | 19 800 000 | 25 100 000 | 33 900 000 | 9 000 | 39 000 | 67 000 |
| | 2011 | 1 496 330 952 | 16 700 000 | 21 100 000 | 28 300 000 | 7 000 | 32 000 | 57 000 |
| | 2012 | 1 514 731 269 | 14 700 000 | 18 400 000 | 24 400 000 | 7 000 | 28 000 | 47 000 |
| | 2013 | 1 532 751 942 | 10 900 000 | 13 700 000 | 18 000 000 | 4 000 | 21 000 | 36 000 |
| | 2014 | 1 550 466 894 | 10 400 000 | 13 200 000 | 17 400 000 | 4 000 | 24 000 | 42 000 |
| | 2015 | 1 567 931 968 | 10 700 000 | 13 600 000 | 18 200 000 | 3 000 | 25 000 | 44 000 |
| | 2016 | 1 585 152 940 | 10 500 000 | 14 000 000 | 19 700 000 | 3 000 | 25 000 | 47 000 |
| | 2017 | 1 602 118 493 | 8 800 000 | 11 300 000 | 15 400 000 | 3 000 | 20 000 | 35 000 |
| | 2018 | 1 618 838 836 | 5 800 000 | 7 900 000 | 10 700 000 | 2 000 | 12 000 | 21 000 |
| Western Pacific | 2010 | 721 038 851 | 1 045 000 | 1 839 000 | 2 779 000 | 800 | 3 800 | 7 500 |
| | 2011 | 726 302 437 | 922 000 | 1 576 000 | 2 340 000 | 600 | 3 300 | 6 600 |
| | 2012 | 731 623 901 | 914 000 | 1 761 000 | 3 009 000 | 700 | 3 600 | 8 000 |
| | 2013 | 736 961 516 | 1 305 000 | 2 027 000 | 2 925 000 | 600 | 4 600 | 9 300 |
| | 2014 | 742 256 202 | 1 588 000 | 2 345 000 | 3 339 000 | 700 | 4 400 | 8 500 |
| | 2015 | 747 456 804 | 1 115 000 | 1 445 000 | 1 852 000 | 500 | 2 800 | 5 000 |
| | 2016 | 752 550 363 | 1 318 000 | 1 733 000 | 2 228 000 | 500 | 3 500 | 6 400 |
| | 2017 | 757 527 287 | 1 392 000 | 1 854 000 | 2 420 000 | 500 | 3 600 | 6 500 |
| | 2018 | 762 325 610 | 1 495 000 | 1 980 000 | 2 588 000 | 500 | 3 600 | 6 500 |
| Total | 2010 | 3 523 638 856 | 231 000 000 | 251 000 000 | 278 000 000 | 541 000 | 585 000 | 649 000 |
| | 2011 | 3 580 209 832 | 222 000 000 | 241 000 000 | 266 000 000 | 499 000 | 536 000 | 588 000 |
| | 2012 | 3 636 820 763 | 214 000 000 | 234 000 000 | 260 000 000 | 474 000 | 508 000 | 560 000 |
| | 2013 | 3 693 546 902 | 205 000 000 | 224 000 000 | 250 000 000 | 446 000 | 477 000 | 531 000 |
| | 2014 | 3 750 515 522 | 202 000 000 | 218 000 000 | 239 000 000 | 434 000 | 463 000 | 504 000 |
| | 2015 | 3 807 816 077 | 203 000 000 | 219 000 000 | 240 000 000 | 416 000 | 446 000 | 491 000 |
| | 2016 | 3 861 786 756 | 210 000 000 | 227 000 000 | 251 000 000 | 398 000 | 427 000 | 473 000 |
| | 2017 | 3 919 580 207 | 211 000 000 | 231 000 000 | 259 000 000 | 390 000 | 416 000 | 462 000 |
| | 2018 | 3 977 632 424 | 206 000 000 | 228 000 000 | 258 000 000 | 384 000 | 405 000 | 452 000 |

# Annex 3 – G. Population at risk and reported malaria cases by place of care, 2018

| WHO region Country/area | Population | | | Number of people living in active foci |
|---|---|---|---|---|
| | UN population | At risk (low + high) | At risk (high) | |
| **AFRICAN** | | | | |
| Algeria | 42 228 415 | – | – | 0 |
| Angola | 30 809 787 | 30 809 787 | 30 809 787 | – |
| Benin | 11 485 035 | 11 485 035 | 11 485 035 | – |
| Botswana | 2 254 067 | 1 494 401 | 94 941 | – |
| Burkina Faso | 19 751 466 | 19 751 466 | 19 751 466 | – |
| Burundi | 11 175 379 | 11 175 379 | 11 175 379 | – |
| Cabo Verde | 543 764 | – | – | 162 814 |
| Cameroon | 25 216 261 | 25 216 261 | 17 903 545 | – |
| Central African Republic | 4 666 375 | 4 666 375 | 4 666 375 | – |
| Chad | 15 477 727 | 15 308 245 | 10 425 023 | – |
| Comoros | 832 322 | 832 322 | 396 019 | – |
| Congo | 5 244 363 | 5 244 363 | 5 244 363 | – |
| Côte d'Ivoire | 25 069 226 | 25 069 226 | 25 069 226 | – |
| Democratic Republic of the Congo | 84 068 092 | 84 068 092 | 81 546 049 | – |
| Equatorial Guinea | 1 308 966 | 1 308 966 | 1 308 966 | – |
| Eritrea | 3 452 797 | 3 452 797 | 2 451 486 | – |
| Eswatini | 1 136 274 | 318 156 | 0 | – |
| Ethiopia | 109 224 410 | 74 272 598 | 29 709 040 | – |
| Gabon | 2 119 275 | 2 119 275 | 2 119 275 | – |
| Gambia | 2 280 092 | 2 280 092 | 2 280 092 | – |
| Ghana | 29 767 108 | 29 767 108 | 29 767 108 | – |
| Guinea | 12 414 292 | 12 414 292 | 12 414 292 | – |
| Guinea-Bissau | 1 874 304 | 1 874 304 | 1 874 304 | – |
| Kenya | 51 392 570 | 51 392 570 | 36 075 015 | – |
| Liberia | 4 818 976 | 4 818 976 | 4 818 976 | – |
| Madagascar | 26 262 313 | 26 262 313 | 23 049 907 | – |
| Malawi | 18 143 215 | 18 143 215 | 18 143 215 | – |
| Mali | 19 077 755 | 19 077 755 | 17 389 755 | – |
| Mauritania | 4 403 312 | 4 403 312 | 2 838 727 | – |
| Mozambique | 29 496 009 | 29 496 009 | 29 496 009 | – |
| Namibia | 2 448 300 | 1 943 338 | 1 130 160 | – |
| Niger | 22 442 831 | 22 442 831 | 22 442 831 | – |
| Nigeria | 195 874 685 | 195 874 685 | 149 605 167 | – |
| Rwanda | 12 301 969 | 12 301 969 | 12 301 969 | – |
| Sao Tome and Principe | 211 032 | 211 032 | 211 032 | – |
| Senegal | 15 854 324 | 15 854 324 | 15 762 845 | – |
| Sierra Leone | 7 650 149 | 7 650 149 | 7 650 149 | – |
| South Africa | 57 792 520 | 5 779 252 | 2 311 701 | – |
| South Sudan[1] | 10 975 924 | 10 975 924 | 10 975 924 | – |
| Togo | 7 889 095 | 7 889 095 | 7 889 095 | – |
| Uganda | 42 729 032 | 42 729 032 | 42 729 032 | – |
| United Republic of Tanzania[2] | 56 313 444 | 56 313 444 | 55 696 563 | – |
|   Mainland | 54 720 096 | 54 720 096 | 54 720 096 | – |
|   Zanzibar | 1 593 348 | 1 593 348 | 976 467 | – |
| Zambia | 17 351 714 | 17 351 714 | 17 351 714 | – |
| Zimbabwe | 14 438 812 | 11 369 510 | 4 131 810 | – |
| **AMERICAS** | | | | |
| Belize | 383 071 | – | – | 17 225 |
| Bolivia (Plurinational State of) | 11 353 140 | 5 150 579 | 283 601 | – |
| Brazil | 209 469 320 | 42 522 271 | 4 817 794 | – |
| Colombia | 49 661 056 | 10 994 461 | 4 989 943 | – |
| Costa Rica | 4 999 443 | – | – | 137 832 |
| Dominican Republic | 10 627 147 | 5 853 645 | 150 374 | – |
| Ecuador | 17 084 359 | – | – | 246 833 |
| El Salvador | 6 420 740 | – | – | 12 700 |
| French Guiana | 282 938 | 156 543 | 26 115 | – |
| Guatemala | 17 247 855 | 13 020 750 | 2 353 125 | – |
| Guyana | 779 007 | 779 007 | 85 021 | – |

| Public sector | | Private sector | | Community level | |
|---|---|---|---|---|---|
| Presumed | Confirmed | Presumed | Confirmed | Presumed | Confirmed |
| 0 | 1 242 [5] | – | – | – | – |
| 777 685 | 5 150 575 [3] | – | – | 0 | 241 294 |
| 280 134 | 1 768 450 [4] | 323 782 | 245 807 | 0 | 207 362 |
| 0 | 585 [5] | 0 | 2 | – | – |
| 1 691 351 | 10 278 970 [4] | 365 492 | 310 030 | 20 825 | 79 954 |
| 182 925 | 4 966 511 [5] | 1 399 | 298 023 | 0 | 679 278 |
| 0 | 21 [5] | 0 | 0 | – | – |
| 1 221 809 | 1 249 705 | 913 574 | 930 111 | 70 741 | 77 817 |
| 23 038 | 972 119 | 27 653 | 147 456 | 9 858 | 959 |
| – | 1 364 706 [3] | – | – | 159 503 | 222 205 |
| 4 069 | 15 613 [5] | 0 | 427 | 881 | 3 642 |
| 207 712 | 116 903 [4] | – | – | – | – |
| 531 449 | 4 766 477 [5] | 0 | 126 327 | 0 | 194 076 |
| 1 236 233 | 16 972 207 [3] | – | – | 0 | 1 372 477 |
| 0 | 8 962 | – | – | – | – |
| 853 | 22 955 [4] | – | – | 1 033 | 23 485 |
| 0 | 656 [5] | 0 | 296 | – | – |
| 244 804 | 962 087 [5] | – | – | – | – |
| 685 559 | 111 719 | – | – | – | – |
| 1 206 | 87 448 [4] | 0 | 1 206 | 0 | 4 294 |
| 6 222 946 | 4 931 448 [5] | 1 919 308 | 1 556 857 | – | – |
| 384 629 | 1 214 996 [5] | 109 156 | 53 260 | 0 | 299 767 |
| 0 | 171 075 | 0 | 5 854 | 0 | 4 318 |
| 8 429 215 | 1 521 566 | 1 738 477 | 465 581 | 128 429 | 330 943 |
| – | – | – | – | – | – |
| – | 972 790 [4] | 262 805 | 51 693 | 105 350 | 108 338 |
| 0 | 5 865 476 [3] | – | – | 0 | 1 045 467 |
| 0 | 2 345 475 [5] | 0 | 51 177 | 0 | 268 623 |
| 145 232 | 30 609 | – | – | – | – |
| 27 629 | 9 292 928 | – | – | 7 229 | 1 011 544 |
| 0 | 36451* | – | – | – | – |
| 311 068 | 3 046 450 [5] | 40 112 | 47 791 | 0 | 93 889 |
| 5 916 631 | 12 953 583 | 498 219 | 1 487 171 | 17 725 | 107 270 |
| 0 | 1 975 926 | 0 | 33 854 | 0 | 2 222 103 |
| 0 | 2 940 [5] | – | – | – | 547 |
| 5 801 | 530 944 [5] | – | – | 1 080 | 143 876 |
| 48 024 | 1 733 831 [3] | 18 871 | 18 230 | 245 840 | 561 180 |
| 6 174 | 10 789 [3] | – | – | 0 | 1 675 |
| 4 598 663 | 98 843 | – | – | – | – |
| 291 076 | 1 090 334 [4] | 0 | 291 076 | 0 | 621 467 |
| 3 136 262 | 5 759 174 [5] | 340 522 | 372 612 | – | – |
| 166 771 | 6 053 714 [2] | 119 178 | 494 052 | 0 | 442 |
| 164 733 | 6 050 382 [4] | 119 178 | 492 692 | – | – |
| 2 038 | 3 332 [4] | 0 | 1 360 | 0 | 442 |
| 156 044 | 5 039 679 [3] | – | – | 710 465 | 393 548 |
| 0 | 184 427 [4] | 0 | 8 630 | 0 | 79 591 |
| | | | | | |
| 0 | 7 [5] | 0 | 2 | – | – |
| 0 | 5 354 [3] | – | – | 0 | 93 |
| 0 | 194 512 [4] | – | – | – | – |
| 0 | 63 143 [5] | – | – | – | – |
| 0 | 108* [4] | 0 | 4 | – | – |
| 0 | 484* | 0 | 84 | 22 | 137 |
| 0 | 1 806 [5] | 0 | 10 | – | – |
| 0 | 2 | 0 | 1 | 0 | 0 |
| – | – | – | – | – | – |
| – | 4 769** | 0 | 3 | – | – |
| 0 | 17 038 | – | 37 | 0 | 2 102 |

# Annex 3 - G. Population at risk and reported malaria cases by place of care, 2018

| WHO region Country/area | Population | | | |
|---|---|---|---|---|
| | UN population | At risk (low + high) | At risk (high) | Number of people living in active foci |
| **AMERICAS** | | | | |
| Haiti | 11 123 183 | 9 937 674 | 2 696 148 | – |
| Honduras | 9 587 523 | 8 684 378 | 2 443 668 | – |
| Mexico | 126 190 782 | – | – | 3 120 973 |
| Nicaragua | 6 465 502 | 2 822 191 | 554 934 | – |
| Panama | 4 176 868 | 4 040 827 | 176 013 | – |
| Peru | 31 989 265 | 12 564 103 | 1 601 383 | – |
| Suriname | 575 987 | 85 073 | 24 456 | – |
| Venezuela (Bolivarian Republic of) | 28 887 117 | 14 443 558 | 5 990 747 | – |
| **EASTERN MEDITERRANEAN** | | | | |
| Afghanistan | 37 171 922 | 28 652 489 | 10 121 171 | – |
| Djibouti | 958 923 | 719 115 | 336 659 | – |
| Iran (Islamic Republic of) | 81 800 204 | 835 180 | 0 | – |
| Pakistan | 212 228 288 | 208 643 752 | 61 370 054 | – |
| Saudi Arabia | 33 702 757 | – | – | 176 408 |
| Somalia | 15 008 225 | 15 008 225 | 7 638 736 | – |
| Sudan | 41 801 532 | 41 801 532 | 36 325 531 | – |
| Yemen | 28 498 683 | 18 373 670 | 10 964 013 | – |
| **SOUTH-EAST ASIA** | | | | |
| Bangladesh | 161 376 713 | 17 352 837 | 2 038 188 | – |
| Bhutan | 754 396 | – | – | 14 876 |
| Democratic People's Republic of Korea | 25 549 606 | – | – | 12 379 473 |
| India | 1 352 642 283 | 1 263 908 949 | 164 089 035 | – |
| Indonesia | 267 670 549 | 267 670 549 | 17 114 855 | – |
| Myanmar | 53 708 318 | 31 966 116 | 8 491 822 | – |
| Nepal | 28 095 712 | 8 155 623 | 1 468 563 | – |
| Thailand | 69 428 454 | 13 174 743 | 1 537 146 | – |
| Timor-Leste | 1 267 975 | 1 192 542 | 429 432 | – |
| **WESTERN PACIFIC** | | | | |
| Cambodia | 16 249 795 | 11 491 692 | 7 820 376 | – |
| China | 1 435 651 150 | 600 418 023 | 200 991 | – |
| Lao People's Democratic Republic | 7 061 498 | 3 674 380 | 3 674 380 | – |
| Malaysia | 31 528 033 | – | – | 3 884 |
| Papua New Guinea | 8 606 324 | 8 606 324 | 8 089 945 | – |
| Philippines | 106 651 394 | 61 936 730 | 7 268 293 | – |
| Republic of Korea | 51 171 700 | 3 582 019 | 0 | – |
| Solomon Islands | 652 856 | 646 327 | 646 327 | – |
| Vanuatu | 292 675 | 292 675 | 254 407 | – |
| Viet Nam | 95 545 959 | 70 416 320 | 6 494 737 | – |
| **REGIONAL SUMMARY** | | | | |
| African | 1 060 267 778 | 925 208 989 | 782 493 367 | 162 814 |
| Americas | 547 304 303 | 131 055 060 | 26 193 322 | 3 535 563 |
| Eastern Mediterranean | 451 170 534 | 314 033 963 | 126 756 164 | 176 408 |
| South-East Asia | 1 960 494 006 | 1 603 421 359 | 195 169 041 | 12 394 349 |
| Western Pacific | 1 753 411 384 | 761 064 490 | 34 449 456 | 3 884 |
| **Total** | **5 772 648 005** | **3 734 783 861** | **1 165 061 350** | **16 273 018** |

UN: United Nations; WHO: World Health Organization.

"–" refers to not applicable or data not available.

\* Corrected for double counting of microscopy and RDT.

\*\* Double counting of microscopy and RDT reported, but proportion is not indicated.

[1] In May 2013, South Sudan was reassigned to the WHO African Region (WHA resolution 66.21, https://apps.who.int/gb/ebwha/pdf_files/WHA66/A66_R21-en.pdf).

[2] Where national data for the United Republic of Tanzania are unavailable, refer to Mainland and Zanzibar.

[3] Figures reported for the public sector include cases detected at the community level.

[4] Figures reported for the public sector include cases detected in the private sector.

[5] Figures reported for the public sector include cases detected at the community level and in the private sector.

[6] Figures include all imported or non-human malaria cases; none of them being indigenous malaria cases.

Note: Reported cases include all presumed and confirmed cases.

| Public sector | | Private sector | | Community level | |
|---|---|---|---|---|---|
| Presumed | Confirmed | Presumed | Confirmed | Presumed | Confirmed |
| - | 8828*[5] | 0 | 2 049 | 0 | 793 |
| 0 | 653* | 0 | 73 | 32 | 152 |
| 0 | 826[5] | 0 | 6 | - | - |
| 0 | 15 934 | - | - | - | - |
| 0 | 715 | 0 | 3 | - | - |
| 0 | 45619* | - | - | - | - |
| 0 | 235[5] | - | 16 | 0 | 17 |
| 0 | 404924*[3] | - | - | - | - |
| 126 370 | 173 493 | 0 | 5 365 | 21 278 | 69 831 |
| 0 | 25 319[4] | - | 474 | - | - |
| 0 | 625*[5] | - | - | - | - |
| 694 738 | 374 510[4] | 0 | 103 693 | - | - |
| 0 | 2 711 | - | - | - | - |
| 9 | 31 021 | - | - | - | - |
| 1 974 469 | 1 606 833[4] | - | - | 4 434 | 31 184 |
| 78 970 | 113 925 | 10 253 | 36 521 | 0 | 3 727 |
| 0 | 1 919 | 0 | 56 | 0 | 8 548 |
| 0 | 54[5] | 0 | 5 | - | - |
| 0 | 3 598 | - | - | - | - |
| 0 | 429 928[3] | - | - | - | 199 496 |
| 0 | 223 468[5] | 0 | 28 759 | 0 | 2 804 |
| 0 | 74 392[3] | 0 | 2 126 | 0 | 59 832 |
| 1 772 | 1 158[5] | 544 | 34 | - | - |
| 428 | 5 389 | 0 | 656 | 0 | 705 |
| 0 | 8*[5] | - | - | 0 | 0 |
| 0 | 42 285 | 0 | 0 | 0 | 20 297 |
| 0 | 2 513 | - | - | - | - |
| 0 | 8 913[3] | 0 | 1 228 | 0 | 1 804 |
| 0 | 4 630[5,6] | 0 | 52[6] | - | - |
| 424 397 | 516 249 | - | - | 0 | 0 |
| 0 | 1 574 | 0 | 295 | 295 | 2 772 |
| 0 | 576 | 0 | 429 | - | - |
| 13 239 | 59 191 | - | - | - | - |
| 0 | 644[3] | - | - | 0 | 150 |
| 0 | 6 661[5] | 0 | 39 | - | - |
| 36 934 992 | 113 681 359 | 6 678 548 | 6 997 523 | 1 478 959 | 10 401 431 |
| 0 | 764 957 | 0 | 2 288 | 54 | 3 294 |
| 2 874 556 | 2 328 437 | 10 253 | 146 053 | 25 712 | 104 742 |
| 2 200 | 739 914 | 544 | 31 636 | 0 | 271 385 |
| 437 636 | 643 236 | 0 | 2 043 | 295 | 25 023 |
| **40 249 384** | **118 157 903** | **6 689 345** | **7 179 543** | **1 505 020** | **10 805 875** |

Data as of 14 February 2020

# Annex 3 - H. Reported malaria cases by method of confirmation, 2010–2018

| WHO region Country/area | | 2010 | 2011 | 2012 | 2013 | 2014 | 2015 | 2016 | 2017 | 2018 |
|---|---|---|---|---|---|---|---|---|---|---|
| **AFRICAN** | | | | | | | | | | |
| Algeria[1] | Presumed and confirmed | 408 | 191 | 887 | 603 | 266 | 747 | 432 | 453 | 1 242 [5] |
| | Microscopy examined | 12 224 | 11 974 | 15 790 | 12 762 | 8 690 | 8 000 | 6 628 | 6 469 | 10 081 |
| | Confirmed with microscopy | 408 | 191 | 887 | 603 | 266 | 747 | 432 | 453 | 1 242 |
| | RDT examined | – | – | – | – | – | 0 | 0 | 0 | 0 |
| | Confirmed with RDT | – | – | – | – | – | 0 | 0 | 0 | 0 |
| | Imported cases | 398 | 190 | 828 | 593 | 260 | 745 | 432 | 453 | 1 242 [3] |
| Angola | Presumed and confirmed | 3 687 574 | 3 501 953 | 3 031 546 | 3 144 100 | 3 180 021 | 3 254 270 | 4 301 146 | 4 500 221 | 5 928 260 |
| | Microscopy examined | 1 947 349 | 1 765 933 | 2 245 223 | 3 025 258 | 3 398 029 | 3 345 693 | 4 183 727 | 7 493 969 | 5 066 780 |
| | Confirmed with microscopy | 1 324 264 | 1 147 473 | 1 056 563 | 1 462 941 | 1 431 313 | 1 396 773 | 2 058 128 | 2 199 810 | 2 442 500 |
| | RDT examined | 639 476 | 833 753 | 1 069 483 | 1 103 815 | 1 855 400 | 3 009 305 | 2 959 282 | 2 931 055 | 5 025 981 |
| | Confirmed with RDT | 358 606 | 484 809 | 440 271 | 536 927 | 867 666 | 1 372 532 | 1 736 125 | 1 675 082 | 2 708 075 |
| | Imported cases | – | – | – | – | – | – | – | – | – |
| Benin | Presumed and confirmed | 1 432 095 | 1 424 335 | 1 513 212 | 1 670 273 | 1 509 221 | 1 495 375 | 1 374 729 | 1 719 171 | 2 048 584 [4] |
| | Microscopy examined | – | 88 134 | 243 008 | 291 479 | 155 205 | 296 264 | 267 405 | 267 492 | 349 191 |
| | Confirmed with microscopy | – | 68 745 | – | 99 368 | 108 714 | 108 061 | 104 601 | 208 823 | 258 519 |
| | RDT examined | – | 475 986 | 825 005 | 1 158 526 | 1 335 582 | 1 486 667 | 1 500 047 | 2 016 767 | 2 016 745 |
| | Confirmed with RDT | – | 354 223 | 705 839 | 979 466 | 935 521 | 1 160 286 | 1 219 975 | 1 487 954 | 1 509 931 |
| | Imported cases | – | – | – | – | – | – | – | – | – |
| Botswana | Presumed and confirmed | 12 196 | 1 141 | 308 | 506 | 1 485 | 340 | 718 | 1 902 | 585 [5] |
| | Microscopy examined | – | – | – | – | – | – | 5 178 | 5 223 | 872 |
| | Confirmed with microscopy | 1 046 | 432 | – | – | – | – | – | – | – |
| | RDT examined | – | – | – | – | – | 1 284 | 7 806 | 7 380 | 13 107 |
| | Confirmed with RDT | – | – | 193 | 456 | 1 346 | 326 | 716 | 1 900 | 585 |
| | Imported cases | – | – | – | 30 | 30 | 48 | 64 | 62 | 51 |
| Burkina Faso | Presumed and confirmed | 5 723 481 | 5 024 697 | 6 970 700 | 7 146 026 | 8 278 408 | 8 286 453 | 9 785 822 | 11 915 816 | 11 970 321 [4] |
| | Microscopy examined | 177 879 | 400 005 | 223 372 | 183 971 | 198 947 | 222 190 | 191 208 | 133 101 | 157 824 |
| | Confirmed with microscopy | 88 540 | 83 857 | 90 089 | 82 875 | 83 259 | 92 589 | 80 077 | 46 411 | 56 989 |
| | RDT examined | 940 985 | 450 281 | 4 516 273 | 4 296 350 | 6 224 055 | 8 290 188 | 11 794 810 | 12 561 490 | 13 061 136 |
| | Confirmed with RDT | 715 999 | 344 256 | 3 767 957 | 3 686 176 | 5 345 396 | 6 922 857 | 9 699 077 | 10 179 048 | 10 221 981 |
| | Imported cases | – | – | – | – | – | – | – | – | – |
| Burundi | Presumed and confirmed | 4 255 301 | 3 298 979 | 2 570 754 | 4 469 007 | 4 831 758 | 5 243 410 | 8 383 389 | 8 133 919 | 5 149 436 [5] |
| | Microscopy examined | 2 825 558 | 2 859 720 | 2 659 372 | 4 123 012 | 4 471 998 | 3 254 670 | 3 941 251 | 3 814 355 | 1 542 232 |
| | Confirmed with microscopy | 1 599 908 | 1 485 332 | 1 484 676 | 2 366 134 | 2 718 391 | 1 964 862 | 2 520 622 | 2 269 831 | 1 148 316 |
| | RDT examined | 273 324 | 181 489 | 1 148 965 | 2 933 869 | 2 903 679 | 5 076 107 | 8 307 007 | 8 058 231 | 7 009 165 |
| | Confirmed with RDT | 163 539 | 86 542 | 666 400 | 1 775 253 | 1 866 882 | 3 194 844 | 5 753 440 | 5 400 346 | 3 818 195 |
| | Imported cases | – | – | – | – | – | – | – | – | – |
| Cabo Verde | Presumed and confirmed | 47 | 36 | – | – | 46 | 28 | 48 | 446 | 21 [5] |
| | Microscopy examined | – | – | 8 715 | 10 621 | 6 894 | 3 117 | 8 393 | 3 857 | 16 623 |
| | Confirmed with microscopy | 47 | – | 36 | 46 | 46 | 28 | 75 | 446 | 21 |
| | RDT examined | – | 26 508 | – | – | – | – | – | – | – |
| | Confirmed with RDT | – | 36 | – | – | – | – | – | – | – |
| | Imported cases | – | 29 | 35 | 24 | 20 | 21 | 27 | 23 | 19 |
| Cameroon | Presumed and confirmed | 1 845 691 | 1 829 266 | 1 589 317 | 1 824 633 | 1 369 518 | 2 321 933 | 1 790 891 | 2 488 993 | 2 471 514 |
| | Microscopy examined | – | 1 110 308 | 1 182 610 | 1 236 306 | 1 086 095 | 1 024 306 | 1 373 802 | 627 709 | 658 017 |
| | Confirmed with microscopy | – | – | – | – | – | 592 351 | 810 367 | 390 130 | 428 888 |
| | RDT examined | – | 120 466 | 93 392 | 591 670 | 1 254 293 | 1 128 818 | 1 740 375 | 1 420 522 | 1 337 354 |
| | Confirmed with RDT | – | – | – | – | – | 570 433 | 864 897 | 801 127 | 820 817 |
| | Imported cases | – | – | – | – | – | – | – | – | – |
| Central African Republic | Presumed and confirmed | 66 484 | 221 980 | 459 999 | 407 131 | 495 238 | 953 535 | 1 400 526 | 1 267 673 | 995 157 |
| | Microscopy examined | – | – | – | 63 695 | 55 943 | 139 241 | 189 481 | 112 007 | 163 370 |
| | Confirmed with microscopy | – | – | – | 36 943 | 41 436 | 106 524 | 144 924 | 28 855 | 117 267 |
| | RDT examined | – | – | 55 746 | 136 548 | 369 208 | 724 303 | 1 249 963 | 483 714 | 1 181 578 |
| | Confirmed with RDT | – | – | 46 759 | 79 357 | 253 652 | 492 309 | 887 840 | 354 454 | 854 852 |
| | Imported cases | – | – | – | – | – | – | – | – | – |

| WHO region Country/area | | 2010 | 2011 | 2012 | 2013 | 2014 | 2015 | 2016 | 2017 | 2018 |
|---|---|---|---|---|---|---|---|---|---|---|
| **AFRICAN** | | | | | | | | | | |
| Chad | Presumed and confirmed | 544 243 | 528 454 | 660 575 | 1 272 841 | 1 513 772 | 1 490 556 | 1 402 215 | 1 962 372 | 1 364 706 [3] |
| | Microscopy examined | 89 749 | – | 69 789 | – | – | – | 1 063 293 | 1 584 525 | 190 006 |
| | Confirmed with microscopy | 75 342 | 86 348 | – | 206 082 | 160 260 | 149 574 | 720 765 | 1 064 354 | 137 501 |
| | RDT examined | 309 927 | 114 122 | – | 621 469 | 1 137 455 | 937 775 | 861 561 | 1 359 070 | 1 751 483 |
| | Confirmed with RDT | 125 106 | 94 778 | – | 548 483 | 753 772 | 637 472 | 574 003 | 898 018 | 1 227 205 |
| | Imported cases | – | – | – | – | – | – | – | – | – |
| Comoros | Presumed and confirmed | 103 670 | 76 661 | 65 139 | 62 565 | 2 465 | 1 517 | 1 333 | 2 274 | 19 682 [5] |
| | Microscopy examined | 87 595 | 63 217 | 125 030 | 154 824 | 93 444 | 89 634 | 71 902 | 130 134 | 90 956 |
| | Confirmed with microscopy | 35 199 | 22 278 | 45 507 | 46 130 | 1 987 | 963 | 559 | 1 325 | 9 197 |
| | RDT examined | 5 249 | 20 226 | 27 714 | 21 546 | 9 839 | 11 479 | 22 219 | 60 691 | 24 567 |
| | Confirmed with RDT | 1 339 | 2 578 | 4 333 | 7 026 | 216 | 337 | 507 | 949 | 6 416 |
| | Imported cases | – | – | – | – | – | – | – | – | – |
| Congo | Presumed and confirmed | 446 656 | 277 263 | 117 640 | 183 026 | 248 159 | 264 574 | 374 252 | 297 652 | 324 615 [4] |
| | Microscopy examined | – | – | – | 69 375 | 88 764 | 87 547 | 202 922 | 153 203 | 178 017 |
| | Confirmed with microscopy | – | 37 744 | 120 319 | 43 232 | 54 523 | 51 529 | 134 612 | 127 939 | 116 903 |
| | RDT examined | – | – | – | 0 | 19 746 | 0 | 60 927 | 0 | 0 |
| | Confirmed with RDT | – | – | – | 0 | 11 800 | 0 | 37 235 | 0 | 0 |
| | Imported cases | – | – | – | – | – | – | – | – | – |
| Côte d'Ivoire | Presumed and confirmed | 1 721 461 | 2 588 004 | 2 795 919 | 4 708 425 | 4 658 774 | 3 606 725 | 3 471 024 | 3 391 967 | 5 297 926 [5] |
| | Microscopy examined | – | 49 828 | 195 546 | 395 914 | 568 562 | 811 426 | 975 507 | 1 221 845 | 1 132 659 |
| | Confirmed with microscopy | 62 726 | 29 976 | 107 563 | 215 104 | 306 926 | 478 870 | 579 566 | 588 969 | 696 124 |
| | RDT examined | – | – | 1 572 785 | 3 384 765 | 4 904 066 | 4 174 097 | 4 202 868 | 5 007 162 | 5 042 040 |
| | Confirmed with RDT | – | – | 1 033 064 | 2 291 849 | 3 405 905 | 2 897 034 | 2 891 458 | 2 685 714 | 4 070 353 |
| | Imported cases | – | – | – | – | – | – | – | – | – |
| Democratic Republic of the Congo | Presumed and confirmed | 9 252 959 | 9 442 144 | 9 128 398 | 11 363 817 | 9 749 369 | 10 878 974 | 15 397 717 | 15 272 767 | 18 208 440 [3] |
| | Microscopy examined | 3 678 849 | 4 226 533 | 4 329 318 | 4 126 129 | 3 533 165 | 2 877 585 | 2 810 067 | 1 981 621 | 1 926 455 |
| | Confirmed with microscopy | 2 374 930 | 2 700 818 | 2 656 864 | 2 611 478 | 2 126 554 | 1 902 640 | 1 847 143 | 1 291 717 | 995 577 |
| | RDT examined | 54 728 | 2 912 088 | 3 327 071 | 6 096 993 | 11 114 215 | 13 574 891 | 18 630 636 | 18 994 861 | 20 671 006 |
| | Confirmed with RDT | 42 850 | 1 861 163 | 2 134 734 | 4 103 745 | 7 842 429 | 9 724 833 | 13 483 698 | 13 885 210 | 15 976 630 |
| | Imported cases | – | – | – | – | – | – | – | – | – |
| Equatorial Guinea | Presumed and confirmed | 78 095 | 37 267 | 20 890 | 25 162 | 19 642 | 8 581 | 7 542 | 7 787 | 8 962 |
| | Microscopy examined | 42 585 | 23 004 | 33 245 | 27 039 | 47 322 | 21 831 | 239 938 | 13 127 | 8 395 |
| | Confirmed with microscopy | 39 636 | 20 601 | 13 196 | 11 235 | 17 685 | 8 564 | 125 623 | 6 800 | 4 135 |
| | RDT examined | 16 772 | 2 899 | 6 826 | 5 489 | 9 807 | 46 227 | 78 841 | 78 090 | 33 174 |
| | Confirmed with RDT | 14 177 | 1 865 | 1 973 | 1 894 | 2 732 | 6 578 | 22 091 | 8 925 | 4 827 |
| | Imported cases | – | – | – | – | – | – | – | – | – |
| Eritrea | Presumed and confirmed | 53 750 | 39 567 | 42 178 | 34 678 | 35 725 | 24 310 | 47 055 | 32 444 | 23 808 [4] |
| | Microscopy examined | 79 024 | 67 190 | 84 861 | 81 541 | 63 766 | 59 268 | 83 599 | 74 962 | 70 465 |
| | Confirmed with microscopy | 13 894 | 15 308 | 11 557 | 10 890 | 10 993 | 8 332 | 24 251 | 14 519 | 10 325 |
| | RDT examined | – | 25 570 | 33 758 | 39 281 | 53 032 | 47 744 | – | 45 144 | 74 917 |
| | Confirmed with RDT | 22 088 | 19 540 | 10 258 | 10 427 | 19 775 | 11 040 | – | 16 967 | 12 630 |
| | Imported cases | – | – | – | – | – | – | – | – | – |
| Eswatini | Presumed and confirmed | 1 722 | 797 | 626 | 669 | – | 651 | 487 | 1 127 | 656 [5] |
| | Microscopy examined | – | – | – | – | – | – | 1 249 | 371 | 1 526 |
| | Confirmed with microscopy | 87 | 130 | 345 | 488 | 711 | 43 | 141 | 68 | 656 |
| | RDT examined | – | – | – | – | – | – | – | 2 841 | 8 311 |
| | Confirmed with RDT | 181 | 419 | 217 | 474 | – | 152 | 209 | 1 059 | – |
| | Imported cases*** | – | 170 | 153 | 234 | 322 | 282 | 221 | 403 | 348 |
| Ethiopia | Presumed and confirmed | 4 068 764 | 3 549 559 | 3 876 745 | 3 316 013 | 2 513 863 | 2 174 707 | 1 962 996 | 1 755 748 | 1 206 891 [5] |
| | Microscopy examined | 2 509 543 | 3 418 719 | 3 778 479 | 8 573 335 | 7 062 717 | 5 679 932 | 6 367 309 | 6 246 949 | 5 668 995 |
| | Confirmed with microscopy | 1 158 197 | 1 480 306 | 1 692 578 | 2 645 454 | 2 118 815 | 1 867 059 | 1 718 504 | 1 530 739 | 962 087 |
| | RDT examined | – | – | – | – | – | – | – | – | – |
| | Confirmed with RDT | – | – | – | – | – | – | – | – | – |
| | Imported cases | – | – | – | – | – | – | – | – | – |

# Annex 3 – H. Reported malaria cases by method of confirmation, 2010–2018

| WHO region Country/area | | 2010 | 2011 | 2012 | 2013 | 2014 | 2015 | 2016 | 2017 | 2018 |
|---|---|---|---|---|---|---|---|---|---|---|
| **AFRICAN** | | | | | | | | | | |
| Gabon | Presumed and confirmed | 185 105 | 178 822 | 188 089 | 185 196 | 185 996 | 217 287 | 161 508 | 157 639 | 797 278 |
| | Microscopy examined | 54 714 | – | 66 018 | 90 185 | 90 275 | 79 308 | 62 658 | 70 820 | 264 676 |
| | Confirmed with microscopy | 12 816 | – | 18 694 | 26 432 | 27 687 | 20 390 | 22 419 | 28 297 | 88 112 |
| | RDT examined | 7 887 | – | 4 129 | 10 132 | 11 812 | 12 761 | 2 738 | 18 877 | 71 787 |
| | Confirmed with RDT | 1 120 | – | 1 059 | 2 550 | 4 213 | 3 477 | 1 496 | 6 947 | 23 607 |
| | Imported cases | – | – | – | – | – | – | – | – | – |
| Gambia | Presumed and confirmed | 194 009 | 261 967 | 271 038 | 279 829 | 166 229 | 249 437 | 155 456 | 75 559 | 88 654 [4] |
| | Microscopy examined | 290 842 | 172 241 | 156 580 | 236 329 | 286 111 | 272 604 | 165 793 | 77 491 | 171 668 |
| | Confirmed with microscopy | 52 245 | 71 588 | 29 325 | 65 666 | 66 253 | 49 649 | 26 397 | 11 343 | 14 510 |
| | RDT examined | 123 564 | – | 705 862 | 614 128 | 317 313 | 609 852 | 677 346 | 508 107 | 533 994 |
| | Confirmed with RDT | 64 108 | 190 379 | 271 038 | 175 126 | 99 976 | 190 733 | 127 377 | 58 588 | 72 938 |
| | Imported cases | – | – | – | – | – | – | – | – | – |
| Ghana | Presumed and confirmed | 3 849 536 | 4 154 261 | 10 676 731 | 7 200 797 | 8 453 557 | 10 186 510 | 10 448 267 | 10 228 988 | 11 154 394 [5] |
| | Microscopy examined | 2 031 674 | 1 172 838 | 4 219 097 | 1 394 249 | 1 987 959 | 2 023 581 | 2 594 918 | 2 495 536 | 2 659 067 |
| | Confirmed with microscopy | 1 029 384 | 624 756 | 2 971 699 | 721 898 | 970 448 | 934 304 | 1 189 012 | 1 089 799 | 1 105 438 |
| | RDT examined | 247 278 | 781 892 | 1 438 284 | 1 488 822 | 3 610 453 | 5 478 585 | 5 532 416 | 5 677 564 | 6 660 205 |
| | Confirmed with RDT | 42 253 | 416 504 | 783 467 | 917 553 | 2 445 464 | 3 385 615 | 3 346 155 | 3 286 140 | 3 826 106 |
| | Imported cases | – | – | – | – | – | – | – | – | – |
| Guinea | Presumed and confirmed | 1 092 554 | 1 189 016 | 1 220 574 | 775 341 | 1 595 828 | 895 016 | 992 146 | 1 335 323 | 1 599 625 [5] |
| | Microscopy examined | – | 43 549 | – | – | 116 767 | 78 377 | 79 233 | 99 083 | 131 715 |
| | Confirmed with microscopy | 20 936 | 5 450 | 191 421 | 63 353 | 82 818 | 52 211 | 53 805 | 64 211 | 77 119 |
| | RDT examined | – | 139 066 | – | – | – | 1 092 523 | 1 423 802 | 2 035 460 | 2 445 164 |
| | Confirmed with RDT | – | 90 124 | 125 779 | 147 904 | 577 389 | 758 768 | 938 341 | 1 271 112 | 1 137 877 |
| | Imported cases | – | – | – | – | – | – | – | – | – |
| Guinea-Bissau | Presumed and confirmed | 140 143 | 174 986 | 129 684 | 132 176 | 98 952 | 142 309 | 150 903 | 143 554 | 171 075 |
| | Microscopy examined | 48 799 | 57 698 | 61 048 | 58 909 | 106 882 | 123 810 | 146 708 | 157 970 | 149 423 |
| | Confirmed with microscopy | 30 239 | 21 320 | 23 547 | 17 733 | 35 546 | 45 789 | 53 014 | 53 770 | 45 564 |
| | RDT examined | 56 455 | 139 531 | 97 047 | 102 079 | 197 536 | 261 868 | 234 488 | 303 651 | 320 217 |
| | Confirmed with RDT | 20 152 | 50 662 | 26 834 | 36 851 | 57 885 | 96 520 | 97 889 | 89 784 | 125 511 |
| | Imported cases | – | – | – | – | – | – | – | – | – |
| Kenya | Presumed and confirmed | 6 071 583 | 11 120 812 | 9 335 951 | 9 750 953 | 9 655 905 | 7 676 980 | 8 322 500 | 7 961 444 | 9 950 781 |
| | Microscopy examined | 2 384 402 | 3 009 051 | 4 836 617 | 6 606 885 | 7 444 865 | 7 772 329 | 6 167 609 | 5 952 353 | 4 282 912 |
| | Confirmed with microscopy | 898 531 | 1 002 805 | 1 426 719 | 2 060 608 | 2 415 950 | 1 025 508 | 1 569 045 | 2 215 665 | 827 947 |
| | RDT examined | – | – | 164 424 | 655 285 | 850 884 | 1 965 661 | 3 588 676 | 3 314 695 | 2 329 005 |
| | Confirmed with RDT | – | – | 26 752 | 274 678 | 392 981 | 473 519 | 1 214 801 | 999 451 | 693 619 |
| | Imported cases | – | – | – | – | – | – | – | – | – |
| Liberia | Presumed and confirmed | 2 675 816 | 2 480 748 | 1 800 372 | 1 483 676 | 1 066 107 | 1 781 092 | 2 343 410 | 1 342 953 | – |
| | Microscopy examined | 335 973 | 728 443 | 772 362 | 818 352 | 1 318 801 | 509 062 | 649 096 | 715 643 | – |
| | Confirmed with microscopy | 212 927 | 577 641 | 507 967 | 496 269 | 302 708 | 305 981 | 381 781 | 425 639 | – |
| | RDT examined | 998 043 | 1 593 676 | 1 276 521 | 1 144 405 | 912 382 | 947 048 | 1 304 021 | 1 045 323 | – |
| | Confirmed with RDT | 709 246 | 1 338 121 | 899 488 | 747 951 | 561 496 | 625 105 | 809 356 | 644 474 | – |
| | Imported cases | – | – | – | – | – | – | – | – | – |
| Madagascar | Presumed and confirmed | 293 910 | 255 814 | 395 149 | 382 495 | 433 101 | 752 176 | 475 333 | 800 661 | 972 790 [4] |
| | Microscopy examined | 24 393 | 34 813 | 38 453 | 42 573 | 37 362 | 39 604 | 33 085 | 34 265 | 43 759 |
| | Confirmed with microscopy | 2 173 | 3 447 | 3 667 | 4 947 | 3 853 | 4 748 | 3 734 | 5 134 | 7 400 |
| | RDT examined | 604 114 | 739 572 | 906 080 | 1 026 110 | 926 998 | 1 488 667 | 1 496 990 | 1 974 518 | 2 290 797 |
| | Confirmed with RDT | 200 277 | 221 051 | 355 753 | 380 651 | 374 110 | 739 355 | 471 599 | 795 527 | 965 390 |
| | Imported cases | – | – | – | – | 712 | 1 167 | 1 212 | – | – |
| Malawi | Presumed and confirmed | 6 851 108 | 5 338 701 | 4 922 596 | 3 906 838 | 5 065 703 | 4 933 416 | 5 165 386 | 5 936 348 | 5 865 476 [3] |
| | Microscopy examined | – | 119 996 | 406 907 | 132 475 | 198 534 | 216 643 | 240 212 | 127 752 | 129 575 |
| | Confirmed with microscopy | – | 50 526 | 283 138 | 44 501 | 77 635 | 75 923 | 96 538 | 46 099 | 34 735 |
| | RDT examined | – | 580 708 | 2 763 986 | 3 029 020 | 5 344 724 | 7 030 084 | 8 661 237 | 9 413 944 | 11 384 109 |
| | Confirmed with RDT | – | 253 973 | 1 281 846 | 1 236 391 | 2 827 675 | 3 585 315 | 4 730 835 | 4 901 344 | 5 830 741 |
| | Imported cases | – | – | – | – | – | – | – | – | – |

| WHO region Country/area | | 2010 | 2011 | 2012 | 2013 | 2014 | 2015 | 2016 | 2017 | 2018 |
|---|---|---|---|---|---|---|---|---|---|---|
| **AFRICAN** | | | | | | | | | | |
| Mali | Presumed and confirmed | 2 171 542 | 1 961 070 | 2 171 739 | 2 327 385 | 2 590 643 | 3 317 001 | 2 311 098 | 2 097 797 | 2 614 104 [5] |
| | Microscopy examined | – | – | – | – | – | – | – | 397 723 | 437 903 |
| | Confirmed with microscopy | – | – | 97 995 | 190 337 | 219 637 | 243 151 | 235 212 | 276 673 | 301 880 |
| | RDT examined | 1 380 178 | 974 558 | – | 1 889 286 | – | 3 389 449 | 3 408 254 | 2 755 935 | 3 019 364 |
| | Confirmed with RDT | 227 482 | 307 035 | 788 487 | 1 176 881 | 1 820 216 | 2 052 460 | 1 921 070 | 1 821 124 | 2 043 595 |
| | Imported cases | – | – | – | – | – | – | – | – | – |
| Mauritania | Presumed and confirmed | 244 319 | 154 003 | 169 104 | 128 486 | 172 326 | 181 562 | 159 225 | 162 572 | 175 841 |
| | Microscopy examined | 5 449 | 3 752 | 1 865 | 5 510 | – | – | – | – | – |
| | Confirmed with microscopy | 909 | 1 130 | 255 | 957 | – | – | – | – | – |
| | RDT examined | 2 299 | 7 991 | 3 293 | 3 576 | 47 500 | 60 253 | 50 788 | 51 515 | 75 889 |
| | Confirmed with RDT | 1 085 | 1 796 | 1 633 | 630 | 15 835 | 22 631 | 29 156 | 20 105 | 30 609 |
| | Imported cases | – | – | – | – | – | – | – | – | – |
| Mayotte | Presumed and confirmed | 396 | 92 | 72 | – | – | – | 18 | 19 | 47 |
| | Microscopy examined | 2 023 | 1 214 | 1 463 | – | – | – | – | – | – |
| | Confirmed with microscopy | 396 | 92 | 72 | 82 | 15 | 11 | 28 | 19 | 47 |
| | RDT examined | – | – | – | – | – | – | – | – | – |
| | Confirmed with RDT | – | – | – | – | – | – | – | – | – |
| | Imported cases*** | 224 | 51 | 47 | 71 | 14 | 10 | 10 | – | 44 |
| Mozambique | Presumed and confirmed | 3 381 371 | 3 344 413 | 3 203 338 | 3 924 832 | 5 485 327 | 5 830 322 | 7 546 091 | 8 993 352 | 9 320 557 |
| | Microscopy examined | 1 950 933 | 2 504 720 | 2 546 213 | 2 058 998 | 2 295 823 | 2 313 129 | 1 886 154 | 1 699 589 | 1 909 051 |
| | Confirmed with microscopy | 644 568 | 1 093 742 | 886 143 | 774 891 | 1 009 496 | 735 750 | 674 697 | 700 282 | 743 435 |
| | RDT examined | 2 287 536 | 2 966 853 | 2 234 994 | 5 215 893 | 9 944 222 | 11 928 263 | 13 567 501 | 14 134 096 | 15 190 949 |
| | Confirmed with RDT | 878 009 | 663 132 | 927 841 | 2 223 983 | 6 108 152 | 6 983 032 | 7 845 679 | 8 220 799 | 8 549 493 |
| | Imported cases | – | – | – | – | – | – | – | – | – |
| Namibia | Presumed and confirmed | 25 889 | 14 406 | 3 163 | 4 745 | 15 914 | 12 050 | 23 568 | 66 141 | 36 451* |
| | Microscopy examined | 14 522 | 13 262 | 7 875 | 1 507 | 1 894 | 1 471 | 1 778 | 1 778 | 1 215 |
| | Confirmed with microscopy | 556 | 335 | 194 | 136 | 222 | 118 | 329 | 364 | 289 |
| | RDT examined | – | 48 599 | – | 32 495 | 185 078 | 207 612 | 308 414 | 616 513 | 394 822 |
| | Confirmed with RDT | – | 1 525 | – | 4 775 | 15 692 | 12 050 | 24 869 | 66 141 | 36 451 |
| | Imported cases*** | – | – | – | – | – | 2 888 | 3 980 | 11 874 | 4 021 |
| Niger | Presumed and confirmed | 3 643 803 | 3 157 482 | 4 592 519 | 4 288 425 | 3 222 613 | 3 817 634 | 5 056 393 | 2 638 580 | 3 358 058 [5] |
| | Microscopy examined | 165 514 | 130 658 | 1 781 505 | 1 799 299 | 2 872 710 | 295 229 | 3 198 194 | 203 583 | 213 795 |
| | Confirmed with microscopy | 49 285 | 68 529 | 1 119 929 | 1 176 711 | 0 | 206 660 | 2 120 515 | 125 856 | 121 657 |
| | RDT examined | 7 426 774 | 1 130 514 | 1 781 505 | 1 799 299 | 2 872 710 | 2 657 057 | 3 066 101 | 3 615 853 | 4 285 516 |
| | Confirmed with RDT | 570 773 | 712 347 | 1 119 929 | 1 176 711 | 1 953 309 | 2 065 340 | 2 027 652 | 2 512 724 | 2 924 793 |
| | Imported cases | – | – | – | – | – | – | – | – | – |
| Nigeria | Presumed and confirmed | 3 873 463 | 4 306 945 | 6 938 519 | 12 830 911 | 16 512 127 | 15 157 491 | 16 740 560 | 18 690 954 | 18 870 214 |
| | Microscopy examined | – | 672 185 | 1 953 399 | 1 633 960 | 1 681 469 | 839 849 | 901 141 | 1 055 444 | 1 428 731 |
| | Confirmed with microscopy | 523 513 | – | – | – | 1 233 654 | 556 871 | 618 363 | 749 118 | 1 023 273 |
| | RDT examined | 45 924 | 242 526 | 2 898 052 | 7 194 960 | 9 188 933 | 8 690 087 | 11 765 893 | 14 808 335 | 15 848 248 |
| | Confirmed with RDT | 27 674 | – | – | – | 6 593 300 | 6 261 971 | 8 616 024 | 10 822 840 | 11 930 310 |
| | Imported cases | – | – | – | – | – | – | – | – | – |
| Rwanda | Presumed and confirmed | 638 669 | 208 498 | 483 470 | 939 076 | 1 610 812 | 2 505 794 | 3 324 678 | 4 413 473 | 1 975 926 |
| | Microscopy examined | 2 708 973 | 1 602 271 | 2 904 793 | 2 862 877 | 4 010 202 | 5 811 267 | 6 603 261 | 6 637 571 | 5 501 455 |
| | Confirmed with microscopy | 638 669 | 208 858 | 422 224 | 879 316 | 1 528 825 | 2 354 400 | 2 916 902 | 2 927 780 | 1 657 793 |
| | RDT examined | – | – | 190 593 | 201 708 | 168 004 | 281 847 | 898 913 | 920 295 | 720 026 |
| | Confirmed with RDT | – | – | 61 246 | 83 302 | 81 987 | 151 394 | 463 666 | 475 403 | 318 133 |
| | Imported cases | – | – | – | – | – | – | – | – | – |
| Sao Tome and Principe | Presumed and confirmed | 3 346 | 8 442 | 12 550 | 7 418 | 1 337 | 2 058 | 2 238 | 2 241 | 2 940 [5] |
| | Microscopy examined | 48 366 | 83 355 | 103 773 | 73 866 | 33 355 | 11 941 | 3 682 | 2 146 | 13 186 |
| | Confirmed with microscopy | 2 233 | 6 373 | 10 706 | 6 352 | 569 | 140 | 33 | 109 | 148 |
| | RDT examined | 9 989 | 33 924 | 23 124 | 34 768 | 58 090 | 72 407 | 117 727 | 94 466 | 156 697 |
| | Confirmed with RDT | 507 | 2 069 | 1 844 | 2 891 | 1 185 | 1 918 | 2 205 | 2 132 | 2 792 |
| | Imported cases*** | – | – | – | – | – | 2 | 4 | 2 | 3 |

# Annex 3 - H. Reported malaria cases by method of confirmation, 2010–2018

| WHO region Country/area | | 2010 | 2011 | 2012 | 2013 | 2014 | 2015 | 2016 | 2017 | 2018 |
|---|---|---|---|---|---|---|---|---|---|---|
| **AFRICAN** | | | | | | | | | | |
| Senegal | Presumed and confirmed | 707 772 | 604 290 | 634 106 | 772 222 | 628 642 | 502 084 | 356 272 | 398 377 | 536 745 [5] |
| | Microscopy examined | 27 793 | 18 325 | 19 946 | 24 205 | 19 343 | 26 556 | 38 748 | 21 639 | 12 881 |
| | Confirmed with microscopy | 17 750 | 14 142 | 15 612 | 20 801 | 12 636 | 17 846 | 9 918 | 10 463 | 3 997 |
| | RDT examined | 651 737 | 555 614 | 524 971 | 668 562 | 697 175 | 1 384 834 | 1 513 574 | 2 011 383 | 2 077 442 |
| | Confirmed with RDT | 325 920 | 263 184 | 265 468 | 325 088 | 252 988 | 474 407 | 339 622 | 385 243 | 526 947 |
| | Imported cases*** | – | – | – | – | – | 352 | 1 905 | 0 | 292 |
| Sierra Leone | Presumed and confirmed | 934 028 | 856 332 | 1 945 859 | 1 715 851 | 1 898 852 | 1 569 606 | 1 845 727 | 1 741 512 | 1 781 855 [3] |
| | Microscopy examined | 718 473 | 46 280 | 194 787 | 185 403 | 66 277 | 75 025 | 120 917 | 10 910 | 20 155 |
| | Confirmed with microscopy | 218 473 | 25 511 | 104 533 | 76 077 | 39 414 | 37 820 | 60 458 | 5 717 | 8 719 |
| | RDT examined | 1 609 455 | 886 994 | 1 975 972 | 2 377 254 | 2 056 722 | 2 176 042 | 2 805 621 | 2 834 261 | 2 827 417 |
| | Confirmed with RDT | 715 555 | 613 348 | 1 432 789 | 1 625 881 | 1 335 062 | 1 445 556 | 1 714 848 | 1 645 519 | 1 725 112 |
| | Imported cases | – | – | – | – | – | – | – | – | 0 |
| South Africa | Presumed and confirmed | 8 060 | 9 866 | 6 846 | 8 851 | 13 988 | 8 976 | 4 323 | 28 295 | 18 638 [3] |
| | Microscopy examined | – | 178 387 | 121 291 | 364 021 | 300 291 | 13 917 | 20 653 | – | – |
| | Confirmed with microscopy | 3 787 | 5 986 | 1 632 | 2 572 | 4 101 | 785 | 1 219 | 9 592 | 2 666 |
| | RDT examined | 276 669 | 204 047 | 30 053 | 239 705 | 240 622 | 17 446 | 42 624 | 56 257 | – |
| | Confirmed with RDT | 4 273 | 3 880 | 3 997 | 6 073 | 7 604 | 3 572 | 3 104 | 18 703 | 8 123 |
| | Imported cases | – | – | – | – | – | 3 568 | 3 075 | 6 234 | 5 742 |
| South Sudan[2] | Presumed and confirmed | 900 283 | 795 784 | 1 125 039 | 1 855 501 | 2 433 991 | 3 789 475 | – | 3 602 208 | 4 697 506 |
| | Microscopy examined | – | – | – | – | 27 321 | 22 721 | 6 954 | 800 067 | 1 204 |
| | Confirmed with microscopy | 900 283 | 112 024 | 225 371 | 262 520 | 18 344 | 11 272 | 2 357 | 335 642 | 634 |
| | RDT examined | – | – | – | – | 102 538 | 26 507 | 10 751 | 2 024 503 | 1 805 912 |
| | Confirmed with RDT | – | – | – | – | 53 033 | 13 099 | 5 262 | 1 152 363 | 98 209 |
| | Imported cases | – | – | – | – | – | – | – | – | – |
| Togo | Presumed and confirmed | 983 430 | 519 450 | 768 287 | 881 611 | 1 113 928 | 1 113 928 | 1 183 265 | 1 209 034 | 1 381 410 [4] |
| | Microscopy examined | 478 354 | 502 977 | 579 507 | 560 096 | 621 119 | 621 119 | 435 164 | 445 035 | 267 028 |
| | Confirmed with microscopy | 224 087 | 237 305 | 260 535 | 272 855 | 310 207 | 305 727 | 231 819 | 209 626 | 108 146 |
| | RDT examined | 575 245 | 390 611 | 660 627 | 882 475 | 1 135 581 | 1 135 581 | 1 410 290 | 1 597 463 | 1 488 587 |
| | Confirmed with RDT | 393 014 | 282 145 | 436 839 | 609 575 | 820 044 | 808 200 | 951 446 | 999 408 | 982 188 |
| | Imported cases | – | – | – | – | – | – | – | – | – |
| Uganda | Presumed and confirmed | 13 208 169 | 12 173 358 | 13 591 932 | 16 541 563 | 13 724 345 | 13 421 804 | 13 657 887 | 12 273 076 | 8 895 436 [5] |
| | Microscopy examined | 3 705 284 | 385 928 | 3 466 571 | 3 718 588 | 2 048 185 | 3 684 722 | 4 492 090 | 5 515 931 | 1 606 330 |
| | Confirmed with microscopy | 1 581 160 | 134 726 | 1 413 149 | 1 502 362 | 578 289 | 1 248 576 | 1 542 091 | 1 694 441 | 458 909 |
| | RDT examined | – | 194 819 | 2 449 526 | 7 387 826 | 7 060 545 | 12 126 996 | 17 473 299 | 16 803 712 | 12 741 670 |
| | Confirmed with RDT | – | 97 147 | 1 249 109 | – | 3 053 650 | 5 889 086 | 7 843 041 | 9 973 390 | 5 300 265 |
| | Imported cases | – | – | – | – | – | – | – | – | – |
| United Republic of Tanzania | Presumed and confirmed | 12 893 535 | 10 164 967 | 8 477 435 | 8 585 482 | 7 403 562 | 7 746 258 | 6 053 868 | 5 597 715 | 6 220 485 [2] |
| | Microscopy examined | 3 637 659 | 5 656 907 | 6 931 025 | 6 804 085 | 727 130 | 673 223 | 1 386 389 | 2 888 538 | 3 015 052 |
| | Confirmed with microscopy | 1 277 024 | 1 813 179 | 1 772 062 | 1 481 275 | 572 289 | 412 702 | 1 262 679 | 916 742 | 831 903 |
| | RDT examined | 136 123 | 1 628 092 | 1 091 615 | 813 103 | 17 740 207 | 16 620 299 | 15 538 709 | 15 257 462 | 19 603 825 |
| | Confirmed with RDT | 1 974 | 337 582 | 214 893 | 71 169 | 107 728 | 3 830 030 | 3 930 841 | 4 437 744 | 5 221 811 |
| | Imported cases*** | | | | 719 | 1 583 | 2 550 | | | 1 754 |
| Mainland | Presumed and confirmed | 12 819 192 | 10 160 478 | 8 474 278 | 8 582 934 | 7 399 316 | 7 741 816 | 6 050 097 | 5 593 544 | 6 215 115 [4] |
| | Microscopy examined | 3 573 710 | 5 513 619 | 6 784 639 | 6 720 141 | 592 320 | 532 118 | 1 285 720 | 2 826 948 | 2 937 666 |
| | Confirmed with microscopy | 1 276 660 | 1 812 704 | 1 771 388 | 1 480 791 | 571 598 | 411 741 | 1 261 650 | 915 887 | 830 668 |
| | RDT examined | – | 1 315 662 | 701 477 | 369 444 | 17 566 750 | 16 416 675 | 15 379 517 | 15 052 571 | 19 338 466 |
| | Confirmed with RDT | – | 333 568 | 212 636 | 69 459 | 106 609 | 3 827 749 | 3 926 855 | 4 435 250 | 5 219 714 |
| | Imported cases | – | – | – | – | – | – | – | – | – |
| Zanzibar | Presumed and confirmed | 74 343 | 4 489 | 3 157 | 2 548 | 4 246 | 4 442 | 3 771 | 4 171 | 5 370 [4] |
| | Microscopy examined | 63 949 | 143 288 | 146 386 | 83 944 | 134 810 | 141 105 | 100 669 | 61 590 | 77 386 |
| | Confirmed with microscopy | 364 | 475 | 674 | 484 | 691 | 961 | 1 029 | 855 | 1 235 |
| | RDT examined | 136 123 | 312 430 | 390 138 | 443 659 | 173 457 | 203 624 | 159 192 | 204 891 | 265 359 |
| | Confirmed with RDT | 1 974 | 4 014 | 2 257 | 1 710 | 1 119 | 2 281 | 3 986 | 2 494 | 2 097 |
| | Imported cases*** | – | – | – | 719 | 1 583 | 2 550 | – | – | 1 754 |

| WHO region Country/area | | 2010 | 2011 | 2012 | 2013 | 2014 | 2015 | 2016 | 2017 | 2018 |
|---|---|---|---|---|---|---|---|---|---|---|
| **AFRICAN** | | | | | | | | | | |
| Zambia | Presumed and confirmed | 4 229 839 | 4 607 908 | 4 695 400 | 5 465 122 | 5 972 933 | 5 094 123 | 5 976 192 | 6 054 679 | 5 195 723 [3] |
| | Microscopy examined | – | – | – | – | – | – | – | – | 180 697 |
| | Confirmed with microscopy | – | – | – | – | – | – | – | – | 49 855 |
| | RDT examined | – | – | – | – | 5 964 354 | 7 207 500 | 8 502 989 | 10 403 283 | 9 718 666 |
| | Confirmed with RDT | – | – | – | – | 4 077 547 | 4 184 661 | 4 851 319 | 5 505 639 | 4 989 824 |
| | Imported cases | – | – | – | – | – | – | – | – | – |
| Zimbabwe | Presumed and confirmed | 648 965 | 319 935 | 276 963 | 422 633 | 535 983 | 391 651 | 280 853 | 316 392 | 184 427 [4] |
| | Microscopy examined | – | 10 004 | – | – | – | – | – | 0 | 2 771 |
| | Confirmed with microscopy | – | – | – | – | – | – | – | 0 | 0 |
| | RDT examined | 513 032 | 470 007 | 727 174 | 1 115 005 | 1 420 894 | 1 384 893 | 1 223 509 | 1 110 705 | 995 715 |
| | Confirmed with RDT | 249 379 | 319 935 | 276 963 | 422 633 | 535 931 | 391 651 | 279 988 | 316 392 | 184 427 |
| | Imported cases*** | – | – | – | – | – | 180 | 358 | 768 | 672 |
| **AMERICAS** | | | | | | | | | | |
| Argentina[1] | Presumed and confirmed | 72 | 18 | 4 | 4 | 4 | 8 | 5 | 15 | 23 |
| | Microscopy examined | 2 547 | 7 872 | 7 027 | 4 913 | 5 691 | 3 862 | 3 479 | 2 114 | 345 |
| | Confirmed with microscopy | 72 | 18 | 4 | 4 | 4 | 11 | 7 | 18 | 23 |
| | RDT examined | – | – | – | 0 | 0 | 0 | 0 | 0 | 0 |
| | Confirmed with RDT | – | – | – | 0 | 0 | 0 | 0 | 0 | 0 |
| | Imported cases | 57 | 18 | 4 | 4 | 4 | 8 | 5 | 15 | 23 |
| Belize | Presumed and confirmed | 150 | 79 | 37 | 26 | 19 | 13 | 5 | 9 | 7 [5] |
| | Microscopy examined | 27 366 | 22 996 | 20 789 | 25 351 | 24 122 | 26 367 | 20 936 | 26 995 | 17 642 |
| | Confirmed with microscopy | 150 | 79 | 37 | 26 | 19 | 13 | 5 | 9 | 7 |
| | RDT examined | – | – | – | – | – | 0 | 0 | 0 | – |
| | Confirmed with RDT | – | – | – | – | – | 0 | 0 | 0 | – |
| | Imported cases | – | 7 | 4 | 4 | 0 | 4 | 1 | 2 | 4 |
| Bolivia (Plurinational State of) | Presumed and confirmed | 13 769 | 7 143 | 7 415 | 7 342 | 7 401 | 6 907 | 5 553 | 4 587 | 5 354 [3] |
| | Microscopy examined | 133 463 | 143 272 | 121 944 | 133 260 | 124 900 | 159 167 | 155 407 | 151 697 | 139 938 |
| | Confirmed with microscopy | 12 252 | 6 108 | 6 293 | 6 272 | 7 401 | 6 907 | 5 553 | 4 334 | 5 261 |
| | RDT examined | 7 394 | 7 390 | 10 960 | 10 789 | – | – | – | – | – |
| | Confirmed with RDT | 1 517 | 1 035 | 1 122 | 1 070 | – | – | – | 253 | 93 |
| | Imported cases | – | – | – | – | – | 33 | 11 | 15 | 12 |
| Brazil | Presumed and confirmed | 334 668 | 267 146 | 242 758 | 178 595 | 144 128 | 143 161 | 129 245 | 194 426 | 194 512 [4] |
| | Microscopy examined | 2 711 432 | 2 476 335 | 2 325 775 | 1 873 518 | 1 744 640 | 1 573 538 | 1 341 639 | 1 656 688 | 1 753 972 |
| | Confirmed with microscopy | 334 667 | 266 713 | 237 978 | 174 048 | 142 744 | 139 844 | 124 210 | 184 877 | 181 923 |
| | RDT examined | – | 1 486 | 23 566 | 19 500 | 11 820 | 16 865 | 23 273 | 39 378 | 46 201 |
| | Confirmed with RDT | – | 433 | 4 780 | 3 719 | 1 384 | 3 318 | 5 034 | 9 549 | 12 589 |
| | Imported cases | – | – | – | 8 905 | 4 847 | 4 915 | 5 068 | 4 867 | 6 819 |
| Colombia | Presumed and confirmed | 117 650 | 64 436 | 60 179 | 51 722 | 40 768 | 55 866 | 83 227 | 54 102 | 63 143 [5,8] |
| | Microscopy examined | 521 342 | 396 861 | 346 599 | 284 332 | 325 713 | 316 451 | 242 973 | 244 732 | 195 286 |
| | Confirmed with microscopy | 117 637 | 60 121 | 50 938 | 44 293 | 36 166 | 48 059 | – | 38 349 | 42 810 |
| | RDT examined | – | 21 171 | 70 168 | 42 723 | 77 819 | 11 983 | 53 118 | 9 648 | 13 252 |
| | Confirmed with RDT | 13 | 4 188 | 9 241 | 7 403 | 4 602 | 3 535 | 5 655 | 5 056 | 3 407 |
| | Imported cases | – | – | – | – | – | 7 785 | 618 | 1 297 | 1 948 |
| Costa Rica | Presumed and confirmed | 114 | 17 | 8 | 6 | 6 | 8 | 13 | 25 | 108* [4] |
| | Microscopy examined | 15 599 | 10 690 | 7 485 | 16 774 | 4 420 | 7 373 | 5 160 | 9 680 | 9 000 |
| | Confirmed with microscopy | 114 | 17 | 8 | 6 | 6 | 8 | 13 | 25 | 108 |
| | RDT examined | – | – | – | 0 | 0 | 0 | 0 | 0 | 700 |
| | Confirmed with RDT | – | – | – | 0 | 0 | 0 | 0 | 0 | 44 |
| | Imported cases | 27 | 7 | 1 | 4 | 5 | 8 | 9 | 13 | 38 |
| Dominican Republic | Presumed and confirmed | 2 482 | 1 616 | 952 | 579 | 496 | 661 | 755 | 324 | 484* |
| | Microscopy examined | 469 052 | 421 405 | 415 808 | 431 683 | 362 304 | 317 257 | 51 329 | 226 988 | 33 420 |
| | Confirmed with microscopy | – | 1 616 | 952 | 579 | 496 | 661 | 484 | 398 | 322 |
| | RDT examined | 26 585 | 56 150 | 90 775 | 71 000 | 54 425 | 7 530 | 22 450 | 38 547 | 42 425 |
| | Confirmed with RDT | 932 | – | – | – | – | – | – | – | 286 |
| | Imported cases | – | – | – | 105 | 37 | 30 | 65 | 57 | 50 |

# Annex 3 - H. Reported malaria cases by method of confirmation, 2010–2018

| WHO region Country/area | | 2010 | 2011 | 2012 | 2013 | 2014 | 2015 | 2016 | 2017 | 2018 |
|---|---|---|---|---|---|---|---|---|---|---|
| **AMERICAS** | | | | | | | | | | |
| Ecuador | Presumed and confirmed | 1 888 | 1 232 | 558 | 378 | 242 | 686 | 1 191 | 1 380 | 1 806 [5] |
| | Microscopy examined | 481 030 | 460 785 | 459 157 | 397 628 | 370 825 | 261 824 | 311 920 | 306 894 | 237 995 |
| | Confirmed with microscopy | 1 888 | 1 232 | 558 | 378 | 242 | 686 | 1 191 | 1 380 | 1 589 |
| | RDT examined | 7 800 | – | – | – | – | – | – | – | 6 782 |
| | Confirmed with RDT | – | – | – | – | – | – | – | – | 217 |
| | Imported cases | – | 14 | 14 | 10 | – | 59 | 233 | 105 | 153 |
| El Salvador[7] | Presumed and confirmed | 24 | 15 | 21 | 7 | 8 | 9 | 14 | 4 | 2 |
| | Microscopy examined | 115 256 | 100 883 | 124 885 | 103 748 | 106 915 | 89 267 | 81 904 | 70 022 | 52 216 |
| | Confirmed with microscopy | 24 | – | 21 | 7 | 8 | 9 | 14 | 4 | 2 |
| | RDT examined | – | 1 | – | – | 0 | 0 | 0 | 0 | 0 |
| | Confirmed with RDT | – | 1 | – | – | 0 | 0 | 0 | 0 | 0 |
| | Imported cases | 7 | 6 | 6 | 1 | 2 | 7 | 1 | 3 | 2 |
| French Guiana | Presumed and confirmed | 1 608 | 1 209 | 900 | 877 | 448 | 434 | 258 | 597 | – |
| | Microscopy examined | 14 373 | 14 429 | 13 638 | 22 327 | 14 651 | 11 558 | 9 430 | – | – |
| | Confirmed with microscopy | – | 505 | 401 | – | 242 | 297 | 173 | 468 | – |
| | RDT examined | – | – | – | – | – | – | – | – | – |
| | Confirmed with RDT | 944 | 704 | 499 | 551 | 206 | 137 | 58 | 129 | – |
| | Imported cases | – | – | – | – | – | 60 | 41 | 43 | – |
| Guatemala | Presumed and confirmed | 7 198 | 6 817 | 5 346 | 6 214 | 4 931 | 5 538 | 4 854 | 3 744 | 4 769** |
| | Microscopy examined | 235 075 | 195 080 | 186 645 | 153 731 | 250 964 | 295 246 | 333 535 | 372 158 | 438 833 |
| | Confirmed with microscopy | 7 198 | 6 817 | 5 346 | 6 214 | – | – | 4 854 | 3 744 | 3 021 |
| | RDT examined | 2 000 | – | 0 | 0 | 50 025 | 6 500 | 74 859 | 0 | 75 300 |
| | Confirmed with RDT | 0 | – | 0 | 0 | – | 1 298 | – | 0 | 1 748 |
| | Imported cases | – | – | – | – | 1 | 2 | 1 | 2 | 3 |
| Guyana | Presumed and confirmed | 22 935 | 29 471 | 31 610 | 31 479 | 12 354 | 9 984 | 11 108 | 13 936 | 17 038 |
| | Microscopy examined | 212 863 | 201 693 | 196 622 | 205 903 | 142 843 | 132 941 | 110 891 | 100 096 | 99 806 |
| | Confirmed with microscopy | 22 935 | – | – | 31 479 | 12 354 | 9 984 | – | 13 734 | 15 599 |
| | RDT examined | – | 35 | – | 0 | 0 | 0 | 5 409 | – | – |
| | Confirmed with RDT | – | 35 | 55 | 0 | 0 | 0 | 1 461 | 202 | 1 439 |
| | Imported cases | – | – | – | – | – | – | 411 | – | – |
| Haiti | Presumed and confirmed | 84 153 | 32 969 | 25 423 | 26 543 | 17 696 | 17 583 | 21 430 | 19 135 | 8 828* [5] |
| | Microscopy examined | 270 427 | 184 934 | 167 726 | 165 823 | 134 766 | 69 659 | 61 428 | 62 539 | 59 803 |
| | Confirmed with microscopy | 84 153 | – | – | 20 957 | 10 893 | 5 224 | 4 342 | 2 119 | 1 586 |
| | RDT examined | – | – | 46 | 5 586 | 126 637 | 233 081 | 245 133 | 232 741 | 228 491 |
| | Confirmed with RDT | – | – | – | – | 6 803 | 12 359 | 18 115 | 17 739 | 7 526 |
| | Imported cases | – | – | – | – | – | – | – | – | – |
| Honduras | Presumed and confirmed | 9 685 | 7 618 | 6 439 | 5 428 | 3 380 | 3 575 | 4 097 | 1 287 | 653* |
| | Microscopy examined | 152 961 | 152 451 | 155 165 | 144 436 | 151 420 | 150 854 | 167 836 | 148 160 | 142 780 |
| | Confirmed with microscopy | – | 7 465 | – | 5 364 | – | 3 555 | 3 695 | 1 251 | 653 |
| | RDT examined | 4 000 | 4 000 | 4 000 | 237 | 1 427 | 3 052 | 14 930 | 17 376 | 18 620 |
| | Confirmed with RDT | – | 45 | 10 | 64 | 102 | 20 | 401 | 35 | 229 |
| | Imported cases*** | – | – | – | – | 2 | 0 | 3 | 10 | 21 |
| Mexico | Presumed and confirmed | 1 226 | 1 124 | 833 | 499 | 666 | 551 | 596 | 765 | 826 [5] |
| | Microscopy examined | 1 192 081 | 1 035 424 | 1 025 659 | 1 017 508 | 900 578 | 867 853 | 798 568 | 644 174 | 548 247 |
| | Confirmed with microscopy | 1 233 | 1 130 | 842 | 499 | – | 551 | 596 | 765 | 826 |
| | RDT examined | – | – | – | 0 | 0 | 0 | 0 | 0 | 0 |
| | Confirmed with RDT | – | – | – | 0 | 0 | 0 | 0 | 0 | 0 |
| | Imported cases | 7 | 6 | 9 | 4 | 10 | 34 | 45 | 29 | 23 |
| Nicaragua | Presumed and confirmed | 692 | 925 | 1 235 | 1 194 | 1 163 | 2 307 | 6 284 | 10 949 | 15 934 |
| | Microscopy examined | 535 914 | 521 904 | 536 278 | 519 993 | 605 357 | 604 418 | 553 615 | 660 452 | 831 077 |
| | Confirmed with microscopy | 692 | 925 | 1 235 | 1 194 | 1 163 | 2 307 | 6 284 | 10 949 | 15 934 |
| | RDT examined | 18 500 | 14 201 | 16 444 | 19 029 | 0 | – | 800 | 2 680 | 44 905 |
| | Confirmed with RDT | 0 | – | 0 | – | 0 | – | – | – | 0 |
| | Imported cases | – | – | – | 34 | 21 | 29 | 12 | 3 | 17 |

| WHO region Country/area | | 2010 | 2011 | 2012 | 2013 | 2014 | 2015 | 2016 | 2017 | 2018 |
|---|---|---|---|---|---|---|---|---|---|---|
| **AMERICAS** | | | | | | | | | | |
| Panama | Presumed and confirmed | 418 | 354 | 844 | 705 | 874 | 562 | 811 | 689 | 715 |
| | Microscopy examined | 141 038 | 116 588 | 107 711 | 93 624 | 80 701 | 64 511 | 50 772 | 38 270 | 23 383 |
| | Confirmed with microscopy | 418 | 354 | 844 | 705 | 874 | 562 | 811 | 689 | 715 |
| | RDT examined | – | 0 | 0 | 0 | 0 | 0 | 0 | 0 | – |
| | Confirmed with RDT | – | 0 | 0 | 0 | 0 | 0 | 0 | 0 | – |
| | Imported cases | – | – | – | 9 | 10 | 16 | 42 | 40 | 31 |
| Paraguay[1] | Presumed and confirmed | 27 | 10 | 15 | 11 | 8 | 8 | 10 | 5 | – |
| | Microscopy examined | 62 178 | 48 611 | 31 499 | 24 806 | 24 832 | 6 687 | 3 192 | 8 014 | – |
| | Confirmed with microscopy | 27 | 10 | 15 | 11 | 8 | 8 | – | 5 | – |
| | RDT examined | – | – | – | – | – | 0 | 1 | 1 267 | – |
| | Confirmed with RDT | – | – | – | – | – | 0 | 1 | 0 | – |
| | Imported cases | 9 | 9 | 15 | 11 | 8 | 8 | 10 | 5 | – |
| Peru | Presumed and confirmed | 31 545 | 25 005 | 31 436 | 48 719 | 65 252 | 63 865 | 56 623 | 55 367 | 45 619* |
| | Microscopy examined | 744 627 | 702 894 | 758 723 | 863 790 | 864 413 | 865 980 | 566 230 | 388 699 | 304 785 |
| | Confirmed with microscopy | – | – | 31 436 | 48 719 | 65 252 | 66 609 | 56 623 | 55 367 | 45 619 |
| | RDT examined | 23 | 58 | 562 | 858 | 1 634 | 0 | – | 13 924 | 160 000 |
| | Confirmed with RDT | 1 | 34 | – | – | – | – | – | 2 325 | 1 000 |
| | Imported cases | – | – | – | – | 0 | 0 | 0 | – | 176 |
| Suriname | Presumed and confirmed | 1 771 | 795 | 569 | 729 | 729 | 376 | 327 | 551 | 235[5] |
| | Microscopy examined | 16 533 | 15 135 | 17 464 | 13 693 | 17 608 | 15 083 | 14 946 | 12 536 | 11 799 |
| | Confirmed with microscopy | 1 574 | 751 | 306 | 530 | – | 345 | 315 | 412 | 218 |
| | RDT examined | 541 | 1 025 | 4 008 | 6 043 | 15 489 | 153 | 8 498 | 9 498 | 8 037 |
| | Confirmed with RDT | 138 | 20 | 50 | 199 | 303 | 31 | 12 | 139 | 17 |
| | Imported cases | – | – | – | 204 | – | 274 | 252 | 414 | 199 |
| Venezuela (Bolivarian Republic of) | Presumed and confirmed | 45 155 | 45 824 | 52 803 | 78 643 | 91 918 | 137 996 | 242 561 | 411 586 | 404 924*[3] |
| | Microscopy examined | 400 495 | 382 303 | 410 663 | 476 764 | 522 617 | 625 174 | 852 556 | 1 144 635 | 699 130 |
| | Confirmed with microscopy | 45 155 | 45 824 | 52 803 | 78 643 | 91 918 | 137 996 | 240 613 | 411 586 | 404 924 |
| | RDT examined | – | – | – | – | – | – | – | – | 48 117 |
| | Confirmed with RDT | – | – | – | – | – | – | – | – | 48 117 |
| | Imported cases | – | – | – | 1 677 | 1 210 | 1 594 | 2 974 | 2 942 | 2 127 |
| **EASTERN MEDITERRANEAN** | | | | | | | | | | |
| Afghanistan | Presumed and confirmed | 392 463 | 482 748 | 391 365 | 319 742 | 295 050 | 366 526 | 384 943 | 326 625 | 299 863 |
| | Microscopy examined | 524 523 | 531 053 | 511 408 | 507 145 | 514 466 | 538 789 | 598 556 | 611 904 | 665 200 |
| | Confirmed with microscopy | 69 397 | 77 549 | 54 840 | 46 114 | 83 920 | 103 377 | 151 528 | 194 866 | 104 960 |
| | RDT examined | – | 0 | 0 | 0 | – | – | 94 975 | 161 925 | 216 240 |
| | Confirmed with RDT | – | 0 | 0 | 0 | – | – | 38 631 | 53 823 | 68 533 |
| | Imported cases | – | – | – | – | – | – | – | – | – |
| Djibouti | Presumed and confirmed | 1 010 | 230 | 27 | 1 684 | 9 439 | 9 557 | 13 804 | 14 671 | 25 319[4] |
| | Microscopy examined | – | 124 | 1 410 | 7 189 | 39 284 | 10 502 | 19 492 | 24 504 | – |
| | Confirmed with microscopy | 1 010 | – | 22 | 1 684 | 9 439 | 1 764 | 2 280 | 1 283 | – |
| | RDT examined | – | – | – | – | – | – | – | 50 104 | 104 800 |
| | Confirmed with RDT | – | – | 3 | – | – | 7 709 | 11 524 | 13 388 | 25 319 |
| | Imported cases | – | – | – | – | – | – | – | – | – |
| Iran (Islamic Republic of)[7] | Presumed and confirmed | 3 031 | 3 239 | 1 629 | 1 373 | 1 238 | 799 | 705 | 939 | 625[5] |
| | Microscopy examined | 614 817 | 530 470 | 479 655 | 385 172 | 468 513 | 610 337 | 418 125 | 383 397 | 477 914 |
| | Confirmed with microscopy | 3 031 | 3 239 | 1 629 | 1 373 | 1 243 | 799 | 705 | 939 | 625 |
| | RDT examined | – | – | 0 | – | – | – | – | – | 64 061 |
| | Confirmed with RDT | – | – | 0 | – | – | – | – | – | 436 |
| | Imported cases | 1 184 | 1 607 | 854 | 879 | 874 | 656 | 620 | 881 | 622 |
| Pakistan | Presumed and confirmed | 4 281 356 | 4 065 802 | 4 285 449 | 3 472 727 | 3 666 257 | 3 776 244 | 2 121 958 | 2 209 768 | 1 069 248[4] |
| | Microscopy examined | 4 281 346 | 4 168 648 | 4 497 330 | 3 933 321 | 4 343 418 | 4 619 980 | 5 046 870 | 4 539 869 | 4 324 570 |
| | Confirmed with microscopy | 220 870 | 287 592 | 250 526 | 196 078 | 193 952 | 137 401 | 154 541 | 132 580 | 119 099 |
| | RDT examined | 279 724 | 518 709 | 410 949 | 628 504 | 779 815 | 691 245 | 1 296 762 | 1 821 139 | 2 207 613 |
| | Confirmed with RDT | 19 721 | 46 997 | 40 255 | 85 677 | 81 197 | 64 612 | 169 925 | 237 237 | 255 411 |
| | Imported cases | – | – | – | – | – | – | – | – | – |

# Annex 3 - H. Reported malaria cases by method of confirmation, 2010–2018

| WHO region Country/area | | 2010 | 2011 | 2012 | 2013 | 2014 | 2015 | 2016 | 2017 | 2018 |
|---|---|---|---|---|---|---|---|---|---|---|
| **EASTERN MEDITERRANEAN** | | | | | | | | | | |
| Saudi Arabia | Presumed and confirmed | 1 941 | 2 788 | 3 406 | – | 2 305 | 2 620 | 5 382 | 3 151 | 2 711 |
| | Microscopy examined | 944 723 | 1 062 827 | 1 186 179 | 1 309 783 | 1 249 752 | 1 306 700 | 1 267 933 | 1 073 998 | 1 015 953 |
| | Confirmed with microscopy | 1 941 | 2 788 | 3 406 | 2 513 | 2 305 | 2 620 | 5 382 | 3 151 | 2 711 |
| | RDT examined | – | – | 0 | – | – | – | – | – | – |
| | Confirmed with RDT | – | – | 0 | – | – | – | – | – | – |
| | Imported cases | 1 912 | 2 719 | 3 324 | 2 479 | 2 275 | 2 537 | 5 110 | 2 974 | 2 650 |
| Somalia | Presumed and confirmed | 24 553 | 41 167 | 23 202 | 9 135 | 26 174 | 39 169 | 58 021 | 37 156 | 31 030 |
| | Microscopy examined | 20 593 | 26 351 | – | – | – | – | – | – | – |
| | Confirmed with microscopy | 5 629 | 1 627 | – | – | – | – | – | – | – |
| | RDT examined | 200 105 | 35 236 | 37 273 | 67 464 | 64 480 | 100 792 | 183 360 | 226 894 | 253 211 |
| | Confirmed with RDT | 18 924 | 1 724 | 6 817 | 7 407 | 11 001 | 20 953 | 35 628 | 35 138 | 31 021 |
| | Imported cases | – | – | – | – | – | – | – | – | – |
| Sudan | Presumed and confirmed | 1 465 496 | 1 214 004 | 964 698 | 989 946 | 1 207 771 | 1 102 186 | 897 194 | 1 562 821 | 3 581 302 [4] |
| | Microscopy examined | – | – | – | – | – | 3 586 482 | 3 236 118 | 2 426 329 | 6 668 355 |
| | Confirmed with microscopy | 625 365 | 506 806 | 526 931 | 592 383 | 579 038 | 586 827 | 378 308 | 588 100 | 1 251 544 |
| | RDT examined | 1 653 300 | 2 222 380 | 2 000 700 | 1 800 000 | 788 281 | – | 632 443 | 422 841 | 1 080 601 |
| | Confirmed with RDT | 95 192 | – | – | – | 489 468 | – | 187 707 | 132 779 | 355 289 |
| | Imported cases | – | – | – | – | – | – | – | – | – |
| Yemen | Presumed and confirmed | 198 963 | 142 152 | 165 687 | 149 451 | 122 812 | 104 831 | 144 628 | 114 004 | 192 895 |
| | Microscopy examined | 645 463 | 645 093 | 685 406 | 723 691 | 643 994 | 561 644 | 960 860 | 1 070 020 | 419 415 |
| | Confirmed with microscopy | 78 269 | 60 751 | 71 300 | 63 484 | 51 768 | 42 052 | 45 886 | 28 936 | 64 233 |
| | RDT examined | 97 289 | 108 110 | 150 218 | 157 457 | 141 519 | 121 464 | 174 699 | 560 449 | 219 250 |
| | Confirmed with RDT | 28 428 | 30 203 | 41 059 | 39 294 | 34 939 | 34 207 | 52 815 | 85 068 | 53 419 |
| | Imported cases | – | – | – | – | – | – | – | – | – |
| **EUROPEAN** | | | | | | | | | | |
| Armenia[1] | Presumed and confirmed | 1 | 0 | 4 | 0 | 1 | 1 | 1 | 2 | – |
| | Microscopy examined | 31 026 | – | – | – | – | 1 213 | 465 | 350 | – |
| | Confirmed with microscopy | 1 | – | – | – | – | 2 | 2 | 2 | – |
| | RDT examined | – | – | – | – | – | 0 | 0 | 0 | – |
| | Confirmed with RDT | – | – | – | – | – | 0 | 0 | 0 | – |
| | Imported cases | 1 | 0 | 4 | 0 | 1 | 1 | 1 | 2 | – |
| Azerbaijan[7] | Presumed and confirmed | 52 | 8 | 4 | 4 | 2 | 1 | 1 | 1 | – |
| | Microscopy examined | 456 652 | 449 168 | 497 040 | 432 810 | 399 925 | 405 416 | 465 860 | 373 562 | – |
| | Confirmed with microscopy | 52 | 8 | 4 | 4 | 2 | 1 | 1 | 1 | – |
| | RDT examined | – | – | – | – | – | 0 | 0 | 0 | – |
| | Confirmed with RDT | – | – | – | – | – | 0 | 0 | 0 | – |
| | Imported cases | 2 | 4 | 1 | 4 | 2 | 1 | 1 | 1 | – |
| Georgia[7] | Presumed and confirmed | 0 | 6 | 5 | 7 | 6 | 5 | 7 | 8 | – |
| | Microscopy examined | 2 368 | 2 032 | 1 046 | 192 | 440 | 294 | 318 | 416 | – |
| | Confirmed with microscopy | 0 | 6 | 5 | 7 | 6 | 5 | 7 | 8 | – |
| | RDT examined | – | – | – | – | – | 0 | 0 | 0 | – |
| | Confirmed with RDT | – | – | – | – | – | 0 | 0 | 0 | – |
| | Imported cases | 0 | 6 | 5 | 7 | 5 | 5 | 7 | 8 | – |
| Kyrgyzstan[1] | Presumed and confirmed | 6 | 5 | 3 | 4 | 0 | 1 | 6 | 2 | – |
| | Microscopy examined | 30 190 | 27 850 | 18 268 | 54 249 | 35 600 | 75 688 | 62 537 | 8 459 | – |
| | Confirmed with microscopy | 6 | 5 | 3 | 4 | 0 | 1 | 6 | 2 | – |
| | RDT examined | – | – | – | – | – | 0 | 0 | 0 | – |
| | Confirmed with RDT | – | – | – | – | – | 0 | 0 | 0 | – |
| | Imported cases | 3 | 5 | 3 | 4 | 0 | 1 | 6 | 2 | – |
| Tajikistan[7] | Presumed and confirmed | 112 | 78 | 33 | 14 | 7 | 5 | 1 | 3 | – |
| | Microscopy examined | 173 523 | 173 367 | 209 239 | 213 916 | 200 241 | 188 341 | 198 766 | 191 284 | – |
| | Confirmed with microscopy | 112 | 78 | 33 | 14 | 7 | 5 | 1 | 3 | – |
| | RDT examined | – | – | – | – | – | – | 34 570 | 41 218 | – |
| | Confirmed with RDT | – | – | – | – | – | – | – | 1 | 3 |
| | Imported cases | 1 | 25 | 15 | 11 | 5 | 5 | 1 | 3 | – |

| WHO region Country/area | | 2010 | 2011 | 2012 | 2013 | 2014 | 2015 | 2016 | 2017 | 2018 |
|---|---|---|---|---|---|---|---|---|---|---|
| **EUROPEAN** | | | | | | | | | | |
| Turkey[7] | Presumed and confirmed | 90 | 132 | 376 | 285 | 249 | 221 | 209 | 214 | – |
| | Microscopy examined | 507 841 | 421 295 | 337 830 | 255 125 | 189 854 | 211 740 | 144 499 | 115 557 | – |
| | Confirmed with microscopy | 78 | 128 | 376 | 285 | 249 | 221 | 209 | 214 | – |
| | RDT examined | – | – | – | – | – | – | – | – | – |
| | Confirmed with RDT | – | – | – | – | – | – | – | – | – |
| | Imported cases | 81 | 128 | 376 | 251 | 249 | 221 | 209 | 214 | – |
| Turkmenistan[1] | Presumed and confirmed | 0 | 0 | 0 | 0 | 0 | 0 | 0 | 0 | – |
| | Microscopy examined | 81 784 | – | – | – | – | 83 675 | 85 536 | 84 264 | – |
| | Confirmed with microscopy | 0 | – | – | – | – | 0 | 0 | 0 | – |
| | RDT examined | – | – | – | – | – | 0 | 0 | 0 | – |
| | Confirmed with RDT | – | – | – | – | – | 0 | 0 | 0 | – |
| | Imported cases | 0 | 0 | 0 | 0 | 0 | 0 | 0 | 0 | – |
| Uzbekistan[1] | Presumed and confirmed | 5 | 1 | 1 | 3 | 1 | 0 | 0 | 0 | – |
| | Microscopy examined | 921 364 | 886 243 | 805 761 | 908 301 | 812 347 | 800 912 | 797 472 | 655 112 | – |
| | Confirmed with microscopy | 5 | 1 | 1 | 3 | 1 | 0 | 0 | 0 | – |
| | RDT examined | – | – | – | – | – | 0 | 0 | 0 | – |
| | Confirmed with RDT | – | – | – | – | – | 0 | 0 | 0 | – |
| | Imported cases | 3 | 1 | 1 | 3 | 1 | 0 | 0 | 0 | – |
| **SOUTH-EAST ASIA** | | | | | | | | | | |
| Bangladesh | Presumed and confirmed | 91 227 | 51 773 | 9 901 | 3 864 | 10 216 | 6 608 | 5 063 | 5 133 | 1 919 |
| | Microscopy examined | 308 326 | 270 253 | 253 887 | 74 755 | 78 719 | 69 093 | 65 845 | 70 267 | 57 557 |
| | Confirmed with microscopy | 20 519 | 20 232 | 4 016 | 1 866 | 3 249 | 1 612 | 1 022 | 1 077 | 377 |
| | RDT examined | 152 936 | 119 849 | 35 675 | 19 171 | 46 482 | 53 713 | 73 128 | 80 251 | 75 990 |
| | Confirmed with RDT | 35 354 | 31 541 | 5 885 | 1 998 | 6 967 | 4 996 | 3 765 | 3 835 | 1 542 |
| | Imported cases*** | – | – | – | – | – | 129 | 109 | 19 | 41 |
| Bhutan | Presumed and confirmed | 487 | 207 | 82 | – | – | 104 | 74 | 62 | 54 [5] |
| | Microscopy examined | 54 709 | 44 481 | 42 512 | 31 632 | 33 586 | 26 149 | 23 442 | 22 885 | 19 778 |
| | Confirmed with microscopy | 436 | 194 | 82 | 45 | 48 | 84 | 59 | 51 | 49 |
| | RDT examined | – | – | – | – | – | 47 938 | 95 399 | 19 250 | 113 720 |
| | Confirmed with RDT | – | – | – | – | – | 20 | 15 | 0 | 5 |
| | Imported cases | – | – | 0 | 23 | 0 | 70 | 59 | 51 | 48 |
| Democratic People's Republic of Korea | Presumed and confirmed | 15 392 | 18 104 | 23 537 | 15 673 | 11 212 | 7 409 | 5 113 | 4 626 | 3 598 |
| | Microscopy examined | 25 147 | 26 513 | 39 238 | 71 453 | 38 201 | 29 272 | 22 747 | 16 835 | 28 654 |
| | Confirmed with microscopy | 13 520 | 16 760 | 21 850 | 14 407 | 10 535 | 7 010 | 4 890 | 4 463 | 3 446 |
| | RDT examined | – | – | 0 | 0 | 0 | 61 348 | 182 980 | 172 499 | 657 050 |
| | Confirmed with RDT | – | – | 0 | 0 | 0 | 12 | 143 | 140 | 252 |
| | Imported cases | – | – | 0 | 0 | 0 | 205 | 0 | 0 | 0 |
| India | Presumed and confirmed | 1 599 986 | 1 310 656 | 1 067 824 | 881 730 | 1 102 205 | 1 169 261 | 1 087 285 | 844 558 | 429 928 [3] |
| | Microscopy examined | 108 679 429 | 108 969 660 | 109 033 790 | 113 109 094 | 124 066 331 | 121 141 970 | 124 933 348 | 110 769 742 | 111 123 775 |
| | Confirmed with microscopy | 1 599 986 | 1 310 656 | 1 067 824 | 881 730 | 1 102 205 | 1 169 261 | 1 087 285 | 306 768 | 230 432 |
| | RDT examined | 10 600 000 | 10 500 384 | 13 125 480 | 14 782 104 | 14 562 000 | 19 699 260 | 19 606 260 | 15 208 057 | 13 489 707 |
| | Confirmed with RDT | – | – | – | – | – | – | – | 537 790 | 199 496 |
| | Imported cases | – | – | – | – | – | – | – | – | – |
| Indonesia | Presumed and confirmed | 465 764 | 422 447 | 417 819 | 343 527 | 252 027 | 217 025 | 218 450 | 261 617 | 223 468 [5] |
| | Microscopy examined | 1 335 445 | 962 090 | 1 429 139 | 1 447 980 | 1 300 835 | 1 224 504 | 1 092 093 | 1 045 994 | 1 111 931 |
| | Confirmed with microscopy | 465 764 | 422 447 | 417 819 | 343 527 | 252 027 | 217 025 | 218 450 | 261 617 | 190 782 |
| | RDT examined | 255 734 | 250 709 | 471 586 | 260 181 | 249 461 | 342 946 | 365 765 | 395 685 | 362 705 |
| | Confirmed with RDT | – | – | – | – | – | – | – | – | 32 686 |
| | Imported cases*** | – | – | – | – | – | – | – | – | 11 |
| Myanmar | Presumed and confirmed | 693 124 | 567 452 | 481 204 | 333 871 | 205 658 | 182 616 | 110 146 | 85 019 | 74 392 [3] |
| | Microscopy examined | 275 374 | 312 689 | 265 135 | 138 473 | 151 258 | 99 025 | 122 078 | 107 242 | 58 126 |
| | Confirmed with microscopy | 103 285 | 91 752 | 75 192 | 26 509 | 12 010 | 6 782 | 6 717 | 4 648 | 2 577 |
| | RDT examined | 729 878 | 795 618 | 1 158 420 | 1 162 083 | 1 415 837 | 2 564 707 | 3 063 167 | 3 261 455 | 3 041 650 |
| | Confirmed with RDT | 317 523 | 373 542 | 405 394 | 307 362 | 193 648 | 175 986 | 103 429 | 80 371 | 71 815 |
| | Imported cases | – | – | – | – | – | 345 | – | – | – |

# Annex 3 - H. Reported malaria cases by method of confirmation, 2010–2018

| WHO region Country/area | | 2010 | 2011 | 2012 | 2013 | 2014 | 2015 | 2016 | 2017 | 2018 |
|---|---|---|---|---|---|---|---|---|---|---|
| **SOUTH-EAST ASIA** | | | | | | | | | | |
| Nepal | Presumed and confirmed | 96 383 | 71 752 | 71 410 | 38 113 | 25 889 | 19 375 | 10 185 | 3 269 | 2 930 [5] |
| | Microscopy examined | 102 977 | 95 011 | 152 780 | 100 336 | 127 130 | 63 946 | 84 595 | 163 323 | 160 904 |
| | Confirmed with microscopy | 3 115 | 1 910 | 1 659 | 1 197 | 1 469 | 1 112 | 1 009 | 1 293 | 1 158 |
| | RDT examined | 17 887 | 25 353 | 22 472 | 32 989 | 48 444 | 49 649 | 52 432 | 48 625 | 93 378 |
| | Confirmed with RDT | 779 | 1 504 | 433 | 777 | – | 725 | – | 329 | 0 |
| | Imported cases*** | – | 1 069 | 592 | – | 667 | 521 | 502 | 670 | 539 |
| Thailand | Presumed and confirmed | 32 480 | 24 897 | 32 569 | 41 362 | 37 921 | 14 755 | 11 522 | 7 342 | 5 817 |
| | Microscopy examined | 1 695 980 | 1 354 215 | 1 130 757 | 1 830 090 | 1 756 528 | 1 358 953 | 1 302 834 | 1 117 648 | 908 540 |
| | Confirmed with microscopy | 22 969 | 14 478 | 32 569 | 33 302 | 37 921 | 14 135 | 11 301 | 7 154 | 5 171 |
| | RDT examined | 81 997 | 96 670 | – | 97 495 | – | 10 888 | 158 173 | 31 898 | 12 580 |
| | Confirmed with RDT | 9 511 | 10 419 | – | 8 300 | – | 0 | 221 | 188 | 218 |
| | Imported cases | – | – | – | – | – | 9 890 | 5 724 | 4 020 | 1 618 |
| Timor-Leste[7] | Presumed and confirmed | 119 072 | 36 064 | 6 458 | 1 240 | 406 | 101 | 107 | 26 | 8* [5] |
| | Microscopy examined | 109 806 | 82 175 | 64 318 | 56 192 | 30 515 | 30 237 | 35 947 | 37 705 | 45 976 |
| | Confirmed with microscopy | 40 250 | 19 739 | 5 208 | 1 025 | 347 | 80 | 94 | 17 | 8 |
| | RDT examined | 85 643 | 127 272 | 117 599 | 121 991 | 86 592 | 90 817 | 114 385 | 91 470 | 108 840 |
| | Confirmed with RDT | 7 887 | – | – | – | 0 | 0 | 0 | – | – |
| | Imported cases | – | – | – | – | – | – | 0 | 13 | 8 |
| **WESTERN PACIFIC** | | | | | | | | | | |
| Cambodia | Presumed and confirmed | 47 910 | 51 611 | 45 553 | 24 130 | 26 278 | 29 957 | 23 492 | 36 932 | 42 285 |
| | Microscopy examined | 90 175 | 86 526 | 80 212 | 54 716 | 48 591 | 49 357 | 42 802 | 38 188 | 42 834 |
| | Confirmed with microscopy | 14 277 | 13 792 | 10 124 | 4 598 | 5 288 | 7 423 | 3 695 | 5 908 | 8 318 |
| | RDT examined | 103 035 | 130 186 | 108 974 | 94 600 | 92 525 | 114 323 | 123 893 | 130 057 | 123 804 |
| | Confirmed with RDT | 35 079 | 43 631 | 30 352 | 16 711 | 19 864 | 26 507 | 19 797 | 31 024 | 33 967 |
| | Imported cases | – | – | – | – | – | – | – | – | – |
| China[7] | Presumed and confirmed | 7 855 | 4 498 | 2 716 | 4 127 | | 3 116 | 3 143 | 2 675 | 2 513 |
| | Microscopy examined | 7 115 784 | 9 189 270 | 6 918 657 | 5 554 960 | 4 403 633 | 4 052 588 | 3 194 915 | 2 409 280 | 1 904 290 |
| | Confirmed with microscopy | 4 990 | 3 367 | 2 603 | 4 086 | 2 921 | 3 088 | 3 129 | 2 666 | 2 513 |
| | RDT examined | – | – | – | – | – | – | – | – | – |
| | Confirmed with RDT | – | – | – | – | – | – | – | – | – |
| | Imported cases | – | – | 2 343 | 3 823 | 2 864 | 3 055 | 3 125 | 2 663 | 2 510 |
| Lao People's Democratic Republic | Presumed and confirmed | 23 047 | 17 904 | 46 819 | 41 385 | 38 754 | 36 056 | 11 753 | 9 336 | 8 913 [3] |
| | Microscopy examined | 150 512 | 213 578 | 223 934 | 202 422 | 133 916 | 110 084 | 89 998 | 110 450 | 89 622 |
| | Confirmed with microscopy | 4 524 | 6 226 | 13 232 | 10 036 | 8 018 | 4 167 | 1 597 | 1 549 | 1 091 |
| | RDT examined | 127 790 | 77 825 | 145 425 | 133 337 | 160 626 | 173 919 | 133 464 | 163 856 | 197 259 |
| | Confirmed with RDT | 16 276 | 11 306 | 32 970 | 28 095 | 40 053 | 31 889 | 9 626 | 7 779 | 7 822 |
| | Imported cases*** | – | – | – | – | – | 0 | – | – | 16 |
| Malaysia[7] | Presumed and confirmed | – | – | – | – | 3 923 | 2 311 | 2 302 | 4 114 | 4 630 [5,6] |
| | Microscopy examined | 1 619 074 | 1 600 439 | 1 566 872 | 1 576 012 | 1 443 958 | 1 066 470 | 1 153 108 | 1 046 163 | 1 070 356 |
| | Confirmed with microscopy | 6 650 | 5 306 | 4 725 | 3 850 | 3 923 | 2 311 | 2 302 | 4 114 | 4 630 |
| | RDT examined | – | – | – | – | – | – | 0 | 0 | 0 |
| | Confirmed with RDT | – | – | – | – | – | – | 0 | 0 | 0 |
| | Imported cases | 897 | 1 168 | 840 | 891 | 776 | 435 | 444 | 423 | 506 |
| Papua New Guinea | Presumed and confirmed | 1 379 787 | 1 151 343 | 878 371 | 1 125 808 | 644 688 | 553 103 | 728 798 | 881 697 | 940 646 |
| | Microscopy examined | 198 742 | 184 466 | 156 495 | 139 972 | 83 257 | 112 864 | 146 242 | 139 910 | 121 766 |
| | Confirmed with microscopy | 75 985 | 70 603 | 67 202 | 70 658 | 68 114 | 64 719 | 80 472 | 70 449 | 59 652 |
| | RDT examined | 20 820 | 27 391 | 228 857 | 468 380 | 475 654 | 541 760 | 772 254 | 857 326 | 967 566 |
| | Confirmed with RDT | 17 971 | 13 457 | 82 993 | 209 336 | 213 068 | 233 068 | 398 025 | 407 891 | 456 597 |
| | Imported cases | – | – | – | – | – | – | – | – | – |
| Philippines | Presumed and confirmed | 19 106 | 9 617 | 8 154 | 7 720 | 4 972 | 8 301 | 6 690 | 3 827 | 1 574 |
| | Microscopy examined | 301 031 | 327 060 | 332 063 | 317 360 | 287 725 | 224 843 | 255 302 | 171 424 | 122 502 |
| | Confirmed with microscopy | 18 560 | 9 552 | 7 133 | 5 826 | 3 618 | 5 694 | 2 860 | 874 | 569 |
| | RDT examined | – | – | – | 1 523 | 28 598 | 35 799 | 66 536 | 113 140 | 156 913 |
| | Confirmed with RDT | – | – | – | 688 | 1 285 | 2 572 | 3 820 | 2 953 | 1 005 |
| | Imported cases*** | – | – | – | – | 68 | 18 | 55 | 69 | 79 |

| WHO region Country/area | | 2010 | 2011 | 2012 | 2013 | 2014 | 2015 | 2016 | 2017 | 2018 |
|---|---|---|---|---|---|---|---|---|---|---|
| **WESTERN PACIFIC** | | | | | | | | | | |
| Republic of Korea | Presumed and confirmed | – | – | – | – | 638 | 699 | 673 | 515 | 576 |
| | Microscopy examined | – | – | – | – | – | 247 | 673 | 515 | 576 |
| | Confirmed with microscopy | 1 772 | 838 | 555 | 443 | 638 | 699 | 673 | 515 | 576 |
| | RDT examined | – | – | – | – | – | – | – | – | – |
| | Confirmed with RDT | – | – | – | – | – | – | – | – | – |
| | Imported cases | 55 | 64 | 46 | 50 | 78 | 71 | 67 | 79 | 75 |
| Solomon Islands | Presumed and confirmed | 95 006 | 80 859 | 57 296 | 53 270 | 51 649 | 50 916 | 84 513 | 68 676 | 72 430 |
| | Microscopy examined | 212 329 | 182 847 | 202 620 | 191 137 | 173 900 | 124 376 | 152 690 | 89 061 | 89 169 |
| | Confirmed with microscopy | 35 373 | 23 202 | 21 904 | 21 540 | 13 865 | 14 793 | 26 187 | 15 978 | 17 825 |
| | RDT examined | 17 300 | 17 457 | 13 987 | 26 216 | 26 658 | 40 750 | 92 109 | 133 560 | 142 115 |
| | Confirmed with RDT | 4 331 | 3 455 | 2 479 | 4 069 | 4 539 | 9 205 | 28 244 | 36 505 | 41 366 |
| | Imported cases | – | – | – | – | – | – | – | – | – |
| Vanuatu | Presumed and confirmed | 16 831 | 5 764 | 3 309 | 2 381 | 982 | 697 | 2 147 | 1 072 | 644 [3] |
| | Microscopy examined | 29 180 | 19 183 | 16 981 | 15 219 | 18 135 | 4 870 | 6 704 | 9 187 | 5 935 |
| | Confirmed with microscopy | 4 013 | 2 077 | 733 | 767 | 190 | 15 | 225 | 120 | 53 |
| | RDT examined | 10 246 | 12 529 | 16 292 | 13 724 | 17 435 | 9 794 | 14 501 | 21 126 | 20 996 |
| | Confirmed with RDT | 4 156 | 2 743 | 2 702 | 1 614 | 792 | 408 | 1 643 | 952 | 591 |
| | Imported cases*** | – | – | – | – | – | 0 | 9 | 1 | 12 |
| Viet Nam | Presumed and confirmed | 54 297 | 45 588 | 43 717 | 35 406 | 27 868 | 19 252 | 10 446 | 8 411 | 6 661 [5] |
| | Microscopy examined | 2 760 119 | 2 791 917 | 2 897 730 | 2 684 996 | 2 357 536 | 2 204 409 | 2 082 986 | 2 009 233 | 1 674 897 |
| | Confirmed with microscopy | 17 515 | 16 612 | 19 638 | 17 128 | 15 752 | 9 331 | 4 161 | 4 548 | 4 813 |
| | RDT examined | 7 017 | 491 373 | 514 725 | 412 530 | 416 483 | 459 332 | 408 055 | 603 161 | 492 270 |
| | Confirmed with RDT | – | – | – | – | – | – | – | 1 594 | 1 848 |
| | Imported cases*** | – | – | – | – | – | – | – | – | 1 681 |

| | 2010 | 2011 | 2012 | 2013 | 2014 | 2015 | 2016 | 2017 | 2018 |
|---|---|---|---|---|---|---|---|---|---|
| **REGIONAL SUMMARY** (presumed and confirmed malaria cases) | | | | | | | | | |
| African | 103 145 240 | 100 204 662 | 110 881 358 | 124 426 890 | 128 466 431 | 131 302 726 | 142 439 487 | 149 021 618 | 150 887 242 |
| Americas | 677 230 | 493 823 | 469 385 | 439 700 | 392 491 | 450 098 | 568 967 | 773 483 | 764 980 |
| Eastern Mediterranean | 6 368 813 | 5 952 130 | 5 835 463 | 4 944 058 | 5 331 046 | 5 401 932 | 3 626 635 | 4 269 135 | 5 202 993 |
| European | 266 | 230 | 426 | 317 | 266 | 234 | 225 | 230 | 0 |
| South-East Asia | 3 113 915 | 2 503 352 | 2 110 804 | 1 659 380 | 1 645 534 | 1 617 254 | 1 447 945 | 1 211 652 | 742 114 |
| Western Pacific | 1 643 839 | 1 367 184 | 1 085 935 | 1 294 227 | 799 752 | 704 408 | 873 957 | 1 017 255 | 1 080 872 |
| **Total** | **114 949 303** | **110 521 381** | **120 383 371** | **132 764 572** | **136 635 520** | **139 476 652** | **148 957 216** | **156 293 373** | **158 678 201** |

Data as of 14 February 2020

RDT: rapid diagnostic test; WHO: World Health Organization.

"–" refers to not applicable or data not available.

* Corrected for double counting of microscopy and RDT.

** Double counting of microscopy and RDT reported, but proportion is not indicated.

*** Case investigation is less than 100%.

[1] Certified malaria free countries are included in this listing for historical purposes.

[2] In May 2013, South Sudan was reassigned to the WHO African Region (WHA resolution 66.21, https://apps.who.int/gb/ebwha/pdf_files/WHA66/A66_R21-en.pdf).

[3] Figures reported for the public sector include cases detected at the community level.

[4] Figures reported for the public sector include cases detected in the private sector.

[5] Figures reported for the public sector include cases detected at the community level and in the private sector.

[6] Figures include all imported or non-human malaria cases; none of them being indigenous malaria cases.

[7] There are no indigenous cases.

[8] Incomplete laboratory data. This country has no presumed cases reported.

Note: Imported cases also include introduced cases.

# Annex 3 – I. Reported malaria cases by species, 2010–2018

| WHO region Country/area | | 2010 | 2011 | 2012 | 2013 | 2014 | 2015 | 2016 | 2017 | 2018 |
|---|---|---|---|---|---|---|---|---|---|---|
| **AFRICAN** | | | | | | | | | | |
| Algeria | Suspected | 12 224 | 11 974 | 15 790 | 12 762 | 8 690 | 8 000 | 6 628 | 6 469 | 10 081 |
| | Indigenous: P. falciparum | – | – | – | – | 0 | 0 | 0 | 0 | 0 |
| | Indigenous: P. vivax | – | – | – | – | – | 0 | 0 | 0 | 0 |
| | Indigenous: mixed | – | – | – | – | – | 0 | 0 | 0 | 0 |
| | Indigenous: other species | – | – | – | – | – | 0 | 0 | 0 | 0 |
| Angola | Suspected | 4 591 529 | 4 469 357 | 4 849 418 | 5 273 305 | 6 134 471 | 6 839 963 | 7 649 902 | 11 050 353 | 10 870 446 |
| Benin | Suspected | 1 432 095 | 1 565 487 | 1 875 386 | 2 041 444 | 1 955 773 | 2 009 959 | 1 817 605 | 2 306 653 | 2 646 070 |
| | Total: P. falciparum | – | 68 745 | 0 | – | 1 044 235 | 1 268 347 | 1 324 576 | 1 696 777 | 1 768 450 |
| | Total: P. vivax | – | 0 | 0 | 0 | 0 | 0 | 0 | 0 | 0 |
| | Total: mixed cases | – | 0 | 0 | 0 | 0 | 0 | 0 | 0 | 0 |
| | Total: other species | – | 0 | 0 | 0 | 0 | 0 | 0 | 0 | 0 |
| Botswana | Suspected | 12 196 | 1 141 | 308 | 506 | 1 485 | 1 298 | 12 986 | 12 605 | 13 979 |
| | Indigenous: P. falciparum | 1 046 | 432 | 193 | 456 | 1 346 | 188 | 333 | 1 713 | 534 |
| | Indigenous: P. vivax | 0 | 0 | 0 | 0 | 0 | 0 | 0 | 4 | 0 |
| | Indigenous: mixed | 0 | 0 | 0 | 0 | 0 | 0 | 13 | 0 | 0 |
| | Indigenous: other species | 0 | 0 | 0 | 0 | 0 | 0 | 0 | 0 | 0 |
| Burkina Faso | Suspected | 6 037 806 | 5 446 870 | 7 852 299 | 7 857 296 | 9 272 755 | 9 783 385 | 11 992 686 | 14 384 948 | 14 910 311 |
| Burundi | Suspected | 5 590 736 | 4 768 314 | 4 228 015 | 7 384 501 | 7 622 162 | 8 414 481 | 12 357 585 | 12 336 328 | 8 734 322 |
| Cabo Verde | Suspected | 47 | 26 508 | 8 715 | 10 621 | 6 894 | 3 117 | 8 393 | 3 857 | 16 623 |
| | Indigenous: P. falciparum | – | – | – | – | 26 | 7 | 48 | 423 | 2 |
| | Indigenous: P. vivax | – | – | – | – | 0 | 0 | 0 | 0 | 0 |
| | Indigenous: mixed | – | – | – | – | 0 | 0 | 0 | 0 | 0 |
| | Indigenous: other species | – | – | – | – | 0 | 0 | 0 | 0 | 0 |
| Cameroon | Suspected | 1 845 691 | 3 060 040 | 2 865 319 | 3 652 609 | 3 709 906 | 3 312 273 | 3 229 804 | 3 345 967 | 3 217 180 |
| | Total: P. falciparum | – | – | – | – | – | 592 351 | 1 675 264 | 1 191 257 | 1 249 705 |
| | Total: P. vivax | – | – | – | – | – | 0 | 0 | 0 | 0 |
| | Total: mixed cases | – | – | – | – | – | 0 | 0 | 0 | 0 |
| | Total: other species | – | – | – | – | – | 0 | 0 | 0 | 0 |
| Central African Republic | Suspected | 66 484 | 221 980 | 468 986 | 491 074 | 625 301 | 1 218 246 | 1 807 206 | 1 480 085 | 1 367 986 |
| | Total: P. falciparum | – | – | – | – | 295 088 | 598 833 | 1 032 764 | 383 309 | 972 119 |
| | Total: P. vivax | – | – | – | – | 0 | 0 | 0 | 0 | 0 |
| | Total: mixed cases | – | – | – | – | 0 | 0 | 0 | 0 | 0 |
| | Total: other species | – | – | – | – | 0 | 0 | 0 | 0 | 0 |
| Chad | Suspected | 743 471 | 528 454 | 730 364 | 1 272 841 | 1 737 195 | 1 641 285 | 2 032 301 | 2 943 595 | 1 941 489 |
| Comoros | Suspected | 159 976 | 135 248 | 168 043 | 185 779 | 103 545 | 101 330 | 94 388 | 190 825 | 119 592 |
| | Total: P. falciparum | 33 791 | 21 387 | 43 681 | 45 669 | 2 203 | 1 300 | 1 066 | 2 274 | 15 613 |
| | Total: P. vivax | 528 | 334 | 637 | 72 | 0 | 0 | 0 | 0 | 0 |
| | Total: mixed cases | 0 | 0 | 0 | 363 | 0 | 0 | 0 | 0 | 0 |
| | Total: other species | 880 | 557 | 0 | 363 | 0 | 0 | 0 | 0 | 0 |
| Congo | Suspected | 446 656 | 277 263 | 117 640 | 209 169 | 290 346 | 300 592 | 466 254 | 322 916 | 385 729 |
| | Total: P. falciparum | | 37 744 | 120 319 | 43 232 | 66 323 | 51 529 | 171 847 | 127 939 | 116 903 |
| | Total: P. vivax | | 0 | 0 | 0 | 0 | 0 | 0 | 0 | 0 |
| | Total: mixed cases | | 0 | 0 | 0 | 0 | 0 | 0 | 0 | 0 |
| | Total: other species | | 0 | 0 | 0 | 0 | 0 | 0 | 0 | 0 |
| Côte d'Ivoire | Suspected | 1 721 461 | 2 607 856 | 3 423 623 | 5 982 151 | 6 418 571 | 5 216 344 | 5 178 375 | 6 346 291 | 6 706 148 |
| | Total: P. falciparum | – | – | – | 2 506 953 | 3 712 831 | 3 375 904 | 3 471 024 | 3 274 683 | 4 766 477 |
| | Total: P. vivax | – | – | – | 0 | 0 | 0 | 0 | 0 | 0 |
| | Total: mixed cases | – | – | – | 0 | 0 | 0 | 0 | 0 | 0 |
| | Total: other species | – | – | – | 0 | 0 | 0 | 0 | 0 | 0 |
| Democratic Republic of the Congo | Suspected | 10 568 756 | 12 018 784 | 11 993 189 | 14 871 716 | 14 647 380 | 16 452 476 | 21 507 579 | 21 072 322 | 23 833 694 |
| | Total: P. falciparum | 0 | 0 | 0 | 0 | – | – | – | – | – |
| | Total: P. vivax | 0 | 0 | 0 | 0 | – | – | – | – | – |
| | Total: mixed cases | 0 | 0 | 0 | 0 | – | – | – | – | – |
| | Total: other species | 0 | 0 | 0 | 0 | – | – | – | – | – |

| WHO region Country/area | | 2010 | 2011 | 2012 | 2013 | 2014 | 2015 | 2016 | 2017 | 2018 |
|---|---|---|---|---|---|---|---|---|---|---|
| **AFRICAN** | | | | | | | | | | |
| Equatorial Guinea | Suspected | 83 639 | 40 704 | 45 792 | 44 561 | 57 129 | 68 058 | 318 779 | 91 217 | 43 533 |
| | Total: *P. falciparum* | 53 813 | 22 466 | 15 169 | 13 129 | 17 452 | – | – | – | – |
| | Total: *P. vivax* | 0 | 0 | 0 | 0 | 0 | – | – | – | – |
| | Total: mixed cases | 0 | 0 | 0 | 0 | 0 | – | – | – | – |
| | Total: other species | 0 | 0 | 0 | 0 | 0 | – | – | – | – |
| Eritrea | Suspected | 96 792 | 97 479 | 138 982 | 134 183 | 121 755 | 111 950 | 106 403 | 121 064 | 146 235 |
| | Total: *P. falciparum* | 9 785 | 10 263 | 12 121 | 12 482 | 23 787 | 14 510 | 20 704 | 21 849 | 16 553 |
| | Total: *P. vivax* | 3 989 | 4 932 | 9 204 | 7 361 | 6 780 | 4 780 | 2 999 | 9 185 | 6 108 |
| | Total: mixed cases | 63 | 94 | 346 | 1 391 | 166 | 70 | 543 | 429 | 268 |
| | Total: other species | 57 | 19 | 0 | 83 | 35 | 12 | 5 | 23 | 26 |
| Eswatini | Suspected | 1 722 | 797 | 626 | 669 | 711 | 651 | 1 386 | 3 212 | 9 837 |
| | Indigenous: *P. falciparum* | 87 | 130 | 345 | 487 | 710 | 157 | 63 | 668 | 271 |
| | Indigenous: *P. vivax* | 0 | 0 | 0 | 0 | 1 | 0 | 0 | 0 | 0 |
| | Indigenous: mixed | 0 | 0 | 0 | 0 | 0 | 0 | 0 | 0 | 0 |
| | Indigenous: other species | 0 | 0 | 0 | 1 | 0 | 0 | 0 | 0 | 0 |
| Ethiopia | Suspected | 5 420 110 | 5 487 972 | 5 962 646 | 9 243 894 | 7 457 765 | 5 987 580 | 6 611 801 | 6 471 958 | 5 913 799 |
| | Total: *P. falciparum* | 732 776 | 814 547 | 946 595 | 1 687 163 | 1 250 110 | 1 188 627 | 1 142 235 | 1 059 847 | 859 675 |
| | Total: *P. vivax* | 390 252 | 665 813 | 745 983 | 958 291 | 868 705 | 678 432 | 576 269 | 470 892 | 102 412 |
| | Total: mixed cases | 73 801 | 0 | 0 | 0 | 0 | 0 | 0 | 0 | 0 |
| | Total: other species | 0 | 0 | 0 | 0 | 0 | 0 | 0 | 0 | 0 |
| Gabon | Suspected | 233 770 | 178 822 | 238 483 | 256 531 | 256 183 | 285 489 | 202 989 | 212 092 | 1 022 022 |
| | Total: *P. falciparum* | 2 157 | – | – | 26 432 | 26 117 | – | 23 915 | 35 244 | 111 719 |
| | Total: *P. vivax* | 720 | – | – | 0 | 0 | – | 0 | 0 | 0 |
| | Total: mixed cases | 55 | – | – | 0 | 0 | – | 0 | 0 | 0 |
| | Total: other species | 0 | – | – | 0 | 1 570 | – | 0 | 0 | 0 |
| Gambia | Suspected | 492 062 | 261 967 | 862 442 | 889 494 | 603 424 | 891 511 | 844 821 | 591 226 | 706 868 |
| | Total: *P. falciparum* | 64 108 | 190 379 | 271 038 | 240 792 | 99 976 | 240 382 | 153 685 | 69 931 | 87 448 |
| | Total: *P. vivax* | 0 | 0 | 0 | 0 | 0 | 0 | 0 | 0 | 0 |
| | Total: mixed cases | 0 | 0 | 0 | 0 | 0 | 0 | 0 | 0 | 0 |
| | Total: other species | 0 | 0 | 0 | 0 | 0 | 0 | 0 | 0 | 0 |
| Ghana | Suspected | 5 056 851 | 5 067 731 | 12 578 946 | 8 444 417 | 10 636 057 | 13 368 757 | 14 040 434 | 14 026 149 | 15 542 218 |
| | Total: *P. falciparum* | 926 447 | 593 518 | 3 755 166 | 1 629 198 | 3 415 912 | 4 319 919 | 4 421 788 | 4 266 541 | 4 808 163 |
| | Total: *P. vivax* | 0 | 0 | 0 | 0 | 0 | 0 | 0 | 0 | 0 |
| | Total: mixed cases | 0 | 0 | 0 | 0 | 0 | 0 | 83 654 | 82 153 | 0 |
| | Total: other species | 102 937 | 31 238 | 0 | 0 | 0 | 0 | 29 725 | 27 245 | 27 635 |
| Guinea | Suspected | 1 092 554 | 1 276 057 | 1 220 574 | 775 341 | 1 595 828 | 1 254 937 | 1 503 035 | 2 134 543 | 2 961 508 |
| | Total: *P. falciparum* | 20 936 | 5 450 | 191 421 | 63 353 | 660 207 | 810 979 | 992 146 | 1 335 323 | 1 214 996 |
| | Total: *P. vivax* | 0 | 0 | 0 | 0 | 0 | 0 | 0 | 0 | 0 |
| | Total: mixed cases | 0 | 0 | 0 | 0 | 0 | 0 | 0 | 0 | 0 |
| | Total: other species | 0 | 0 | 0 | 0 | 0 | 0 | 0 | 0 | 0 |
| Guinea-Bissau | Suspected | 195 006 | 300 233 | 237 398 | 238 580 | 309 939 | 385 678 | 381 196 | 461 621 | 469 640 |
| | Total: *P. falciparum* | – | – | – | – | – | 96 520 | 97 889 | 89 784 | 125 511 |
| | Total: *P. vivax* | – | – | – | – | – | 0 | 0 | 0 | 0 |
| | Total: mixed cases | – | – | – | – | – | 0 | 0 | 0 | 0 |
| | Total: other species | – | – | – | – | – | 0 | 0 | 0 | 0 |
| Kenya | Suspected | 7 557 454 | 13 127 058 | 12 883 521 | 14 677 837 | 15 142 723 | 15 915 943 | 15 294 939 | 14 013 376 | 15 041 132 |
| | Total: *P. falciparum* | 898 531 | 1 002 805 | 1 453 471 | 2 335 286 | 2 808 931 | 1 499 027 | 2 783 846 | 3 215 116 | 1 521 566 |
| | Total: *P. vivax* | 0 | 0 | 0 | 0 | 0 | 0 | 0 | 0 | 0 |
| | Total: mixed cases | 0 | 0 | 0 | 0 | 0 | 0 | 0 | 0 | 0 |
| | Total: other species | 0 | 0 | 0 | 0 | 0 | 0 | 0 | 0 | 0 |
| Liberia | Suspected | 3 087 659 | 2 887 105 | 2 441 800 | 2 202 213 | 2 433 086 | 2 306 116 | 3 105 390 | 2 033 806 | – |
| | Total: *P. falciparum* | 212 927 | 577 641 | 1 407 455 | 1 244 220 | 864 204 | 2 086 600 | 1 191 137 | 1 760 966 | – |
| | Total: *P. vivax* | 0 | 0 | 0 | 0 | 0 | 0 | 0 | 0 | – |
| | Total: mixed cases | 0 | 0 | 0 | 0 | 0 | 0 | 0 | 0 | – |
| | Total: other species | 0 | 0 | 0 | 0 | 0 | 0 | 0 | 0 | – |
| Madagascar | Suspected | 719 967 | 805 701 | 980 262 | 1 068 683 | 1 019 498 | 1 536 344 | 1 530 075 | 2 008 783 | 2 334 556 |

# Annex 3 – I. Reported malaria cases by species, 2010–2018

| WHO region Country/area | | 2010 | 2011 | 2012 | 2013 | 2014 | 2015 | 2016 | 2017 | 2018 |
|---|---|---|---|---|---|---|---|---|---|---|
| **AFRICAN** | | | | | | | | | | |
| Malawi | Suspected | 6 851 108 | 5 734 906 | 6 528 505 | 5 787 441 | 7 703 651 | 8 518 905 | 9 239 462 | 10 530 601 | 11 513 684 |
| | Total: P. falciparum | – | – | 1 564 984 | 1 280 892 | 2 905 310 | 3 585 315 | 4 730 835 | 4 901 344 | 5 830 741 |
| | Total: P. vivax | – | – | 0 | 0 | 0 | 0 | 0 | 0 | 0 |
| | Total: mixed cases | – | – | 0 | 0 | 0 | 0 | 0 | 0 | 0 |
| | Total: other species | – | – | 0 | 0 | 0 | 0 | 0 | 0 | 0 |
| Mali | Suspected | 3 324 238 | 2 628 593 | 2 171 739 | 2 849 453 | 2 590 643 | 4 410 839 | 3 563 070 | 3 333 079 | 3 725 896 |
| Mauritania | Suspected | 239 795 | 191 726 | 209 955 | 190 446 | 203 991 | 233 362 | 192 980 | 214 087 | 221 121 |
| Mayotte | Suspected | 2 023 | 1 214 | 1 463 | 82 | 15 | – | 12 | – | – |
| | Indigenous: P. falciparum | – | – | – | – | – | – | – | – | – |
| | Indigenous: P. vivax | – | – | – | – | – | – | – | – | – |
| | Indigenous: mixed | – | – | – | – | – | – | – | – | – |
| | Indigenous: other species | – | – | – | – | – | – | – | – | – |
| Mozambique | Suspected | 6 097 263 | 7 059 112 | 6 170 561 | 8 200 849 | 12 240 045 | 14 241 392 | 15 453 655 | 15 905 956 | 17 127 629 |
| | Total: P. falciparum | 878 009 | 663 132 | 927 841 | 2 998 874 | 7 117 648 | 7 718 782 | 8 520 376 | 8 921 081 | 9 292 928 |
| | Total: P. vivax | 0 | 0 | 0 | 0 | 0 | 0 | 0 | 0 | 0 |
| | Total: mixed cases | 0 | 0 | 0 | 0 | 0 | 0 | 0 | 0 | 0 |
| | Total: other species | 0 | 0 | 0 | 0 | 0 | 0 | 0 | 0 | 0 |
| Namibia | Suspected | 39 855 | 74 407 | 10 844 | 34 002 | 186 972 | 209 083 | 310 192 | 618 291 | 400 337 |
| | Total: P. falciparum | 556 | 335 | 194 | 136 | 15 914 | 12 050 | 329 | 364 | 280 |
| | Total: P. vivax | 0 | 0 | 0 | 0 | 0 | 0 | 0 | 0 | 0 |
| | Total: mixed cases | 0 | 0 | 0 | 0 | 0 | 0 | 0 | 0 | 0 |
| | Total: other species | 0 | 0 | 0 | 0 | 0 | 0 | 0 | 0 | 0 |
| Niger | Suspected | 10 616 033 | 3 637 778 | 5 915 671 | 5 533 601 | 7 014 724 | 4 497 920 | 7 172 521 | 3 819 436 | 4 810 919 |
| | Total: P. falciparum | 601 455 | 757 449 | 2 185 060 | 2 306 354 | 3 828 486 | 2 267 867 | 3 961 178 | 2 638 580 | 3 046 450 |
| | Total: P. vivax | 0 | 0 | 0 | 0 | 0 | 0 | 0 | 0 | 0 |
| | Total: mixed cases | 17 123 | 21 370 | 22 399 | 46 068 | 78 102 | 0 | 0 | 0 | 0 |
| | Total: other species | 0 | 0 | 0 | 0 | 0 | 4 133 | 186 989 | 0 | 0 |
| Nigeria | Suspected | 3 873 463 | 5 221 656 | 11 789 970 | 21 659 831 | 19 555 575 | 17 388 046 | 20 173 207 | 22 982 775 | 23 193 610 |
| | Total: P. falciparum | 523 513 | – | – | – | – | – | – | – | – |
| | Total: P. vivax | 0 | – | – | – | – | – | – | – | – |
| | Total: mixed cases | 0 | – | – | – | – | – | – | – | – |
| | Total: other species | 0 | – | – | – | – | – | – | – | – |
| Rwanda | Suspected | 2 708 973 | 1 602 271 | 3 095 386 | 3 064 585 | 4 178 206 | 6 093 114 | 7 502 174 | 7 557 866 | 6 221 481 |
| | Total: P. falciparum | 638 669 | 208 858 | 483 470 | 962 618 | 1 623 176 | – | – | 2 927 780 | 1 657 793 |
| | Total: P. vivax | 0 | 0 | 0 | 0 | 0 | – | – | 0 | 0 |
| | Total: mixed cases | 0 | 0 | 0 | 0 | 0 | – | – | 0 | 0 |
| | Total: other species | 0 | 0 | 0 | 0 | 0 | – | – | 0 | 0 |
| Sao Tome and Principe | Suspected | 58 961 | 117 279 | 126 897 | 108 634 | 91 445 | 84 348 | 121 334 | 96 612 | 169 883 |
| | Total: P. falciparum | 2 219 | 6 363 | 10 700 | 9 242 | 1 754 | 2 057 | 2 238 | 2 241 | 2 940 |
| | Total: P. vivax | 14 | 4 | 1 | 1 | 0 | 0 | 0 | 0 | 0 |
| | Total: mixed cases | 0 | 0 | 0 | 0 | 0 | 0 | 0 | 0 | 0 |
| | Total: other species | 0 | 6 | 0 | 0 | 0 | 1 | 0 | 0 | 0 |
| Senegal | Suspected | 739 714 | 628 096 | 655 294 | 802 227 | 741 835 | 1 421 221 | 1 559 054 | 2 035 693 | 2 096 124 |
| | Total: P. falciparum | 343 670 | 277 326 | 281 080 | 345 889 | 265 624 | 492 253 | 349 540 | 395 706 | 530 944 |
| | Total: P. vivax | 0 | 0 | 0 | 0 | 0 | 0 | 0 | 0 | 0 |
| | Total: mixed cases | 0 | 0 | 0 | 0 | 0 | 0 | 0 | 0 | 0 |
| | Total: other species | 0 | 0 | 0 | 0 | 0 | 0 | 0 | 0 | 0 |
| Sierra Leone | Suspected | 2 327 928 | 1 150 747 | 2 579 296 | 2 576 550 | 2 647 375 | 2 337 297 | 2 996 959 | 2 935 447 | 2 895 596 |
| | Total: P. falciparum | 218 473 | 25 511 | 1 537 322 | 1 701 958 | 1 374 476 | 1 483 376 | 1 775 306 | 1 651 236 | 1 733 831 |
| | Total: P. vivax | 0 | 0 | 0 | 0 | 0 | 0 | 0 | 0 | 0 |
| | Total: mixed cases | 0 | 0 | 0 | 0 | 0 | 0 | 0 | 0 | 0 |
| | Total: other species | 0 | 0 | 0 | 0 | 0 | 0 | 0 | 0 | 0 |

| WHO region Country/area | | 2010 | 2011 | 2012 | 2013 | 2014 | 2015 | 2016 | 2017 | 2018 |
|---|---|---|---|---|---|---|---|---|---|---|
| **AFRICAN** | | | | | | | | | | |
| South Africa | Suspected | 276 669 | 382 434 | 152 561 | 603 932 | 543 196 | 35 982 | 63 277 | 56 257 | – |
| | Indigenous: P. falciparum | – | – | – | – | – | 554 | 1 113 | 21 442 | 9 540 |
| | Indigenous: P. vivax | – | – | – | – | – | 0 | 0 | 0 | 0 |
| | Indigenous: mixed | – | – | – | – | – | 1 | 0 | 0 | 0 |
| | Indigenous: other species | – | – | – | – | – | 0 | 0 | 0 | 0 |
| South Sudan[1] | Suspected | 900 283 | 795 784 | 1 125 039 | 1 855 501 | 2 492 473 | 3 814 332 | 17 705 | 4 938 773 | 6 405 779 |
| | Total: P. falciparum | – | 112 024 | – | – | – | 24 371 | 7 619 | 1 488 005 | 3 242 |
| | Total: P. vivax | – | 0 | – | – | – | 0 | 0 | 0 | 0 |
| | Total: mixed cases | – | 0 | – | – | – | 0 | 0 | 0 | 0 |
| | Total: other species | – | 0 | – | – | – | 0 | 0 | 0 | 0 |
| Togo | Suspected | 1 419 928 | 893 588 | 1 311 047 | 1 442 571 | 1 756 700 | 1 756 701 | 1 845 454 | 2 042 498 | 2 046 691 |
| | Total: P. falciparum | 224 080 | 237 282 | 260 526 | 272 847 | 1 130 234 | 1 113 910 | 1 174 116 | 1 208 957 | 1 090 110 |
| | Total: P. vivax | 0 | 0 | 0 | 0 | 0 | 0 | 0 | 0 | 0 |
| | Total: mixed cases | 0 | 0 | 0 | 8 | 0 | 0 | 0 | 0 | 0 |
| | Total: other species | 7 | 23 | 0 | 8 | 17 | 17 | 9 149 | 77 | 224 |
| Uganda | Suspected | 15 294 306 | 12 340 717 | 16 845 771 | 26 145 615 | 19 201 136 | 22 095 860 | 26 238 144 | 22 319 643 | 17 484 262 |
| | Total: P. falciparum | 1 565 348 | 231 873 | 2 662 258 | 1 502 362 | 3 631 939 | 7 137 662 | 9 385 132 | 11 667 831 | 5 759 174 |
| | Total: P. vivax | 15 812 | 0 | 0 | 0 | 0 | 0 | 0 | 0 | 0 |
| | Total: mixed cases | 47 435 | 0 | 0 | 0 | 0 | 0 | 0 | 0 | 0 |
| | Total: other species | 0 | 0 | 0 | 0 | 0 | 0 | 0 | 0 | 0 |
| United Republic of Tanzania | Suspected | 15 388 319 | 15 299 205 | 14 513 120 | 14 650 226 | 25 190 882 | 20 797 048 | 17 786 690 | 18 389 229 | 22 785 648 |
| | Total: P. falciparum | 2 338 | 4 489 | 2 730 | 2 194 | 1 810 | 414 983 | 5 015 | 1 733 | 2 240 |
| | Total: P. vivax | 0 | 0 | 0 | 0 | 0 | 0 | 0 | 0 | 0 |
| | Total: mixed cases | 0 | 0 | 212 837 | 69 511 | 106 764 | 175 | 89 | 1 606 | 1 020 |
| | Total: other species | 0 | 0 | 0 | 0 | 0 | 0 | 0 | 10 | 26 |
| Mainland | Suspected | 15 116 242 | 14 843 487 | 13 976 370 | 14 122 269 | 24 880 179 | 20 451 119 | 17 526 829 | 18 121 926 | 22 440 865 |
| | Total: P. falciparum | – | – | 0 | 0 | 0 | 411 741 | – | – | – |
| | Total: P. vivax | – | – | 0 | 0 | 0 | 0 | – | – | – |
| | Total: mixed cases | – | – | 212 636 | 69 459 | 106 609 | 0 | – | – | – |
| | Total: other species | – | – | 0 | 0 | 0 | 0 | – | – | – |
| Zanzibar | Suspected | 272 077 | 455 718 | 536 750 | 527 957 | 310 703 | 345 929 | 259 861 | 267 303 | 344 783 |
| | Total: P. falciparum | 2 338 | 4 489 | 2 730 | 2 194 | 1 810 | 3 242 | 5 015 | 1 733 | 2 240 |
| | Total: P. vivax | 0 | 0 | 0 | 0 | 0 | 0 | 0 | 0 | 0 |
| | Total: mixed cases | 0 | 0 | 201 | 52 | 155 | 175 | 89 | 1 606 | 1 020 |
| | Total: other species | 0 | 0 | 0 | 0 | 0 | 0 | 0 | 10 | 26 |
| Zambia | Suspected | 4 229 839 | 4 607 908 | 4 695 400 | 5 465 122 | 7 859 740 | 8 116 962 | 9 627 862 | 10 952 323 | 10 055 407 |
| | Total: P. falciparum | – | – | – | – | 4 077 547 | 4 184 661 | 4 851 319 | 5 505 639 | 5 039 679 |
| | Total: P. vivax | – | – | – | – | 0 | 0 | 0 | 0 | 0 |
| | Total: mixed cases | – | – | – | – | 0 | 0 | 0 | 0 | 0 |
| | Total: other species | – | – | – | – | 0 | 0 | 0 | 0 | 0 |
| Zimbabwe | Suspected | 912 618 | 480 011 | 727 174 | 1 115 005 | 1 420 946 | 1 384 893 | 1 224 374 | 1 110 705 | 998 486 |
| | Total: P. falciparum | 249 379 | 319 935 | 276 963 | 422 633 | 535 931 | 391 651 | 279 988 | 316 392 | 184 427 |
| | Total: P. vivax | 0 | 0 | 0 | 0 | 0 | 0 | 0 | 0 | 0 |
| | Total: mixed cases | 0 | 0 | 0 | 0 | 0 | 0 | 0 | 0 | 0 |
| | Total: other species | 0 | 0 | 0 | 0 | 0 | 0 | 0 | 0 | 0 |

# Annex 3 – I. Reported malaria cases by species, 2010–2018

| WHO region Country/area | | 2010 | 2011 | 2012 | 2013 | 2014 | 2015 | 2016 | 2017 | 2018 |
|---|---|---|---|---|---|---|---|---|---|---|
| **AMERICAS** | | | | | | | | | | |
| Argentina[2] | Suspected | 2 547 | 7 872 | 7 027 | 4 913 | 5 691 | 3 862 | 3 479 | 2 114 | 345 |
| | Indigenous: P. falciparum | 0 | – | – | – | 0 | 0 | 0 | 0 | 0 |
| | Indigenous: P. vivax | 14 | – | – | – | 0 | 0 | 0 | 0 | 0 |
| | Indigenous: mixed | – | – | – | – | 0 | 0 | 0 | 0 | 0 |
| | Indigenous: other species | – | – | – | – | 0 | 0 | 0 | 0 | 0 |
| Belize | Suspected | 27 366 | 22 996 | 20 789 | 25 351 | 24 122 | 26 367 | 20 936 | 26 995 | 17 642 |
| | Indigenous: P. falciparum | – | 0 | 0 | 0 | 0 | 0 | 0 | 0 | 1 |
| | Indigenous: P. vivax | – | 72 | 33 | 20 | 19 | 9 | 4 | 5 | 2 |
| | Indigenous: mixed | – | – | – | 0 | 0 | 0 | 0 | 2 | 0 |
| | Indigenous: other species | – | 0 | 0 | 0 | 0 | 0 | 0 | 0 | 0 |
| Bolivia (Plurinational State of) | Suspected | 140 857 | 150 662 | 132 904 | 144 049 | 124 900 | 159 167 | 155 407 | 151 697 | 139 938 |
| | Indigenous: P. falciparum | 1 557 | 526 | 385 | 959 | 325 | 77 | 4 | 0 | 0 |
| | Indigenous: P. vivax | 13 694 | 7 635 | 8 141 | 6 346 | 7 060 | 6 785 | 5 535 | 2 849 | 5 342 |
| | Indigenous: mixed | 35 | 17 | 11 | 37 | 16 | 12 | 3 | 0 | 0 |
| | Indigenous: other species | 0 | 0 | 0 | 0 | 0 | 0 | 0 | 0 | 0 |
| Brazil | Suspected | 2 711 433 | 2 477 821 | 2 349 341 | 1 893 018 | 1 756 460 | 1 590 403 | 1 364 917 | 1 695 805 | 1 800 173 |
| | Indigenous: P. falciparum | – | – | – | 26 178 | 21 295 | 14 762 | 13 160 | 18 614 | 17 852 |
| | Indigenous: P. vivax | – | – | – | 141 391 | 117 009 | 122 746 | 110 340 | 169 887 | 168 499 |
| | Indigenous: mixed | – | – | – | 2 090 | 939 | 683 | 669 | 1 032 | 1 331 |
| | Indigenous: other species | – | – | – | 31 | 28 | 38 | 8 | 26 | 11 |
| Colombia | Suspected | 521 342 | 418 032 | 416 767 | 327 055 | 403 532 | 332 706 | 296 091 | 265 077 | 225 464 |
| | Indigenous: P. falciparum | – | – | – | – | – | 27 875 | 47 232 | 29 558 | 29 953 |
| | Indigenous: P. vivax | – | – | – | – | – | 19 002 | 32 635 | 22 132 | 30 063 |
| | Indigenous: mixed | – | – | – | – | – | 739 | 2 742 | 1 115 | 1 179 |
| | Indigenous: other species | – | – | – | – | – | 0 | 0 | 0 | 0 |
| Costa Rica | Suspected | 15 599 | 10 690 | 7 485 | 16 774 | 4 420 | 7 373 | 5 160 | 9 680 | 9 700 |
| | Indigenous: P. falciparum | – | – | – | 0 | 0 | 0 | 0 | 0 | 9 |
| | Indigenous: P. vivax | 110 | 10 | – | 0 | 0 | 0 | 4 | 12 | 61 |
| | Indigenous: mixed | – | – | – | 0 | 0 | 0 | 0 | 0 | 0 |
| | Indigenous: other species | – | – | – | 0 | 0 | 0 | 0 | 0 | 0 |
| Dominican Republic | Suspected | 495 637 | 477 555 | 506 583 | 502 683 | 416 729 | 324 787 | 302 600 | 265 535 | 76 007 |
| | Indigenous: P. falciparum | 2 480 | 1 614 | 950 | 473 | 459 | 631 | 690 | 341 | 433 |
| | Indigenous: P. vivax | 0 | 0 | 0 | 0 | 0 | 0 | 0 | 0 | 0 |
| | Indigenous: mixed | 0 | 0 | 0 | 0 | 0 | 0 | 0 | 0 | 0 |
| | Indigenous: other species | 0 | 0 | 0 | 0 | 0 | 0 | 0 | 0 | 0 |
| Ecuador | Suspected | 488 830 | 460 785 | 459 157 | 397 628 | 370 825 | 261 824 | 311 920 | 306 894 | 244 777 |
| | Indigenous: P. falciparum | – | – | – | – | – | 184 | 403 | 309 | 149 |
| | Indigenous: P. vivax | – | – | – | – | – | 434 | 788 | 963 | 1 504 |
| | Indigenous: mixed | – | – | – | – | – | 0 | 0 | 3 | 0 |
| | Indigenous: other species | – | – | – | – | – | 0 | 0 | 0 | 0 |
| El Salvador | Suspected | 115 256 | 100 884 | 124 885 | 103 748 | 106 915 | 89 267 | 81 904 | 70 022 | 52 216 |
| | Indigenous: P. falciparum | – | – | – | 0 | 0 | 0 | 0 | 0 | 0 |
| | Indigenous: P. vivax | – | – | – | 6 | 6 | 2 | 13 | 0 | 0 |
| | Indigenous: mixed | – | – | – | 0 | 0 | 0 | 0 | 0 | 0 |
| | Indigenous: other species | – | – | – | 0 | 0 | 0 | 0 | 0 | 0 |

| WHO region Country/area | | 2010 | 2011 | 2012 | 2013 | 2014 | 2015 | 2016 | 2017 | 2018 |
|---|---|---|---|---|---|---|---|---|---|---|
| **AMERICAS** | | | | | | | | | | |
| French Guiana | Suspected | 14 373 | 14 429 | 13 638 | 22 327 | 14 651 | 11 558 | 9 457 | 597 | – |
| | Total: P. falciparum | 987 | 584 | 382 | 304 | 136 | 84 | 72 | 70 | – |
| | Total: P. vivax | 476 | 339 | 257 | 220 | 129 | 230 | 119 | 400 | – |
| | Total: mixed cases | 561 | 496 | 381 | 348 | 182 | 120 | 67 | 127 | – |
| | Total: other species | 5 | 5 | 2 | 0 | 1 | 0 | 0 | 0 | – |
| Guatemala | Suspected | 237 075 | 195 080 | 186 645 | 153 731 | 300 989 | 301 746 | 408 394 | 372 158 | 514 133 |
| | Indigenous: P. falciparum | 30 | 64 | 54 | 101 | 24 | 43 | 4 | 0 | 3 |
| | Indigenous: P. vivax | 7 163 | 6 707 | 5 278 | 6 062 | 4 838 | 5 487 | 4 849 | 1 781 | 3 018 |
| | Indigenous: mixed | 5 | 3 | 14 | 51 | 67 | 8 | – | – | 0 |
| | Indigenous: other species | 0 | 0 | 0 | 0 | 0 | 0 | – | 0 | 0 |
| Guyana | Suspected | 212 863 | 201 728 | 196 622 | 205 903 | 142 843 | 132 941 | 116 300 | 100 096 | 99 806 |
| | Total: P. falciparum | 11 244 | 15 945 | 16 722 | 13 655 | 3 943 | 3 219 | 4 200 | 5 141 | 6 032 |
| | Total: P. vivax | 8 402 | 9 066 | 11 244 | 13 953 | 7 173 | 6 002 | 7 144 | 7 645 | 9 853 |
| | Total: mixed cases | 3 157 | 4 364 | 3 607 | 3 770 | 1 197 | 731 | 966 | 1 078 | 1 089 |
| | Total: other species | 132 | 96 | 92 | 101 | 41 | 32 | 57 | 72 | 64 |
| Haiti | Suspected | 270 427 | 184 934 | 167 772 | 176 995 | 261 403 | 302 740 | 302 044 | 295 572 | 288 294 |
| | Total: P. falciparum | 84 153 | 32 969 | 25 423 | 20 957 | 17 696 | 17 583 | 22 457 | 19 858 | 9 112 |
| | Total: P. vivax | 0 | 0 | 0 | 0 | 0 | 0 | 0 | 0 | 0 |
| | Total: mixed cases | 0 | 0 | 0 | 0 | 0 | 0 | 0 | 0 | 0 |
| | Total: other species | 0 | 0 | 0 | 0 | 0 | 0 | 0 | 0 | 0 |
| Honduras | Suspected | 156 961 | 156 559 | 159 165 | 144 673 | 152 847 | 153 906 | 182 767 | 165 536 | 161 400 |
| | Indigenous: P. falciparum | 866 | 585 | 560 | 1 113 | 564 | 404 | – | 99 | 55 |
| | Indigenous: P. vivax | 8 759 | 7 044 | 5 865 | 4 269 | 2 881 | 1 250 | – | 773 | 564 |
| | Indigenous: mixed | 120 | 34 | 24 | 46 | 37 | 7 | – | – | 1 |
| | Indigenous: other species | 0 | 0 | 0 | 0 | 0 | 0 | – | 0 | – |
| Mexico | Suspected | 1 192 081 | 1 035 424 | 1 025 659 | 1 017 508 | 900 580 | 867 853 | 798 568 | 644 174 | 548 247 |
| | Indigenous: P. falciparum | – | – | – | 0 | 0 | 0 | 0 | 0 | 0 |
| | Indigenous: P. vivax | – | – | – | 495 | 656 | 517 | 551 | 736 | 803 |
| | Indigenous: mixed | – | – | – | 0 | 0 | 0 | 0 | 0 | 0 |
| | Indigenous: other species | – | – | – | 0 | 0 | 0 | 0 | 0 | 0 |
| Nicaragua | Suspected | 554 414 | 536 105 | 552 722 | 539 022 | 605 357 | 604 418 | 554 415 | 663 132 | 875 982 |
| | Indigenous: P. falciparum | – | – | – | 208 | 155 | 338 | 1 285 | 1 836 | 1 319 |
| | Indigenous: P. vivax | – | – | – | 954 | 985 | 1 937 | 4 965 | 9 080 | 14 553 |
| | Indigenous: mixed | – | – | – | 0 | 2 | 4 | 22 | 33 | 45 |
| | Indigenous: other species | – | – | – | 0 | 0 | 0 | 0 | 0 | 0 |
| Panama | Suspected | 141 038 | 116 588 | 107 711 | 93 624 | 80 701 | 64 511 | 50 772 | 38 270 | 23 383 |
| | Indigenous: P. falciparum | – | – | – | – | 0 | 0 | 21 | 1 | 0 |
| | Indigenous: P. vivax | – | – | – | – | 864 | 546 | 748 | 648 | 684 |
| | Indigenous: mixed | – | – | – | – | 0 | 0 | 0 | 0 | 0 |
| | Indigenous: other species | – | – | – | – | 0 | 0 | 0 | 0 | 0 |
| Paraguay | Suspected | 62 178 | 48 611 | 31 499 | 24 806 | 24 832 | 6 687 | 3 193 | 9 281 | – |
| | Indigenous: P. falciparum | – | – | – | – | – | 0 | 0 | 0 | – |
| | Indigenous: P. vivax | 18 | 1 | – | – | – | 0 | 0 | 0 | – |
| | Indigenous: mixed | – | – | – | – | – | 0 | 0 | 0 | – |
| | Indigenous: other species | – | – | – | – | – | 0 | 0 | 0 | – |
| Peru | Suspected | 744 650 | 702 952 | 759 285 | 864 648 | 866 047 | 867 980 | 566 230 | 402 623 | 464 785 |
| | Indigenous: P. falciparum | 2 291 | 2 929 | 3 399 | 7 890 | 10 416 | 12 569 | 15 319 | 13 173 | 9 438 |
| | Indigenous: P. vivax | 29 169 | 21 984 | 28 030 | 40 829 | 54 819 | 49 287 | 41 287 | 42 044 | 36 005 |
| | Indigenous: mixed | 83 | 89 | 102 | 213 | 0 | 0 | 0 | 0 | 0 |
| | Indigenous: other species | 3 | 3 | 7 | 11 | 17 | 9 | 17 | 2 | 0 |

# Annex 3 – I. Reported malaria cases by species, 2010–2018

| WHO region Country/area | | 2010 | 2011 | 2012 | 2013 | 2014 | 2015 | 2016 | 2017 | 2018 |
|---|---|---|---|---|---|---|---|---|---|---|
| **AMERICAS** | | | | | | | | | | |
| Suriname | Suspected | 17 133 | 16 184 | 21 685 | 19 736 | 33 425 | 15 236 | 23 444 | 22 034 | 19 836 |
| | Indigenous: P. falciparum | 638 | 310 | 115 | 322 | 165 | 17 | 6 | 1 | 5 |
| | Indigenous: P. vivax | 817 | 382 | 167 | 322 | 78 | 61 | 69 | 17 | 23 |
| | Indigenous: mixed | 83 | 21 | 11 | 85 | 158 | 3 | 1 | 1 | 1 |
| | Indigenous: other species | 36 | 17 | 2 | 0 | 0 | 0 | 0 | 0 | 0 |
| Venezuela (Bolivarian Republic of) | Suspected | 400 495 | 382 303 | 410 663 | 476 764 | 522 617 | 625 174 | 932 556 | 1 144 635 | 747 247 |
| | Indigenous: P. falciparum | 10 629 | 9 724 | 10 978 | 22 777 | 21 074 | 24 018 | 46 503 | 69 076 | 71 504 |
| | Indigenous: P. vivax | 32 710 | 34 651 | 39 478 | 50 938 | 62 850 | 100 880 | 179 554 | 316 401 | 307 622 |
| | Indigenous: mixed | 286 | 909 | 2 324 | 4 882 | 6 769 | 11 491 | 14 531 | 26 080 | 25 789 |
| | Indigenous: other species | 60 | 6 | 23 | 46 | 15 | 13 | 25 | 29 | 9 |
| **EASTERN MEDITERRANEAN** | | | | | | | | | | |
| Afghanistan | Suspected | 847 589 | 936 252 | 847 933 | 787 624 | 743 183 | 801 938 | 939 389 | 932 096 | 932 614 |
| | Total: P. falciparum | 6 142 | 5 581 | 1 231 | 1 877 | 3 000 | 4 004 | 6 369 | 6 907 | 6 437 |
| | Total: P. vivax | 63 255 | 71 968 | 53 609 | 43 369 | 58 362 | 82 891 | 132 407 | 154 468 | 166 583 |
| | Total: mixed cases | 0 | 0 | 0 | 0 | 0 | 0 | 311 | 403 | 473 |
| | Total: other species | 0 | 0 | 0 | 0 | 0 | 0 | 0 | 0 | 0 |
| Djibouti | Suspected | 1 010 | 354 | 1 410 | 7 189 | 39 284 | 10 586 | 19 492 | 74 608 | 104 800 |
| | Total: P. falciparum | 1 010 | – | 20 | 0 | – | – | 11 781 | 9 290 | 16 130 |
| | Total: P. vivax | 0 | – | 0 | 0 | – | – | 2 041 | 5 381 | 9 189 |
| | Total: mixed cases | 0 | – | 0 | 0 | – | – | 0 | 0 | 0 |
| | Total: other species | 0 | – | 0 | 0 | – | – | 0 | 0 | 0 |
| Iran (Islamic Republic of) | Suspected | 614 817 | 530 470 | 479 655 | 385 172 | 468 513 | 630 886 | 418 125 | 383 397 | 541 975 |
| | Indigenous: P. falciparum | – | – | – | – | – | 8 | 0 | 2 | 0 |
| | Indigenous: P. vivax | – | – | – | – | – | 157 | 79 | 55 | 0 |
| | Indigenous: mixed | – | – | – | – | – | 1 | 2 | 0 | 0 |
| | Indigenous: other species | – | – | – | – | – | 0 | 0 | 0 | 0 |
| Pakistan | Suspected | 8 601 835 | 8 418 570 | 8 902 947 | 7 752 797 | 8 514 341 | 8 885 456 | 8 072 464 | 8 122 212 | 7 123 228 |
| | Total: P. falciparum | 73 857 | 73 925 | 95 095 | 46 067 | 33 391 | 30 075 | 42 011 | 54 467 | 55 639 |
| | Total: P. vivax | 143 136 | 205 879 | 228 215 | 283 661 | 232 332 | 163 872 | 257 962 | 300 623 | 314 572 |
| | Total: mixed cases | 0 | 0 | 2 901 | 10 506 | 9 426 | 8 066 | 24 493 | 14 787 | 4 299 |
| | Total: other species | 0 | 0 | 0 | 0 | 0 | 0 | 0 | 0 | 0 |
| Saudi Arabia | Suspected | 944 723 | 1 062 827 | 1 186 179 | 1 309 783 | 1 249 752 | 1 306 700 | 1 267 933 | 1 073 998 | 1 015 953 |
| | Indigenous: P. falciparum | – | – | 82 | – | – | 83 | 270 | 172 | 57 |
| | Indigenous: P. vivax | – | – | – | – | – | 0 | 2 | 5 | 4 |
| | Indigenous: mixed | – | – | – | – | – | 0 | 0 | 0 | 0 |
| | Indigenous: other species | – | – | – | – | – | 0 | 0 | 0 | 0 |
| Somalia | Suspected | 220 698 | 99 403 | 53 658 | 69 192 | 79 653 | 119 008 | 205 753 | 228 912 | 253 220 |
| | Total: P. falciparum | 5 629 | – | – | – | – | – | – | – | – |
| | Total: P. vivax | 0 | – | – | – | – | – | – | – | – |
| | Total: mixed cases | 0 | – | – | – | – | – | – | – | – |
| | Total: other species | 0 | – | – | – | – | – | – | – | – |
| Sudan | Suspected | 2 398 239 | 2 929 578 | 2 438 467 | 2 197 563 | 1 207 771 | 4 101 841 | 4 199 740 | 3 691 112 | 9 723 425 |
| | Total: P. falciparum | – | – | – | – | – | – | 333 009 | 580 145 | 1 286 915 |
| | Total: P. vivax | – | – | – | – | – | – | 82 175 | 58 335 | 143 314 |
| | Total: mixed cases | – | – | – | – | – | – | 32 557 | 82 399 | 187 270 |
| | Total: other species | – | – | – | – | – | – | 24 105 | 0 | 0 |
| Yemen | Suspected | 835 018 | 804 401 | 888 952 | 927 821 | 821 618 | 711 680 | 1 181 486 | 1 630 469 | 713 908 |
| | Total: P. falciparum | 77 271 | 59 689 | 109 504 | 102 369 | 86 428 | 75 898 | 45 469 | 109 849 | 112 823 |
| | Total: P. vivax | 966 | 478 | 398 | 408 | 267 | 334 | 347 | 1 833 | 970 |
| | Total: mixed cases | 30 | 7 | 0 | 0 | 12 | 27 | 70 | 2 322 | 63 |
| | Total: other species | 2 | 33 | 0 | 0 | 0 | 0 | 0 | 0 | 69 |

| WHO region Country/area | | 2010 | 2011 | 2012 | 2013 | 2014 | 2015 | 2016 | 2017 | 2018 |
|---|---|---|---|---|---|---|---|---|---|---|
| **EUROPEAN** | | | | | | | | | | |
| Armenia | Suspected | 31 026 | 0 | 821 860 | 825 443 | – | – | – | 350 | – |
| | Indigenous: P. falciparum | 0 | 0 | 0 | 0 | 0 | 0 | 0 | 0 | – |
| | Indigenous: P. vivax | 0 | 0 | 0 | 0 | 0 | 0 | 0 | 0 | – |
| | Indigenous: mixed | 0 | 0 | 0 | 0 | 0 | 0 | 0 | 0 | – |
| | Indigenous: other species | 0 | – | – | – | – | 0 | 0 | 0 | – |
| Azerbaijan | Suspected | 456 652 | 449 168 | 497 040 | 432 810 | 399 925 | 405 416 | 465 860 | 373 562 | – |
| | Indigenous: P. falciparum | 0 | 0 | 0 | 0 | 0 | 0 | 0 | 0 | – |
| | Indigenous: P. vivax | 50 | 4 | 3 | 0 | 0 | 0 | 0 | 0 | – |
| | Indigenous: mixed | 0 | 0 | 0 | 0 | 0 | 0 | 0 | 0 | – |
| | Indigenous: other species | 0 | 0 | 0 | 0 | 0 | 0 | 0 | 0 | – |
| Georgia | Suspected | 2 368 | 2 032 | 1 046 | 192 | 440 | 294 | 318 | 416 | – |
| | Indigenous: P. falciparum | 0 | 0 | 0 | 0 | 0 | 0 | 0 | 0 | – |
| | Indigenous: P. vivax | 0 | 1 | 1 | 0 | 0 | 0 | 0 | 0 | – |
| | Indigenous: mixed | 0 | 0 | 0 | 0 | 0 | 0 | 0 | 0 | – |
| | Indigenous: other species | 0 | 0 | 0 | 0 | 0 | 0 | 0 | 0 | – |
| Kyrgyzstan[2] | Suspected | 30 190 | 27 850 | 18 268 | 54 249 | 35 600 | – | – | – | – |
| | Indigenous: P. falciparum | 0 | 0 | 0 | 0 | 0 | 0 | 0 | 0 | – |
| | Indigenous: P. vivax | 3 | 0 | 0 | 0 | 0 | 0 | 0 | 0 | – |
| | Indigenous: mixed | 0 | 0 | 0 | 0 | 0 | 0 | 0 | 0 | – |
| | Indigenous: other species | 0 | 0 | 0 | 0 | 0 | 0 | 0 | 0 | – |
| Tajikistan | Suspected | 173 523 | 173 367 | 209 239 | 213 916 | 200 241 | 188 341 | 233 336 | 232 502 | – |
| | Indigenous: P. falciparum | 0 | 0 | 0 | 0 | 0 | 0 | 0 | 0 | – |
| | Indigenous: P. vivax | 111 | 65 | 18 | 7 | 2 | 0 | 0 | 0 | – |
| | Indigenous: mixed | 0 | 0 | 0 | 0 | 0 | 0 | 0 | 0 | – |
| | Indigenous: other species | 0 | 0 | 0 | 0 | 0 | 0 | 0 | 0 | – |
| Turkey | Suspected | 507 841 | 421 295 | 337 830 | 255 125 | 189 854 | 221 | 144 499 | 115 557 | – |
| | Indigenous: P. falciparum | 0 | 0 | 0 | 0 | 0 | 0 | 0 | 0 | – |
| | Indigenous: P. vivax | 9 | 4 | 219 | 34 | 5 | 0 | 0 | 0 | – |
| | Indigenous: mixed | 0 | 0 | 0 | 0 | 0 | 0 | 0 | 0 | – |
| | Indigenous: other species | 0 | 0 | 0 | 0 | 0 | 0 | 0 | 0 | – |
| Turkmenistan[2] | Suspected | 81 784 | – | – | – | – | 83 675 | 85 536 | 84 264 | – |
| | Indigenous: P. falciparum | 0 | 0 | 0 | 0 | 0 | 0 | 0 | 0 | – |
| | Indigenous: P. vivax | 0 | 0 | 0 | 0 | 0 | 0 | 0 | 0 | – |
| | Indigenous: mixed | 0 | 0 | 0 | 0 | 0 | 0 | 0 | 0 | – |
| | Indigenous: other species | 0 | 0 | 0 | 0 | 0 | 0 | 0 | 0 | – |
| Uzbekistan[2] | Suspected | 921 364 | 886 243 | 805 761 | 908 301 | 812 347 | 800 912 | 797 472 | 655 112 | – |
| | Indigenous: P. falciparum | 0 | 0 | 0 | 0 | 0 | 0 | 0 | 0 | – |
| | Indigenous: P. vivax | 3 | 0 | 0 | 0 | 0 | 0 | 0 | 0 | – |
| | Indigenous: mixed | 0 | 0 | 0 | 0 | 0 | 0 | 0 | 0 | – |
| | Indigenous: other species | 0 | 0 | 0 | 0 | 0 | 0 | 0 | 0 | – |
| **SOUTH-EAST ASIA** | | | | | | | | | | |
| Bangladesh | Suspected | 461 262 | 390 102 | 309 179 | 93 926 | 125 201 | 122 806 | 138 973 | 150 518 | 133 547 |
| | Total: P. falciparum | 52 012 | 49 084 | 9 428 | 3 597 | 8 981 | 5 351 | 3 509 | 4 224 | 1 609 |
| | Total: P. vivax | 3 824 | 2 579 | 396 | 262 | 489 | 488 | 427 | 522 | 280 |
| | Total: mixed cases | 37 | 110 | 36 | 5 | 746 | 769 | 851 | 166 | 30 |
| | Total: other species | 0 | 0 | 0 | 0 | 0 | 0 | 0 | 0 | 0 |

# Annex 3 – I. Reported malaria cases by species, 2010–2018

| WHO region Country/area | | 2010 | 2011 | 2012 | 2013 | 2014 | 2015 | 2016 | 2017 | 2018 |
|---|---|---|---|---|---|---|---|---|---|---|
| **SOUTH-EAST ASIA** | | | | | | | | | | |
| Bhutan | Suspected | 54 760 | 44 494 | 42 512 | 31 632 | 33 586 | 74 087 | 118 841 | 42 146 | 133 498 |
| | Indigenous: P. falciparum | – | – | – | – | – | 13 | 1 | 0 | 1 |
| | Indigenous: P. vivax | – | – | – | – | – | 21 | 13 | 11 | 5 |
| | Indigenous: mixed | – | – | – | – | – | 0 | 1 | 0 | 0 |
| | Indigenous: other species | – | – | – | – | – | 0 | 0 | 0 | 0 |
| Democratic People's Republic of Korea | Suspected | 27 019 | 27 857 | 40 925 | 72 719 | 38 878 | 91 007 | 205 807 | 189 357 | 685 704 |
| | Total: P. falciparum | 0 | 0 | 0 | 0 | 0 | 0 | 0 | 0 | 0 |
| | Total: P. vivax | 13 520 | 16 760 | 21 850 | 14 407 | 10 535 | 7 022 | 5 033 | 4 603 | 3 598 |
| | Total: mixed cases | 0 | 0 | 0 | 0 | 0 | 0 | 0 | 0 | 0 |
| | Total: other species | 0 | 0 | 0 | 0 | 0 | 0 | 0 | 0 | 0 |
| India | Suspected | 119 279 429 | 119 470 044 | 122 159 270 | 127 891 198 | 138 628 331 | 140 841 230 | 144 539 608 | 125 977 799 | 124 613 482 |
| | Total: P. falciparum | 830 779 | 662 748 | 524 370 | 462 079 | 720 795 | 774 627 | 706 257 | 525 637 | 204 733 |
| | Total: P. vivax | 765 622 | 645 652 | 534 129 | 417 884 | 379 659 | 390 440 | 375 783 | 315 028 | 222 730 |
| | Total: mixed cases | 3 585 | 2 256 | 0 | 1 767 | 1 751 | 4 194 | 5 245 | 3 893 | 2 465 |
| | Total: other species | 0 | 0 | 0 | 0 | 0 | 0 | 0 | 0 | 0 |
| Indonesia | Suspected | 1 591 179 | 1 212 799 | 1 900 725 | 1 708 161 | 1 550 296 | 1 567 450 | 1 457 858 | 1 441 679 | 1 474 636 |
| | Total: P. falciparum | 220 077 | 200 662 | 199 977 | 170 848 | 126 397 | 103 315 | 118 844 | 143 926 | 101 736 |
| | Total: P. vivax | 187 583 | 187 989 | 187 583 | 150 985 | 107 260 | 94 267 | 81 748 | 95 694 | 70 867 |
| | Total: mixed cases | 21 964 | 31 535 | 29 278 | 20 352 | 16 410 | 13 105 | 16 751 | 18 899 | 16 068 |
| | Total: other species | 2 547 | 2 261 | 981 | 1 342 | 1 960 | 1 387 | 1 106 | 1 818 | 1 902 |
| Myanmar | Suspected | 1 277 568 | 1 210 465 | 1 423 555 | 1 300 556 | 1 567 095 | 2 663 732 | 3 185 245 | 3 368 697 | 3 099 776 |
| | Total: P. falciparum | 70 941 | 59 604 | 314 650 | 223 303 | 138 311 | 110 539 | 62 917 | 50 730 | 37 566 |
| | Total: P. vivax | 29 944 | 28 966 | 135 386 | 99 037 | 61 830 | 65 590 | 43 748 | 32 070 | 31 389 |
| | Total: mixed cases | 2 054 | 3 020 | 30 419 | 12 255 | 5 511 | 6 632 | 3 476 | 2 214 | 1 474 |
| | Total: other species | 346 | 162 | 103 | 25 | 6 | 14 | 5 | 5 | 3 |
| Nepal | Suspected | 213 353 | 188 702 | 243 432 | 168 687 | 200 631 | 131 654 | 146 705 | 214 265 | 256 912 |
| | Total: P. falciparum | 550 | 219 | 612 | 273 | 195 | 250 | 137 | 103 | 47 |
| | Total: P. vivax | 2 349 | 1 631 | 1 480 | 1 659 | 1 154 | 1 516 | 846 | 1 173 | 1 106 |
| | Total: mixed cases | 216 | 30 | 0 | 22 | 120 | 71 | 26 | 17 | 5 |
| | Total: other species | 0 | 0 | 0 | 0 | 0 | 0 | 0 | 0 | 0 |
| Sri Lanka[2] | Suspected | 1 001 107 | 985 060 | 948 250 | 1 236 580 | 1 069 817 | 1 156 151 | 1 090 760 | 1 104 796 | 1 149 897 |
| | Indigenous: P. falciparum | 6 | 3 | 4 | – | – | 0 | 0 | 0 | 0 |
| | Indigenous: P. vivax | 668 | 119 | 19 | – | – | 0 | 0 | 0 | 0 |
| | Indigenous: mixed | – | – | – | – | – | 0 | 0 | 0 | 0 |
| | Indigenous: other species | 0 | 0 | 0 | – | – | 0 | 0 | 0 | 0 |
| Thailand | Suspected | 1 777 977 | 1 450 885 | 1 130 757 | 1 927 585 | 1 756 528 | 1 370 461 | 1 461 007 | 1 149 546 | 921 548 |
| | Indigenous: P. falciparum | – | – | – | – | – | 3 291 | 1 609 | 846 | 447 |
| | Indigenous: P. vivax | – | – | – | – | – | 4 655 | 5 765 | 4 802 | 3 575 |
| | Indigenous: mixed | – | – | – | – | – | 57 | 40 | 36 | 34 |
| | Indigenous: other species | – | – | – | – | – | 19 | 14 | 10 | 21 |
| Timor-Leste | Suspected | 266 386 | 225 858 | 182 857 | 178 200 | 117 107 | 121 054 | 150 333 | 129 175 | 154 816 |
| | Indigenous: P. falciparum | – | – | – | – | – | – | 46 | 5 | 0 |
| | Indigenous: P. vivax | – | – | – | – | – | – | 8 | 3 | 0 |
| | Indigenous: mixed | – | – | – | – | – | – | 28 | 8 | 0 |
| | Indigenous: other species | – | – | – | – | – | – | 0 | 0 | 0 |
| **WESTERN PACIFIC** | | | | | | | | | | |
| Cambodia | Suspected | 193 210 | 216 712 | 194 263 | 152 137 | 142 242 | 163 680 | 166 695 | 168 245 | 166 638 |
| | Total: P. falciparum | 8 213 | 7 054 | 14 896 | 7 092 | 8 332 | 17 830 | 12 156 | 20 328 | 10 525 |
| | Total: P. vivax | 4 794 | 5 155 | 19 575 | 11 267 | 10 356 | 13 146 | 9 816 | 15 207 | 30 680 |
| | Total: mixed cases | 1 270 | 1 583 | 4 971 | 2 418 | 6 464 | 2 954 | 1 520 | 1 397 | 1 080 |
| | Total: other species | 0 | 0 | 0 | 0 | 0 | 0 | 0 | 0 | 0 |

| WHO region Country/area | | 2010 | 2011 | 2012 | 2013 | 2014 | 2015 | 2016 | 2017 | 2018 |
|---|---|---|---|---|---|---|---|---|---|---|
| **WESTERN PACIFIC** | | | | | | | | | | |
| China | Suspected | 7 118 649 | 9 190 401 | 6 918 770 | 5 555 001 | 4 403 633 | 4 052 616 | 3 194 929 | 2 409 280 | 1 904 295 |
| | Indigenous: P. falciparum | – | – | – | – | – | 1 | 0 | 0 | 0 |
| | Indigenous: P. vivax | – | – | – | – | – | 26 | 3 | 0 | 0 |
| | Indigenous: mixed | – | – | – | – | – | 0 | 0 | 0 | 0 |
| | Indigenous: other species | – | – | – | – | – | 6 | 0 | 0 | 0 |
| Lao People's Democratic Republic | Suspected | 280 549 | 291 775 | 369 976 | 339 013 | 294 542 | 284 003 | 223 992 | 274 314 | 286 881 |
| | Total: P. falciparum | 4 393 | 5 770 | 37 692 | 24 538 | 23 928 | 14 430 | 4 255 | 4 550 | 4 726 |
| | Total: P. vivax | 122 | 442 | 7 634 | 12 537 | 22 625 | 20 804 | 6 795 | 4 590 | 4 077 |
| | Total: mixed cases | 8 | 0 | 769 | 956 | 1 517 | 822 | 173 | 193 | 110 |
| | Total: other species | 1 | 14 | 0 | 1 | 1 | 0 | 0 | 0 | 0 |
| Malaysia | Suspected | 1 619 074 | 1 600 439 | 1 566 872 | 1 576 012 | 1 443 958 | 1 066 470 | 1 153 108 | 1 046 163 | 1 070 356 |
| | Indigenous: P. falciparum | – | – | – | – | – | 110 | 67 | 18 | 0 |
| | Indigenous: P. vivax | – | – | – | – | – | 84 | 178 | 59 | 0 |
| | Indigenous: mixed | – | – | – | – | – | 22 | 9 | 1 | 0 |
| | Indigenous: other species | – | – | – | – | – | 26 | 12 | 7 | 0 |
| Papua New Guinea | Suspected | 1 505 393 | 1 279 140 | 1 113 528 | 1 454 166 | 922 417 | 909 940 | 1 168 797 | 1 400 593 | 1 513 776 |
| | Total: P. falciparum | 56 735 | 59 153 | 58 747 | 119 469 | 120 641 | 118 452 | 183 686 | 163 160 | 174 818 |
| | Total: P. vivax | 13 171 | 9 654 | 7 108 | 7 579 | 78 846 | 62 228 | 95 328 | 113 561 | 138 006 |
| | Total: mixed cases | 4 089 | 1 164 | 0 | 1 279 | 79 574 | 115 157 | 197 711 | 200 186 | 201 658 |
| | Total: other species | 1 990 | 632 | 0 | 1 279 | 2 125 | 1 950 | 1 772 | 1 433 | 1 767 |
| Philippines | Suspected | 301 577 | 327 125 | 333 084 | 320 089 | 316 323 | 280 222 | 321 838 | 284 564 | 282 385 |
| | Total: P. falciparum | 11 824 | 6 877 | 4 774 | 4 968 | 3 760 | 4 781 | 5 320 | 3 160 | 1 370 |
| | Total: P. vivax | 2 885 | 2 380 | 2 189 | 1 357 | 834 | 760 | 826 | 538 | 129 |
| | Total: mixed cases | 214 | 166 | 0 | 83 | 235 | 196 | 391 | 83 | 26 |
| | Total: other species | 175 | 127 | 0 | 67 | 74 | 87 | 142 | 46 | 49 |
| Republic of Korea | Suspected | 1 772 | 838 | 555 | 443 | 638 | 699 | 0 | 0 | 576 |
| | Indigenous: P. falciparum | – | – | – | – | – | 0 | 0 | 0 | 0 |
| | Indigenous: P. vivax | – | – | – | – | – | 628 | 602 | 436 | 501 |
| | Indigenous: mixed | – | – | – | – | – | 0 | 0 | 0 | 0 |
| | Indigenous: other species | – | – | – | – | – | 0 | 0 | 0 | 0 |
| Solomon Islands | Suspected | 284 931 | 254 506 | 249 520 | 245 014 | 233 803 | 192 044 | 274 881 | 238 814 | 244 523 |
| | Total: P. falciparum | 22 892 | 14 454 | 14 748 | 13 194 | 9 835 | 10 478 | 16 607 | 15 400 | 15 771 |
| | Total: P. vivax | 12 281 | 8 665 | 9 339 | 11 628 | 7 845 | 12 150 | 33 060 | 30 169 | 35 072 |
| | Total: mixed cases | 200 | 83 | 232 | 446 | 724 | 1 370 | 4 719 | 6 917 | 8 341 |
| | Total: other species | 0 | 0 | 0 | 0 | 0 | 0 | 46 | 33 | 7 |
| Vanuatu | Suspected | 48 088 | 32 656 | 33 273 | 28 943 | 35 570 | 14 938 | 21 484 | 30 313 | 26 931 |
| | Total: P. falciparum | 1 545 | 770 | 1 257 | 1 039 | 279 | 150 | 186 | 273 | 49 |
| | Total: P. vivax | 2 265 | 1 224 | 1 680 | 1 342 | 703 | 273 | 1 682 | 799 | 595 |
| | Total: mixed cases | 193 | 81 | 470 | 0 | 0 | 0 | 0 | 0 | 0 |
| | Total: other species | 10 | 2 | 0 | 0 | 0 | 0 | 0 | 0 | 0 |
| Viet Nam | Suspected | 2 803 918 | 3 312 266 | 3 436 534 | 3 115 804 | 2 786 135 | 2 673 662 | 2 497 326 | 2 614 663 | 2 167 376 |
| | Total: P. falciparum | 12 763 | 10 101 | 11 448 | 9 532 | 8 245 | 4 327 | 2 323 | 2 858 | 2 966 |
| | Total: P. vivax | 4 466 | 5 602 | 7 220 | 6 901 | 7 220 | 4 756 | 1 750 | 1 608 | 1 751 |
| | Total: mixed cases | 0 | 0 | 0 | 0 | 287 | 234 | 73 | 70 | 83 |
| | Total: other species | 0 | 0 | 0 | 0 | 0 | 14 | 15 | 12 | 13 |

Data as of 14 February 2020

P.: Plasmodium; WHO: World Health Organization.

"–" refers to not applicable or data not available.

[1] In May 2013, Sudan was reassigned to the WHO African Region (WHA resolution 66.21, https://apps.who.int/gb/ebwha/pdf_files/WHA66/A66_R21-en.pdf).

[2] Certified malaria free countries are included in this listing for historical purposes.

Note: Indigenous cases are reported for countries with elimination programmes and/or with >99% of total confirmed cases investigated. For countries in the WHO Region of the Americas, the number of Total: P. falciparum, Total: P. vivax, Total: mixed cases and Total: other species are indigenous cases for all years apart from Dominican Republic and Venezuela (Bolivarian Republic of) (2013 onwards), Argentina, Guatemala and Peru (2014 onwards) and Bolivia (Plurinational State of), Honduras and Suriname (2015 onwards). Indigenous cases are reported for Botswana and Eswatini from 2015 onwards. Suspected cases include indigenous and imported cases. For countries with only suspected cases shown, no species breakdown was provided.

# Annex 3 - J. Reported malaria deaths, 2010–2018

| WHO region Country/area | 2010 | 2011 | 2012 | 2013 | 2014 | 2015 | 2016 | 2017 | 2018 |
|---|---|---|---|---|---|---|---|---|---|
| **AFRICAN** | | | | | | | | | |
| Algeria[1] | 1 | 0 | 0 | 0 | 0 | 0 | 0 | 0 | 0 |
| Angola | 8 114 | 6 909 | 5 736 | 7 300 | 5 714 | 7 832 | 15 997 | 13 967 | 11 814 |
| Benin | 964 | 1 753 | 2 261 | 2 288 | 1 869 | 1 416 | 1 646 | 2 182 | 2 138 |
| Botswana | 8 | 8 | 3 | 7 | 22 | 5 | 3 | 17 | 9 |
| Burkina Faso | 9 024 | 7 001 | 7 963 | 6 294 | 5 632 | 5 379 | 3 974 | 4 144 | 4 294 |
| Burundi | 2 677 | 2 233 | 2 263 | 3 411 | 2 974 | 3 799 | 5 853 | 4 414 | 2 481 |
| Cabo Verde | 1 | 1 | 0 | 0 | 1 | 0 | 1 | 1 | 0 |
| Cameroon | 4 536 | 3 808 | 3 209 | 4 349 | 4 398 | 3 440 | 2 639 | 3 195 | 3 256 |
| Central African Republic | 526 | 858 | 1 442 | 1 026 | 635 | 1 763 | 2 668 | 3 689 | 1 292 |
| Chad | 886 | 1 220 | 1 359 | 1 881 | 1 720 | 1 572 | 1 686 | 2 088 | 1 948 |
| Comoros | 53 | 19 | 17 | 15 | 0 | 1 | 0 | 3 | 8 |
| Congo | – | 892 | 623 | 2 870 | 271 | 435 | 733 | 229 | 131 |
| Côte d'Ivoire | 1 023 | 1 389 | 1 534 | 3 261 | 4 069 | 2 604 | 3 340 | 3 222 | 3 133 |
| Democratic Republic of the Congo | 23 476 | 23 748 | 21 601 | 30 918 | 25 502 | 39 054 | 33 997 | 27 458 | 18 030 |
| Equatorial Guinea | 30 | 52 | 77 | 66 | – | 28 | 109 | – | – |
| Eritrea | 27 | 12 | 30 | 6 | 15 | 12 | 21 | 8 | 5 |
| Eswatini | 8 | 1 | 3 | 4 | 4 | 5 | 3 | 20 | 2 |
| Ethiopia | 1 581 | 936 | 1 621 | 358 | 213 | 662 | 510 | 356 | 158 |
| Gabon | 182 | 74 | 134 | 273 | 159 | 309 | 101 | 218 | 591 |
| Gambia | 151 | 440 | 289 | 262 | 170 | 167 | 79 | 54 | 60 |
| Ghana | 3 859 | 3 259 | 2 855 | 2 506 | 2 200 | 2 137 | 1 264 | 599 | 428 |
| Guinea | 735 | 743 | 979 | 108 | 1 067 | 846 | 867 | 1 174 | 1 267 |
| Guinea-Bissau | 296 | 472 | 370 | 418 | 357 | 477 | 191 | 296 | 244 |
| Kenya | 26 017 | 713 | 785 | 360 | 472 | 15 061 | 603 | – | – |
| Liberia | 1 422 | – | 1 725 | 1 191 | 2 288 | 1 379 | 1 259 | 758 | – |
| Madagascar | 427 | 398 | 552 | 641 | 551 | 841 | 443 | 370 | 927 |
| Malawi | 8 206 | 6 674 | 5 516 | 3 723 | 4 490 | 3 799 | 4 000 | 3 613 | 2 967 |
| Mali | 3 006 | 2 128 | 1 894 | 1 680 | 2 309 | 1 544 | 1 344 | 1 050 | 1 001 |
| Mauritania | 60 | 66 | 106 | 46 | 19 | 39 | 315 | 67 | – |
| Mayotte | 0 | 0 | 0 | 0 | 0 | 0 | 0 | – | – |
| Mozambique | 3 354 | 3 086 | 2 818 | 2 941 | 3 245 | 2 467 | 1 685 | 1 114 | 968 |
| Namibia | 63 | 36 | 4 | 21 | 61 | 45 | 65 | 104 | 82 |
| Niger | 3 929 | 2 802 | 2 825 | 2 209 | 2 691 | 2 778 | 2 226 | 2 316 | 3 576 |
| Nigeria | 4 238 | 3 353 | 7 734 | 7 878 | 6 082 | – | – | – | – |
| Rwanda | 670 | 380 | 459 | 409 | 496 | 516 | 715 | 376 | 341 |
| Sao Tome and Principe | 14 | 19 | 7 | 11 | 0 | 0 | 1 | 1 | 0 |
| Senegal | 553 | 472 | 649 | 815 | 500 | 526 | 325 | 284 | 555 |
| Sierra Leone | 8 188 | 3 573 | 3 611 | 4 326 | 2 848 | 1 107 | 1 345 | 1 298 | 1 949 |
| South Africa | 83 | 54 | 72 | 105 | 174 | 110 | 34 | 301 | 69 |
| South Sudan[2] | 1 053 | 406 | 1 321 | 1 311 | – | – | – | 3 483 | 1 191 |
| Togo | 1 507 | 1 314 | 1 197 | 1 361 | 1 205 | 1 205 | 847 | 995 | 905 |
| Uganda | 8 431 | 5 958 | 6 585 | 7 277 | 5 921 | 6 100 | 5 635 | 5 111 | 3 302 |
| United Republic of Tanzania | 15 867 | 11 806 | 7 820 | 8 528 | 5 373 | 6 313 | 5 046 | 3 685 | 2 753 |
|   Mainland | 15 819 | 11 799 | 7 812 | 8 526 | 5 368 | 6 311 | 5 045 | 3 684 | 2 747 |
|   Zanzibar | 48 | 7 | 8 | 2 | 5 | 2 | 1 | 1 | 6 |
| Zambia | 4 834 | 4 540 | 3 705 | 3 548 | 3 257 | 2 389 | 1 827 | 1 425 | 1 209 |
| Zimbabwe | 255 | 451 | 351 | 352 | 406 | 200 | 351 | 527 | 192 |
| **AMERICAS** | | | | | | | | | |
| Argentina[1] | 0 | 0 | 0 | 0 | 0 | 0 | 0 | 0 | 0 |
| Belize | 0 | 0 | 0 | 0 | 0 | 0 | 0 | 0 | 0 |
| Bolivia (Plurinational State of) | 0 | 0 | 0 | 0 | 1 | 0 | 0 | 0 | 0 |
| Brazil | 76 | 70 | 60 | 40 | 36 | 35 | 35 | 34 | 44 |
| Colombia | 42 | 23 | 24 | 10 | 17 | 18 | 36 | 19 | 9 |
| Costa Rica | 0 | 0 | 0 | 0 | 0 | 0 | 0 | 0 | 0 |
| Dominican Republic | 15 | 10 | 8 | 5 | 4 | 3 | 1 | 1 | 1 |
| Ecuador | 0 | 0 | 0 | 0 | 0 | 0 | 0 | 0 | 0 |
| El Salvador[3] | 0 | 0 | 0 | 0 | 0 | 0 | 0 | 0 | 0 |
| French Guiana | 1 | 2 | 2 | 3 | 0 | 0 | 0 | 0 | – |
| Guatemala | 0 | 0 | 0 | 1 | 1 | 1 | 0 | 0 | 0 |
| Guyana | 24 | 36 | 35 | 14 | 11 | 12 | 13 | 11 | 6 |
| Haiti | 8 | 5 | 6 | 10 | 9 | 15 | 13 | 12 | 12 |
| Honduras | 3 | 2 | 1 | 1 | 2 | 0 | 0 | 1 | 1 |
| Mexico | 0 | 0 | 0 | 0 | 0 | 0 | 0 | 0 | 0 |
| Nicaragua | 1 | 1 | 2 | 0 | 0 | 1 | 2 | 1 | 3 |
| Panama | 1 | 0 | 1 | 0 | 0 | 0 | 0 | 0 | 0 |

| WHO region Country/area | 2010 | 2011 | 2012 | 2013 | 2014 | 2015 | 2016 | 2017 | 2018 |
|---|---|---|---|---|---|---|---|---|---|
| **AMERICAS** | | | | | | | | | |
| Paraguay[1] | 0 | 0 | 0 | 0 | 0 | 0 | 0 | 0 | 0 |
| Peru | 0 | 1 | 7 | 4 | 4 | 5 | 7 | 10 | 4 |
| Suriname | 1 | 1 | 0 | 1 | 1 | 0 | 0 | 1 | 0 |
| Venezuela (Bolivarian Republic of) | 18 | 16 | 10 | 6 | 5 | 8 | 105 | 333 | 257 |
| **EASTERN MEDITERRANEAN** | | | | | | | | | |
| Afghanistan | 22 | 40 | 36 | 24 | 32 | 49 | 47 | 10 | 1 |
| Djibouti | 0 | 0 | 0 | 17 | 28 | 23 | 5 | – | – |
| Iran (Islamic Republic of)[3] | 0 | 0 | 0 | 0 | 0 | 0 | 0 | 0 | 0 |
| Pakistan | – | 4 | 260 | 244 | 56 | 34 | 33 | 113 | 102 |
| Saudi Arabia | 0 | 0 | 0 | 0 | 0 | 0 | 0 | 0 | 0 |
| Somalia | 6 | 5 | 10 | 23 | 14 | 27 | 13 | 20 | 31 |
| Sudan | 1 023 | 612 | 618 | 685 | 823 | 868 | 698 | 1 534 | 3 129 |
| Yemen | 92 | 75 | 72 | 55 | 23 | 14 | 65 | 37 | 57 |
| **EUROPEAN** | | | | | | | | | |
| Armenia[1] | 0 | 0 | 0 | 0 | 0 | 0 | 0 | 0 | 0 |
| Azerbaijan[3] | 0 | 0 | 0 | 0 | 0 | 0 | 0 | 0 | 0 |
| Georgia[3] | 0 | 0 | 0 | 0 | 0 | 0 | 0 | 0 | 0 |
| Kyrgyzstan[1] | 0 | 0 | 0 | 0 | 0 | 0 | 0 | 0 | 0 |
| Tajikistan[3] | 0 | 0 | 0 | 0 | 0 | 0 | 0 | 0 | 0 |
| Turkey[3] | 0 | 0 | 0 | 0 | 0 | 0 | 0 | 0 | 0 |
| Turkmenistan[1] | 0 | 0 | 0 | 0 | 0 | 0 | 0 | 0 | 0 |
| Uzbekistan[1] | 0 | 0 | 0 | 0 | 0 | 0 | 0 | 0 | 0 |
| **SOUTH-EAST ASIA** | | | | | | | | | |
| Bangladesh | 37 | 36 | 11 | 15 | 45 | 9 | 17 | 13 | 7 |
| Bhutan | 2 | 1 | 1 | 0 | 0 | 0 | 0 | 0 | 0 |
| Democratic People's Republic of Korea | 0 | 0 | 0 | 0 | 0 | 0 | 0 | 0 | 0 |
| India | 1 018 | 754 | 519 | 440 | 562 | 384 | 331 | 194 | 96 |
| Indonesia | 432 | 388 | 252 | 385 | 217 | 157 | 161 | 47 | 34 |
| Myanmar | 788 | 581 | 403 | 236 | 92 | 37 | 21 | 30 | 19 |
| Nepal | 6 | 2 | 0 | 0 | 0 | 0 | 3 | 0 | 0 |
| Sri Lanka[1] | 0 | 0 | 0 | 0 | 0 | 0 | 0 | 0 | 0 |
| Thailand | 80 | 43 | 37 | 47 | 38 | 33 | 27 | 15 | 8 |
| Timor-Leste[3] | 58 | 16 | 6 | 3 | 1 | 0 | 0 | 0 | 0 |
| **WESTERN PACIFIC** | | | | | | | | | |
| Cambodia | 151 | 94 | 45 | 12 | 18 | 10 | 3 | 1 | 0 |
| China[3] | 19 | 33 | 0 | 0 | 0 | 0 | 0 | 0 | 0 |
| Lao People's Democratic Republic | 24 | 17 | 44 | 28 | 4 | 2 | 1 | 2 | 6 |
| Malaysia[4] | *13* | *12* | *12* | *10* | *4* | *4* | *2* | *10* | *12* |
| Papua New Guinea | 616 | 523 | 381 | 307 | 203 | 163 | 306 | 273 | 216 |
| Philippines | 30 | 12 | 16 | 12 | 10 | 20 | 7 | 3 | 1 |
| Republic of Korea | *1* | *2* | 0 | 0 | 0 | 0 | 0 | 0 | 0 |
| Solomon Islands | 34 | 19 | 18 | 18 | 23 | 13 | 20 | 27 | 7 |
| Vanuatu | 1 | 1 | 0 | 0 | 0 | 0 | 0 | 0 | 0 |
| Viet Nam | 21 | 14 | 8 | 6 | 6 | 3 | 2 | 5 | *1* |
| **REGIONAL SUMMARY** | | | | | | | | | |
| African | 150 335 | 104 057 | 104 105 | 116 354 | 99 380 | 118 362 | 103 748 | 94 212 | 73 276 |
| Americas | 190 | 167 | 156 | 95 | 91 | 98 | 212 | 423 | 337 |
| Eastern Mediterranean | 1 143 | 736 | 996 | 1 048 | 976 | 1 015 | 861 | 1 714 | 3 320 |
| European | 0 | 0 | 0 | 0 | 0 | 0 | 0 | 0 | 0 |
| South-East Asia | 2 421 | 1 821 | 1 229 | 1 126 | 955 | 620 | 560 | 299 | 164 |
| Western Pacific | 910 | 727 | 524 | 393 | 268 | 215 | 341 | 321 | 243 |
| **Total** | **154 999** | **107 508** | **107 010** | **119 016** | **101 670** | **120 310** | **105 722** | **96 969** | **77 340** |

Data as of 26 November 2019

[1] Certified malaria free countries are included in this listing for historical purposes.
[2] In May 2013, South Sudan was reassigned to the WHO African Region (WHA resolution 66.21, https://apps.who.int/gb/ebwha/pdf_files/WHA66/A66_R21-en.pdf).
[3] There is no indigenous malaria deaths.
[4] In Malaysia, there is no local transmission of human malaria in 2018. Malaria deaths are imported non-human malaria.

Note: Deaths reported before 2000 can be probable and confirmed or only confirmed deaths depending on the country. Indigenous malaria deaths are in italics.

# Notes